WE 805

Commissioning Editor: Rita Demetriou-Swanwick
Development Editor: Ailsa Laing
Project Manager: Beula Christopher
Designer: Charles Gray
Illustration Manager: Bruce Hogarth
Illustrator: Graeme Chambers

Neck and Arm Pain Syndromes

Evidence-informed screening, diagnosis and management

Edited by

César Fernández de las Peñas, PT, DO, PhD
Head, Division of Physical Therapy, Department of Physiotherapy, Faculty of Health Sciences, University Rey Juan Carlos, Madrid, Spain

Joshua A Cleland, PT, PhD
Professor, Franklin Pierce University, Concord, New Hampshire

Peter A Huijbregts, PT, MSc, MHSc, DPT, OCS, FAAOMPT, FCAMT
Assistant Professor, University of St. Augustine for Health Sciences, St. Augustine, Florida

ELSEVIER
CHURCHILL
LIVINGSTONE

ELSEVIER
CHURCHILL
LIVINGSTONE

Two of the cover photos used with kind permission from Evidence in Motion

ISBN 978-0-7020-3528-9

British Library Cataloguing in Publication Data
A catalogue record for this book is available from the British Library

Library of Congress Cataloging in Publication Data
A catalog record for this book is available from the Library of Congress

Notices
Knowledge and best practice in this field are constantly changing. As new research and experience broaden our understanding, changes in research methods, professional practices, or medical treatment may become necessary.

Practitioners and researchers must always rely on their own experience and knowledge in evaluating and using any information, methods, compounds, or experiments described herein. In using such information or methods they should be mindful of their own safety and the safety of others, including parties for whom they have a professional responsibility.

With respect to any drug or pharmaceutical products identified, readers are advised to check the most current information provided (i) on procedures featured or (ii) by the manufacturer of each product to be administered, to verify the recommended dose or formula, the method and duration of administration, and contraindications. It is the responsibility of practitioners, relying on their own experience and knowledge of their patients, to make diagnoses, to determine dosages and the best treatment for each individual patient, and to take all appropriate safety precautions.

To the fullest extent of the law, neither the Publisher nor the authors, contributors, or editors, assume any liability for any injury and/or damage to persons or property as a matter of products liability, negligence or otherwise, or from any use or operation of any methods, products, instructions, or ideas contained in the material herein.

ELSEVIER

your source for books,
journals and multimedia
in the health sciences

www.elsevierhealth.com

Working together to grow
libraries in developing countries

www.elsevier.com | www.bookaid.org | www.sabre.org

ELSEVIER   BOOK AID
            International   Sabre Foundation

The
Publisher's
policy is to use
**paper manufactured
from sustainable forests**

Printed in China

Contents

Contents

Preface

The most obvious reason for producing a book on neck and arm pain syndromes is the frequency with which these complaints occur. A Dutch general population study noted 1-year prevalence for neck pain of 31.4% (Picavet & Schouten 2003). In that same study, 30.3% of people reported shoulder, 11.2% elbow, and 17.5% wrist or hand pain over the course of a year (Picavet & Schouten 2003). Radhakrishnan et al (1994) reported an annual incidence of cervical radicular symptoms of 83.2 per 100 000 in a US general population study. Closely related in a functional and anatomical sense and discussed in this text as often relevant to management of neck and arm pain, the reported 1-year prevalence for thoracic spine pain was found to range between 3.5–34.8% (Briggs et al 2009). Reported 1-year prevalence of upper extremity musculoskeletal disorders ranged from 2.3–41% (Huisstede et al 2006). In 1992, in the province of Ontario in Canada, these disorders constituted up to 24% of lost-time workers' compensation claims and in the US in 1989 the total workers' compensation costs for such disorders was estimated at $563 million (Webster & Snook 1994, Polanyi et al 1997). More data on the epidemiology of neck and arm pain syndromes is provided in Chapter 1 and the pathology-specific chapters throughout this text and underlines the relevance of this textbook.

More relevant even to the readers of this book are those people with neck and arm pain that go on to seek out health care services for the diagnosis and management of their complaints. In the Netherlands, a family physician in an average-sized practice can expect to see 147 new cases of non-traumatic arm, neck, and shoulder complaints each year (Feleus et al 2008). At almost four times the incidence of consultations for wrist, hand/finger, or tennis elbow complaints, Bot et al (2005) reported neck followed by shoulder symptoms as the most frequent reason for general practice visits for neck and upper extremity complaints. Boissonnault (1999) reported on US outpatient physical therapy clinics noting that 16% of patients had cervical, 11% shoulder, and 0.04% wrist and hand-related diagnoses. Occupational therapists, chiropractors, osteopaths, massage therapists, and acupuncturists are other groups that will likely see patients with neck and arm pain in their clinical practice. In-depth knowledge and adequate skills with regard to screening, diagnosis, and management of these patients is relevant to these professionals, especially as direct-access increasingly becomes the norm.

The practice paradigm we have chosen for this book is the evidence-informed paradigm. It has been more than 30 years since a group of clinical epidemiologists at McMaster University introduced the evidence-based practice paradigm to replace the traditional medical paradigm (Guyatt 2002). The defining characteristic of the traditional paradigm was that the diagnosis and management were guided mainly by a patho-physiologic rationale and by knowledge provided by respected authorities in the field. With its emphasis on expert opinion, this traditional medical paradigm has been called the authority-based or also, somewhat tongue-in-cheek, the eminence-based medicine paradigm (Poolman et al 2007). However, the evidence-based practice paradigm has met and continues to meet with considerable resistance from the clinical field. Its early definition as the 'conscientious, explicit and judicious use of current best evidence in making decisions about the care of individual patients' (Sackett et al 1996), seemed to mirror the often-heard criticisms of over-reliance on research evidence at the expense of clinical expertise and experience and disregard of social context. And although evidence-based practice has evolved to where it now adopts a more inclusive view of evidence (which recognizes not only the value of different research designs but also of clinical expertise, patient values and preferences, and even contextual factors in the clinical decision-making process (Rycroft-Malone 2008)), the evidence-*informed* paradigm has been suggested as more appropriate, in which the clinician takes the evidence from research into account when making a clinical decision with regard to patient management, but where evidence does not dictate the decision (Bohart 2005, Pencheon 2005).

Throughout this text, chapter authors integrate clinical experience and expertise and reasoning based on a pathophysiologic rationale with current best evidence, thereby in effect combining the best of the traditional and evidence-based paradigms in a new paradigm truly representative of what clinicians do in everyday clinical practice. We believe that this approach has made for a textbook that truly provides practicing clinicians with what they need to know for real-life screening, diagnosis and management of patients with neck and arm pain syndromes.

Spain, USA & Canada, 2009

César Fernández-de-las-Peñas
Joshua A Cleland
Peter A Huijbregts

REFERENCES

Bohart, A., 2005. Evidence-based psychotherapy means evidence-informed, not evidence-driven. J. Contemp. Psychother. 35, 39–53.

Boissonnault, W.G., 1999. Prevalence of comorbid conditions, surgeries, and medication use in a physical therapy outpatient population: A multicentered study. J. Orthop. Sports Phys. Ther. 29, 506–525.

Bot, S.D.M., Van der Waal, J.M., Terwee, C.B., et al., 2005. Incidence and prevalence of complaints of the neck and upper extremity in general practice. Ann. Rheumat. Dis. 64, 118–123.

Briggs, A.M., Smith, A.J., Straker, L.M., Bragge, P., 2009. Thoracic spine pain in the general population: Prevalence, incidence and associated factors in children, adolescents and adults: A systematic review. BMC Musculoskelet. Disord. 10, 77.

Feleus, A., Bierma-Zeinstra, S.M., Miedema, H.S., Bernsen, R.M., Verhaar, J.A., Koes, B., 2008. Incidence of non-traumatic complaints of arm, neck and shoulder in general practice. Man. Ther. 13, 426–433.

Guyatt, G., 2002. Preface. In: Guyatt, G., Rennie, D. (Eds.), User's guide to the medical literature: A manual for evidence-based clinical practice. AMA Press, Chicago, pp. xiii–xvi.

Huisstede, B.M.A., Bierma-Zeinstra, S.M.A., Koes, B.W., Verhaar, J.A.N., 2006. Incidence and prevalence of upper-extremity musculoskeletal disorders: A critical appraisal of the literature. BMC Musculoskelet. Disord. 7, 7.

Pencheon, D., 2005. What's next for evidence-based medicine? Evidence-Based Health Care & Public Health 9, 319–321.

Picavet, H.S., Schouten, J.S., 2003. Musculoskeletal pain in the Netherlands: Prevalences, consequences and risk groups, the DMC (3) study. Pain 102, 167–178.

Polanyi, M.F., Cole, D.C., Beaton, D.E., et al., 1997. Upper limb work-related musculoskeletal disorders among newspaper employees: Cross-sectional survey results. Am. J. Ind. Med. 32, 620–628.

Poolman, R.W., Petrisor, B.A., Marti, R.K., Kerkhoffs, G.M., Zlowodzki, M., Bhandari, M., 2007. Misconceptions about practicing evidence-based orthopaedic surgery. Acta Orthop. Scand. 78, 2–11.

Radhakrishnan, K., Litchy, W.J., O'Fallon, W.M., Kurland, L.T., 1994. Epidemiology of cervical radiculopathy. A population-based study from Rochester, Minnesota, 1976–1990. Brain 117, 325–335.

Rycroft-Malone, J., 2008. Evidence-informed practice: From individual to context. J. Nurs. Manag. 16, 404–408.

Sackett, D., Rosenberg, W.M.C., Gray, J.A.M., Haynes, R.B., Richardson, W.S., 1996. Evidence based medicine: what it is and what it isn't. Br. Med. J. 312, 71–72.

Webster, B.S., Snook, S.H., 1994. The cost of compensable upper extremity cumulative trauma disorders. J. Occup. Med. 36, 713–717.

In Memoriam

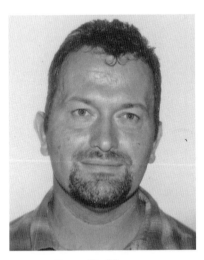

Peter Huijbregts

We are greatly saddened by the sudden loss of our close friend and colleague Peter Huijbregts, who passed away on November 6th 2010. This is a great tragedy and a terrible loss to his family and friends, the profession of physical therapy, and indeed to society in general. We are also saddened by the countless individuals who will never have a chance to be personally influenced by him. Peter was one of those individuals you never forgot if you were fortunate enough to have him cross your path.

We were aware of Peter's substantial contribution to the physical therapy profession well before we had an opportunity to meet and work with him personally. We first became friends during his tenure as Editor for the *Journal of Manual and Manipulative Therapy*. Since that time he has had a huge influence on both our professional lives. We have been fortunate enough to work with him as co-editors on this textbook, as well as on many peer-reviewed publications.

Peter was wonderfully articulate and never at a loss for words. We can recall numerous late evenings spent at national conferences enjoying conversations with Peter, who would frequently mention his love for his wife Rap, and his two children, Arun Joseph and Annika Dani. Peter had a terrific passion for both his personal and his professional life.

He was always up for discussing the historical origins of manual therapy or the current evidence supporting the effectiveness of interventions. We will never forget his sense of humour – many times Peter entertained the room with his wit and comedy.

Peter has had a remarkable influence on many professionals who have been fortunate enough to encounter him. His passing will leave a huge void in the manual therapy community around the world.

Peter was truly a great gentleman, a wise scholar and an inspiring man.

We will miss him greatly.

César and Josh

Contributors

Hilmir Agustsson, MHSc, DPT, MTC, CFC
Assistant Professor
Lead Course Writer
University of St. Augustine
St. Augustine, Florida

Steven C Allen, PT, MSc, OCS, FAAOMPT
Clinic Director
Liberty Lake Physical Therapy
Therapeutic Associates, Inc.
Liberty Lake, Washington

Lars Arendt-Nielsen, Dr. Med. Sci., PhD, FRSM
Professor
Center for Sensory-Motor Interaction
Department of Health Science and Technology
Aalborg University
Aalborg, Denmark

Carel Bron, PT, MT
Physical Therapist and Manual Therapist
Private Practice for Physical Therapy for Neck,
Shoulder and Arm Disorders
Groningen, The Netherlands

Joshua A Cleland, PT, PhD
Professor
Franklin Pierce University
Concord, New Hampshire

Amy E Cook, PT, MS
Contract Physical Therapist
North Canton, Ohio

Chad E Cook, PT, PhD, MBA
Professor and Chair
Division of Physical Therapy
Walsh University
North Canton, Ohio

Douglas S Creighton, PT, DPT, OCS, FAAOMPT
Assistant Professor
Oakland University
Rochester, Michigan

Arthur de Gast, MD, PhD
Orthopedic surgeon
Head Clinical Orthopedic Research Center midden-Nederland
Department of Orthopedics
Diakonessenhuis Utrecht/Zeist Doorn
The Netherlands

Bryan S Dennison, PT, DPT, MPT, OCS, CSCS, FAAOMPT
Summit Physical Therapy
Mammoth Lakes, California
Affiliate Faculty
Rueckert-Hartman College for Health Professions
Regis University
Denver, Colorado

Andrew Dilley, BSc, PhD
Lecturer in Anatomy
Brighton and Sussex Medical School
University of Sussex
Brighton, UK

Jan Dommerholt, PT, DPT, MPS, DAAPM
Bethesda Physiocare / Myopain Seminars
Bethesda, Maryland

William Egan, PT, DPT, OCS, FAAOMPT
Clinical Assistant Professor
Department of Physical Therapy
College of Health Professions
Temple University
Philadelphia, Pennsylvania

Contributors

César Fernández de las Peñas, PT, DO, PhD
Head, Division of Physical Therapy
Department of Physiotherapy
Faculty of Health Sciences
University Rey Juan Carlos
Madrid, Spain

Timothy Flynn, PT, PhD, OCS, FAAOMPT
Distinguished Professor
Rocky Mountain University of Health Professions
Provo, Utah

Jo L M Franssen, PT
Physical Therapist
Private Practice for Physical Therapy for Neck,
Shoulder and Arm Disorders
Groningen, The Netherlands

B Jane Freure, BSc(PT), MManipTher(AU), FCAMT,
Dip. Sport PT
Physiotherapist
D3 Physiotherapy
St Joseph's Health Care
Ontario, Canada

Gary Fryer, PhD, BSc(Osteopathy), ND
Senior Lecturer
Osteopathic Medicine Unit
School of Biomedical and Health Sciences
Victoria University
Melbourne, Australia
Research Associate Professor
A.T. Still Research Institute
A.T. Still University of Health Sciences
Kirksville, Missouri

Hong-You Ge, MD, PhD
Associate Professor
Center for Sensory–Motor Interaction
Department of Health Science and Technology
Aalborg University
Aalborg, Denmark

Paul E Glynn, PT, DPT, OCS, FAAOMPT
Supervisor of Staff Development and Clinical Research
Newton-Wellesley Hospital
Newton Lower Falls, Massachusetts
Founder and Owner of Physical Therapy in Collaboration
Sudbury, Massachusetts
Adjunct Faculty
Regis University
Denver, Colorado

Jane Greening, MCSP, MSc, PhD, FMACP
Visiting Research Fellow
Brighton and Sussex Medical School
University of Sussex
Brighton, UK

Ruby Grewal, MD, MSc, FRCSC
Assistant Professor
Department of Surgery
University of Western Ontario
Hand and Upper Limb Center
Ontario, Canada

Wayne Hing, PhD, MSc(Hons), ADP(OMT), DipMT,
DipPhys, FNZCP
Associate Professor
Auckland University of Technology
Auckland, New Zealand

Peter A Huijbregts, PT, MSc, MHSc, DPT, OCS, FAAOMPT,
FCAMT [Deceased]
Assistant Professor
University of St. Augustine for Health Sciences
St. Augustine, Florida

Ana Isabel-de-la-Llave-Rincón, PT, MSc, PhD
Professor of Physical Therapy
Department of Physical Therapy
Occupational Therapy
Rehabilitation and Physical Medicine Faculty of Health Sciences
University of Rey Juan Carlos
Madrid, Spain

Mark A Jones, BSc (Psych), CertPhysTher,
GradDipAdvManipTher, MAppSc
Senior Lecturer, Program Director
Graduate Programs in Musculoskeletal
and Sports Physiotherapy
School of Health Sciences
University of South Australia
Adelaide, Australia

Freddy M Kaltenborn, PT, OMT, ATC, PhD(Hon)
Physical therapist, Orthopaedic Manipulative therapist, Athletic
trainer certificate, Chiropractor, Osteopath
Scheidegg, Germany

Traudi Baldauf Kaltenborn, PT, OMT
Physical therapist, Orthopaedic manipulative therapist
Scheidegg, Germany

Carol Kennedy, BScPT, MClSc(manip), FCAMPT
Partner
Treloar Physiotherapy Clinic
British Columbia, Canada

Shane Koppenhaver, PT, PhD, OCS, FAAOMPT
Assistant Professor
US Army/Baylor University Doctoral Program in
Physical Therapy
San Antonio, Texas

John R Krauss, PT, PhD, OCS, FAAOMPT
Associate Professor
Oakland University
Rochester, Michigan

Michael H Leal, PT, DPT, MPT, OCS
Staff Physical Therapist
Presbyterian Intercommunity Hospital
Whittier, California
Adjunct Faculty
Department of Physical Therapy
Azusa Pacific University
Azusa, California
Affiliate Faculty
Rueckert-Hartman College for Health Professions
Regis University
Denver, Colorado

Adriaan Louw, PT, M.App.Sc(Physio), GCRM, CSMT
Senior Instructor
International Spine and Pain Institute and Neuro Orthopaedic
Institute
Story City, Iowa

Joy C MacDermid, BSc, BScPT, MSc, PhD
Associate Professor
School of Rehabilitation Science
McMaster University
Hamilton, Ontario
Co-director of Clinical Research
Hand and Upper Limb Centre
London, Ontario, Canada

Mary E Magarey, PhD, FACP, GradDipAdvManipTher
Specialist Musculoskeletal and Sports Physiotherapist
Senior Lecturer and Coordinator (Sports)
Graduate Programs in Musculoskeletal and
Sports Physiotherapy
School of Health Sciences
University of South Australia
Adelaide, Australia

Johnson McEvoy, BSc, MSc, DPT, MISCP, MCSP, PT
United Physiotherapy Clinic
Head Physiotherapist Irish Boxing Team
External Lecturer BSc (Sports Science)
University of Limerick
Limerick, Ireland

Jack Miller, BSc, PT, DipMT(NZ), MClSc, FCAMT
Adjunct Clinical Professor
Faculty of Health Science
School of Physical Therapy
University of Western Ontario
London, Canada
Lecturer
Faculty of Medicine
Department of Rehabilitation Medicine

University of Toronto
Toronto, Canada

Paul Mintken, PT, DPT, OCS, FAAOMPT
Assistant Professor
Physical Therapy Program
School of Medicine
University of Colorado
Denver, Colorado

Kieran O'Sullivan, BScPT(Hons), MManipTher
Specialist Musculoskeletal Physiotherapist
Lecturer in Physiotherapy
University of Limerick
Limerick, Ireland

Luca Padua, MD, PhD
Professor of Neurology
Department of Neurosciences
Institute of Neurology
Catholic University
Rome, Italy
Don C Gnocchi Foundation
Milan, Italy

Costanza Pazzaglia, MD
Postgraduate Student
Department of Neurosciences
Institute of Neurology
Università Cattolica del Sacro Cuore
Rome, Italy
Don C Gnocchi Foundation
Milan, Italy

Erland Pettman, PT, OMT, FCAMT
Associate Professor
Post-professional Program
Department of Physical Therapy
Andrews University
Berrien Springs, Michigan

Andrzej Pilat, PT
Director
Myofascial Therapy School "Tupimek"
Postgraduate Program Physiotherapy School ONCE
Universiad Autónoma
Madrid, Spain

Ellen J Pong, OT, PT, BA, MOT, DPT
Physical and Occupational Therapist
Sacred Heart Rehabilitation at Pace
Online Instructor
University of St. Augustine for Health Sciences
St. Augustine, Florida

Janette W Powell, PT, MHSc, OCS, STC
Supervisor of Performance Medicine
Cirque du Soleil 'O'
Las Vegas, Nevada

Contributors

Emilio Puentedura, PT, DPT, GDMT, OCS, FAAOMPT
Assistant Professor
Department of Physical Therapy
University of Nevada Las Vegas
Las Vegas, Nevada
Senior Instructor
International Spine and Pain Institute and Neuro
Orthopaedic Institute
Story City, Iowa

Caroline A Quartly, MD, FRCPC, BScPT,
GradDipManTher (Aus), FAANEM
Physical Medicine and Rehabilitation Electromyography
Vancouver Island Health Authority
British Columbia, Canada

Chris A Sebelski, PT, DPT, OCS
Assistant Professor
Department of Physical Therapy and Athletic Training
Saint Louis University
Saint Louis, Missouri

Ian Shrier, MD, PhD, Dip Sport Med, FACSM
Associate Professor
Centre for Clinical Epidemiology and Community Studies
Lady Davis Institute for Medical Research
Jewish General Hospital
McGill University
Montreal, Canada

David G Simons, MD [Deceased]
Volunteer Clinical Professor
Rehabilitation Medicine at Emory University
Adjunct Professor
Physical Therapy Department
Georgia State University
Atlanta, Georgia

Helen Slater, PhD, FACP, MappSc, BAppSc
Specialist Musculoskeletal Physiotherapist
School of Physiotherapy
Curtin University
Perth, Australia

Michele Sterling, PhD, MPHTY, GradDipManipPhysio,
BPHTY, FACP
Associate Professor
NHMRC Research Fellow

Associate Director
Centre for National Research on Disability
and Rehabilitation Medicine
The University of Queensland
Herston, Australia

Susan W Stralka, PT, DPT, MS, ACHE
CEO/Administrator
Baptist Rehabilitation Hospital – Germantown
Clinical Instructor
University of Tennessee Health Sciences Center
College of Allied Health
Department of Physical Therapy
Memphis, Tennessee

Louise Thwaites, MBBS, BSc, MD, MLCOM, MRCP
Musculoskeletal Physician
Horsham, West Sussex, UK

Russell S VanderWilde, MD
Orthopedic Surgeon
Northwest Orthopedic Specialists
Spokane, Washington

Bill Vicenzino, PhD, MSc, BPhty, GradDipSportsPhty
Professor of Sports Physiotherapy
Head of Physiotherapy
School of Health and Rehabilitation Sciences
University of Queensland
Brisbane, Australia

Karen Walker-Bone, BM, FRCP, PhD
Senior Lecturer (Honorary Consultant) in Rheumatology and
Clinical Academic Sub-Dean
Brighton and Sussex Medical School
Brighton, East Sussex, UK

David M Walton, PT, PhD
Assistant Professor
School of Physical Therapy
The University of Western Ontario
London, Ontario, Canada

C Joseph Yelvington, PT, BA
Physical Therapist
Sacred Heart Rehabilitation at Pace
Pace, Florida

Chapter | 1 |

Epidemiology

Louise Thwaites, Karen Walker-Bone

CHAPTER CONTENTS

INTRODUCTION

In the 21st century, upper extremity pain syndromes are common and cause substantial pain and disability. Upper extremity pain can arise from a very wide range of clinical conditions; however this text focuses on pain arising from non-traumatic non-articular soft tissues, i.e. excluding pain resulting from acute trauma, malignancy and chronic rheumatic diseases (Box 1.1). Non-articular soft tissue disorders include some relatively well defined 'specific' patho-anatomical conditions such as lateral epicondylalgia, de Quervain's tenosynovitis and carpal tunnel syndrome. Upper extremity pain may also be referred from pathology occurring in the cervical spine (cervico-brachial disorders). Frequently also, upper extremity pain arises in the absence of distinct patho-anatomical physical signs and is labelled as 'non-specific' regional pain.

It has been estimated that at a given point in time 20–53% of the adult population in Western countries experience upper extremity pain symptoms. Over a lifetime this is > 70% (Walker-Bone et al 2003a, Huisstede et al 2006). These disorders occur commonly in the working population, causing considerable morbidity and sickness absence and thereby a significant economic impact (Silverstein et al 1998). In the developed world, musculoskeletal disorders represent the majority of occupational ill-health and upper extremity pain is second only to back pain as a cause of work related illness (Palmer 2006). In the UK, according to one estimate, at least 4 million working days are lost annually due to upper limb disorders (Jones & Clegg 1998). This compares with an estimated 52 million working days lost to low back pain (Macfarlane et al 2009). Using recent criteria for examining work-relatedness of upper extremity disorders, of the order of 70–95% of

© 2011 Elsevier Ltd.
DOI: 10.1016/B978-0-7020-3528-9.00001-7

> Box 1.1 **Causes of upper extremity pain**
>
> | Outside the scope of this text | Within the scope of this text |
> |---|---|
> | **Rheumatological conditions** | **Specific non-articular conditions** |
> | Inflammatory arthritis e.g. rheumatoid arthritis, ankylosing spondylitis | Adhesive capsulitis |
> | | Rotator cuff syndrome |
> | | Sub-acromial bursitis |
> | Osteoarthritis | Acromio-clavicular joint |
> | Systemic Lupus | dysfunction |
> | Erythematosus (SLE) | Lateral epicondylitis |
> | Fibromyalgia syndrome | Medial epicondylitis |
> | Polymyalgia rheumatica/ | Tenosynovitis |
> | temporal arteritis | De Quervain's disease |
> | | Carpal tunnel syndrome |
> | **Systemic conditions** | |
> | Malignancy (primary or | **Non-specific pain** |
> | secondary) | **syndromes** |
> | Stroke | Occupational cervico-brachial |
> | Myocardial infarction and | disorder |
> | coronary artery syndromes | Cumulative trauma disorder |
> | Multiple sclerosis | (CTD) |
> | Diabetes mellitus | Repetitive strain injury (RSI) |
> | Diaphragmatic irritation | Work-related upper limb |
> | (liver disease, splenic | disorder (WRULD) |
> | disease) | Work-related upper extremity |
> | | musculoskeletal disorder |
> | **Acute trauma** | (WRUEMSD) |
> | Fracture /dislocation | Non-specific forearm pain |

upper extremity musculoskeletal disorders in general working populations could be classified as 'work related' (Roquelaure et al 2006) but this may not imply a causal relationship.

Given these rates of occurrence and the associated levels of disability, it could be reasonably expected that the epidemiology of these conditions would be thoroughly investigated and understood. Unfortunately, for many reasons, this is not currently the case. In fact, high-quality epidemiological research in this field has been hampered in several different ways resulting in the confusion and controversy which beset this field. In order to understand the available epidemiological data which make up the majority of this chapter, we will briefly explain the epidemiological issues in the next section.

EPIDEMIOLOGICAL ISSUES

Terminology

As with other branches of medicine, much of the terminology for specific upper extremity disorders is historical, dating back from the original publications of the findings

associated with an individual clinical syndrome (e.g. 'lawn tennis arm' (Morris 1882)). Some conditions have eponyms (de Quervain's tenosynovitis) and others presumed views of the patho-anatomical basis of the pain (tendonitis, epicondylitis, tenosynovitis). Recently there have been attempts to standardize some of these terms aiming to better suit our modern view of the underlying patho-physiology (Hutson 2006). For example in non-rheumatological tendon pain (tendonitis), there is growing evidence that true inflammation is rarely present. Instead histopathological studies suggest that repetitive mechanical overload produces degenerative changes within the tendon substance leading to eventual collagen fibril micro-failure. A similar pathological picture is seen in tendons as they pass through the synovial lined fibro-osseous tunnels at the wrist. Thus technically 'tendinosis' would be a much more accurate clinical term then tendonitis, reserving this latter term and 'tenosynovitis' for use only in the presence of true synovial inflammation (e.g. in rheumatoid arthritis). However, it should be borne in mind that histology is rarely available in the diagnosis or management of these conditions in practice and the clinician may be faced with patients presenting with a secondary inflammatory reaction visible in the paratenons overlying degenerate tendons. It is unsurprising therefore that terms that may be technically inaccurate continue to prevail in clinical practice.

Non-specific pain

Upper extremity pain frequently occurs in the absence of clinical signs that fit into the conventional anatomical–pathological model ('non-specific' pain). As long ago as 1713, Ramazzini described an upper extremity disorder related to 'constant sitting, perpetual motion of the hand in the same manner and the attention and application of the mind' (Ramazzini 1940). Since then, upper extremity pain has been described occurring among different groups of workers many times (e.g. writer's cramp (British Civil Service 1830s) and telegraphists' cramp among telegraphers (UK 1908)). In the last half of the 20th century, occupational cervico-brachial disorders (Japan), cumulative trauma disorders (CTDs) (USA), repetitive strain injury (RSI) (Australia) and work-related upper limb disorders (WRULD) (UK) were terms used in different countries for syndromes similar to each other occurring in groups of workers. These terms were used similarly to describe pain at different sites in the neck and upper limb with no confirmed patho-anatomical abnormality and they were overlapping but non-identical in their use (Robinson & Walker-Bone 2009). It is now widely believed that terms with implied causation such as these have impacted negatively on research in this field (Helliwell 1995). For one thing, these tautological terms imply blame or even negligence by an employer and so this is now a field where much of the investigation has moved into the law courts rather than the research laboratories. Secondly, if a pain has, because of its nomenclature, been attributed to a type of occupation, it is very difficult to systematically investigate any other possible aetiology as the individual affected already has fixed preconceptions.

Classification criteria

In clinical practice, diagnostic criteria are used to separate types of disease with different cause, treatment or prognosis. It is an absolute requirement of epidemiological research that the problem under study is clearly defined. We have already seen that non-specific pains are widely classified using different systems in different countries. However, even amongst the specific upper extremity conditions, classification criteria may differ widely and few have a 'gold standard' diagnostic test. Therefore, case definitions used in epidemiological studies have historically used textbook definitions or authors' personal opinions. In a systematic review of studies investigating incidence and prevalence of upper extremity disorders, Huisstede et al (2008) found variation in point prevalence from 1% to 53% largely due to disparity of case definitions. Without consistent and clear classification, reliable data regarding disease burden and its health and socioeconomic impact are impossible to obtain. This in turn impacts upon treatment and prevention strategies and future research.

In 1996 Buchbinder et al (1996) examined existing classification schemes for soft tissue disorders of the neck and upper limb. They found major inadequacies such as failure to be comprehensive, overlap of categories and consequently suggested criteria by which future classification systems might be better assessed. In an attempt to improve consensus over classification several multidisciplinary groups convened and produced their own classifications systems (Harrington et al 1998, Sluiter et al 2001). However these have been criticised for reflecting the opinions of workshop participants without clear definitions of extent or duration of symptoms and without any formal testing. A systematic review of 117 articles showed very few attempts to establish the validity of classification systems with only one showing rigorous testing of validity and reliability (Walker-Bone et al 2003b).

The Southampton examination schedule was developed from the multidisciplinary UK workshop consensus statement on classification of musculoskeletal disorders of the upper limb and tested in both hospital and general populations (Fig 1.1) (Palmer et al 2000, Walker-Bone et al 2002). Overall findings showed a valid reproducible system for the examination of upper limb disorders which was suitable for use in large scale epidemiological research, although performing better in hospital subjects (Palmer et al 2000) with the most clear-cut clinical presentations as compared with community subjects (Walker-Bone et al 2002).

More recently a 'complaints of the arm, neck and/or shoulder' (CANS) classification was proposed by a group

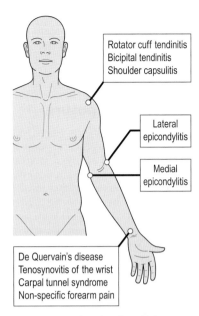

Fig 1.1 Upper extremity disorders for which consensus criteria were developed by the HSE Delphi Workshop.

comprising 11 medical and paramedical disciplines. They aimed to obtain consensus and establish a group of specific and non-specific conditions defined as musculoskeletal complaints of the arm, neck and shoulder not caused by acute trauma or any systemic disease (CANS). A final group of 23 conditions, categorized as specific disorders, was produced. All other conditions were classified as non-specific disorders (Huisstede et al 2007).

Study design

Neck and upper limb disorders are often episodic and recurrent and therefore most studies examine prevalence, rather than incidence, using a cross-sectional design. Investigators often choose different case definitions: 'neck pain lasting > 1 day in the past 7 days' (1-week prevalence) is one possible case definition which will yield a different prevalence estimate from: 'neck pain lasting > 6 months in the past year' (1-year prevalence of chronic neck pain) and also from 'neck pain ever' (lifetime prevalence of neck pain). Many of the studies have eschewed the difficulties of classification and chosen instead to measure the prevalence of self-reported pain at different sites of the neck and/or upper limb, using this as the outcome (Walker-Bone et al 2003b).

Population

Many of the available epidemiological studies are centred on workplace or occupational groups, rather than population samples. This choice of setting incurs the risk of results biased by the 'healthy worker' effect in which those most severely affected are off sick or medically retired and not in the workplace. Many studies have been done using workers' compensation claims which again may underestimate the true occurrence of disorders and bias the results towards only the most severe types of conditions causing the worst levels of disability (Roquelaure et al 2006).

Measurement of exposure

Measurement of exposure to different types of occupational risk is also fraught with difficulty. Exposures to different types of physical risk factors are often multifaceted (e.g. force and vibration or pulling and pushing) thus difficult to define and objectively measure as they involve complex, physical actions, repetitions and varying degrees of force. Direct observation and video surveillance are preferred methods for quantifying these but are time-consuming and expensive, so not practicable for large studies. Surrogate markers such as job title or occupation classification are used, but are less sensitive. Thus subjective retrospective reporting of exposure is frequently used; however this relies on subject's recall, estimation of times, forces and other physical factors and may be influenced by the subject's own personal hypotheses regarding aetiology of their symptoms. Some investigators have attempted to overcome these by using a combination of subjective reporting and direct observation validation (Andersen et al 2007).

To summarize, there is little doubt that upper extremity pain is common, recurrent and disabling. There are several weaknesses inherent in our knowledge and understanding of the occurrence, risk factors and impact of these conditions which have arisen because of methodological hindrances. For this reason, discrepancies have arisen and controversy remains about even basic aspects. The reader must put the following section into this context.

OCCURRENCE OF UPPER EXTREMITY DISORDERS

Prevalence of upper extremity pain

The results of epidemiological surveys suggest that neck pain may affect 10–17% of adults at any point in time and as many as 71% during a lifetime and that pain in the upper limb has a point prevalence between 7–26% (Walker-Bone et al 2004b). Many of the studies are poorly comparable due to wide variation in the case definition and population characteristics. Shoulder pain lasting > 1 day in the past month, for example, was estimated to affect 13% of men and 15% of women aged 53 years (Bergenudd et al 1988) whereas in a different study, 26% of men and 19% of women aged 31–74 years reported current shoulder pain and restricted movement (Allander 1974). Point prevalence and period prevalence estimates for the occurrence of upper extremity pain,

Table 1.1 Population-based prevalence estimates for the occurrence of upper extremity regional pain (updated from Walker-Bone et al 2003a)

	Case definition	Size of population sampled	Age (years)	Prevalence estimate men (%)	Prevalence estimate women (%)	Prevalence estimate all (%)
NECK PAIN						
Period prevalence	Pain lasting > 1 week in past month	5752	>16	11	17	14
	Neck pain, tenderness or stiffness in past year	537	18–65	–	–	12
	Troublesome neck pain in the past year	7648	18–67	29	40	34
	Pain lasting > 1 day in past year	800	>30	15	17	–
	Pain lasting > 1 day in past week (Walker-Bone et al 2004b)	9698	25–64	21	26	24
Point prevalence	Currently suffering from neck pain	10,532	20–65	10	18	–
	Pain lasting > 1 month	1806	25–74	15	19	17

Table 1.1 Population-based prevalence estimates for the occurrence of upper extremity regional pain (updated from Walker-Bone et al 2003a)—cont'd

	Case definition	Size of population sampled	Age (years)	Prevalence estimate men (%)	Prevalence estimate women (%)	Prevalence estimate all (%)
SHOULDER PAIN						
Period prevalence	Pain lasting > 1 week in past month	5752	> 16	14	17	16
	Pain lasting > 1 day in past month	574	53	13	15	14
	Pain lasting > 1 day in past week (Walker-Bone et al 2004)	9698	25–64	21	26	24
Point prevalence	Current pain lasting > 3 months	1806	25–74	–	–	7
	Current pain and restricted movement	15,268	31–74	26	19	20
	Current shoulder pain	644	> 70	–	–	26
ELBOW PAIN						
Period prevalence	Pain lasting > 1 week in past month	5752	> 16	6	6	6
	Pain lasting > 1 day in past week (Walker-Bone et al 2004)	9698	25–64	12	10	11
Point prevalence	Pain lasting > 3 months in elbow/forearm	1806	25–74	8	12	11
WRIST/HAND PAIN						
Period prevalence	Pain in the hand lasting > 1 week in the past month	5752	> 16	12	20	–
	Pain lasting > 1 day in past week (Walker-Bone et al 2004)	9698	25–64	19	23	21
Point prevalence	Current pain in hand/wrist lasting > 3 months	1806	25–74	9	17	13

together with their case definitions, are summarized in Table 1.1. Although few specific conclusions can be drawn, these data tend to suggest that all these complaints are common and generally reported more often by women than men and tend to be more frequent proximally (neck/shoulder) than distally, although hand/wrist pain is more frequent than elbow pain. These findings from general population studies have been replicated in working populations. Recently-published French

workforce data showed 12-month prevalence of upper extremity musculoskeletal symptoms of 35% in women compared to 27% in men (Roquelaure et al 2006) and similar Danish data estimated the prevalence rates of chronic upper extremity symptoms as 11.3% among women as compared with 7.7% among men (Huisstede et al 2008).

In general, where studies compared different types of workers, prevalence rates are higher in those who are current workers than among the non-working general population (8.1 vs 6.1% in Holland) and rates vary according to specific occupational groups. For example 50% of college students in the USA experienced upper extremity musculoskeletal symptoms (Menendez et al 2008). Similarly high prevalence rates have been reported in computer workers (Tornqvist et al 2009) and textile workers (Huisstede et al 2006). In a recent Danish study of working adults, the overall prevalence of moderately severe neck and shoulder pain was 37%, but was 49% in kitchen and cleaning workers compared with 22% in skilled workers (Andersen et al 2007). In French workers undergoing routine medical examinations, disorders were most common in those working in manufacturing industries and public administration (Roquelaure et al 2006). Highest prevalence rates were in unskilled industrial and agricultural workers, drivers and male public service

employees and female personal care workers. This correlates with occupations at highest risk for compensation claims in the USA (Silverstein et al 1998).

Although most data on upper extremity symptoms comes from the Developed World, one study amongst office workers in Sudan using the CANS classification system has shown similar prevalence rates to those seen in Western populations (Eltayeb et al 2008).

Prevalence of specific upper extremity disorders

There are relatively few population based surveys aimed at determining anatomical locations or specific causes of upper extremity pain. Differences in diagnostic and classification procedures discussed add difficulty in interpretation. Table 1.2 summarizes the results of the available

Table 1.2 Population-based occurrence of specific upper extremity musculoskeletal disorders

	Case definition (reference for original data in parentheses)	Size of population sampled	Age (years)	Prevalence estimate men (%)	Prevalence estimate women (%)	Prevalence estimate all (%)
SHOULDER						
Rotator cuff disorder	Pain in the shoulder region accompanied by pain on resisted abduction, external rotation or internal rotation (Chard et al 1991)	644	> 70 years	–	–	15
Rotator cuff tendinitis	Pain in the deltoid region and pain on resisted active movement (Walker-Bone et al 2004b)	9698	25–64	4.5	6.1	–
Adhesive capsulitis	Pain in the deltoid area and equal restriction of active and passive glenohumeral movement with a capsular pattern (Walker-Bone et al 2004b)	9698	25–64	8.2	10.1	–
Acromio-clavicular joint dysfunction	Pain over the acromio-clavicular joint and tenderness over the joint and a positive AC stress test (Walker-Bone et al 2004b)	9698	25–64	1.0	1.0	–
ELBOW						
Lateral epicondylitis	History of pain in the elbow region for > 1 month, tenderness over lateral epicondyle and pain increased when hand pronated against resistance and increased pain on carrying (Allander 1974)	15,268	31–74	–	–	2.5

Table 1.2 Population-based occurrence of specific upper extremity musculoskeletal disorders—cont'd

	Case definition (reference for original data in parentheses)	Size of population sampled	Age (years)	Prevalence estimate men (%)	Prevalence estimate women (%)	Prevalence estimate all (%)
Lateral epicondylitis	Lateral epicondylar pain and tenderness and pain on resisted extension of the wrist (Walker-Bone et al 2004b)	9698	25–64	1.3	1.1	–
Lateral epicondylitis	Not stated (Verhaar 1994)	708	20–80	–	–	4.4
Medial epicondylitis	Medial epicondylar pain and tenderness and pain on resisted flexion of the wrist (Walker-Bone et al 2004b)	9698	25–64	0.6	1.1	
WRIST / HAND						
De Quervain's disease	Pain over the radial styloid and tender swelling of the first extensor compartment and either pain reproduced by resisted thumb extension or positive Finkelstein's test (Walker-Bone et al 2004b)	9698	25–64	0.5	1.3	–
Tenosynovitis	Pain on movement localized to the tendon sheaths in the wrist and reproduction of the pain on resisted active movement (Walker-Bone et al 2004b)	9698	25–64	1.1	2.2	–
Carpal tunnel syndrome	Pain or paraesthesia or sensory loss in the median nerve distribution and one of: Phalen's test positive, Tinel's test positive, nocturnal exacerbation of symptoms, motor loss with wasting of abductor pollicis brevis (Walker-Bone et al 2004b)	9698	25–64	1.2	0.9	–
Carpal tunnel syndrome	Clinical diagnosis of CTS (Atroshi et al 1999)	2466	25–74	3	5	4
Carpal tunnel syndrome	Electrophysiological diagnosis of CTS (Atroshi et al 1999)	2466	25–74	4	5	5
Carpal tunnel syndrome	Clinical and electrophysiological diagnosis of CTS (Atroshi et al 1999)	2466	25–74	2	3	3
Carpal tunnel syndrome	Electrophysiological diagnosis of CTS (de Krom et al 1992)	715	25–74	1	6	5
Carpal tunnel syndrome	Electrophysiological motor latency > 4.5ms (Ferry et al 1998)	820	18–75	8	6	7

population-based prevalence studies for specific conditions, together with the case definitions utilized. Shoulder conditions appear to occur most frequently, in line with the relative frequency of shoulder pain followed by carpal tunnel syndrome and epicondylitis. Most data are available regarding carpal tunnel syndrome, probably because of its relative frequency and the availability of nerve conduction studies allowing more readily defined endpoints. The incidence of carpal tunnel syndrome has been estimated at approximately 1 per 1000 of the general population with higher rates among women than men (1.5 per 1000) (Walker-Bone et al 2004b). Rates of prevalence range from 0.9% to 5% depending upon the case definition utilized.

In contrast, specific conditions have been much more commonly studied in different occupational settings, often comparing the prevalence of one or more specific upper extremity diagnoses in groups of workers with different types of occupational exposure (e.g. rates of prevalence of epicondylitis were compared between meat packers and cutters and those working in administration in meat factories) (Vikari-Juntura 1983). In 1993, all published studies were collated and critically appraised in a detailed review by the US NIOSH organization in 1993 (Bernard 1997). Similar methodological shortcomings were reported in the occupation-based studies to those already described above.

In a recent French study, data collected by a regional network of occupational physicians showed > 50% of a sample of 2685 working adults experienced non-specific upper extremity musculoskeletal symptoms in the preceding year, with approximately 30% experiencing symptoms in the preceding week (Roquelaure et al 2006). Altogether, the 12-month prevalence of 'specific' upper limb musculoskeletal disorders (rotator cuff syndrome, lateral epicondylitis, ulnar tunnel syndrome, carpal tunnel syndrome, de Quervain's disease, and flexor-extensor peritendinitis or tenosynovitis of the forearm-wrist defined according to specific criteria) was 13%.

It is noteworthy that several recent studies have demonstrated that concurrent pain at different anatomical locations is common (Walker-Bone et al 2004a). In a recent study 33% of Dutch adults reported pain at two different anatomical sites in the upper extremity, with a further 8.5% experiencing pain at three separate sites (Huisstede et al 2008). In addition 'specific' and 'non-specific' causes of pain commonly occur together, for example features of hypersensitivity and allodynia have been shown to occur with lateral epicondylitis and myofascial trigger points are widespread in other arm pain syndromes (Huisstede et al 2008, De la Llave-Rincón et al 2009).

HEALTH CARE UTILIZATION AND IMPACT

Upper extremity disorders result in considerable disability and morbidity. Regional musculoskeletal pain syndromes are one of the commonest reasons for presentation in primary care or rheumatology clinics (Turk & Rudy 1990). Chronic symptoms are associated with higher healthcare use and higher levels of disability. Dutch population data show that in individuals meeting the CANS criteria for chronic symptoms (pain lasting more than 3 months in the last 12 months) 58% reported use of healthcare in the last 12 months – 81% of these patients consulted their general practitioner, 59% a medical specialist and 54% a physiotherapist (Huisstede et al 2008). Comparable data were seen for respondents to a British population-based study, such that 39% of those with pain had seen a doctor in the preceding 12 months, 11% a physiotherapist, 10% a chiropractor and 24% had been prescribed medication for their complaint (Walker-Bone 2002). In the Dutch study healthcare users reported more sickness absence than non-healthcare users; 37.2% reported sickness absence due to upper extremity symptoms, compared to 9.3% non-healthcare users and 12.4% reported sickness absence for more than 4 weeks. Healthcare users also reported more recurrent and constant pain and more limitation in daily life due to their symptoms (48.9% compared to 8.5%).

In comparing specific and non-specific upper extremity disorders in the UK, specific diagnoses were also associated with higher healthcare use although self-prescribed medication was similar among people with specific and non-specific diagnoses. Upper extremity pain was associated with significant impact on daily life activities such that 69% of subjects with upper extremity pain reported difficulty with their work, hobbies, or housework (Table 1.3). In total, 59% reported difficulty sleeping caused by their pain. In this study, specific upper limb conditions were more disabling than non-specific pain (Walker-Bone et al 2004b). For example inability to carry shopping bags was seen in 11.5% of people with specific shoulder diagnoses compared with only 6.1% of people classified to have non-specific shoulder pain (Walker-Bone 2002).

RISK FACTORS FOR UPPER EXTREMITY DISORDERS

Gender

As with other musculoskeletal pain, women generally report more upper extremity pain than men at all anatomical sites. Women also tend to consult in primary care more frequently with other symptoms, which may reflect a gender difference in the threshold for seeking help. Alternatively, women may be more vulnerable to factors causing musculoskeletal pain, either because of their physical size and strength or constitutional differences such as hormonal factors (Walker-Bone et al 2003a). Fewer data are available comparing prevalence rates of the specific

Table 1.3 Disability associated with upper extremity pain (adapted from Walker-Bone 2002)

	No difficulty (%)	Some difficulty (%)	Impossible to do (%)
Impact of regional pain at different sites on ability to perform normal daily activities (e.g. work, hobbies, housework)			
Neck pain	30	59	11
Shoulder pain	28	48	11
Elbow pain	29	58	12
Wrist/hand pain	28	58	13
Pain at any site	31	56	13
Impact of pain at any site on sleeping	41	55	4
Impact of pain at any site on driving	34	46	5
Impact of pain at any site on dressing	30	58	8
Impact of pain at any site on carrying bags	67	34	3
NB. Not all rows add up to 100(%) as not all respondents completed every question			

conditions between men and women but there is some evidence that women are more commonly affected by tenosynovitis, de Quervain's disease, shoulder capsulitis and carpal tunnel syndrome. The available studies suggest that epicondylitis is more common among men than women.

Age

Musculoskeletal pain is reported more frequently with age in both genders with a peak in the middle years (50–60 years) and a modest reduction in prevalence in the subsequent decades. The pattern with specific conditions is less well studied but there is evidence of a similar age curve for lateral epicondylitis, CTS among women and possibly de Quervain's disease and tenosynovitis.

Anthropometry

Obesity is associated with an increased frequency of reporting of neck and upper extremity pain and disability caused by painful conditions also increases with body mass index. Carpal tunnel syndrome is strongly associated with obesity such that in one US survey, the risk of CTS increased by 8% for every 1 unit increase in BMI.

Hand dominance

Often used as a surrogate for occupational stressors, hand dominance has been included in some of the more recent workplace studies (Shiri et al 2007). In particular, epicondylitis has been demonstrated to occur more frequently in the dominant, as compared with non-dominant arm.

Hormonal factors

Carpal tunnel syndrome occurs more frequently during pregnancy and lactation and early after the menopause (Walker-Bone et al 2003a). Hysterectomy without oophorectomy has been found to lead to a doubling of the risk of carpal tunnel syndrome when compared with hysterectomy and oophorectomy. Both the oral contraceptive pill and hormone replacement therapy have also been associated with an increased risk of carpal tunnel syndrome. Case reports also suggest that de Quervain's disease is more common during pregnancy or early post-partum. These relationships imply a hormonal component, perhaps related to oedema of the non-articular tissues but the underlying mechanism has not been elucidated.

Occupational risk factors: physical/mechanical factors

Occupational and physical factors have been shown to be risk factors for upper extremity pain disorders and the difficulties in accurately estimating these have already been discussed. Many epidemiological studies have investigated these factors and this literature has been the subject of several comprehensive reviews, all of which comment on the heterogeneity of design, variation in assessment of outcomes and exposures, mode of analysis and presentation. Few stand up to rigorous methodological examination (Buchbinder et al 1996).

Similar to low back pain, mechanical load, repetitive work and abnormal working postures are associated with the development of upper extremity symptoms (Macfarlane et al 2000). Lifting heavy loads, standing for long periods or pushing/pulling are more likely to be associated with low back pain than upper extremity symptoms (Andersen et al 2007). Nevertheless standing for long periods has been shown to be associated with the development of any regional musculoskeletal pain (HR 1.6, 95% CI 1.2–2.3) (Andersen et al 2007).

Results of systematic reviews have suggested strong evidence that neck pain is associated with sustained and abnormal posture, e.g. prolonged sitting with the neck or trunk held in flexion or rotation or a combination of both (Bernard 1997). There is also evidence that neck and neck/shoulder symptoms are increased when work involves forceful and/or repetitive tasks. To date, there is no convincing evidence that vibration increases the risk of neck or neck/shoulder problems. Likewise physical factors also increase the risk of shoulder symptoms, with exposure to intensive and/or repetitive shoulder work, especially overhead, being particularly high risk. The risk seems maximal where an occupation involves combinations of these exposures, e.g. working overhead with a heavy tool. Elbow conditions are associated with exposure to high forces in the workplace. The risk appears maximal when a worker is exposed to combinations of repetition, force and abnormal postures as part of their daily work. Repetitious movements may increase the risk of carpal tunnel syndrome, as may forceful work and exposure to vibration (Bernard 1997). Once again however, the evidence is strongest that occupations involving combinations of force, vibration and repetition are most likely to increase the risk of carpal tunnel syndrome (Abbas et al 1998). When a job involves exposure to awkward forearm, wrist and finger postures, this too may play a role.

Hand/wrist tendonitis or tenosynovitis has been observed in a wide range of different occupational groups ranging from tobacco packers to factory workers during World War II, automobile assembly workers, scissor manufacturers and textile workers (Walker-Bone et al 2003a). It appears that the exposure to high forces, repetitious tasks and sustained abnormal finger/wrist postures are the most risky. The underlying mechanism is poorly researched but it may well represent a physiological/mechanical response of the tendon to chronic mechanical stressors.

Occupational risk factors: psychosocial

Psychosocial factors such as perceived workload, psychological stress and support are increasingly found to be important determinant risks for upper extremity disorders but again exposure is difficult to accurately measure and lacks any standard measurement system, thus is usually estimated from subjective reports. A recent initiative by the European League against Rheumatism (EULAR) aimed to establish whether reviews of risk factors for work related musculoskeletal disorders reached consistent conclusions (Macfarlane et al 2009). The resulting paper looked at four regional pain syndromes, two of which were of the upper extremity and reported that the most consistent conclusions related to psychosocial exposures i.e. high work demands and low job demands – such as monotonous or insufficient use of skills and low work control (Bongers et al 1993). In a prospective study of risk factors for non-specific forearm pain, Macfarlane et al (2000) found that psychosocial factors were important predictors of the development of upper extremity symptoms. For example psychological distress (OR 1.8, 95% CI 0.8–4.0) and aspects of illness behaviour (OR 6.6, 95% CI 1.5–29) compared with the physical factors of repetitive tasks (OR 2.9, 95% CI 1.2–7.3). Similarly North Staffordshire data shows that little job control and little supervisor support are risk factors (OR 1.6, 95% CI 1.3–1.8 and OR 1.3, 95% CI 1.1–1.5) respectively) (Sim et al 2006).

CONCLUSIONS

Upper extremity pain syndromes are common both in the general population and the work-place and are associated with high levels of morbidity and disability. Until recently epidemiological research has been hampered by lack of clear case definitions; however, increasing use of standardized classification schemes allows more meaningful analysis to occur and for comparisons to be made between settings and over time. Nevertheless, many disorders are still classified as 'non-specific' although knowledge is increasing regarding the aetiology of many of these conditions. Many upper extremity pain syndromes can be classified as work-related and are associated with potentially modifiable workplace factors. Many of these are physical but increasing evidence points to psychosocial factors as being significant. This suggests that interventions in the workplace based solely upon mechanical exposures (e.g. ergonomic keyboards and workstations) may not be 100% successful unless attention is also paid to psychosocial risk factors such as control over work, job demands and support in the workplace.

REFERENCES

Abbas, M.A., Afifi, A.A., Zhang, Z.W., Kraus, J.F., 1998. Meta-analysis of published studies of work-related carpal tunnel syndrome. Int J Occup Environ Health. 4 (3), 160–167.

Allander, E., 1974. Prevalence, incidence and remission rates of some rheumatic diseases and syndromes. Scand. J. Rheumatol. 3, 145–153.

Andersen, J.H., Haahr, J.P., Frost, P., 2007. Risk factors for more severe regional musculoskeletal symptoms: a two-year prospective study of a general working population. Arthritis Rheum. 56, 1355–1364.

Atroshi, I., Gummesson, C., Johnsson, R., Ornstein, E., Ranstam, J., Rosen, I., 1999. Prevalence of carpal tunnel syndrome in the general population. JAMA 282, 153–158.

Bergenudd, H., Lindgarde, F., Nilsson, B., Petersson, C.J., 1988. Shoulder pain in middle age. Clin. Orthop. 231, 234–238.

Bernard, B.P. (Ed.), 1997. Musculoskeletal disorders (MSDs) and workplace factors. US Department of Health and Human Services, Cincinnati (OH).

Bongers, P.M., Ijmker, S., van den Heuvel, S., Blatter, B.M., 2006. Epidemiology of work related neck and upper limb problems: psychosocial and personal risk factors (part I) and effective interventions from a bio behavioural perspective (part II). J Occup Rehabil. 16 (3), 279–302.

Buchbinder, R., Goel, V., Bombardier, C., Hogg-Johnson, S., 1996. Classification systems of soft tissue disorders of the neck and upper limb: do they satisfy methodological guidelines? J. Clin. Epidemiol. 49, 141–149.

Chard, M.D., Hazelman, R., Hazelman, B.L., King, R.H., Reiss, B. B., 1991. Shoulder disorders in the elderly: a community survey. Arthritis Rheum. 34, 766–769.

De la Llave-Rincón, A.I., Fernández-de-las-Peñas, C., Fernández-Carnero, J., Padua, L., Arendt-Nielsen, L., Pareja, J.A., 2009. Bilateral hand/wrist heat and cold hyperalgesia, but not hypoesthesia in unilateral carpal tunnel syndrome. Exp. Brain Res. 198, 455–463.

De Krom, M., Knipschild, P.G., Kester, A. D.M., Thus, C.T., Boekkooi, P.F., Spaans, F., 1992. Carpal tunnel syndrome: prevalence in the general population. J. Clin. Epidemiol. 45, 373–376.

Eltayeb, S.M., Staal, J.B., Hassan, A.A., Awad, S.S., de Bie, R.A., 2008. Complaints of the arm, neck and shoulder among computer office workers in Sudan: a prevalence study with validation of an Arabic risk factors questionnaire. Environ. Health 7, 33.

Ferry, S., Silman, A., Pritchard, T., Keenan, J., Croft, P., 1998. The association between different patterns of hand symptoms and objective evidence of median nerve compression. Arthritis Rheum 41, 720–724.

Harrington, J.M., Carter, J.T., Birrell, L., Gompertz, D., 1998. Surveillance case definitions for work related upper limb pain syndromes. Occup. Environ. Med. 55, 264–271.

Helliwell, P., 1995. Diagnostic criteria for work-related upper limb disorders. Br. J. Rheumatol. 35, 1195–1196.

Huisstede, B.M., Bierma-Zeinstra, S.M., Koes, B.W., Verhaar, J.A., 2006. Incidence and prevalence of upper-extremity musculoskeletal disorders. A systematic appraisal of the literature. BMC Musculoskelet. Disord. 7, 7.

Huisstede, B.M., Miedema, H.S., Verhagen, A.P., Koes, B.W., Verhaar, J.A., 2007. Multidisciplinary consensus on the terminology and classification of complaints of the arm, neck and/or shoulder. Occup. Environ. Med. 64, 313–319.

Huisstede, B.M., Wijnhoven, H.A., Bierma-Zeinstra, S.M., Koes, B.W., Verhaar, J.A., Picavet, S., 2008. Prevalence and characteristics of complaints of the arm, neck, and/or shoulder (CANS) in the open population. Clin. J. Pain 24, 253–259.

Hutson, M., 2006. Textbook of Musculoskeletal Medicine 3.5 Upper limb disorders. In: Hutson, E., Ellis, R. (Eds.), Oxford University Press.

Jones, J.R.H.J.T., Clegg, T.A., 1998. Self-reported work-related illness in 1995. HMSO, London.

Macfarlane, G.J., Hunt, I.M., Silman, A.J., 2000. Role of mechanical and psychosocial factors in the onset of forearm pain: prospective population based study. Br. Med. J. 321, 676–679.

Macfarlane, G.J., Pallewatte, N., Paudyal, P., et al., 2009. Evaluation of work-related psychosocial factors and regional musculoskeletal pain: results from a EULAR Task Force. Ann. Rheum. Dis. 68, 885–891.

Menendez, C.C., Amick 3rd., B.C., Chang, C.H., et al., 2008. Computer use patterns associated with upper extremity musculoskeletal symptoms. J. Occup. Rehabil. 18, 166–174.

Morris, H., 1882. Riders sprain. Lancet 2, 557.

Palmer, K.C., 2006. Work related disorders of the upper limb. Topical Reviews 10, 1–7.

Palmer, K., Walker-Bone, K., Linaker, C., et al., 2000. The Southampton examination schedule for the diagnosis of musculoskeletal disorders of the upper limb. Ann. Rheum. Dis. 59, 5–11.

Ramazzini, B., 1940. De morbis artificum. [(First published 1713)]. University of Chicago, Chicago.

Robinson, H., Walker-Bone, K., 2009. Occupation and disorders of the neck and upper limb. Rheumatology in Practice 7, 7–10.

Roquelaure, Y., Ha, C., Leclerc, A., Touranchet, A., et al., 2006. Epidemiologic surveillance of upper-extremity musculoskeletal disorders in the working population. Arthritis Rheum. 55, 765–778.

Shiri, R., Varonen, H., Heliövaara, M., Viikari-Juntura, E., 2007. Hand dominance in upper extremity musculoskeletal disorders. J. Rheumatol. 34, 1076–1082.

Silverstein, B., Welp, E., Nelson, N., Kalat, J., 1998. Claims incidence of work-related disorders of the upper extremities: Washington State, 1987 through 1995. Am J Pub Health 88, 1827–1833.

Sim, J., Lacey, R.J., Lewis, M., 2006. The impact of workplace risk factors on the occurrence of neck and upper limb pain: a general population study. BMC Public Health 6, 234.

Sluiter, J.K., Rest, K.M., Frings-Dresen, M. H., 2001. Criteria document for evaluating the work-relatedness of upper-extremity musculoskeletal disorders. Scand. J. Work Environ. Health 27, 1–102.

Tornqvist, E.W., Hagberg, M., Hagman, M., Risberg, E.H., Toomingas, A., 2009. The influence of working conditions and individual factors on the incidence of neck and upper limb symptoms among professional computer users. Int. Arch. Occup. Environ. Health 82, 689–702.

Turk, D.C., Rudy, T.E., 1990. Neglected factors in chronic pain treatment outcome studies–referral patterns, failure to enter treatment, and attrition. Pain 1, 7–25.

Verhaar, J.A.N., 1994. Tennis elbow. Int Orthop 18, 263–267.

Viikari-Juntura, E., 1983. Neck and upper limb disorders among slaughterhouse workers. Scand. J. Work Environ. Health 9, 283–290.

Walker-Bone, K., 2002. Prevalence of and risk factors for musculoskeletal disorders of the neck and upper limb. PhD Thesis, University of Southampton.

Walker-Bone, K., Byng, P., Linaker, C., et al., 2002. Reliability of the Southampton examination schedule for the diagnosis of upper limb disorders in the general population. Ann. Rheum. Dis. 61, 1103–1106.

Walker-Bone, K.E., Palmer, K.T., Reading, I., Cooper, C., 2003a. Soft-tissue rheumatic disorders of the neck and upper limb: prevalence and risk factors. Seminars in Arthritis Rheumatism 33, 185–203.

Walker-Bone, K.E., Palmer, K.T., Reading, I., Cooper, C., 2003b. Criteria for assessing pain and nonarticular soft-tissue rheumatic disorders of the neck and upper limb. Semin. Arthritis Rheum. 33, 168–184.

Walker-Bone, K., Reading, I., Coggon, D., Cooper, C., Palmer, K.T., 2004a. The anatomical pattern and determinants of pain in the neck and upper limbs: an epidemiologic study. Pain 109, 45–51.

Walker-Bone, K., Palmer, K., Reading, I., Coggon, D., Cooper, C., 2004b. Prevalence and impact of musculoskeletal disorders of the upper limb in the general population. Arthritis Rheum. 51, 642–651.

Chapter | 2 |

History taking

Peter A Huijbregts

INTRODUCTION

In all health care professions including physical therapy there are five elements to patient management. An examination is usually followed by evaluation of the examination findings, establishing a diagnosis, producing a prognosis and a plan of care, and finally, performing the interventions (APTA 2001). In physical therapy the examination usually consists of history taking, systems review, and tests and measures and serves to provide data used in the clinical reasoning process. During this clinical reasoning process the clinician develops in an ongoing manner multiple competing diagnostic hypotheses. Data acquired during the examination are then used to support or refute the various hypotheses. This hypothesis testing process guides the format and content of the ongoing examination process until the clinician decides that sufficient information is obtained to make a diagnostic or management decision (Jones 1995).

Within the profession of physical therapy there are many distinct approaches to patient management. The specific information that a clinician looks for, the order in which it is obtained, and the emphasis that is given to the data collected, varies depending on which philosophy the individual clinician subscribes to. However, all approaches end up testing hypotheses related to (Jones 1995):

1. Source of the symptoms
2. Contributing factors including environmental, behavioural, emotional, psychosocial, systemic/pathologic, and musculoskeletal factors
3. Precautions or contraindications to examination and management
4. Management
5. Prognosis

Irrespective of management philosophy, the need to test the above-mentioned types of hypotheses leads to a consistent content of the history component of examination with history items related to six categories (Boissonnault & Janos 1995) (Box 2.1):

1. Patient profile
2. Location and description of symptoms
3. Symptom behaviour
4. Symptom history
5. Medical history
6. Review of systems

In the examination, history taking and physical examination are inextricably linked. History taking allows the clinician to gather information that is used in the subsequent physical examination to establish the patient's concordant or comparable signs. A concordant sign consists of pain or other symptoms reproduced upon physical examinations that are indicated by the patient as his or her chief complaint, i.e. the reason to seek out therapy (Laslett et al 2003). Without this information derived from history taking the clinician would be unable during the examination

© 2011 Elsevier Ltd.
DOI: 10.1016/B978-0-7020-3528-9.00002-9

Box 2.1 **History taking content**

Patient profile
- Age
- Sex
- Ethnic origin
- Marital status
- Social situation
- Occupation
- Leisure time activities

Location and description of symptoms
- Chief complaint
- Presence and location of pain, sensory abnormalities, strength deficits, range of motion deficits, inflammatory symptoms
- Character of symptoms

Symptom behaviour
- Constant, episodic, or intermittent
- Aggravating factors
- Easing factors
- Diurnal variation

Symptom history
- Nature/mechanism of onset
- Symptom change since onset
- Treatment received

Medical history
- Current and past illnesses
- Hospitalizations
- Family medical history
- Medication use
- Substance abuse
- Nutritional status
- Medical tests and results (imaging, blood work, urinalysis, electrodiagnosis, cerebrospinal fluid analysis, biopsies, etc.)

Review of systems
- Gastrointestinal system
- Urogenital system
- Cardiovascular system
- Pulmonary system
- Musculoskeletal system
- Neurologic system
- Integumentary system
- Psychosocial factors

to distinguish between concordant and discordant signs. Discordant signs are findings on physical examination seemingly implicating a source of symptoms that are, however, in no way related to the chief complaint (Cook 2007).

During history taking the clinician also should seek to get an impression of patient communication ability, affect, cognition, language, and learning style (APTA 2001). In addition, the history allows the clinician to gain insight into the patients' understanding of their own health problem, underlying pathology or dysfunction, mechanism of injury or aetiology, and contributing factors. It provides information on patient goals (that may or may not be realistic or attainable with interventions within the physical therapy scope of practice) and patient motivation and willingness to change (Brouwer et al 1999).

Data collection in the history also establishes a baseline against which to compare the results of the treatment (Cook 2007). Baseline data can of course consist of answers to questions asked during the history and findings on physical examination tests, however the often dichotomous (and even most continuous) variables of this nature usually lack the sufficient responsiveness required of an outcome measure. Therefore, outcomes are preferably collected using reliable, valid, and responsive questionnaire-type outcomes. These outcome measures can be generic, i.e. collect data on general health status, such as the Short Form (SF)-36 (Ware et al 1993), or they can be more specific to a condition. Examples of condition-specific outcome

measures relevant to patients with neck and arm pain include the Neck Disability Index (Vernon & Mior 1991) and the DASH (Disabilities of the Arm, Shoulder, and Hand) tools (Hudak et al 1996). Subsequent chapters will discuss various relevant condition-specific outcome measures. Some validated measures collected as part of history taking serve a prognostic purpose: the Tampa Scale of Kinesiophobia (TSK) is a good example of such a prognostic tool relevant to patients with neck pain (Vlaeyen et al 1995).

In addition to data collection, the history (and subsequent physical examination) also serves another important purpose. A skilfully applied funnel sequence where open-ended questions are followed by specific closed-ended follow-up questions, paraphrasing by the therapist of information provided by the patient to establish effective and accurate communication, appropriate intonation, and attentive non-verbal communication, including appropriate therapist body posture and facial expression, all allow the clinician to establish a professional relationship based on mutual cooperation, respect, and trust (Goodman & Snyder 1995, Brouwer et al 1999).

PATIENT PROFILE

During this portion of the history the clinician collects and records demographic data on patient age, sex, ethnic origin, marital status, social situation, occupation and leisure time activities. Various pathologies are more common based on age and sex (Table 2.1). There is strong evidence for older age as a poor prognostic indicator with regard to mechanical neck pain (McLean et al 2007, Carroll et al 2008a). Sex also seems to affect prognosis for some neck and arm pain syndromes. Women are at a greater risk than men for developing persistent problems after cervical whiplash injury (OR 1.54, 95% CI 1.16–2.06) (Walton et al 2009), whereas men are at higher risk of persistent arm and especially elbow pain (OR 1.9, 95% CI 1.2–3.2) (Ryall et al 2007).

Ethnicity may also predispose patients to certain diseases with, for example, with sickle cell disease (and its musculoskeletal presentation) more prominent in the Black population and skin cancer more prominent in the White population (Boissonnault & Janos 1995). White, Asian, or Hispanic ethnic origin predisposes women to osteoporosis, whereas Black women are less likely to be osteopenic (Huijbregts 2001, Siris et al 2001, South-Paul 2001).

Information on marital status and social situation (including questions on the available support network, adaptations in home and work situation, durable medical equipment availability, and disposable income) helps the therapist establish realistic goals but may also indicate areas relevant to intervention. Questions on leisure time activities and occupation can identify causative or contributing factors but also establish loading requirements and thus appropriate rehabilitation goals. Occupational exposure to industrial toxins (asbestos, lead, agricultural pesticides, or arsenic), extreme temperatures, repetitive or sustained postures and movements, or excessive emotional or mental pressure may predispose patients to pathology. For example, exposure to silica, coal dust, flour dust, or asbestos can lead to pulmonary pathology (Boissonnault & Janos 1995, Goodman & Snyder 1995). Occupational variables can also affect prognosis. Prognosis with regard to neck pain is better for white-collar than for blue-collar workers and worse if patients have little influence on their own work situation (Carroll et al 2008c).

LOCATION AND DESCRIPTION OF SYMPTOMS

Although the patient's chief complaint often revolves around pain and pain-related functional limitations, symptoms that need to be investigated with regard to location and description also include sensory abnormalities, strength deficits, range of motion deficits, and inflammatory symptoms. The subsequent chapters will address location and description of symptoms relevant to the respective neuro-musculoskeletal dysfunctions discussed in those chapters in more detail.

Inherent in testing competing hypotheses with regard to the source of symptoms is ruling out various conditions that can result in a similar presentation. These conditions are not limited to the mechanical neuro-musculoskeletal dysfunctions with an indication for physical therapy management but also include visceral or other systemic pathology that may indicate a need for referral or at the very least affect physical therapy management and prognosis. Note that the role of the physical therapist is not to establish a specific disease-level medical diagnosis but rather to screen for disease using a systems approach (Boissonnault & Janos 1995).

Although in physical therapy clinical practice we certainly encounter patients with cutaneous pain related to the skin and other superficial structures, deep somatic, true visceral, and neuropathic pain are more relevant to physical therapy differential diagnosis. Neuropathic pain results from a primary lesion or dysfunction in the peripheral or central nervous system. Painful neuropathies are characterized by spontaneous and/or abnormal stimulus-evoked pain related to the presence of allodynia, whereby pain is caused by normally innocuous stimuli, and/or hyperalgesia in which case pain intensity evoked by normally painful stimuli is increased (Merskey & Bogduk 1994). Deep somatic pain can originate in bone, muscle, tendon, capsule and ligaments, periosteum, arteries, and nerve connective tissue structures (Boissonnault & Janos 1995). It can also be the result of visceral pathology with irritation of the parietal peritoneum. True visceral pain is a deep pain felt at the site of nociceptive stimulation of the affected internal organ (McCowin et al 1991, Goodman & Snyder 1995). The predominant clinical presentation of both deep somatic and visceral pain is the associated referred pain pattern. Related to convergence of a greater number of primary afferent neurons on a lesser number of secondary afferent neurons and subsequent cortical misinterpretation of the true location of nociceptive afferent input, the patient will report referred pain more superficially in tissues that are segmentally related to the dysfunctional tissue or organ (Van der El 2010).

Referred pain patterns have been established for muscles and will be discussed in detail in Chapter 32, as will neuropathic (including radicular) pain. Chapter 7 (Mechanical neck pain) discusses referral patterns established for cervical zygapophyseal joints, dorsal rami, and disks (Fukui et al 1996, Grubb et al 2000, Cooper et al 2007). Most relevant for suggesting possible visceral pathology in patients presenting with neck, thoracic, and arm pain are the referral patterns related to the cardiovascular, pulmonary, and gastrointestinal systems although a thorough examination even of patients with predominant neck and arm symptoms cannot a priori exclude pathology in other systems. Figure 2.1, therefore, provides visceral referral patterns to the neck, arm, and trunk from all systems (Boissonnault & Janos 1995).

Although serious gastrointestinal disease rarely causes pain without concomitant digestive symptoms it is important to know that both a peptic ulcer and oesophagitis can

Table 2.1 Some age and sex-related medical conditions (Boissonnault & Bass 1990a,b, Goodman & Snyder 1995, Huijbregts 2001, South-Paul 2001)

Diagnosis	Age (years)	Sex
Musculoskeletal		
Rotator cuff degeneration	30+	
Spinal stenosis	60+	Men > women
Costochondritis	40+	Women > men
Neurologic		
Guillain–Barré syndrome	Any age (history of infection)	
Multiple sclerosis	15–50	
Neurogenic claudication	40–60+	
Systemic		
AIDS/HIV	20–49	Men > women
Coronary artery disease	40+	Men > women
Mitral valve prolapse	Young	Women > men
Bürger disease	20–40 (smokers)	Men > women
Aortic aneurysm	40–70	Men > women
Breast cancer	45–70	Women > men
Hodgkin lymphoma	20–40; 50–60	Men > women
Osteoid osteoma	10–20	Men > women
Pancreatic cancer	50–70	Men > women
Skin cancer	Rarely before puberty	Men = women
Gallbladder disease	40+	Women > men
Gout	40–59	Men > women
Gynaecologic conditions	20–45	Women
Prostatitis	40+	Men
Primary biliary cirrhosis	40-60	Women > men
Reiter syndrome	20-40	Men > women
Rheumatic fever	4–8; 18–30	Women > men
Shingles	60+	
Spontaneous pneumothorax	20–40	Men > women
Thyroiditis	30–50	Women > men
Vascular claudication	40–60+	
Osteoporosis	50+	Women > men

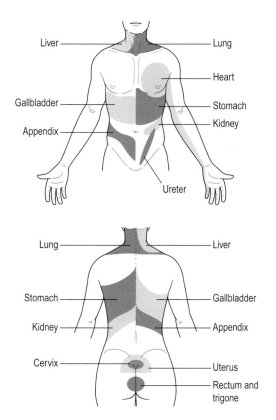

Fig 2.1 Visceral referral patterns.

Table 2.2 Diagnostic accuracy data pain location and description in the diagnosis of acute myocardial infarction (adapted from Swap & Nagurney 2005).

Pain descriptor	Positive likelihood ratio (95% CI)
Increased likelihood of myocardial infarction:	
Radiation to right arm or shoulder	4.7 (1.9–12)
Radiation to both arms or shoulders	4.1 (2.5–6.5)
Radiation to left arm	2.7 (1.7–3.1)
Worse than previous angina or similar	1.8 (1.6–2.0)
Described as pressure	1.3 (1.2–1.5)
Decreased likelihood of myocardial infarction:	
Described as pleuritic	0.2 (0.1–0.3)
Described as sharp	0.3 (0.2–0.5)
Inframammary location	0.8 (0.7–0.9)

cause pain in the upper and mid-abdomen, mid-thoracic region, anterior chest, neck, and bilateral shoulders. The mechanism for referral from the stomach and oesophagus to the neck and shoulders is related to irritation of the adjacent diaphragm with its segmental innervation derived from C3 to C5 through the phrenic nerve. The liver and pancreas normally refer to the right upper and mid-thoracic spine or to the thoracolumbar and upper abdominal region, respectively, but again through irritation of the diaphragm can also cause neck and shoulder pain, with the liver referring the right side of the anterior, lateral, and posterior neck (Boissonnault & Bass 1990a). The gallbladder generally refers to the right costal margin or epigastrium but in some patients also refers pain to the bilateral or unilateral infrascapular region (Vestergaard et al 1998). Grieve (1994) noted that a hiatal hernia can present with widespread chest and bilateral shoulder pain.

Cardiovascular pathology can also be the cause of pain in patients with neck and arm symptoms. Pain originating in the heart can refer to the face, jaw, neck, the precordial region, epigastrium, and less commonly the posterior thorax. Upper extremity referral can be bilateral or unilateral but is most commonly in a left C8 distribution (Boissonnault & Bass 1990b, Grieve 1994). Swap & Nagurney

(2005) provided diagnostic accuracy data for history items related to pain description and location in the clinical diagnosis of acute myocardial infarction (Table 2.2). Diffuse throbbing or aching pain in the mid-back, abdomen, chest, and left shoulder may indicate a symptomatic aortic aneurysm (Boissonnault & Bass 1990b). A sudden tearing chest pain radiating into the neck, dorsal trunk, abdomen, and legs may indicate a dissection of the ascending aorta or aortic arch (Grieve 1994). Pain from internal carotid artery dissection is felt in the ipsilateral fronto-temporal and peri-orbital region, whereas pain from vertebral artery dissection is reported in the ipsilateral occipital region (Triano & Kawchuk 2006). Figures 2.2 and 2.3 shows pain referral patterns for major vascular structures.

The pulmonary system produces local thoracic and chest pain but can also cause referred pain to the neck and shoulders. As with serious gastrointestinal pathology, noted pulmonary pathology in addition to pain will generally present with other symptoms including stridor, coughing, wheezing, dyspnoea, hoarseness, fever, or a sore throat. Pleurisy originating in the parietal pleura refers to the scapular, axillary, and nipple regions (Boissonnault & Bass 1990b, Grieve 1994). A Pancoast tumour of the apex of the lung may cause neck, shoulder, and upper extremity pain in a C8–T1 distribution mimicking thoracic outlet syndrome or low cervical radiculopathy (Boissonnault & Bass 1990b,c).

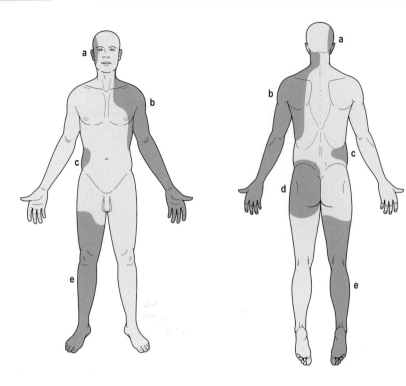

Fig 2.2 Vascular referral patterns: (a) common carotid artery, (b) subclavian artery, (c) descending aorta, (d) internal iliac artery, (e) external iliac artery.

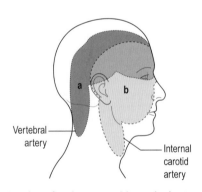

Fig 2.3 Vascular referral patterns: (a) vertebral artery, (b) internal carotid artery.

boring, colicky, coming in waves, or deep aching as possibly indicative of visceral problems. Cramping or colicky pain may be related to the rhythmic contraction and relaxation of the smooth muscle wall of a hollow viscus that may last up to a few minutes per cycle. Throbbing, cramping, or aching pain may also be suggestive of cardiovascular involvement, as is pain described as pressure, tightness, or heaviness (Boissonnault & Janos 1995). Tearing pain has been associated with aortic dissection (Grieve 1994). A stabbing, pulsating, aching, thunderclap-like headache may indicate cervical (vertebral and internal carotid) artery dissection (Triano & Kawchuk 2006). Clinicians should note, however, the overlap of at least a number of these pain descriptors with pain of myofascial or other somatic aetiology.

With both visceral and deep somatic structures causing the same poorly localized, vague, and deep aching somatic pain the description or character of pain is less relevant in the differential diagnosis between mechanical neuro-musculoskeletal dysfunction and visceral pathology (Boissonnault & Bass 1990a, Goodman & Snyder 1995). However, some pain descriptors have been suggested or shown to have diagnostic value. Pressure-like pain is indicative of acute myocardial infarction, whereas pain described as sharp or pleuritic decreases the likelihood of this condition (Swap & Nagurney 2005). Goodman & Snyder (1995) suggested pain characterized as knife-like,

SYMPTOM BEHAVIOUR

Symptom behaviour can be defined as a change in location, intensity, and/or quality of symptoms related to aggravating and easing factors (Boissonnault & Janos 1995). When investigating symptom behaviour the clinician seeks to find out whether symptoms are intermittent, episodic, or constant, if there is a 24-hour or diurnal pattern to the symptoms, and to get information about aggravating or easing factors.

Physical therapists should expect that pain associated with mechanical neuro-musculoskeletal dysfunction is aggravated and eased by postures and activities. This is not to say that the pain and symptoms from mechanical dysfunction are always intermittent, especially in the acute stage where inflammation is predominant, symptoms can be constant, although intensity will still be affected by postures or activities (Boissonnault & Janos 1995). Episodic symptoms are suggestive of systemic disease, especially a progressive pattern with periods where cyclically the patient feels better and then again worse should raise the clinician's index of suspicion with regard to systemic etiology (Goodman & Snyder 1995).

A diurnal pattern when not related to consistent mechanical aggravation (as may sometimes occur with occupational demands) also suggests systemic pathology. Examples are the pain related to a duodenal ulcer that will consistently start some two hours after eating (Boissonnault & Bass 1990a). Particularly ominous in this regard is night pain. In this context, we do not think of the pain that wakes up the patient but is easily relieved by changing positions. Various studies have reported an association of this type of night pain with osteoarthritis especially of the lumbar, hip, and knee joints (Acheson et al 1969, Siegmeth & Noyelle 1988, Foldes et al 1992, Jonsson & Stromqvist 1993). Night pain becomes relevant as a red flag indicating the need for medical referral if the patient reports that this pain is the worst pain over a 24-hour period and/or if this night pain results in the patient being unable or requiring considerable effort to get back to sleep (Boissonnault & Janos 1995, Goodman & Snyder 1995).

Symptoms of visceral pathology can often be elicited and relieved by factors that are clearly not mechanical in nature. We discussed above the pain from a duodenal ulcer occurring some two hours after eating. Duodenal pain can often be relieved by again eating or by taking antacid medication. Gastrointestinal pathology should be suspected if the patient reports that ingestion of certain foods or food in general precipitates or alleviates symptoms. Pain in the right costal margin or epigastrium and the infrascapular region(s) after eating high-fat food may implicate the gallbladder as the source of pain symptoms (Boissonnault & Bass 1990a). Pain decreased with fasting, after a bowel movement, or after vomiting also implicates the gastrointestinal system. Ingestion of caffeine, especially when combined with smoking raises the blood pressure for some two hours, which may lead to cardiovascular symptomatology in hypertensive patients. Alcohol consumption and fever increase the systolic thrust and may elicit pain originating in arteries. Increased metabolic demand not related to physical activity as occurs with emotion or exposure to extreme temperatures may elicit cardiovascular symptoms (Goodman & Snyder 1995).

Associating symptoms aggravated with postures and activities solely with benign mechanical dysfunction is,

however, a dangerous oversimplification of the clinical picture (Grieve 1994). Activity-related cardiovascular symptoms including vascular claudication and pain due to coronary ischaemia in patients with coronary artery disease or pulmonary system pain from the pleura and trachea with respiratory movement require no further explanation. Perhaps less obvious is pain due to distension of a hollow organ aggravated by increased intra-abdominal pressure and relieved by positions that reduce pressure or support the painful organ. For example, the pain from acute gallbladder distension decreases with slight trunk flexion, whereas flexion and ipsilateral sidebending may relieve kidney pain. Seated flexion or bringing the knees to the chest in supine may decrease pancreatic pain. Bending over increases the systolic thrust and may aggravate pain arising from arteries (Goodman & Snyder 1995). The pain from pericarditis is aggravated by coughing or changing position and relieved by leaning forward.

Pain with swallowing or breathing may be related to the mechanical compression of the oesophagus or bronchi caused by an aortic aneurysm. Although dyspnea would lead a clinician to suspect cardiovascular or pulmonary pathology, a patient report of nocturnal shortness of breath relieved by sitting up or sleeping with multiple pillows (orthopnea) should raise even greater suspicion. Swap & Nagurney (2005) provided diagnostic accuracy data for history items related to (non) mechanical symptom behaviour in the clinical diagnosis of acute myocardial infarction (Table 2.3). One system often overlooked when screening for pathology using a systems approach is the musculoskeletal system: systemic inflammatory

Table 2.3 Diagnostic accuracy data symptom behaviour (and associated symptoms) in the diagnosis of acute myocardial infarction (adapted from Swap & Nagurney 2005).

Symptom behaviour	Positive likelihood ratio (95% CI)
Increased likelihood of myocardial infarction:	
Associated with exertion	2.4 (1.5–3.8)
Associated with diaphoresis	2.0 (1.9–2.2)
Associated with nausea or vomiting	1.9 (1.7–2.3)
Decreased likelihood of myocardial infarction:	
Described as positional	0.3 (0.2–0.5)
Reproducible with palpation	0.3 (0.2–0.4)
Not associated with exertion	0.8 (0.6–0.9)

conditions, infection, and fractures are all likely to be aggravated and eased mechanically and may thereby be mistaken for benign mechanical dysfunctions (Boissonnault & Bass 1990c).

An inventory of pain symptom behaviour also serves the purpose of identifying limitations in activities and restrictions in participation resulting from dysfunction or pathology. This way the clinician gets an impression of severity, which is the subjective identification of how significantly the patient has been affected by this current health problem. In addition, questioning the patient with regard to symptom behaviour also provides the clinician with information on irritability. Irritability or reactivity is a concept that tries to quantify how stable a condition is. In other words, how quickly does a stable presentation degenerate in the presence of aggravating factors? Irritability is a three-dimensional concept. The clinician not only collects information on aggravating factors (1) but also on duration and severity of a condition once aggravated (2) and on what the patient needs to do to again relieve or decrease symptoms (3) (Cook 2007).

SYMPTOM HISTORY

In the symptom history portion the therapist constructs a chronological description of the current health problem including information on onset, changes in symptoms since onset, and treatment received for the current problem (Boissonnault & Janos 1995). This allows determination of the stage of the health problem, which reflects the patient's interpretation of current complaints and impairments as compared to a given point in the past. Health problems can be worse, better, or the same with regard to symptoms and impact on function leading the clinician to characterize a condition as stabilized, stagnated, or progressed (for better or worse). Together with information on severity and irritability gained from the symptom behaviour portion, knowledge with regard to the stage of a condition determines precautions with regard to subsequent examination and guides management (Cook 2007). If the stage, severity, and irritability of a condition do not match the expected normal course of a mechanical dysfunction of traumatic aetiology where an acute inflammatory stage with moderate to high severity and high irritability is followed by a progressively less irritable and severe sub-acute and/or chronic stabilized, stagnated, or improved presentation, systemic pathology may be suspected. Likewise, a cyclical or episodic presentation should raise suspicion with regard to non-mechanical problems.

Although clinicians might associate an insidious, slow progressive onset more with systemic pathology and a clear traumatic mechanism of acute injury with mechanical dysfunction, the clinician needs to consider systemic pathology even when complaints seem to have been brought on acutely by trauma. For example, pathological fractures in bones weakened by osteoporosis, osteomalacia, infection, and tumours may result from similar traumatic mechanisms that can also cause mechanical neuro-musculoskeletal dysfunctions (Boissonnault & Janos 1995). Acute-onset monoarthritis has to be considered infective until proven otherwise (Woolf & Åkesson 2008). In contrast, mechanical dysfunctions related to overuse or chronic pain syndromes associated with peripheral and central sensitization are characterized by an insidious onset and a slow progressive presentation.

Collecting information on the nature and the results of previous treatments provides guidance with regard to management. After all, replicating previously unsuccessful treatment makes little sense. However, when the patient reports no improvement despite seemingly appropriate previous treatments again the index of suspicion for systemic pathology is raised (Goodman & Snyder 1995).

MEDICAL HISTORY

In the medical history portion the physical therapist collects information on the patient's current and past illnesses, hospitalizations, family medical history, medication use, substance abuse, nutritional status, and medical tests and results.

Current illnesses may affect physical therapy diagnosis, prognosis, and management (Boissonnault & Janos 1995). Cardiovascular and pulmonary pathology of course often affect exercise tolerance. Although less acutely, gastrointestinal pathology, especially if it results in malabsorption, also limits how much we can have a patient exercise. Knowledge of past and concurrent illnesses affects diagnosis. A medical history of previous cancer with a presentation not indicative of mechanical dysfunction should raise the clinician's index of suspicion. Metastases from primary tumours in the prostate, lung, breast, kidney, and colon preferentially occur in the spine (Boissonnault & Bass 1990c). In fact, patients with breast cancer have an 85% lifetime incidence of bony metastases, especially in the thoracic spine (Greenhalgh & Selfe 2004). A history of, for example, rheumatic fever increases the risk of valvular heart disease (Boissonnault & Bass 1990b). Previous surgery, even in the absence of constitutional symptoms, carries an increased risk of iatrogenic infection up to several months after the surgery. Cancer, certain cardiovascular conditions, diabetes, osteoporosis, and kidney disease all have a familial tendency (Boissonnault & Bass 1990a). A thorough questioning with regard to medication often not only uncovers additional concurrent pathology but the therapist also needs to be aware of adverse effects of medication that may mimic mechanical dysfunction or predispose the patient to pathology. The depth and breadth of knowledge required for the therapist to elicit and be able to interpret a comprehensive medical history is well illustrated when, for example, reviewing the various causes described for secondary osteoporosis as one of the relevant pathologies to be considered in patients complaining of neck, trunk, and arm pain (Box 2.2).

The medical history may also provide less ominous prognostic indicators. Concurrent chronic pain at sites other than the arm increases the risk of arm pain continuing up to 12 months after initial onset (OR 1.6–2.4 based on the site of pain) (Ryall et al 2007). Shoulder pain concomitant with neck pain indicates a poorer prognosis for resolution of the neck pain (McLean et al 2007). Concomitant neck pain is a predictor of shoulder pain at six weeks, whereas concomitant low back pain is a predictor for continued shoulder pain at six months (Kuijpers

et al 2006). Concomitant low back pain also serves as a poor prognostic indicator in patients with neck pain (Hill et al 2004, Hoving et al 2004). Previous neck pain indicates a poorer prognosis for occupational neck pain (Carroll et al 2008c) and a higher risk of chronic pain postwhiplash injury (OR 1.7, 95% CI 1.17–2.48) (Walton et al 2009).

Although patients are less likely to freely discuss this, the therapist needs to also be attentive of indications of substance abuse. Excessive alcohol use not only increases the risk of osteoporosis but also of cirrhosis and neurodegenerative conditions. It can also cause osteonecrosis and subsequent pathologic fractures. The therapist also needs to be aware of an alcohol-related altered perception of pain and fatigue and interaction of alcohol with numerous medications (Goodman & Snyder 1995, Huijbregts 2000, Huijbregts & Vidal 2004). As an example of

---

Box 2.2 **Secondary causes of osteoporosis (Huijbregts 2001, South-Paul 2001)**

Nutritional deficiencies
- Excessive consumption of phosphates, oxalates, alkalis, fatty acids, dietary fibres, proteins, refined sugar, caffeine, alcohol, and sodium
- Insufficient intake calcium and/or vitamin D

Endocrine diseases
- Acromegaly
- Anorexia nervosa
- Athletic amenorrhea
- Cystic fibrosis
- Delayed puberty
- Diabetes mellitus (untreated)
- Female hypogonadism
- Growth hormone deficiencies
- Haemochromatosis
- Hypercortisolism (Cushing disease)
- Hyperparathyroidism
- Hyperprolactinaemia
- Hyperthyroidism
- Hypothalamic amenorrhea
- Idiopathic hypogonadotropic hypogonadism
- Klinefelter syndrome
- Male hypogonadism
- Oophorectomy
- Premature and primary ovarian failure
- Primary gonadal failure

Gastrointestinal diseases
- Alactasia
- Chronic obstructive jaundice
- Malabsorption syndromes
- Primary biliary cirrhosis and other cirrhoses

- Subtotal gastrectomy

Bone marrow disorders
- Disseminated carcinoma
- Haemolytic anemias
- Leukemia
- Lymphoma
- Multiple myeloma
- Systemic mastocytosis

Connective tissue diseases
- Ehlers–Danlos syndrome
- Glycogen storage diseases
- Homocystinuria
- Hypophosphatasia
- Marfan syndrome
- Osteogenesis imperfecta

Medication
- Anticonvulsants
- Chemotherapy
- Cyclosporine
- Glucocorticoids
- GnRH agonists
- Heparin
- Methothrexate
- Phenobarbital
- Phenothiazines
- Thyroxine

Miscellaneous
- Immobilization
- Rheumatoid arthritis
- Smoking

the effects of illicit drugs, cocaine and amphetamines increase the production of adrenaline causing systemic vasoconstriction resulting in increased blood pressure and possibly seizures, dysrhythmia, and tachycardia. Cocaine use has also been associated with an increased risk of stroke, aortic rupture, pulmonary edema, and clotting disorders (Goodman & Snyder 1995). Intravenous drug use increases the chances of bloodborne infections (Boissonnault & Bass, 1990c). Cardiovascular health risks of smoking need no further discussion but smoking also increases the risk of gastrointestinal pathology and osteoporosis (Boissonnault & Bass 1990a, Huijbregts 2001, South-Paul 2001). Smoking also generally retards musculoskeletal healing. For example, a current smoking habit is a poor prognostic indicator for continued arm pain at 12 months (OR 3.3, 95% CI 1.6–6.6) (Ryall et al 2007).

Nutritional status affects diagnosis and prognosis and the therapist needs to have at least a basic knowledge base in this area. General malnutrition in the sense of insufficient dietary glucose and protein intake retards musculoskeletal healing but high-protein diets used to combat malnutrition especially in the elderly can cause dehydration, which also impairs healing (Posthauer 2006). Amino acid deficiencies (arginine, methionine, and glutamine) negatively affect the course of the normal inflammatory process. Deficiencies in the trace minerals manganese, copper, calcium, magnesium, and iron decrease collagen synthesis. Deficiencies in zinc and vitamins A, B, C, and E impair the immune response relevant to musculoskeletal healing (Arnold & Barbul 2006, Broughton et al 2006, Campos et al 2008). If nutritional deficiencies are suggested in the history a nutritional wellness assessment by the therapist and if indicated a referral to a dietitian are indicated (Fair 2010).

Finally, the therapist should ask the patient about medical diagnostic procedures that may have been done, e.g. imaging, blood work, urinalysis, electrodiagnosis, cerebrospinal fluid analysis, and biopsies. Knowing which tests have already been done with knowledge of their findings is obviously helpful in diagnosis and management.

SYSTEMS REVIEW

Screening for systemic pathology occurs as part of the history and physical examination but also throughout the management process, where we continuously monitor the patients' condition and also their response to seemingly appropriate treatment (Cook 2007). We discussed how therapists screen for medical disease at the systems level, unlike medical physicians who seek to diagnose patients at the disease-level (Boissonnault & Janos 1995). Despite this distinction the therapist needs to have considerable acumen with regard to knowledge of pathology to optimally screen even at the systems level.

The medical screening or systems review portion of the history (and physical examination) serves a number of purposes. First and foremost, by way of ruling out systemic pathology it allows for sufficient confidence that a patient presentation is in fact based on a mechanical neuro-musculoskeletal dysfunction and, therefore, may pose an indication for physical therapy management. Second, the systems review may raise the index of suspicion with regard to a systemic etiology of the patient presentation and indicate the need for referral for medical-surgical evaluation. Starting a systems review with a list of general health status indicators either as part of the patient–therapist face-to-face encounter or in the form of an intake questionnaire reviewed prior to the examination by the clinician can indicate the need for a more in-depth systems review (Box 2.3). A number of these general health status indicators have been discussed above and some return in more specific systems-based questions. Fever and night sweats are characteristic symptoms of systemic disease. Weight loss of 10% over a 4-week period not related to lifestyle changes (diet, exercise) may indicate diabetes, hyperthyroidism, depression, anorexia nervosa, or neoplastic disease. However, an unexplained weight gain may also be relevant in that it can be the result of congestive heart failure and again neoplastic disease or hyperthyroidism (Goodman & Snyder 1995). The need for a more in-depth systems review becomes greater if, as the history taking progresses, other portions of the history as discussed above also yield indicators of systemic etiology or contribution to patient

---

Box 2.3 Checklist for review of general health status (Boissonnault & Janos 1995, Goodman & Snyder 1995)

- Fever/chills
- Unexplained perspiration
- Night sweats
- Recent infection
- Unexplained weight change
- Malaise
- Nausea/vomiting
- Bowel dysfunction
- Numbness
- Weakness
- Pallor
- Dizziness/lightheadedness
- Syncope
- Night pain
- Difficulty breathing
- Difficulty urinating
- Urinary frequency changes
- Sexual dysfunction

presentation. Although no such list can ever be comprehensive, Table 2.4 provides suggestions for more specific systems-based questions. Positive findings on any of the questions in the systems-based review should again prompt further investigation. Table 2.5 provides an example for further investigation of indicators for the need for urgent medical referral (red flags) in the case of a patient report of headache (Huijbregts 2009).

The third and final purpose of medical screening is to also provide the clinician with information on systemic pathology that can affect prognosis/rehabilitation potential or that dictates choice and progression of physical therapy interventions (Boissonnault & Janos 1995).

Relevant to the differential diagnosis of a multitude of symptoms suggestive of visceral pathology and within the context of screening for psychosocial factors in

Table 2.4 Suggested questions systems review (Boissonnault & Bass 1990a, Goodman & Snyder 1995, Flynn et al 2008)

System	Questions
Cardiovascular	Do you ever experience chest pain (angina)? Do you experience excessive unexplained fatigue? Do you have shortness of breath? Do you ever note chest palpitations? Have you noted lightheadedness? Have you ever fainted? Do you experience widespread leg pains? Have you noted swelling in the feet, ankles, or perhaps the hands?
Pulmonary	Do you ever experience chest pain? Do you have shortness of breath? Have you been coughing more lately? Have you noticed a change in your breathing? Do you have difficulty catching your breath when lying flat; do you have to sleep propped up on multiple pillows?
Gastrointestinal	Have you had difficulty swallowing? Have you noticed intolerance to specific foods? Have you had abdominal pain? Has your stool been black in color? Have you had rectal bleeding? Has your stool been different in consistency (diarrhoea, tarry stool)? Have you been constipated?
Genitourinary	Any difficulty urinating? Have you noted blood in your urine? Have you noted an increased frequency with regard to urination? Have you noted an increased urgency with regard to urination? Have you noted an increased difficulty with initiating urination? Have you noted decreased force with urination? Have there been episodes of impotence? Have there been any changes with regard to menstruation? Have you experienced pain with intercourse? Have you noted incontinence for urine and/or stool?
Integumentary	Have you recently experienced any rashes? Have you noticed any enlargement or bleeding of moles? Have you noted any itching or burning of the skin? Have you noticed any areas of blistering?
Neurologic	Have you been experiencing headaches or vision changes? Have you noted dizziness or vertigo? Have you been experiencing seizures or unconsciousness? Do you ever experience weakness or paraesthesiae?

Table 2.5 Red flag indicators in the history taking of patients with headaches indicating the need for urgent referral (adapted from Huijbregts 2009).

Factor	'Red flag' indicators
Demographics	New onset of headache or change in existing headache pattern in patients over 50
Location of pain	Persistent unilateral location of headaches
Onset and course of headache	New-onset headache Onset of a new headache type Unexplained change for the worse in pattern of existing headache Progressively worsening headache Abrupt, split-second onset of headache: thunderclap headache
Character and intensity of headache	New pain level, especially when described as worst-ever Cluster-type headache
Aggravating and easing factors	Headache aggravated or brought on by physical exertion, coughing, sneezing, straining or sexual activity Noted effect of position changes on pain No response to seemingly appropriate treatment
Neurological symptoms	Seizures, confusion, changes in alertness, apathy, clumsiness, unexplained inappropriate behaviour, brain stem symptoms, bowel and bladder symptoms, neck flexion stiffness, aura preceding the headache (especially one with quick diffusion), or weakness (not consistent with an existing diagnosis of migraine headaches or other pathology explaining these symptoms) Pre-syncope or syncope starting off headache
Otolaryngological symptoms	Associated eye pain and simultaneous vision changes
Systemic symptoms	Fever, weight loss, temporal artery tenderness, profuse vomiting (especially when not associated with nausea), photophobia, phonophobia, or developing rash (not consistent with an existing diagnosis of migraine headaches) Headache that awakens a patient from night sleep (especially in children)
Medical history	Medical history of cancer and human immunodeficiency virus infection Head or neck injury Uncontrolled hypertension
Medication history	Use of anticoagulant medication in combination with even minor trauma
Family history	Absence of a family history of migraine in children with migraine-like symptoms

patients with neck and arm pain is the diagnosis of panic disorder (Box 2.4) (Huijbregts & Vidal 2004). Psychosocial factors often serve as prognostic indicators. Depression is an independent risk factor for developing subsequent low back or neck pain (Carroll et al 2004) but also predicts poorer outcome after cervical whiplash injury (Carroll et al 2008b). Passive coping and fear of movement also serve as poor prognostic indicators after whiplash injury (Carroll et al 2008b) and fear of movement is also a consistent impediment to recovery from sub-acute neck pain both at the 12- and 52-week mark (Pool et al 2010). Fear of movement can be quantified using the Tampa Scale of Kinesiophobia tool (Vlaeyen et al 1995). It will also serve the clinician well to be familiar with the presentation of depression (Box 2.5). Arroll et al (2003) reported a sensitivity of 97% and a specificity of 67% in the clinical diagnosis of depression in primary care for the following two questions:

1. During the last month have you often been bothered by feeling down, depressed, or hopeless?
2. During the last month have you often been bothered by little interest or pleasure in doing things?

Box 2.4 Diagnosis of panic disorder (adapted from Huijbregts & Vidal 2004)

Signs and symptoms (diagnosis requires four):
- Sweating
- Rapid heart rate, palpitations, pounding heart
- Tremor
- Shortness of breath
- Feeling of choking
- Chest pain
- Nausea/abdominal distress
- Dizziness
- Lightheadedness
- Feeling of unreality
- Fear of losing control
- Fear of dying
- Paraesthesiae
- Hot flashes

Associated signs and symptoms
- Insomnia
- Anxiety
- Depression
- Chronic fatigue
- Gastro-oesophageal reflux

Box 2.5 Symptoms associated with depression (adapted from Goodman & Snyder 1995)

- Persistent sadness or feelings of emptiness
- Sense of hopelessness
- Frequent or unexplained crying spells
- Problems with sleeping
- Feelings of guilt
- Loss of interest or pleasure in normal activities
- Fatigue or decreased energy
- Difficulty in concentrating, remembering, and decision-making
- Appetite loss (or overeating)

Although as therapists we tend to concentrate on mechanical dysfunction of the musculoskeletal system, in our systems review we should not overlook the possibility of musculoskeletal pathology including fractures, and infectious, inflammatory, and neoplastic disease. Indicators for neoplastic disease have been discussed above. Chapter 9 discusses cervical myelopathy as a differential diagnostic possibility in patients with neck and arm pain.

In this era of direct access to physical therapy services, therapists need to be able to screen for the presence of fractures. With regard to cervical spine injuries, both the NEXUS (National Emergency X-radiography Utilization Study) and the Canadian C-spine Rule need to be considered (Eyre 2006). The NEXUS rule recommends cervical plain-film radiography unless all five criteria below are met:

1. Absence of posterior midline cervical spine tenderness
2. No evidence of intoxication
3. Normal level of alertness/consciousness
4. Absence of focal neurological deficit
5. Absence of distracting injuries

Although the NEXUS rule has shown a sensitivity of 99.6% and a specificity of 12.9% and also 100% sensitivity in separate studies in a geriatric and a pediatric population, with distracting injuries defined as long bone fractures, degloving injuries, and extensive burns and lacerations, it was obviously developed and validated in an emergency room and not in a primary care physical therapy setting (Eyre 2006). The Canadian C-spine Rule, although suffering from the same spectrum bias and thereby expected to overestimate sensitivity and underestimate specificity when applied in a physical therapy primary care setting (Cook et al 2007), still seems more relevant to therapists (Fig 2.4). When compared in nine Canadian emergency departments the Canadian C-spine rule showed 99.4% sensitivity and 45.1% specificity versus 90.7% sensitivity and 36.8% specificity for the NEXUS rule (Eyre 2006).

We discussed osteoporosis in the medical history portion above (see Box 2.2). Cadarette et al (2000) developed the Osteoporosis Risk Assessment Instrument (ORAI) (Table 2.6). Screening women with a score ≥ 9 yielded a sensitivity of 93.3% (95% CI 86.3–97.0%) and a specificity of 46.4% (95% CI 41.0–51.8) for osteopenia. The sensitivity for a diagnosis of osteoporosis was 94.4% (95% CI 83.7–98.6%). A score < 9 on this instrument would thus seem to reduce the likelihood of a suspected osteoporotic fracture in female patients.

We discussed surgery as a risk factor for subsequent bloodborne or haematogenous infection. Recent infection was an item included in our general health status checklist (see Box 2.3). Risk factors for, for example, diskitis also include intravenous drug use and immunosuppression (as occurs for example in patients with AIDS and HIV). Infection can also lead to vertebral osteomyelitis. Risk factors for pyogenic (bacterial) osteomyelitis include (Vincent & Benson 1991, Heggeness et al 1993):

- Intravenous drug use
- Diabetes
- Urinary tract infection
- Stab wounds
- Gunshot wounds
- Sickle cell disease

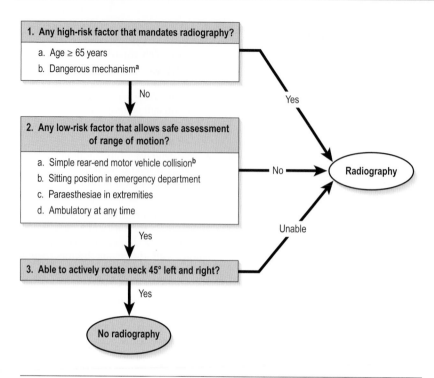

1. **Any high-risk factor that mandates radiography?**
   a. Age ≥ 65 years
   b. Dangerous mechanism[a]

No ↓   Yes →

2. **Any low-risk factor that allows safe assessment of range of motion?**
   a. Simple rear-end motor vehicle collision[b]
   b. Sitting position in emergency department
   c. Paraesthesiae in extremities
   d. Ambulatory at any time

No → **Radiography**

Yes ↓   Unable →

3. **Able to actively rotate neck 45° left and right?**

Yes ↓

No radiography

[a] A dangerous mechanism is considered to be a fall from an elevation ≥3 ft or 5 stairs, an axial load to the head (e.g. diving), a motor vehicle collision at high speed (>100 km/hr), or with rollover or ejection

[b] A simple rear-end motor vehicle collision excludes being pushed into oncoming traffic, being hit by a bus or a large truck, a rollover, and being hit by a high-speed vehicle

Fig 2.4 Canadian cervical-spine rule.

Table 2.6 Scoring system ORAI (adapted from Cadarette et al 2000)

Variable	Score
Age (years):	
≥ 75	15
65–74	9
55–64	5
45–54	0
Weight (kg):	
< 60	9
60–69	3
≥ 70	0
Current estrogen use:	
Yes	0
No	2

- Immunodeficiency
- Pre-existing paraplegia
- Non-operatively treated thoracolumbar fractures
- Metal implants
- Polymethylmethacrylate
- Urology or dental procedures in patients with metal implants without antibiotic prophylaxis

The most common systemic inflammatory diseases relevant to patients with neck and arm pain include rheumatoid arthritis and seronegative spondylarthropathies. Pathological changes in spondylarthropathies involve joints but also entheses or insertions of ligaments, tendons, and capsule to the bone. Especially these enthesopathies and initially the spinal articular manifestations may be mistaken for mechanical dysfunctions in patients with neck and arm pain. Table 2.7 provides information on clinical findings in patients with inflammatory joint disease (Katz & Liang 1991, McCowin et al 1991).

Table 2.7 Clinical findings in seronegative spondylarthropathies (Katz & Liang 1991, McCowin et al 1991)

Disease	Clinical presentation
Ankylosing spondylitis	Affects sacroiliac, zygapophyseal, and costovertebral joints Pain in heels, ischial tuberosities, iliac crests, humeral epicondyles, and shoulders Nocturnal pain Morning pain and stiffness Asymmetric peripheral arthritis yet often symmetric arthritis in both hips Uveitis with pain and photophobia
Psoriatic arthritis	Asymmetric oligoarthritis, symmetric polyarthritis Back or peripheral joint initial symptom Unilateral sacroiliac involvement More frequent in patients with psoriatic skin involvement
Enteropathic arthritis	Occurs in patients with Crohn disease or ulcerative colitis Morning pain and stiffness Affects sacroiliac, zygapophyseal, and costovertebral joints May include periostitis, osteonecrosis, septic hip arthritis, granulomatous inflammation of the bone, synovium, and muscle May include ulceration of the perineum, oropharynx, and rectum Erythema nodosum and pyoderma gangrenosum
Reiter syndrome	Can develop after or during infection elsewhere in body Lumbopelvic and lower limb arthritis Genitourinary symptoms: mucopurulent discharge, dysuria, vaginitis, cervicitis Ocular disease: conjunctivitis or iritis Systemic symptoms: fever, anorexia, weight loss, fatigue Heel pain, Achilles tendonitis, dactylitis Mucocutaneous lesions of oropharynx, soles, palms, and nails

CONCLUSION

History taking is inextricably linked to physical examination in the examination phase of patient management. Although various approaches to patient management within physical therapy differ with regard to the specific information they seek to collect during history taking, the order in which they collect these data and the importance they place on them, clinicians can still identify six consistent and distinct categories in all history taking. Within this chapter we have addressed this general content of history taking with specific attention to the systems review component and to screening for systemic pathology in patients with neck and arm pain during the patient history. Subsequent chapters will address in more detail history findings specific to the dysfunctions discussed. With a paucity of data on diagnostic accuracy relevant to history items, history taking still heavily relies on extrapolation of basic science knowledge, experience, and authority-based knowledge. Rather than devaluing the role of the history within the evidence-informed paradigm as a result of this absence of diagnostic accuracy research, this chapter has sought to indicate the depth and breadth of knowledge required from the clinician when the goal is to elicit from the patient a comprehensive and clinically useful history.

REFERENCES

Acheson, R.M., Chan, Y.K., Payne, M., 1969. New Haven survey of joint diseases: The interrelationships between morning stiffness, nocturnal pain and swelling of the joints. J. Chronic Dis. 21, 533–542.

American Physical Therapy Association, 2001. Guide to physical therapist practice, second ed. Physical Therapy 81, 9–744.

Arnold, M., Barbul, A., 2006. Nutrition and wound healing. Plast. Reconstr. Surg. 117, 42S–58S.

Arroll, B., Khin, N., Kerse, N., 2003. Screening for depression in primary care with two verbally asked questions: Cross-sectional study. Br. Med. J. 327, 144–146.

Boissonnault, W.G., Bass, C., 1990a. Pathological origins of trunk and neck pain: Part I. Pelvic and abdominal visceral disorders. J. Orthop. Sports Phys. Ther. 12, 192–207.

Boissonnault, W.G., Bass, C., 1990b. Pathological origins of trunk and neck pain: Part II. Disorders of the cardiovascular and pulmonary systems. J. Orthop. Sports Phys. Ther. 12, 208–215.

Boissonnault, W.G., Bass, C., 1990c. Pathological origins of trunk and neck pain: Part III. Diseases of the musculoskeletal system. J. Orthop. Sports Phys. Ther. 12, 216–221.

Boissonnault, W.G., Janos, S.C., 1995. Screening for medical disease: Physical therapy assessment and treatment principles. In: Boissonnault, W.G. (Ed.), Examination in physical therapy practice. second ed. Churchill Livingstone, New York, pp. 1–30.

Broughton, G., Janis, J.E., Attinger, C.E., 2006. Wound healing: An overview. Plast. Reconstr. Surg. 117, 1eS–32eS.

Brouwer, T., Boiten, J.C., Uilenreef-Tobi, F.C., Helders, P.J.M., Lindner, K., 1999. Diagnostiek in de fysiotherapie: Proces en werkwijze, second ed. Elsevier/Bunge, Maarssen.

Cadarette, S.M., Jaglal, S.B., Kreiger, N., McIsaac, W.J., Darlington, G.A., Tu, J.V., 2000. Development and validation of the osteoporosis risk assessment instrument to facilitate selection of women for bone densitometry. Can. Med. Assoc. J. 162, 1289–1294.

Campos, A.C.L., Groth, A.K., Branco, A.B., 2008. Assessment and nutritional aspects of wound healing. Curr. Opin. Clin. Nutr. Metab. Care 11, 281–288.

Carroll, L.J., Cassidy, J.D., Côté, P., 2004. Depression as a risk factor for the onset of an episode of troublesome neck and low back pain. Spine 107, 134–139.

Carroll, L.J., Hogg-Johnson, S., Van der Velde, G., et al., 2008a. Course and prognostic factors for neck pain in the general population. Spine 33 (4S), S75–S82.

Carroll, L.J., Holm, L.W., Hogg-Johnson, S., et al., 2008b. Course and prognostic factors for neck pain in whiplash-associated disorders (WAD). Spine 33 (4S), S83–S92.

Carroll, L.J., Hogg-Johnson, S., Côté, P., et al., 2008c. Course and prognostic factors for neck pain in workers. Spine 33 (4S), S93–S100.

Cook, C.E., 2007. Orthopaedic manual therapy: An evidence-based approach. Pearson Prentice Hall, Upper Saddle River.

Cook, C., Cleland, J., Huijbregts, P.A., 2007. Creation and critique of studies of diagnostic accuracy: Use of the STARD and QUADAS methodological quality assessment tools. Journal of Manual and Manipulative Therapy 15, 93–102.

Cooper, G., Bailey, B., Bogduk, N., 2007. Cervical zygapophysial joint pain maps. Pain Med. 8, 344–353.

Eyre, A., 2006. Overview and comparison of the NEXUS and Canadian C-spine rules. Am. J. Med. 8, 12–15.

Fair, S.E., 2010. Wellness and physical therapy. Jones & Bartlett, Sudbury.

Flynn, T.W., Cleland, J.A., Whitman, J.M., 2008. User's guide to the musculoskeletal examination: Fundamentals for the evidence-based clinician. Evidence in Motion, Buckner.

Foldes, K., Balint, P., Gaal, M., Buchanan, W.W., Balint, G.P., 1992. Nocturnal pain correlates with effusions in diseased hip. J. Rheumatol. 19, 1756–1758.

Fukui, S., Osheto, K., Shiotani, M., Ohno, K., Karasawa, H., Naganuma, Y., Yuda, Y., 1996. Referred pain distribution of the cervical zygapophyseal joints and cervical dorsal rami. Pain 68, 79–83.

Goodman, C.C., Snyder, T.E.K., 1995. Differential diagnosis in physical therapy, second ed. W B Saunders Company, Philadelphia.

Greenhalgh, S., Margaret, S.J., 2004. A tragic case of spinal red flags and red herrings. Physiotherapy 90, 73–76.

Grieve, G.P., 1994. The masqueraders. In: Boyling, J.D., Palastanga, N. (Eds.), Grieve's modern manual therapy. second ed. Churchill Livingstone, Edinburgh, pp. 841–856.

Grubb, S.A., Kelly, C.K., Bogduk, N., 2000. Cervical discography: Clinical implications from 12 years of experience. Spine 25, 182–1389.

Heggeness, M.H., Esses, S.I., Errico, T., Yuan, H., 1993. Late infection of spinal instrumentation by hematogenous seeding. Spine 18, 492–496.

Hill, J., Lewis, M., Papageorgiou, A.C., et al., 2004. Predicting persistent neck pain: A 1-year follow-up of a population cohort. Spine 29, 1648–1654.

Hoving, J.L., De Vet, H.C.W., Twisk, J.W.R., et al., 2004. Prognostic factors for neck pain in general practice. Pain 110, 639–645.

Hudak, P.L., Amadio, P.C., Bombardier, C., 1996. The Upper Extremity Collaborative Group (UECG): Development of an upper extremity outcome measure: The DASH (Disabilities of the Arm, Shoulder, and Hand). Am. J. Ind. Med. 29, 602–608.

Huijbregts, P.A., 2000. Osteonecrosis of the humeral head: A literature review and two case studies. Journal of Manual and Manipulative Therapy 8, 175–182.

Huijbregts, P.A., 2001. Osteoporosis: Diagnosis and conservative management. Journal of Manual and Manipulative Therapy 9, 143–153.

Huijbregts, P.A., 2009. Clinical reasoning in the diagnosis: History taking in patients with headache. In: Fernández-de-las-Peñas, C., Arendt-Nielsen, L., Gerwin, R. (Eds.), Diagnosis and management of tension-type and cervicogenic headache. Jones & Bartlett Publishers, Sudbury, pp. 133–152.

Huijbregts, P., Vidal, P., 2004. Dizziness in orthopaedic physical therapy: Classification and pathophysiology. Journal of Manual and Manipulative Therapy 12, 199–214.

Jones, M.A., 1995. Clinical reasoning process in manipulative therapy. In: Boyling, J.D., Palastanga, N. (Eds.), Grieve's modern manual therapy. second ed. Churchill Livingstone, Edinburgh, pp. 471–490.

Jonsson, B., Stromqvist, B., 1993. Symptoms and signs in degeneration of the lumbar spine: A prospective, consecutive study of 300 operated patients. J. Bone Joint Surg 75B, 381–385.

Katz, J.N., Liang, M.H., 1991. Differential diagnosis and

conservative treatment of rheumatic disorders. In: Frymoyer, J.W. (Ed.), The adult spine: Principles and practice. Raven Press, New York, pp. 699–718.

Kuijpers, T., Van der Windt, D.A.W.M., Boeke, A.J.P., Twisk, J.W.R., Vergouwe, Y., Bouter, L.M., Van der Heijden, G.J.M.G., 2006. Clinical prediction rules for the prognosis of shoulder pain in general practice. Pain 120, 276–285.

Laslett, M., Young, S.B., Aprill, C.N., McDonald, B., 2003. Diagnosing painful sacroiliac joints: A validity study of a McKenzie evaluation and sacroiliac provocation tests. Aus. J. Physiother. 49, 89–97.

McCowin, P.R., Borenstein, D., Wiesel, S.W., 1991. The current approach to the medical diagnosis of low back pain. Orthop. Clin. North Am. 22, 315–325.

McLean, S.M., May, S., Klaber-Moffett, J., Sharp, D.M., Gardiner, E., 2007. Prognostic factors for progressive non-specific neck pain: A systematic review. Physical Therapy Reviews 12, 207–220.

Merskey, H., Bogduk, N., 1994. Classification of chronic pain: Descriptions of chronic pain syndromes and definitions of pain terms. IASP Press, Seattle, pp. 209–213.

Pool, J.J., Ostelo, R.W., Knol, D., Bouter, L.M., De Vet, H.C., 2010. Are psychological factors prognostic indicators of outcome in patients with sub-acute neck pain? Man. Ther. 15, 111–116.

Posthauer, M.E., 2006. Hydration: Does it play a role in wound healing? Adv. Skin Wound Care 19, 74–76.

Ryall, C., Coggon, D., Peveler, R., Poole, J., Palmer, K.T., 2007. A prospective cohort study of arm pain in primary care and physiotherapy: Prognostic determinants. Rheumatology 46, 508–515.

Siegmeth, B., Noyelle, R.M., 1988. Night pain and morning stiffness in osteoarthritis: A crossover study of flurbiprofen and diclofenac sodium. Journal of Internal Medicine Research 16, 182–188.

Siris, E.S., Miller, P.D., Barrett-Connor, E., et al., 2001. Identification and fracture outcomes of undiagnosed low bone mineral density in postmenopausal women. J. Am. Med. Assoc. 286 (22), 2815–2822.

South-Paul, J.E., 2001. Osteoporosis: Part I. Evaluation and assessment. Am. Fam. Physician. 63 (5), 897–904.

Swap, C.J., Nagurney, J.T., 2005. Value and limitations of chest pain history in the evaluation of patients with suspected acute coronary syndromes. J. Am. Med. Assoc. 294, 2623–2629.

Triano, J.J., Kawchuk, G. (Eds.), 2006. Current concepts: Spinal manipulation and cervical arterial incidents. NCIMC, Clive.

Van der El, A., 2010. Orthopaedic manual therapy diagnosis: Spine and temporomandibular joints. Jones & Bartlett, Sudbury.

Vernon, H., Mior, S., 1991. The Neck Disability Index: a study of reliability and validity. J. Manipulative Physiol. Ther. 14, 409–415.

Vestergaard-Middelfart, H., Jensen, P., Højgaard, L., Funch-Jensen, P., 1998. Pain patterns after distension of the gallbladder in patients with acute cholecystitis. Scand. J. Gastroenterol. 33, 982–987.

Vincent, K.A., Benson, D.R., 1991. Differential diagnosis and conservative management of infectious diseases. In: Frymoyer, J.W. (Ed.), The adult spine: Principles and practice. Raven Press, New York, pp. 763–785.

Vlaeyen, J., Kole-Snijders, A., Boeren, R., Van Eek, H., 1995. Fear of movement /(re) injury in chronic low back pain and its relation to behavioral performance. Pain 62, 363–372.

Walton, D.M., Pretty, J., MacDermid, J.C., Teasell, R.W., 2009. Risk factors for persistent problems following whiplash injury: Results of a systematic review and meta-analysis. J. Orthop. Sports Phys. Ther. 39, 334–350.

Ware, J.E., Snow, K.K., Kosinki, M., Gandek, B., 1993. The MOS 36-item Short-Form Health Survey (SF-36): Manual and interpretation guide. The Health Institute, New England Medical Center, Boston.

Woolf, A.D., Åkesson, K., 2008. Primer: History and examination in the assessment of musculoskeletal problems. Nat. Clin. Pract. Rheumatol. 4, 26–33.

Chapter 3

Physical examination

Shane Koppenhaver, Timothy Flynn

INTRODUCTION

The physical examination should be a continuation of a comprehensive history. No matter how thorough the physical examination is, it can never substitute for a thorough patient history. Upon completion of an inclusive history, the examiner should have an appreciation of the severity of symptoms, potential irritability of the condition (once provoked, how long do symptoms take to ease?), the stage of the process (acute, sub-acute, chronic), and a reasonable hypothesis, or several competing hypotheses, about the likely pathology or treatment classification, and an initial prognostic assessment. Therefore, the physical examination focuses on testing the initial hypotheses formed during the patient history and gaining the additional information necessary to establish an appropriate treatment plan and patient prognosis. It should be systematic yet adaptable to the individual patient findings that support or refute the examiner's primary and alternative hypotheses.

A comprehensive physical examination consists of both global screening of the neuromotor and vascular systems along with region-specific procedures. Screening tests refer to a group of tests that can be used to decrease the likelihood of a particular condition being present. Therefore a screening test should be highly sensitive and have small negative likelihood ratios (−LRs). A sensitive test is one in which the examiner is very confident will be positive if the condition is present (i.e. false negative results should be rare). The real value in a screening test is that a negative result, when using a highly sensitive test with a very small −LR, dramatically lowers the probability that the patient has the condition (i.e. they can confidently 'rule it out'). Typically screening tests will have an increased number of false positives (since they are highly sensitive) and thus a positive screening test should alert the clinician to perform a more thorough investigation to rule in or rule out the condition. On the other hand, region-specific procedures are generally deductive in nature, should be highly specific, and have large positive likelihood ratios (+LRs). A specific test is only positive when the condition is present (i.e. false positive results should be rare). Therefore, a positive result when using a highly specific test with a very large +LR, dramatically increases the probability of the patient having the condition (i.e. the clinician can confidently 'rule it in'). It is imperative that clinicians understand diagnostic properties of the clinical examination tests they perform. For example, frequently clinicians will get a positive test result

© 2011 Elsevier Ltd.
DOI: 10.1016/B978-0-7020-3528-9.00003-0

when utilizing a sensitive test (−LR is small) and immediately label the patient with that disorder without considering the possibility of a false positive test result.

The screening portion of a cervical or upper extremity physical examination is a continuation of the review of systems that occurs during that patient history. While some elements should be routinely performed on all patients with neck and/or upper extremity symptoms, the inclusion of other components will be driven by findings from the history and other physical examination. Most inclusively a comprehensive screening examination will consist of:

- Observation
- Screening for medical conditions
- Screening for severe injuries to the cervical spine
- Screening for neurologic deficits
- 'Clearing' the cervical spine (in other words removing the cervical spine as a prime contributor to the patient's complaints)

The region-specific portion of a cervical or upper extremity physical examination should also be tailored by the history and other findings during the physical examination. A comprehensive region-specific examination, however, will always consist of:

- Active movements
- Passive movements (with and without overpressure)
- Palpation
- Clinical special tests

Because the screening portion of the cervical and upper extremity physical examination is basically the same regardless of the specific location of primary symptoms it will be the focus of this general physical examination chapter. Although the region-specific portion of any examination should include the same general components, the specific evaluative procedures depend on the location of primary symptoms and the potential joints and soft tissues involved. However, emerging evidence demonstrates that many neck and arm pain syndromes are appropriately managed with cervical and upper thoracic spine manual techniques (Hurwitz et al 2002, Cleland et al 2005, 2007, Boyles et al 2009) and require a cervical screening prior to performing manual interventions in this area. Subsequent chapters will focus on the relevant pathology-specific examination procedures for specific disorders.

OBSERVATION AND SCREENING FOR MEDICAL CONDITIONS

The initial questions that should be at the forefront of a musculoskeletal practitioner's mind during the physical examination is whether or not the patient's symptoms are consistent with neuro-musculoskeletal pathology and whether the patient may require immediate referral to another specialist. Many visceral pathologies can cause symptoms that can be confused with neuro-musculoskeletal conditions. Screening for visceral pathology is primarily done with a comprehensive and detailed patient history as discussed in Chapter 2. However symptoms from neuro-musculoskeletal pathology should also be able to be reproduced and/or exacerbated during a comprehensive neuro-musculoskeletal physical exam. When patients report symptoms of moderate to severe intensity that the examiner is unable to reproduce and/or exacerbate during the physical exam, the examiner should be highly suspicious of underlying medical pathology.

Signs of non-neuro-musculoskeletal pathology can be noted during the initial observation portion of the physical examination. For this reason, the clothing over any region of symptoms should be removed and the area should be closely inspected for any abnormalities. Primary skin lesions (e.g. macule, papule, patch, wheal, cyst) may be immediately discoverable during observation. While most primary skin lesions are not emergent, a musculoskeletal practitioner may be the first medical provider to discover the lesion, and at a minimum the patient should be told to discuss the lesion with their primary care provider. Primary skin lesions that are associated with a fever, difficulty breathing or swallowing, or tenderness with mucosal involvement, however, may be life threatening and require immediate emergent referral (Cole & Gray-Miceli 2002).

During observation, providers may additionally discover signs of fever, an abdominal mass, or atraumatic swelling. The presence of a pulsatile abdominal mass may represent an abdominal aortic aneurysm and requires immediate emergent referral. Atraumatic swelling, especially joint effusion, may signify an infectious or malignant process and should prompt further examination and/or immediate referral to another specialist.

Vascular disorders of the cervical arterial system (vertebro-basilar and carotid arteries) can present as head and neck pain. Occlusion of these arteries may lead to ischaemia with symptoms ranging from dizziness, diplopia, dysarthria, dysphagia, drop attacks, nausea, nystagmus, facial numbness, ataxia, vomiting, hoarseness, loss of short-term memory, vagueness, hypotonia/limb weakness, ahidrosis (lack of facial sweating), hearing disturbances, malaise, perioral dysthesia, photophobia, papillary changes, clumsiness and agitation to permanent neurological damage and death (Kerry & Taylor 2009). Damage to the arterial system, particularly the vertebro-basilar artery, has been linked to cervical manipulation (Ernst 2007). Several screening procedures have been advocated to identify patients at risk for vertebro-basilar insufficiency. The tests usually involve cervical postures that put stress on the vertebro-basilar system and monitor for signs and symptoms suggestive of such compromise (e.g. dizziness, diplopia, dysarthria, nystagmus, etc.)

Table 3.1 Important physical examination procedures for differentiating vasculogenic head and neck pain

Test	Purpose	Evidence status	Limitation and advantages
Functional positional test, cervical rotation	Affects flow in contralateral vertebral artery. Limited effect on internal carotid artery.	Poor sensitivity, variable specificity. Blood flow studies support effect on vertebral artery flow.	Only assesses posterior circulation. Results should be interpreted with caution. Recommended by existing protocols. Cannot predict propensity for injury.
Functional positional test, cervical extension	Affects flow in internal carotid arteries. Limited effect on vertebral arteries.	No specific diagnostic utility evidence available. Blood flow studies support effect on internal carotid artery flow.	Primarily assesses anterior circulation
Blood pressure examination	Measure of cardiovascular health	Correlates to cervical arterial atherosclerotic pathology.	Reliability dependent on equipment, environment, and experience. Continuous, not categorical, measure.
Cranial nerve examination	Identifies specific cranial nerve dysfunction resulting from ischaemia or vessel compression	No specific diagnostic utility evidence available.	Reliability dependent on experience
Eye examination	Assists in diagnosis of possible neural deficit related to internal carotid artery dysfunction	No specific diagnostic utility evidence available.	Eye symptoms may be early warning of serious underlying pathology
Handheld Doppler ultrasound	Direct assessment of blood flow velocity	Limited manual therapy specific evidence. Existing studies suggest good to requires further study.	Reliability dependent on equipment, environment, and experience

Reprinted from Manual Therapy, 11(4), Kerry and Taylor, Cervical arterial dysfunction assessment and manual therapy, 243–253.

(Childs et al 2005). Unfortunately no studies have demonstrated the ability of such tests to effectively identify patients with vertebro-basilar insufficiency or those at risk of having a cerebrovascular accident. Table 3.1 provides a summary of physical examination procedures designed to differentiate vascular head and neck pain. Kerry & Taylor (2009) have provided prudent advice to clinicians by encouraging them to develop a high index of suspicion for cervical vascular pathology, particularly in cases of cervical trauma. However, the clinician must balance this 'alertness' with the knowledge that chronic-pain and psychological issues are common factors in this patient group and should, therefore, be sensitive to the possible impact of reinforcing biomedical beliefs about a chronic-pain episode.

At a minimum screening for cervical artery dysfunctions should include a detailed historical exam (when the patient reports trauma and/or signs or symptoms consistent with compromise to the vascular system), and the physical exam portion of screening should include routine physical assessment using incrementally greater movements and loads of the cervical spine (Childs et al 2005). When 'clearing' the cervical spine the examiner should constantly observe the patient's response during cervical range of motion, especially during rotation and combined extension, rotation, and side-bending motions (Fig 3.1). In addition to assessing for nystagmus, the examiner also notes the presence of dizziness, lightheadedness, impaired sensation to the face, blurred vision, or other signs or symptoms consistent with compromise to the vertebro-basilar complex.

SCREENING FOR SEVERE INJURIES TO THE CERVICAL SPINE

The Canadian C-Spine Rule and the NEXUS Low-Risk Criteria are clinical decision rules that indicate when to order cervical spine radiographs to rule out cervical fractures (Stiell et al 2003) and have been detailed in Chapter 2. Both criteria are excellent at ruling out clinically important cervical spine fractures (Stiell et al 2003) and the Canadian C-Spine Rule has been shown to be superior to physician judgment in ordering radiography (Bandiera et al 2003).

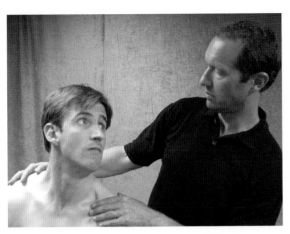

Fig 3.1 Observing eyes during combined extension, rotation, and side-bending motion (from Flynn et al 2008, with permission).

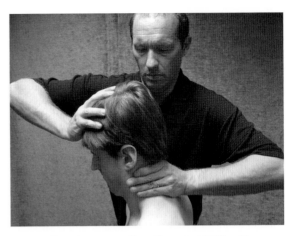

Fig 3.2 Sharp-Purser test (from Flynn et al 2008, with permission).

Although potentially less severe than a cervical fracture, upper cervical spine instability should be screened for in the presence of any predisposing factors, especially before administering any mechanical treatment (mobilization, manipulation, traction) of the upper cervical spine. Upper cervical spine instability has been associated with trauma and infection and is also commonly reported in patients with rheumatoid arthritis because of the chronic inflammation and subsequent tissue degeneration (Sizer et al 2007). Additionally, people with congenital disorders such as Down syndrome (Riaz et al 2007), Marfan syndrome (Demetracopoulos & Sponseller 2007) and other skeletal dysplasias (Song & Maher 2007) are at increased risk of experiencing upper cervical spine instability.

Several clinical tests have been purported to screen for upper cervical spine instability by testing for laxity of the transverse ligament of the atlas (TLA), of which the TLA test and the Sharp-Purser test are perhaps the most widely known. To perform the TLA test, the examiner grasps the cranium of a sitting patient with one hand while stabilizing C2 against C3 in an anterior inferior direction. The examiner then translates the cranium and C1 in a posterior direction. The test is repeated in each lateral direction and considered positive when symptoms are reproduced during the test (Sizer et al 2007). The Sharp-Purser test is performed on a patient while sitting with the neck in a semi-flexed position. With one hand on the patient's forehead and the index finger of the other hand on the spinous process of axis, the examiner applies posterior pressure through the patient's forehead (Fig 3.2). A sliding motion of the head posteriorly in relation to axis indicates a positive test for atlanto-axial instability. While the diagnostic utility of the TLA test remains unknown, the single study (Uitvlugt & Indenbaum 1988) to investigate the Sharp-Purser test found

it to be highly specific in identifying upper cervical spine instability as defined by radiographic evidence of an atlantodens interval of greater than 3 mm. The resulting +LR of 17.3 and −LR of 0.32 suggest that the Sharp-Purser test may be very helpful in both ruling in and ruling out upper cervical spine instability (Uitvlugt & Indenbaum 1988).

Furthermore, as with most screening tests, the paucity of studies investigating tests for upper cervical spine instability should not prevent clinicians from performing them or, perhaps more importantly, using robust clinical reasoning during screening for such disorders. The importance of clinical reasoning and upper cervical ligament testing has been well documented in case studies (Elliott & Cherry 2008, Mintken et al 2008) which illustrate potential effects of upper cervical spine instability as well as how positive outcomes can be obtained if properly diagnosed.

SCREENING FOR NEUROLOGICAL DEFICITS

In addition to screening for more serious neurological diseases, musculoskeletal providers should attempt to screen for radiculopathies and myelopathies. Radiculopathies are disorders of the spinal nerve roots as they exit the spinal column. They are most commonly caused by disc herniation or other space-occupying lesions and result in inflammation and/or impingement of the nerve root (Wainner et al 2003). Patients with cervical radiculopathy may or may not experience pain, which if present, commonly presents in the neck, upper extremity, and thoracic regions (Slipman et al 1998). Additionally cervical radiculopathy commonly causes unilateral upper extremity strength, sensation, and reflex deficits that are isolated to the distribution of the affected nerve root(s). Myelopathies, on the other hand, are disorders of the spinal cord and are discussed in detail in Chapter 9. Although symptoms often begin as merely neck pain or a 'stiff neck', myelopathies of the mid-cervical spine (C3–C5) commonly cause more distal pain and symptoms of numb and/or 'clumsy' hands. Myelopathies of the lower cervical spine (C6–T1), in addition, typically include weakness and proprioceptive losses in the legs that can result in gait disturbances (Sizer et al 2007).

Myelopathies and radiculopathies can often be difficult to distinguish from one another. Moreover, they are not mutually exclusive as many patients have disorders that affect both the nerve roots and the spinal cord. That being said, the two most obvious discriminators between the conditions are the presence of bilateral or unilateral symptoms and the finding of upper motor or lower motor symptoms. Patients with simple (single unilateral level) radiculopathies classically present with unilateral lower motor symptoms whereas patients with myelopathies typically present with bilateral symptoms that include upper motor neuron signs. Moreover, a radiculopathy affecting a single nerve root can theoretically be identified by the pattern and location of dermatomal and myotomal symptoms.

Nerve root examination

Traditional neurologic screening consists of sensation, muscle stretch reflex, and manual muscle testing. Although considered a key component of any standard neuromusculoskeletal examination for decades, very little evidence exists regarding the diagnostic utility of traditional neurologic screening. The one study to investigate the diagnostic utility of neurologic testing did so by comparing findings to a diagnosis of cervical radiculopathy via needle electromyography and nerve conduction studies (Wainner et al 2003). Although findings from this study suggest overall that neurologic testing may be only moderately helpful in identifying cervical radiculopathy, it is important to note the challenges of performing such research. First of all, there is no universally agreed definition of radiculopathy. Some sources define it solely by the clinical exam (Magee 2008) whereas others use imaging or electrophysiologic findings as the criterion standard (Rubinstein et al 2007). Additionally, there is wide individual anatomic variation in nerve root innervations (Magee 2008), which means operational definitions of what constitutes positive findings for each nerve root may greatly affect the reported diagnostic utilities of the tests. Lastly, the symptoms associated with radiculopathies have been reported to be highly variable and somewhat unpredictable (Slipman et al 1998, Cook 2007), which will naturally decrease the ability of even a highly reliable test to identify such underlying pathologies.

Therefore, we advocate sensation, muscle stretch reflex, and manual muscle test screening be routinely performed as a part of every cervical and upper extremity musculoskeletal examination. In addition to being prudent from a neurologic screening perspective, sensation, muscle stretch reflex, and manual muscle testing is largely considered the standard of care and, therefore, should be performed also from a legal/ethical perspective. Finally, the results of the neurological screening can be used as interim outcome measures to judge patient's response to treatment.

Sensation

Although light touch and pin-prick are the most common testing procedures, sensation can be tested by various other methods including two-point discrimination, vibration, and temperature testing. In general, dermatomal patterns of sensory changes are thought to be associated with radiculopathies and multiple level and/or bilateral patterns of dermatomal changes are associated with myelopathies (Sizer et al 2007). Although there is some individual anatomic variation in dermatomal nerve root innervations (Magee 2008), Figure 3.3 illustrates a typical dermatomal map from the cervical spine. Wainner et al (2003) tested pin-prick sensation graded as normal or abnormal, and found poor diagnostic utility for identifying cervical radiculopathy at all dermatomal levels. With the exception of the C5 dermatome, decreased sensation demonstrated +LR point estimates of < 1 and −LR estimates of > 1. However, the fact that both +LR and −LR confidence intervals included 1 for all dermatomal levels indicates that the presence of decreased sensation in isolation is not a robust measure of the probability of having cervical radiculopathy. Nonetheless, a sensory screen provides a baseline level of patient presentation and should drive the examiner's subsequent testing, particularly if there is multi-segmental or bilateral loss of sensation.

Myotomes

Like sensation, manual muscle testing has also been reported using various methods. Most commonly, isometric strength is tested by providing manual resistance to the muscle in the midrange of joint range of motion. The patient is instructed to 'not let me move you' as the examiner exerts enough force to surpass (break) the patient's maximal isometric resistance. The patient's maximum resistance is generally graded on a scale from 0 to 5 (see page 40) with some clinicians adding + or − to further delineate the scale. Although all muscles are innervated by multiple nerve roots, muscles that are primarily innervated by each cervical level are selected to screen the cervical nerve roots and are listed in Table 3.2 and the testing of each muscle is illustrated in Figures 3.4–3.11.

Fig 3.3 Typical cervical dermatomes

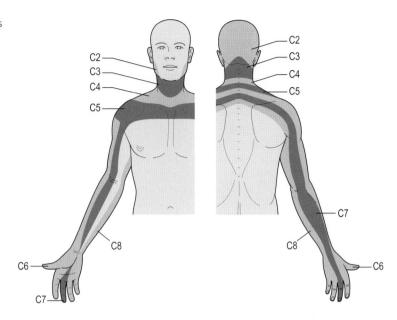

Table 3.2 Manual muscle testing for the cervical nerve roots

Nerve root	Primary muscles innervated	Test procedure
C1 & C2	Muscles that flex the neck	The examiner stabilizes the trunk with one hand and applies a posteriorly directed force through the patient's forehead while matching the resistance
C3	Muscles that side-bend the neck	The examiner stabilizes the shoulder with one hand and applies a force away from the side to be tested while the patient is instructed to match the resistance
C4	Muscles that elevate the shoulders	The patient is instructed to elevate their shoulders. The examiner applies an inferiorly directed force through the shoulders while the patient is instructed to match the resistance.
C5	Deltoids	The patient is instructed to abduct their shoulders to 90 degrees. The examiner applies a force into adduction while the patient resists.
C6	Biceps and extensor carpi radialis brevis and longus	The patient's elbow is flexed to 90 degrees and the forearm supinated. The examiner applies a force into extension while the patient resists. The patient's elbow is flexed to 90 degrees, forearm pronated, and wrist extended and radially deviated. The examiner applies a force into flexion and ulnar deviation while the patient resists.
C7	Triceps and flexor carpi radialis	The patient's elbow is flexed to 90 degrees and the examiner applies a force into elbow flexion while the patient resists. The patient's elbow is flexed to 90 degrees with the wrist flexed and radially deviated with forearm supinated. The examiner applies a force into wrist extension and ulnar deviation while the patient resists.
C8	Abductor pollicis brevis	The examiner places the thumb in abduction. The examiner applies a resistance through the proximal phalanx in the direction of abduction while the patient resists.
T1	First dorsal interossei	The examiner separates the index and middle finger and applies a force against the lateral aspect of proximal phalanx of the index finger into adduction

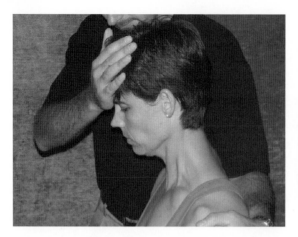

Fig 3.4 Cervical flexion (C1 & 2) (from Flynn et al 2008, with permission)

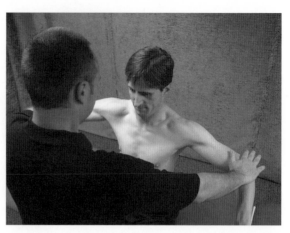

Fig 3.7 Shoulder abduction (C5) (from Flynn et al 2008, with permission)

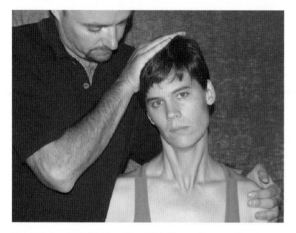

Fig 3.5 Cervical side-bending (C3) (from Flynn et al 2008, with permission)

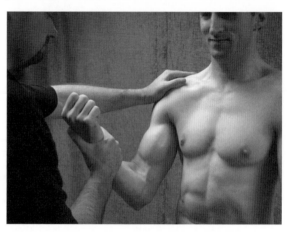

Fig 3.8 Elbow flexion (C6) (from Flynn et al 2008, with permission)

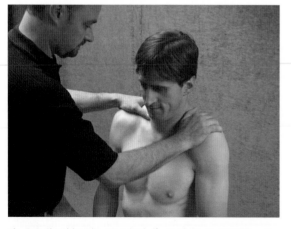

Fig 3.6 Shoulder elevation (C4) (from Flynn et al 2008, with permission)

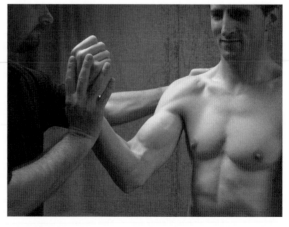

Fig 3.9 Elbow extension (C7) (from Flynn et al 2008, with permission)

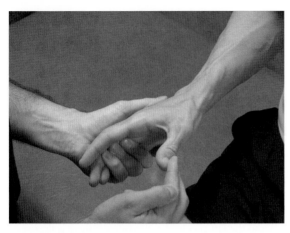

Fig 3.10 Thumb abduction (C8) (from Flynn et al 2008, with permission)

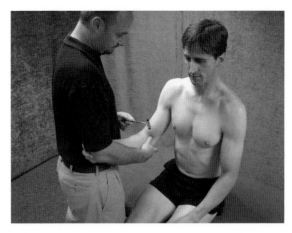

Fig 3.12 Testing biceps muscle stretch reflex (from Flynn et al 2008, with permission)

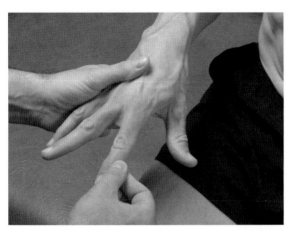

Fig 3.11 Finger abduction (T1) (from Flynn et al 2008, with permission)

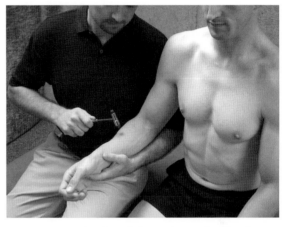

Fig 3.13 Testing brachioradialis muscle stretch reflex (from Flynn et al 2008, with permission)

- 5 (Normal): Complete range of motion against gravity with full resistance
- 4 (Good): Complete range of motion against gravity with some resistance
- 3 (Fair): Complete range of motion against gravity
- 2 (Poor): Complete range of motion gravity eliminated
- 1 (Trace): Evidence of slight muscle contraction
- 0 (Zero): No evidence of muscle contraction

Wainner et al (2003) tested manual muscle testing dichotomized as either normal or abnormal, and found poor diagnostic utility for identifying cervical radiculopathy. Although the +LR point estimates for the deltoids and biceps were 2.1 and 3.7 respectively, LR confidence intervals for every muscle included 1, indicating that the presence of isolated weakness may not alter the probability of having cervical radiculopathy. However, findings of gross weakness or multi-segmental weakness have not been studied and are likely more strongly suggestive of myelopathy, peripheral nerve injury, or neuromuscular disease.

Reflexes

Attenuated muscle stretch reflexes (MSRs) suggest lower motor neuron problems, most commonly of the spinal nerve roots (i.e. radiculopathy). Hyperactive muscle stretch reflexes can present an increased single response and/or repetitive response (clonus). Generally, the cervical nerve roots are screened by testing the biceps, brachioradialis, and triceps MSRs, which are illustrated in Figures 3.12–3.14. Like myotomes and sensation, MSR

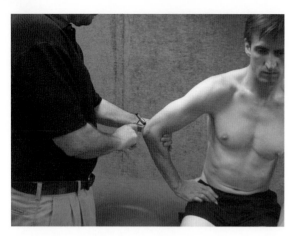

Fig 3.14 Testing triceps muscle stretch reflex (from Flynn et al 2008, with permission)

testing has been reported to be poorly sensitive for identifying (ruling out) cervical radiculopathy (Lauder et al 2000, Wainner et al 2003). Perhaps, this is because many abnormalities of both efferent and afferent pathways via electromyography have been found to be subthreshold during MSR testing (Miller et al 1999). However, two studies (Lauder et al 2000, Wainner et al 2003) found that the presence of a decreased biceps reflex substantially increased the probability of patients having (ruling in) a cervical radiculopathy (+LR = 4.9–10). The findings of the studies conflicted, however, on the utility of a decreased brachioradialis or triceps reflex. Lauder et al (2000) found +LRs of 2.0 for a decreased triceps reflex and 8.0 for a decreased brachioradialis reflex, whereas Wainner et al (2003) found +LRs that did not alter the probability of having cervical radiculopathy. Given the challenges of performing such studies described previously and the lack of the superior evidence-based alternative, sensation testing, manual muscle testing, and reflex testing are recommended for all patients with neck and upper extremity disorders.

Upper motor neuron examination

Although probably not required for all patients that present with neck and/or upper extremity pain, further neurologic examination should be done when indicated by the history, observation, or traditional neurologic screen. For example if a patient reports subjective complaints of bilateral neurologic involvement, a history of neck trauma, or problems with balance or walking, the examiner should include an upper motor neuron examination as a part of the neurologic screen. Moreover, if the examiner witnesses problems with coordination or gait disturbances during visual observation or clonus during muscle stretch reflex

testing, he/she may suspect disturbances of the corticospinal and spinocerebellar tracts within the spinal cord and further testing is also indicated. Whereas disruptions of the spinal nerve roots generally cause attenuation of motor reflexes, disorders of the central nervous system usually cause a disruption of the upper motor neuron's regulatory control over the motor reflexes and they become hyper-reflexive. Although no studies to our knowledge have investigated the diagnostic utility of tests of the upper motor neuron system, the following are a prudent set of procedures that have been advocated to identify upper motor neuron problems.

- Hoffman's Reflex (Fig 3.15) is tested with the patient seated with the head in a neutral position. The examiner flicks the distal phalanx of the middle finger and the test is considered positive if there is flexion of the interphalangeal joint of the thumb, with or without flexion of the index finger proximal or distal interphalangeal joints.
- Babinski Sign (Fig 3.16) is tested with the patient supine. The examiner strokes the plantar surface of the foot with a fingernail or instrument from posterior lateral toward the ball of the foot. The test is considered positive if the great toe extends and the other toes fan out.
- Clonus (Fig 3.17) is generally assessed for the gastrocnemius and soleus muscles and can be assessed with the patient seated or supine. The examiner rapidly dorsiflexes the ankle and the test is considered positive if the quick stretch results in reflexive twitching of the plantar-flexors.
- Romberg Test (Fig 3.18) is performed with the patient standing with their feet closed together. The patient is then instructed to close the eyes and the test is considered positive if the amount of sway

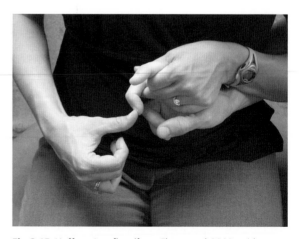

Fig 3.15 Hoffman's reflex (from Flynn et al 2008, with permission)

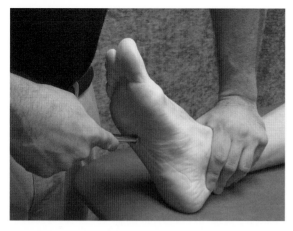

Fig 3.16 Babinski sign (from Flynn et al 2008, with permission)

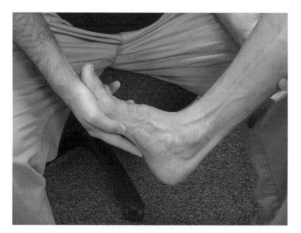

Fig 3.17 Testing for clonus (from Flynn et al 2008, with permission)

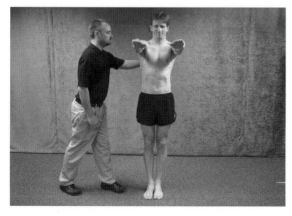

Fig 3.18 Romberg test (from Flynn et al 2008, with permission)

is increased with their eyes closed or if the patient loses balance.

- The scapulo-humeral reflex evaluates from upper motor neuron signs from the upper cervical spine (C1–C4). It is evaluated by striking the superior tip of a patient's lateral acromion process and/or the superior midpoint of the scapular spine with a reflex hammer. A test is considered positive when the patient involuntarily shrugs and/or abducts the shoulder (Shimizu et al 1993, Sizer et al 2007).
- Lhermitte's sign is when cervical flexion causes tingling and/or an 'electrical shock' in the midline of the thoracic spine and is thought to signify the possible presence of spinal cord conditions including multiple sclerosis, tumours, or other space occupying lesions (Sizer et al 2007, Gemici 2010).

Cranial nerve examination

The 12 cranial nerves are peripheral nerves carrying motor and sensory information to the head, face and neck. Like the upper motor neuron screen, a cranial nerve examination is recommended when indicated by the history, observation, or traditional neurologic screen. Some examples of indications are if patients report significant trauma to the head or neck, symptoms such as pain, weakness, or numbness in the head, face, or neck, visual or other sensory disturbances, or trouble with eating, drinking or swallowing. Table 3.3 lists the 12 cranial nerves and a typical examination of each.

CLEARING THE CERVICAL SPINE

Even in the absence of neurologic deficit, it is not uncommon for symptoms anywhere in the upper extremity to originate more proximally, especially from the cervical spine. Therefore, it is recommended that examiners perform a screening examination of the region proximal to the primary area of symptoms, and at a minimum, ensure that distal symptoms are not primarily altered with movements of the cervical spine. The cervical screening examination should consist of active range of motion of cervical flexion, extension, bilateral side-bending, bilateral rotation, and combined extension, side-bending, and rotation (quadrant). If no symptoms are produced with full active range of motion, the examiner should add slow overpressure to each motion (Figs 3.19–3.23).

Two additional examination tests have been identified, that when performed in conjunction with cervical range of motion with overpressure, substantially alter the probability of a patient's symptoms originating from the cervical spine, or more specifically, having cervical radiculopathy. Wainner et al (2003) reported that when patients are found to have a positive upper limb tension test A,

Table 3.3 Cranial nerves and cranial nerve examination

Cranial nerve number	Function	Test
I: Olfactory	Sensory from olfactory epithelium	Assess the ability to smell common scents
II: Optic	Sensory from retina of eyes	Assess peripheral vision by having person read an eye chart
III: Oculomotor	Motor to muscles controlling upward, downward, and medial eye movements, as well as pupil constriction	Assess pupil constriction as a reaction to light
IV: Trochlear	Motor to muscles controlling downward and inward eye movements	Assess the ability to move eye downward and inward by asking patient to follow your finger
V: Trigeminal	Sensory from face and motor to muscles of mastication	Test sensation of face and cheeks as well as corneal reflex. Assess the patient's ability to clench the teeth.
VI: Abducens	Motor to muscles that move eye laterally	Assess patient's ability to move eyes away from midline by asking him to follow your finger with his eyes
VII: Facial	Motor to muscles of facial expression and sensory to anterior tongue	Assess symmetry and smoothness of facial expressions. Test taste on anterior two-thirds of tongue
VIII: Vestibulocochlear	Hearing and balance	Assess by rubbing fingers by each ear. Patient should hear both equally. Can also ask patient to perform balance test.
IX: Glossopharyngeal	Controls gag reflex and sensory to posterior tongue	Assess gag reflex and taste on the posterior tongue
X: Vagus	Controls muscles of pharynx, which facilitate swallowing. Provides sensory to thoracic and abdominal visceral region.	Ask patient to say 'ah' and watch for elevation of soft palate
XI: Accessory	Motor to trapezius and sternocleidomastoid muscles	Muscle testing of trapezius
XII: Hypoglossal	Motor to muscles of the tongue	Ask patient to stick tongue straight out. Tongue will deviate toward injured side.

distraction test, Spurling's test, and cervical rotation less than 60° to the ipsilateral side, their probability of having a cervical radiculopathy was altered from 23% to 90% (+LR = 30.3). If three of the four tests were positive, the probability of having cervical radiculopathy was altered from 23% to 65% (+LR = 6.1). Spurling's test is merely cervical side-bending with overpressure, and is therefore included in the general cervical screening examination. To perform cervical distraction, the examiner grasps under the chin and occiput of a supine patient while slightly flexing the patient's neck and applies distraction force of approximately 14 pounds (Fig 3.24). The test is considered positive if the patient's symptoms are reduced during the manoeuvre. The upper limb tension test A is also performed with patient supine (see Chapter 38). The examiner then performs the following movements in order: 1. scapular depression, 2. shoulder abduction, 3. forearm supination, 4. wrist and finger extension, 5. shoulder lateral rotation, 6. elbow extension, 7. contralateral/ipsilateral cervical side-bending. A positive response is defined by any of the following:

1. Patient symptoms reproduced
2. Side-to-side differences in elbow extension > 10°
3. Contralateral cervical side-bending increases symptoms or ipsilateral side-bending decreases symptoms

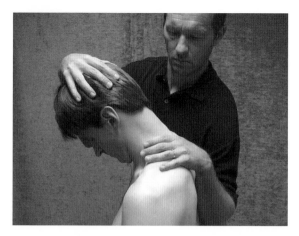

Fig 3.19 Cervical flexion with overpressure (from Flynn et al 2008, with permission)

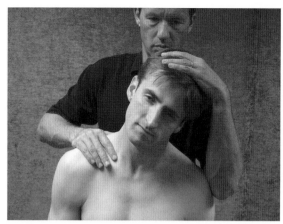

Fig 3.21 Cervical side-bending with overpressure (from Flynn et al 2008, with permission)

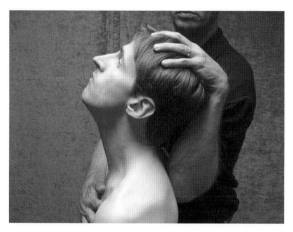

Fig 3.20 Cervical extension with overpressure (from Flynn et al 2008, with permission)

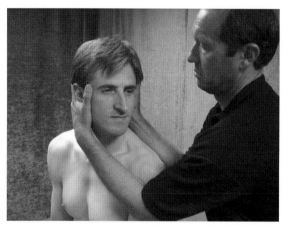

Fig 3.22 Cervical rotation with overpressure (from Flynn et al 2008, with permission)

Used in isolation, the upper limb tension test is helpful to rule out cervical radiculopathy. The diagnostic accuracy has been demonstrated to be substantial (Sensitivity = 0.97 and −LR = 0.12) and thus a negative test substantially reduces the likelihood that a cervical radiculopathy is present.

REGION SPECIFIC EXAMINATION

Like the screening portion, the region-specific portion of the physical examination should be focused on testing hypotheses formed during the patient history. Unlike the screening portion, however, the region-specific portion of the physical examination generally consists of deductive procedures aimed at (1) narrowing in on a patient's concordant sign and (2) gathering knowledge of how specific movements affect the patient's symptoms. As described in Chapter 2, a patient's concordant sign consists of their familiar symptoms that caused them to seek medical care (Laslett et al 2003). During the region-specific examination, concordant signs are distinguished from discordant signs, which are symptoms that are unlike the pain or other symptoms that caused the patient to seek treatment (Laslett et al 2003). Clearly establishing a patient's concordant sign and knowing specifically what movements or procedures primarily reproduce such symptoms is a pragmatic method for establishing a patho-anatomical diagnosis. However, even when establishing a

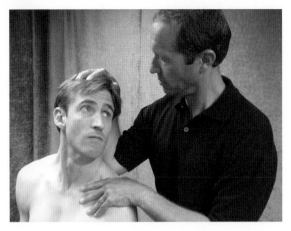

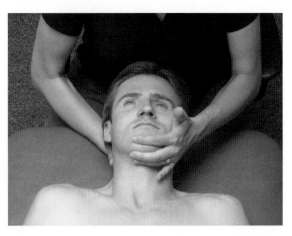

Fig 3.23 Combined cervical extension, rotation, and side-bending with overpressure (from Flynn et al 2008, with permission)

Fig 3.24 Cervical distraction (from Flynn et al 2008, with permission).

specific patho-anatomical diagnosis is not possible, knowledge of a patient's concordant sign and the movements or procedures that specifically reproduce that sign can be used to guide patient management and evaluate treatment effectiveness. As will be detailed in later chapters, immediately reassessing a patient's concordant sign after each treatment procedure is an objective method of evaluating the effectiveness of the procedure and helps guide which treatment procedure to perform next. Therapeutic benefits obtained using this method within a single treatment session, have been shown to be predictive of longer-term clinical benefits (Hahne et al 2004).

The region-specific portion of a cervical or upper extremity physical examination should generally consist of:

- Active movements
- Passive movements
- Palpation
- Clinical special tests

Active movements are physiologic movements performed exclusively by the patient in each motion plane for a selected joint. The goals of active movements are to both identify concordant vs discordant signs and to determine the effect of the specific active movements on those signs. Since all active movements are within complete control of the patient, starting an examination with active movements begins the deductive examination process in a safe and gradually more aggressive manner. Consistent with this concept of incrementally increasing loads, the examiner will follow active movements that do not cause symptoms with overpressure which is manual pressure in each direction at the end range of motion. The overpressure should start gently and be gradually progressed while carefully monitoring the patient's response.

Passive movements include both passive physiologic movements and passive accessory movements performed exclusively by the examiner. Physiologic movements are joint movements that can be performed by the patient actively, such as flexion, extension, and rotation. Accessory movements are joint movements that cannot be performed by the patient and generally occur across joint planes such as anterior or posterior glides. Comparing symptom response during passive physiologic movements to that of active physiologic movement gives the examiner information about the nature of the affected tissue and whether it is likely contractile (e.g. muscle, tendon) or not (e.g. ligament, bone, cartilage, nerve). Additionally, assessing passive physiologic motion allows the examiner to assess true full range of motion without the limitations of muscle function and patient motivation, and permits the examiner to assess the type of resistance encountered at the end of joint motion ('end-feel'). Assessing passive accessory motion is helpful to better localize the tissues and area responsible for the concordant sign. In the spine, for example, passive accessory intervertebral motions help the examiner isolate the side and specific spinal level(s) of primary symptoms. Additionally, many manual practitioners use assessments of both the amount and quality of accessory motion to make treatment decisions on how and where to deliver joint mobilization and/or manipulation. While assessments of joint mobility have consistently been shown to be unreliable (Mootz et al 1989, Binkley et al 1995, Maher et al 1998, Smedmark et al 2000, Hicks et al 2003, Fritz et al 2005, Arab et al 2009), there is some evidence that such assessments are helpful in treatment selection and patient management (Flynn et al 2002, Fritz et al 2005, Hicks et al 2005, Brennan et al 2006).

Palpation is a standard procedure for almost any sort of medical examination. Like passive accessory motion testing, palpation can help further localize the tissues and areas responsible for the concordant sign. Also like passive accessory motion testing, palpation can help differentiate whether an area of symptoms represent the primary source of symptoms or are more likely referred symptoms that are actually originating from another location. For example, pain in the proximal lateral forearm may be caused by local tissues underlying the area (tendinopathy or epicondylalgia) or may be referred from the cervical spine or shoulder.

Clinical special tests are procedures used to further identify specific diagnoses. They include combinations of active and passive movements, resistive tests, functional tests, and are generally both region and diagnosis specific. Hundreds (perhaps thousands) of special tests have been advocated based on clinician experience and biological plausibility. A growing number of special tests have been scrutinized in diagnostic research by comparing their outcomes to those of reference standard tests. Whenever possible, it is recommended that clinicians select special tests and procedures with known diagnostic utility and that have demonstrated high specificity and large +LRs.

REFERENCES

Arab, A.M., Abdollahi, I., Joghataei, M.T., Golafshani, Z., Kazemnejad, A., 2009. Inter- and intra-examiner reliability of single and composites of selected motion palpation and pain provocation tests for sacroiliac joint. Man. Ther. 14, 213–221.

Bandiera, G., Stiell, I.G., Wells, G.A., et al., 2003. The Canadian C-spine rule performs better than unstructured physician judgment. Ann. Emerg. Med. 42, 395–402.

Binkley, J., Stratford, P.W., Gill, C., 1995. Inter-rater reliability of lumbar accessory motion mobility testing. Phys. Ther. 75, 786–792.

Boyles, R.E., Ritland, B.M., Miracle, B.M., et al., 2009. The short-term effects of thoracic spine thrust manipulation on patients with shoulder impingement syndrome. Man. Ther. 14, 375–380.

Brennan, G.P., Fritz, J.M., Hunter, S.J., Thackeray, A., Delitto, A., Erhard, R.E., 2006. Identifying subgroups of patients with 'non-specific' low back pain: results of a randomized clinical trial. Spine 31, 623–631.

Childs, J.D., Flynn, T.W., Fritz, J.M., et al., 2005. Screening for vertebro-basilar insufficiency in patients with neck pain: manual therapy decision-making in the presence of uncertainty. J. Orthop. Sports Phys. Ther. 35, 300–306.

Cleland, J.A., Childs, J.D., Fritz, J.M., Whitman, J.M., Eberhart, S.L., 2007. Development of a clinical prediction rule for guiding treatment of a subgroup of patients with neck pain: use of thoracic spine manipulation, exercise, and patient education. Phys. Ther. 87, 9–23.

Cleland, J.A., Childs, J.D., McRae, M., Palmer, J.A., Stowell, T., 2005. Immediate effects of thoracic manipulation in patients with neck pain: a randomized clinical trial. Man. Ther. 10, 127–135.

Cole, J.M., Gray-Miceli, D., 2002. The necessary elements of a dermatologic history and physical evaluation. Dermatol. Nurs. 14, 377–383.

Cook, C., 2007. Orthopaedic manual therapy: An evidence-based approach. Pearson Prentice Hall, Upper Saddle River.

Demetracopoulos, C.A., Sponseller, P., 2007. Spinal deformities in Marfan syndrome. Orthop. Clin. North Am. 38, 563–572.

Elliott, J.M., Cherry, J., 2008. Upper cervical ligamentous disruption in a patient with persistent whiplash associated disorders. J. Orthop. Sports Phys. Ther. 38, 377.

Ernst, E., 2007. Adverse effects of spinal manipulation: a systematic review. J. R. Soc. Med. 100, 330–338.

Flynn, T., Fritz, J., Whitman, J., et al., 2002. A clinical prediction rule for classifying patients with low back pain who demonstrate short-term improvement with spinal manipulation. Spine 27, 2835–2843.

Flynn, T., Cleland, J., Whitman, J., 2008. Users' Guide to the Musculoskeletal Examination: Fundamentals for the Evidence-Based Clinician. Evidence in Motion, Louisville.

Fritz, J.M., Piva, S.R., Childs, J.D., 2005. Accuracy of the clinical examination to predict radiographic instability of the lumbar spine. Eur. Spine J. 14, 743–750.

Gemici, C., 2010. Lhermitte's sign: Review with special emphasis in oncology practice. Crit. Rev. Oncol. Hematol. 74, 79–86.

Hahne, A.J., Keating, J.L., Wilson, S.C., 2004. Do within-session changes in pain intensity and range of motion predict between-session changes in patients with low back pain? Aust. J. Physiother. 50, 17–23.

Hicks, G.E., Fritz, J.M., Delitto, A., McGill, S.M., 2005. Preliminary development of a clinical prediction rule for determining which patients with low back pain will respond to a stabilization exercise program. Arch. Phys. Med. Rehabil. 86, 1753–1762.

Hicks, G.E., Fritz, J.M., Delitto, A., Mishock, J., 2003. The reliability of clinical examination measures used for patients with suspected lumbar segmental instability. Arch. Phys. Med. Rehabil. 84, 1858–1864.

Hurwitz, E.L., Morgenstern, H., Harber, P., Kominski, G.F., Yu, F., Adams, A.H., 2002. A randomized trial of chiropractic manipulation and mobilization for patients with neck pain: clinical outcomes from the UCLA neck-pain study. Am. J. Public Health 92, 1634–1641.

Kerry, R., Taylor, A.J., 2009. Cervical arterial dysfunction: knowledge and reasoning for manual physical therapists. J. Orthop. Sports Phys. Ther. 39, 378–387.

Laslett, M., Young, S.B., Aprill, C.N., McDonald, B., 2003. Diagnosing painful sacroiliac joints: A validity study of a McKenzie evaluation and sacroiliac provocation tests. Aust. J. Physiother. 49, 89–97.

Lauder, T.D., Dillingham, T.R., Andary, M., et al., 2000. Predicting electrodiagnostic outcome in patients with upper limb symptoms: are the history and physical examination helpful? Arch. Phys. Med. Rehabil. 81, 436–441.

Magee, D., 2008. Orthopedic physical assessment, fifth ed. Saunders, St. Louis.

Maher, C.G., Latimer, J., Adams, R., 1998. An investigation of the reliability and validity of posteroanterior spinal stiffness judgments made using a reference-based protocol. Phys. Ther. 78, 829–837.

Miller, T.A., Pardo, R., Yaworski, R., 1999. Clinical utility of reflex studies in assessing cervical radiculopathy. Muscle Nerve 22, 1075–1079.

Mintken, P.E., Metrick, L., Flynn, T.W., 2008. Upper cervical ligament testing in a patient with os odontoideum presenting with headaches. J. Orthop. Sports Phys. Ther. 38, 465–475.

Mootz, R.D., Keating, J.C.J., Kontz, H.P., Milus, T.B., Jacobs, G.E., 1989.

Intra- and interobserver reliability of passive motion palpation of the lumbar spine. J. Manipulative Physiol. Ther. 12, 440–445.

Riaz, S., Drake, J.M., Hedden, D.M., 2007. Images in spine surgery: atlanto-axial instability in Down syndrome. J. Pak. Med. Assoc. 57, 213–215.

Rubinstein, S.M., Pool, J.J., van Tulder, M.W., Riphagen, I.I., de Vet, H.C., 2007. A systematic review of the diagnostic accuracy of provocative tests of the neck for diagnosing cervical radiculopathy. Eur. Spine J. 16, 307–319.

Shimizu, T., Shimada, H., Shirakura, K., 1993. Scapulohumeral reflex (Shimizu). Its clinical significance and testing maneuver. Spine 18, 2182–2190.

Sizer, P.S.J., Brismee, J.M., Cook, C., 2007. Medical screening for red flags in the diagnosis and management of musculoskeletal spine pain. Pain Pract. 7, 53–71.

Slipman, C.W., Plastaras, C.T., Palmitier, R.A., Huston, C.W., Sterenfeld, E.B., 1998. Symptom provocation of fluoroscopically guided cervical nerve root

stimulation. Are dynatomal maps identical to dermatomal maps? Spine 23, 2235–2242.

Smedmark, V., Wallin, M., Arvidsson, I., 2000. Inter-examiner reliability in assessing passive intervertebral motion of the cervical spine. Man. Ther. 5, 97–101.

Song, D., Maher, C.O., 2007. Spinal disorders associated with skeletal dysplasias and syndromes. Neurosurg. Clin. N. Am. 18, 499–514.

Stiell, I.G., Clement, C.M., McKnight, R.D., et al., 2003. The Canadian C-spine rule versus the NEXUS low-risk criteria in patients with trauma. N. Engl. J. Med. 349, 2510–2518.

Uitvlugt, G., Indenbaum, S., 1988. Clinical assessment of atlanto-axial instability using the Sharp-Purser test. Arthritis Rheum. 31, 918–922.

Wainner, R.S., Fritz, J.M., Irrgang, J.J., Boninger, M.L., Delitto, A., Allison, S., 2003. Reliability and diagnostic accuracy of the clinical examination and patient self-report measures for cervical radiculopathy. Spine 28, 52–62.

Chapter | 4 |

Imaging studies

Hilmir Agustsson

IMAGING IN PHYSICAL THERAPIST PRACTICE

Imaging has not been widely integrated into physical therapist practice; however, there is increasing emphasis on imaging in physical therapy curricula and in textbooks intended for physical therapists (Deyle 2005, Magee 2006). Although minimal competencies for physical therapist imaging have been suggested, the scope of

© 2011 Elsevier Ltd.
DOI: 10.1016/B978-0-7020-3528-9.00004-2

musculoskeletal imaging for physical therapists has not been defined. There, furthermore, seems to be an assumption that the physical therapist's approach to imaging is no different from the medical approach. However, according to the Normative Model of Physical Therapist Professional Education, physical therapists should be able to identify the need for imaging studies and use the results of imaging studies in the management of patients with musculoskeletal problems and other disorders (APTA 2004), which would seem to require an approach to imaging that is unique to the physical therapy evaluation and treatment. Still, apart from case reports that show the 'intersection' of PT practice and imaging (Graber 2005), there are few examples of physical therapists using imaging to aid their clinical decisions (Agustsson 2005).

The need for increased knowledge and physical therapist involvement with imaging partly relates to direct access. Physical therapists are successfully diagnosing and managing musculoskeletal conditions on a direct-access basis (Jette et al 2006), an arrangement that may improve the treatment outcomes and lower costs (Daker-White et al 1999). However, seeing patients without prior medical screening carries increased professional responsibilities, including the ability to appropriately refer patients for imaging, based on history and examination, as well as the ability to screen imaging studies supplied by the patient. Physical therapists may not be ready for such an expansion in the scope of practice; with the exception of therapists in the military that routinely order imaging studies and employ them in clinical practice (Donato et al 2004). Physical therapists in the United States rarely make referrals for imaging, while therapists in many other countries do.

Basic competencies relating to physical therapist imaging have been suggested (Barr 2005). These include being able to:

- Understand the radiographic report and the terminology used to describe findings
- Make appropriate referrals for imaging studies, based on physical examination and history
- Explain findings on imaging studies to patients and discuss diagnostic imaging with other professionals
- Based on the radiographic report or on own evaluation of the images, to recognize precautions and contraindications to treatment and to modify treatment plans accordingly

IMAGING MODALITIES

Imaging modalities include conventional radiography and advanced imaging methods, ultrasound, computed tomography (CT), and magnetic resonance imaging (MRI). The advanced imaging technologies were primarily developed for the purpose of obtaining better soft tissue resolution and more accurate spatial location. The superior spatial location is possible because the cross-sectional imaging methods represent 'slices' of the body, free of superimposition, which makes accurate location of structures possible. While this represents great gains in detail and control over what is being viewed, cross-sectional imaging is challenging to the viewer since it offers limited overview and requires the mental reconstruction of perspective and three-dimensionality.

Conventional radiography

Conventional radiography involves x-rays, that is, electromagnetic radiation of short wavelengths. This method was extensively used for medical diagnosis from the beginning of the 20th century. The radiographic image represents the tissue densities of the body. X-rays pass through the body to the film and the radiation that reaches the film darkens it. The radiograph can therefore be considered a shadowgram, where different shades of gray represent the combined radiodensities of the intervening tissues.

Radiodensities

A structure is said to be radio-dense, relatively white in the image, if it absorbs much of the x-rays passing through the tissues; as in the example of bone. A structure is said to be radiolucent, relatively black in the image, if it has little radiodensity, as in the example of fat (Fig 4.1).

However, in the radiograph, radiodensity is not a fixed characteristic of the imaged tissue. It is the product of combined density and thickness tissues, as well as the superimposition of structures (Fig 4.2). For example, soft tissue is normally radiolucent relative to bone, but when there is increased radiodensity in soft tissues (for instance as a result of haematoma), they may appear to have greater

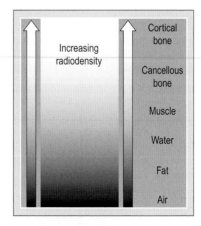

Fig 4.1 Body tissues arranged in order of radio-density.

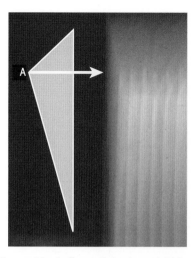

Fig 4.2 The combined effects of density and thickness. When a wooden wedge is stood up on its edge, at point 'A' the x-rays must pass through greater amount of wood before reaching the film. More x-rays are absorbed and the image is brighter at that point. The veins of the wood appear more radio-dense in the image, as they, due to their density, absorb more energy.

density than a thin bone, such as the ilium. Furthermore, radiodensity in the image is affected by the strength of the x-rays, and length of exposure. Short exposure time and low strength increase the apparent radiodensity.

Viewing radiographs

The different radiographic views are often referred to as projections. In the antero-posterior (AP) projection, the x-rays enter the body anteriorly on their way to the image receptor (film or digital plate) situated posteriorly to the patient's body, or body part. Lateral and oblique projections are named according to which side of the body is closest to the film; in the left lateral projections, the film is on the left side of the body; a left posterior oblique radiograph of the cervical spine is made with the film closest to the posterior left side of neck.

Thus, AP images are viewed as if we were facing the patient in the anatomical position, while in the lateral view we look in the direction of the x-rays. So, when looking at a lateral radiograph of the left elbow we look from the lateral to the medial side, since the plate is on the medial side of the elbow. Normally at least two images are needed; projections made at right angles to each other. This aids in mentally constructing a sense of three dimensions and decreases the risk for diagnostic error (Fig 4.3).

Alternative forms of radiography

There are several variants of conventional radiography. In myelography, contrast medium is injected for the purpose of outlining the thecal sac and nerve roots. This increases the radiodensity of the cerebrospinal fluid in the thecal sac and nerve root sleeves, rendering these as radiodense outlines. In arthrography, contrast medium and/or air is injected into a joint space. If both are used (double-

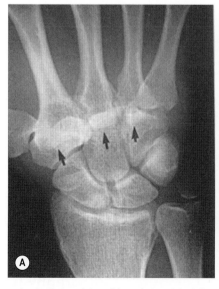
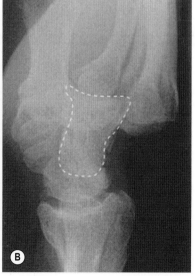

Fig 4.3 Postero-anterior (PA) view (A) and lateral view (B) of the wrist, demonstrating posterior dislocation of the 2nd, 3rd, and 4th metacarpals. In the PA image, areas of increased radio-density (arrows) indicate partial overlap of the trapezium, capitate (dashed outline) and hamate with their corresponding metacarpals indicates their apposition is not normal. However, a lateral view is required to appreciate the severity of the dislocation (from Taylor & Resnick 2000, with permission).

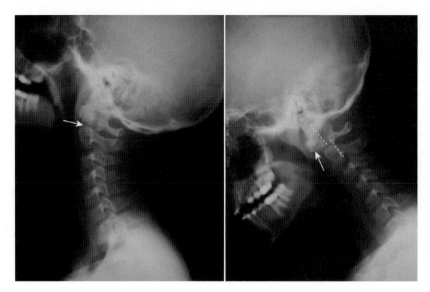

Fig 4.4 A 12-year-old boy fell out a bunk bed and immediately experienced cervical pain and inability to move. Stress radiographs in the lateral view, made in flexion and extension, reveal an area of radiolucency at the root of the odontoid process, indicating fracture (arrow) and anterior translation atlas on the axis in flexion (dashed lines).

contrast arthrogram), the synovial cavity is distended with the radiolucent air, while the joint capsule and intra-articular structures are outlined with the radiodense contrast material. This can help demonstrate damage to joint surfaces and capsule.

Stress radiography, where the joint is radiographed at the extremes of range of motion (ROM), has been employed for the diagnosis of cervical instability (Fig 4.4). In full flexion or extension, excessive translation or increased angulation of an intervertebral space is considered indicative of injury.

Videofluoroscopy offers a real-time view and recording of joint motion and allows visualization of joint position throughout the ROM. This is valuable for the detection of instability that is best seen in the mid-range of a joint's motion (Wong et al 2004), not at the ends of range of motion.

Systematic evaluation of radiographs – ABCs

Conventional radiographs are evaluated in a systematic manner. When the radiologist performs an evaluation of a conventional radiograph, it may look intuitive, however it is well established that the radiologist's competence is grounded in rigorous training and based on a systematic approach. The basic radiographic evaluation is often referred to in terms of the ABCs – *alignment, bone density, cartilage* space, and *soft* tissue.

Alignment refers to the general skeletal architecture; the contour and shape of individual bones, and the position of bone, relative to each other. Fractures, exotoses, and dislocations are examples of disturbed alignment of bones.

Abnormalities in *bone density* may manifest, generally, as loss of density or contrast, altered bone texture, and thin trabeculae – possibly indicative of osteoporosis. Local changes in bone density, such as areas of increased or decreased radiodensity, can indicate osteolytic (bone destroying) or osteoblastic (bone forming) activity associated with tumours. Increased radiodensity near a joint could indicate sclerosis associated with osteoarthritis, while loss of density near a joint is found in rheumatoid arthritis.

Normally, the *cartilage* cannot be seen; it simply presents as a radiolucent area between the articulating bones. The thickness of intervening cartilage is indicated by this space.

While *soft tissues* are normally not clearly seen on conventional radiographs, their visibility has improved with modern digital radiographs. Muscle outlines may be visible on radiographs, allowing for the estimate of asymmetry and wasting, and fat pads, associated with joints, as well as fat planes between muscles may be visible. If fat lines near joints are displaced outwards, this usually indicates intra-articular swelling (Fig 4.5). Similarly, if fat planes between muscles are displaced, this could indicate swelling or the presence of a tumour. Joint capsules, normally not visible, can become visible if distended with fluid and their radiodensity may be increased in case of haemarthrosis.

Computed tomography (CT)

CT, introduced in the 1970s, dramatically improved the ability for diagnosing soft tissue pathology. CT is in many ways similar to conventional radiography; using x-rays for

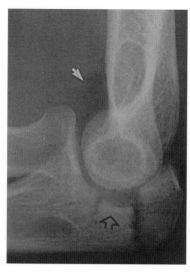

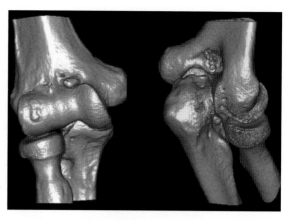

Fig 4.6 Screenshots of a 3D CT video, where the elbow joint is rotated in space while flexing and extending (from Toshiba American Medical Systems, with permission).

Fig 4.5 A lateral radiograph showing a comminuted (multi-fragment) intra-articular fracture of the olecranon. There is posterior displacement of the olecranon process and a depression of the articular surface (open arrow). The fat pad in the coronoid fossa is displaced anteriorly, indicating joint effusion (arrow) (from Taylor & Resnick 2000, with permission).

the purpose of producing images that are based on radiodensities. Images are displayed in shades of gray, but with greater contrast than is possible with radiography.

Acquisition of images

During the acquisition of the images, x-rays are passed through the tissues in a 360-degree arc; literally creating hundreds of projections per slice, while the x-rays are picked up by electronic sensors (detectors) on the side opposite to the x-ray tube. The result is a digital matrix (e.g. 1024 × 1024 pixels) forming cross-sectional images. Each pixel in the matrix represents a definitive radiodensity; largely free of superimposition of other radiodensities. Modern scanners collect information from multiple slices simultaneously (volumetric scanning) and can create images in any plane, as well as producing three-dimensional (3D) images (Fig 4.6). With increasing computing power, it has become possible to show 3D images of joints as high quality videos; a development that is likely to have an impact on the movement sciences.

The quality of images

The slice thickness varies, according to which body part is being imaged. The thorax may be scanned using a slice thickness of 6–8 mm, whereas the wrist may be presented with a slice thickness of only 0.5–2 mm. Image detail varies directly with the number of pixels in the matrix and inversely with slice thickness. Thinner slices provide

greater resolution, but are associated with greater radiation and longer scanning times.

Densities – the setting of the window

In CT images, the shades of grey reflect the exact radiodensity of the tissue. Known values for radiodensities of different tissues are used when setting the 'window' of viewing which radiodensities to emphasize. While any range can be selected, sometimes the selection is simply referred to in terms of a bone window or a soft tissue window. A bone window would allow clear distinction between cancellous and cortical bone, while in a soft tissue window the details of muscle and viscera may be viewed, while different parts of bones may not be discerned, since their radiodensity renders them uniformly white in the image.

Viewing the image

When viewing the axial image, the patient is viewed below. Thus, the spinous processes point down and the left side of the image represents the patient's right. Coronal images are viewed from the front; as if viewing an AP radiograph. Images in the sagittal plane are viewed from the left to the right, for both sides (Fig 4.7). A 'scout' image, made in a different plane, may be used for orientation. For a sagittal slice, a small axial image may show the location of the sagittal slice being viewed. The same viewing principles also apply to MRI.

Imaging characteristics for CT are the same as for a radiograph; cortical bone is white, muscle is grey, fat is dark, and air is black.

Advantages and limitations of CT

CT is usually the imaging modality of choice for evaluating subtle and complex fractures. CT may also be the first

49

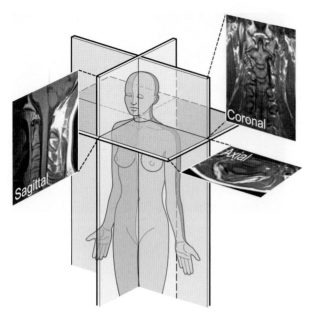

Fig 4.7 The orthogonal planes used for displaying CT and MR images.

imaging choice in serious trauma, since multiple injuries to osseous and soft-tissue structures can be determined from one imaging series. CT excels in the evaluation of spinal stenosis and is the best modality for the evaluation of intra-articular loose bodies. The advantages of CT include shorter scanning times than for MRI or ultrasound and the ability to create high quality 3D images.

The disadvantages of CT include relatively high costs and greater radiation than that of conventional radiographs. A limitation of CT is that it distinguishes tissues and pathologies solely based on differences in radiodensity, thus it may fail to demonstrate a pathology that has the same radiodensity as surrounding, healthy tissue.

Magnetic resonance imaging (MRI)

MRI differs significantly from previous imaging modalities that, in one form or another, produce images based on densities. MRI produces images based on the emission of energy from protons in the body. Still, the MR image is a greyscale representation of the tissues, the image represents a slice of a given thickness, and there are possibilities for selecting a window for viewing – expressed in terms of T1 and T2 weighting. MRI creates detailed images as cross-sectional slices in the three orthogonal planes, as well as having the capability but of being reformatted to any plane.

Acquisition of MR images

MR imaging starts by placing the body in a strong magnetic field, which aligns all hydrogen protons. The alignment of the protons then is disturbed with a radiofrequency pulse delivered at right angles to the main magnetic field. As the protons re-align, they send out information on their location, state and surroundings (Fig 4.8).

The centrepiece of the traditional MRI scanner is a large magnet that has the field strength of 6000 to 60,000 times the strength of the Earth's magnetic field. The bore of the magnet, which is large enough for the human body to slide into, contains a receiver coil (body coil) for recording proton energy emissions. This body coil may be employed when viewing large areas like the spine, but smaller specialized coils may also be placed around the extremity joints, such as the knee, or be placed 'flat' on a joint, such as the TMJ.

T1 and T2 imaging

MRI employs the different energy-emission characteristics of various tissues for selecting which tissues to emphasize. This is done based on imaging parameters referred to as T1- or T2-weighted imaging. Understanding the differences between T1 and T2 images allows us to understand what tissues are being emphasized.

The gradual realignment of protons with the main magnetic field, following the application of the radiofrequency pulse, takes place at different rates for different tissues. Protons that reside in fat give up their energy more freely than protons residing in free water, such as the cerebrospinal fluid (CSF) or synovial fluid. T1 images are made using short imaging times; there is only a brief interval from the application of the radiofrequency pulse to the time the signal is captured. This point in time is referred to as time to echo (TE) (Fig 4.8). Since fat releases energy more rapidly than water, it has high signal intensity (appears bright) in a T1 image. In T2 imaging, the

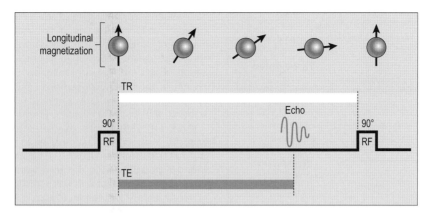

Fig 4.8 The protons, aligned with the main magnetic field, are displaced by RF pulse applied at 90 degrees. Once the RF pulse is turned off, the protons gradually align with the main magnetic field.

signal is captured late in the imaging process (long TE) and since free water releases energy slowly, T2 imaging emphasizes fluid (for example inflammation), while fat will normally appear intermediate to dark (Fig 4.9). Thus, it is the timing of the 'picture' that determines whether a T1 or a T2 image is produced.

Tissue characteristics

The different characteristics of the tissues on T1 and T2 aid tissue recognition and diagnosis. Structures that are indistinguishable in a T1 image can be distinguished by comparing T1 and T2 images. In T1 images it may not be possible to distinguish between dense intra-articular tissues and the surrounding synovial fluid, while in a T2 image the synovial fluid will light up. Table 4.1 outlines the imaging characteristics of normal tissues.

Thus, where in the CT image identification of tissues and diagnosis is based on radiodensities, diagnosis with MRI is most often made with reference to the different presentation on T1 and T2. Table 4.2 details the imaging characteristics of abnormal tissues.

Different forms of MRI

MRI can take several different forms. Using open and upright scanners has solved some problems and opened

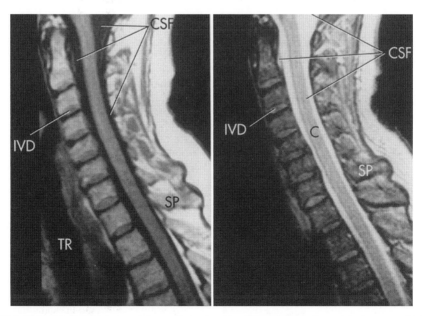

Fig 4.9 Sagittal T1 (left) and T2 (right) images of the cervical spine. The CSF and the nucleus of the inter-vertebral disc are dark on T1, but bright on T2. The bone marrow of the vertebral body is brighter on T1 than on T2 (from Marchiori 1999, with permission).

Table 4.1 Signal intensities of normal tissues on T1-weighted and T2-weighted MRI.

Tissue	T1 weighted	T2 weighted
Cortical bone	Very low	Very low
Cartilage	Intermediate	Low to intermediate
Fat	High	Intermediate
Bone marrow	High	Intermediate
Ligaments – tendons	Low	Low
Muscle	Intermediate	Low to intermediate
Fluid: CSF, synovial fluid	Low	High

Table 4.2 Signal intensities of abnormal tissues on T1-weighted and T2-weighted MRI

Type of abnormality	T1 weighted	T2 weighted
Inflammation	Low	High
Synovial hypertrophy	Low to intermediate	Intermediate to high
Acute haemorrhage	High	Intermediate to low
Subacute haemorrhage	Intermediate to high	Intermediate to high
Chronic haemorrhage	Variable	High
Soft-tissue calcifications	Low	Low
Osteogenic bone tumours	Low	Low
Chondromalacia	Decreased	Increased
Fractures	Low, with a dark band	High, with a dark band
Avascular necrosis	Low	Intermediate to high

new possibilities. Since open scanners do not require the patient to slide into the bore of the scanner, claustrophobia is not a problem. The open-upright configuration allows the patient to be weight-bearing during the examination, which may reveal herniations and instability not evident in the recumbent position. The field strength of open scanners is typically lower than in conventional scanners, thus image acquisition takes longer.

Direct MR arthrography may be considered the gold-standard non-operative joint-imaging technique (Steinbach et al 2002). It combines elements of the standard arthrogram with MR imaging. It is the investigation of choice for labral tears of the shoulder, as well as for ligament tears in the wrist. The injected gadolinium renders a bright signal, which allows the radiologist to see small defects in the capsule, articular surfaces, ligaments, or labra. Indirect MR arthrography is accomplished using intravenous administration of gadolinium, which enhances vascularized or inflamed tissue, but does not render the joint fluid bright.

Comparison of image characteristics of CT and MRI

Telling the MR image and CT image apart is easy, if one principle is kept in mind. CT is really a radiograph, thus tissues that have high density, like cortical bone, appear bright. On MRI images, these same tissues appear dark (Fig 4.10).

Advantages and disadvantages of MRI

MRI clearly displays soft-tissue detail and excels at detecting changes in bone marrow, which makes it invaluable in the diagnosis of bone tumours, stress fractures, and avascular necrosis. It has replaced invasive diagnostic procedures, such as arthroscopy in the detection of meniscal tears and myelography for the diagnosis of disc herniations and other causes of nerve root impingement.

Among the limitations of MRI is its limited ability to image cortical bone, which renders virtually no signal, and the limited differentiation between cortical bone and other dense tissues that also render low signal intensity, such as tendons and ligaments. It is contraindicated in the presence of aneurysmal brain clips and, furthermore, the presence of orthopaedic hardware can cause degradation of the image, although rarely any hazards.

Diagnostic ultrasound

Over the last 15 years, there has been considerable interest in ultrasound imaging among physical therapists, in large part due to landmark studies of muscles associated with lumbar stabilization performed using ultrasound (Hides et al 1994). This has led to fairly widespread clinical use of ultrasound as a form of biofeedback. There, however, are few reports of physical therapists using ultrasound for the purpose of diagnosing musculoskeletal problems. Ultrasound would seem to be an ideal addition to the physical therapists'

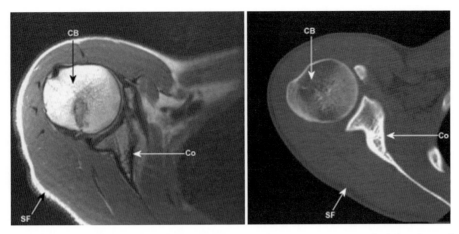

Fig 4.10 Axial T1 MRI (left) and bone window CT (right) of the right shoulder. The subcutaneous fat (SF) and cancellous bone (CB) appear bright in the MR image, but dark on the CT. Conversely, cortical bone is dark in the MR image, but bright on the CT (from Kassarjian et al 2006, with permission).

diagnostic process since it matches the sensitivity and specificity of MRI for the diagnosis of musculoskeletal soft tissues and can be employed during the physical examination – while performing active contractions, passive stretching, or traction.

Generating the image

Ultrasound creates images based on ultrasound reflected from tissues and/or tissue interfaces by comparing emitted and received ultrasound. The emitted ultrasound waves lose energy due to attenuation, absorption, reflection, refraction, and scattering. Reflection is of greatest importance for image creation; differentiation between tissues is made based on the amount of ultrasound reflected. Bone, for example, reflects almost all the incoming ultrasound waves; tendons reflect a significant amount of waves, muscles less, and water almost not at all (van Holsbeeck & Introcaso 2001). The amplitude of the reflected signal determines the brightness of the tissue on the screen of the ultrasound unit (Fig 4.11). Tissues and interfaces that reflect a high proportion of sound

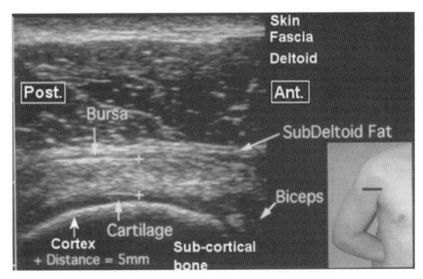

Fig 4.11 Transverse sonogram of the supraspinatus tendon (+ signs), displaying the imaging characteristics of the various tissues. The scanning plane is shown in the inserted photograph (from van Holsbeeck et al 2001, with permission).

waves are referred to as hyperechoic; tissues with low reflectivity as hypoechoic, or even anechoic. Note that reflection is increased at interfaces of tissues with vastly different acoustic properties. The signal characteristics of normal tissues are summarized in Table 4.3.

The reflective characteristics of tissues not only differ based on the acoustic properties of the tissue and the nature of its interface with other tissues; reflection is greatest when waves are reflected off flat surfaces and may differ depending on the incident angle of the ultrasound waves. A tendon that gives rise to a hyperechoic signal when the ultrasound beam is perpendicular to its long axis may appear hypoechoic when the beam is not perpendicular. This phenomenon is called anisotropy (Fig 4.12).

Frequency affects attenuation, as well as the quality of the image. Higher ultrasound frequencies, using shorter wavelengths, have less penetration, but greater resolution. Thus, the ultrasonographer will use the highest frequency that provides the desired depth of penetration.

Diagnosis is not only made on the basis of altered tissue reflectivity, but based on numerous other factors, including the internal architecture of muscles, tendons, and ligaments. The signal characteristics of abnormal tissues are summarized in Table 4.4.

Viewing the image

Ultrasound images are not customarily referred to in terms of the orthogonal planes, as is done with CT and

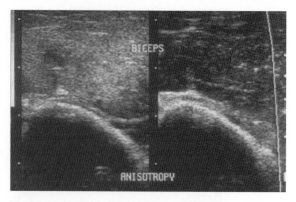

Fig 4.12 Transverse sonogram of the anterior upper arm displaying anisotropy. In the image on the right, the ultrasound beam is tilted 40 degrees away from the axial plane, resulting in decreased signal from muscle and tendons. (from van Holsbeeck et al 2001, with permission).

MR images. Most commonly, the viewing plane is described as longitudinal and transverse with reference to the viewed structures. A longitudinal view of the supraspinatus is a view aligned with the long axis of the muscle (in the oblique coronal plane); a transverse view of the long head of biceps tendon is a view across the tendon in the bicipital groove. Thus, the image represents a plane that is in direct continuation of the ultrasound transducer.

Advantages and disadvantages

As an imaging modality, ultrasound has numerous advantages. For example, the ability to modify the imaging process and stretch tissues or apply resistance while imaging. Ultrasound compares favourably to MRI for soft tissue diagnosis of the musculoskeletal system. The general advantages of ultrasound over MRI include greater resolution, lower cost, and shorter imaging times. For the imaging of muscle, ultrasound is just as accurate as MRI and provides more intricate details of muscle architecture. The intricate architecture of tendons and ligaments is better displayed with ultrasound than with MRI; it can reveal pathology not diagnosed with MRI.

There are some disadvantages. Ultrasound imaging has a narrow field of view and it is very operator-dependent; one examiner cannot replicate exactly the examination of another. Furthermore, structures deep to bone are not visualized and since ultrasound does not cross air interfaces imaging of structures obscured by the lungs or gas in the intestine is difficult. Compared to MRI, ultrasound has limited ability to show intra-articular structures, although it is valuable for demonstrating joint effusion.

Table 4.3 Ultrasound signal characteristics of normal tissue on ultrasound

Tissue	Signal on ultrasound
Bone	Cortex: hyperechoic, smooth, and continuous. Sub-cortical bone: not visible.
Tendons and ligaments	Hyperechoic; distinct parallel fiber pattern; dotted appearance in transverse plane
Muscles	Hypoechoic, with parallel hyperechoic fibrous bands
Bursae	Thin hypoechoic lines
Hyaline cartilage	Hypoechoic layer, next to the hyperechoic cortex.
Nerves	Hyperechoic, relative to muscle, with parallel strands; dotted in transverse plane
Cysts	Anechoic

Table 4.4 Ultrasound signal intensities of abnormal tissue

Abnormality	Signal on ultrasound
Fracture	Break in continuity cortex; uneven surfaces
Tendinopathy	Thickening of the tendon, focal or diffuse; underlying bone may be roughened and irregular
Synovial sheath inflammation	In longitudinal view; a hypoechoic layer superficial and deep to tendon. If chronic, thickening and a brighter signal
Tendon/ligament strains	Thickening and mixed echogenicity (hypoechoic if inflammation or haematoma); partly disrupted fibre pattern
Tendon/ligament rupture	Disruption of structures; filling with hypoechoic haematoma; separation of ends
Muscle strain	Disruption of fibrous bands; hypoechoic haematoma in early stages
Muscle rupture	Retraction of muscle stumps
Bursitis	Increased width (hypoechoic) of bursa; in chronic stages, hyperechoic thickening of bursa walls
Cartilage damage	Early changes: inhomogeneous thickening; later irregularity and disruption
Nerve compression	Flattening; swelling proximal to compression
Distended/ abnormal cyst	Increased volume (hypoechoic); thickened walls; septations; debris

IMAGING OF THE CERVICAL SPINE

Trauma, spondylarthropathy, nerve root impingements, and central stenosis, with associated myelopathy, are commonly encountered clinical problems in the cervical spine.

Choice of imaging modality

Conventional radiography is the imaging examination of choice for demonstrating alignment and evaluating fractures, although CT is the preferred modality for occult fractures. For imaging of trauma, CT may also be the modality of choice because of its sensitivity for both osseous and soft tissue structures and the short scanning times. It is the best modality for demonstrating osteophytosis resulting in the narrowing of the intervertebral foramina or the osseous spinal canal. However, MRI is superior to CT for the differential diagnosis of the causes of radiculopathy or myelopathy and for viewing the spinal cord, nerve roots, and the cervical vessels.

The cervical spine is frequently injured and when these injuries are complicated by pain referred into the upper extremity, this is associated with poor prognosis. Whiplash injury is one of the most common indications for imaging studies of cervical spine.

Conventional radiographs for whiplash

Most patients reporting to emergency rooms following whiplash undergo imaging studies; as a rule, conventional radiography. The value of radiography in the evaluation of whiplash injuries is doubtful. Comparisons of post-mortem cryosections and radiography have demonstrated extremely poor sensitivity for conventional radiographs for demonstrating osseous, discal, and ligamentous lesions (Jónsson et al 1991). However, the validity of the radiographic examination can be greatly improved by using simple clinical decision making rules, such as the Canadian C-spine rules (Stiell et al 2001). These rules state that after cervical injury, the following constitute indications for radiography: 'dangerous' mechanism of injury, age >65 years, extremity paraesthesias, and cervical rotation of less than half the normal range. Others need no radiographic studies.

Following whiplash, the radiographic evaluation is typically normal, except for altered sagittal alignment of the cervical spine (Fig 4.13) (Kristjánsson & Jónsson 2002). Radiography following trauma typically includes an open-mouth AP radiograph of the sub-cranial spine. Faulty alignment in this area should alert the clinician to the possibility of sub-cranial ligamentous injury (Fig 4.14).

Although radiographs may not demonstrate the whiplash injury, they may contain other valuable information. Patients with pre-existing degenerative changes (Watkinson et al 1991) and patients with a small diameter of the spinal canal (Pettersson et al 1995) are more likely to experience prolonged symptoms (Fig 4.15). This may influence patient management.

Dynamic radiography in whiplash

Stress-radiography may show abnormality, in spite of normal findings on static images (Fig 4.16). However, this method has serious limitations and may not be

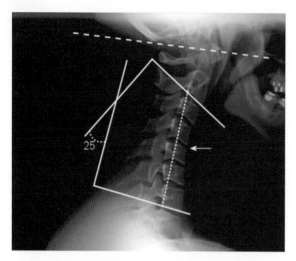

Fig 4.13 A lateral radiograph of the cervical spine of a young woman a week post-whiplash. The neck is held in kyphosis (25°); the posterior vertebral borders of all cervical vertebrae fall behind a line drawn between the inferior posterior vertebral borders of C2 and C7. The head is held in a flexed position, as evidenced by the anteriorly downward-sloping McGregor's plane (dashed line).

justified in the initial stages of whiplash injury. The examination can result in further trauma to the patient and one-third of patients with whiplash injury may not, due to pain, have the active range of motion necessary for detection of instability (Wang et al 1999).

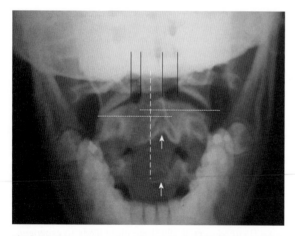

Fig 4.14 AP open-mouth radiograph, showing faulty alignment. The atlas is rotated to the left (black solid lines); the left lateral mass moves away from the midline, opening up a space on that side, while the right lateral mass closes down the space on the right. The spinous processes of C2 and C3 (arrows) are to the left of a vertical line from odontoid (dashed line), indicating right rotation of C2 and C3. The right lateral mass of atlas is lower than the left (dotted lines), indicating right side bending (Courtesy of M. Rocabado).

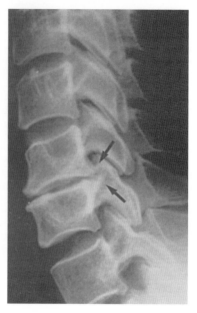

Fig 4.15 Lateral radiograph showing disc space narrowing and marginal osteophytes projecting from posterior vertebral borders and unco-vertebral margins (from Taylor & Resnick 2000, with permission).

Further, stress radiography only shows vertebral positions at the extreme ranges of motion. As a result of this, instability is rarely demonstrated on stress radiographs, giving rise to concerns about false negative findings.

Videofluoroscopy, considered by some to be a valuable alternative to stress radiography, has some of the same limitations in the acute phase of the whiplash injury that apply to stress radiography. However, once videofluoroscopy can be safely applied, it may show abnormal patterns of motion, such as mid-range instability and uneven contribution of cervical segments to the range of motion (Hino et al 1999).

Advanced imaging in whiplash

Many find it surprising that MRI studies for most patients with acute whiplash injury are normal. In all but rare instances, it is impossible to demonstrate evidence of injury, such as oedema, bleeding or other soft tissue pathology, on MRI (Borchgrevink et al 1997). However, in patients in patients with longstanding symptoms, there is a high incidence of ruptures of upper cervical ligaments, such as the alar and transverse ligaments (Krakenes et al 2003). CT is of limited value in the evaluation of the whiplash injury. However, CT scans revealing increased rotation at the atlanto-occipital joint can accurately classify 80% of patients with chronic pain following whiplash injury (Patijn et al 2001).

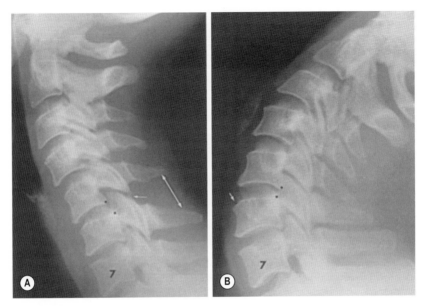

Fig 4.16 Segmental instability, post whiplash injury. A lateral radiograph in the neutral position (A) shows cervical kyphosis and a focal angulation at the C5–6 level, with separation of the spinous processes (double arrow) and loss of apposition at the facet joints (arrow), as well as widening of the posterior C5–6 disc space (black dots). A radiograph during neck extension (B) reveals posterior translation of the C5 (black dots) and a small radiolucent vacuum cleft (arrow) within the anterior fibres of the C5–6 disc. The inter-segmental motion, the widening of the posterior disc space, and vacuum cleft indicate segmental instability (from Taylor & Resnick 2000, with permission).

IMAGING OF THE SHOULDER AND SHOULDER GIRDLE

When imaging the shoulder girdle and shoulder, one must keep in mind the influence of the posture of the cervical and thoracic spines and contribution of the multiple joints of the shoulder girdle to movements of the shoulder joint. Malunion of clavicular fractures will, for example, affect the acromio-clavicular and sterno-clavicular joints and movements in the shoulder girdle (Fig 4.17).

Imaging of the shoulder girdle

Radiographs of the scapula may be used to diagnose fractures and to demonstrate scapulo-humeral relationships. The typical scapular views are the AP, lateral (posterior oblique), and the axillary views. The axillary view, produced by directing the x-ray beam through the shoulder joint in an infero-superior direction, is used to determine the relationship of the humeral head to the glenoid fossa.

Two views are typically employed for the clavicle; the AP and an AP view with a 45-degree caudal tilt. When there is fracture of the clavicle, the AP view typically shows superior displacement of the proximal fragment and inferior displacement of the distal fragment due to the opposing forces of the pull of the sternomastoid and the weight of the arm.

Acromio-clavicular joint separations can be visualized on the standard AP view of the shoulder, or with both joints imaged simultaneously. Weights of 4–7 kg (10–15 pounds) are used to apply stress to the acromio-clavicular joints in order to assess ligamentous integrity. The acromio-clavicular joint space should measure 3–8 mm and the coraco-clavicular distance 10–13 mm. An increase in these distances indicates sprain.

Imaging for the shoulder joint

The shoulder is the most commonly imaged joint of the upper extremity; most often for the evaluation of rotator cuff pathology and suspected fractures of the proximal humerus. Conventional radiographs are important in the evaluation of fractures, but obviously of limited value for the evaluation of rotator cuff pathology, although they can sometimes indicate impingement (Fig 4.18).

Conventional radiography

The standard radiographic examination includes the AP view, in internal rotation and external rotation, axillary view, and lateral view of the scapula. The AP internal rotation, which brings the lesser tuberosity into view may be used to evaluate for the Hill-Sachs fracture. The AP external

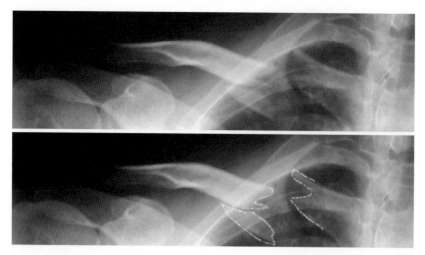

Fig 4.17 Comminuted clavicular fracture in a middle-aged bicyclist, displayed on an AP, caudally directed radiograph. The fracture was treated conservatively, with the middle fragment left in the position outlined in the lower image. No radiographic evaluation was done for a suspected fracture in the distal third of the clavicle. Nine years later, the patient has palpable hypertrophy at the fracture site, as well as the acromio-clavicular joint and at the pseudarthrosis just medial to it.

rotation view best shows the relationship between the humeral head and the glenoid, the size of the sub-acromial space, and the vertical position of the humeral head relative to the glenoid, which may be elevated in case of rotator cuff tear. In this view, the lesser tuberosity is superimposed on the humeral head, but the greater tuberosity is viewed in profile. The axillary view, previously described for radiography of the scapula, is used for the evaluation of fractures or dislocations of the proximal humerus.

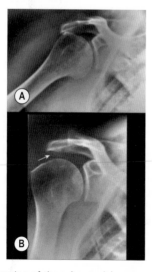

Fig 4.18 Narrowing of the subacromial space accentuated on active abduction (A). Impingement (B). There are osteophytic spurs on the undersurface of the acromion. Impingement of the rotator cuff must be considered likely (from Umans et al 2001, with permission).

Magnetic resonance imaging (MRI)

Advanced imaging is performed on the basis of specific indications, most commonly for the evaluation of rotator cuff pathology. MRI is most commonly performed in modified orthogonal planes: oblique coronal plane and oblique sagittal views. The oblique coronal plane is aligned with the supraspinatus muscle, while the oblique sagittal plane is aligned parallel to the glenoid fossa; showing the coracoacromial arch and the contents of the sub-acromial space. MRI is as accurate as arthrography to diagnose full-thickness tears of the rotator cuff, but can also be used to evaluate partial tears and evaluate degenerative changes in tendons (tendinosis). Biceps tendon pathology and dislocation of the tendon, often associated with rotator cuff pathology, are clearly viewed with MRI. Physical evidence of instability, for example ligamentous laxity or labral tears, may first be detected with MRI. The shoulder joint is the second most common site for avascular necrosis and MRI is the most sensitive imaging method for detecting early changes.

Ultrasound

The key soft tissues around the shoulder are readily accessible to ultrasound and the ability of ultrasound to detect soft tissue pathology rivals or exceeds that of MRI (Fig 4.19). Ultrasound has been used to display intra-tendinous pathology and tears of the rotator cuff, dislocation of the long head of biceps, bursal pathology, and sprains of the acromio-clavicular joint. It is advantageous to be able to perform clinical examination during the sonographic evaluation; including guiding the patient's movement though flexion and abduction while the movements of tendons and bursae are observed.

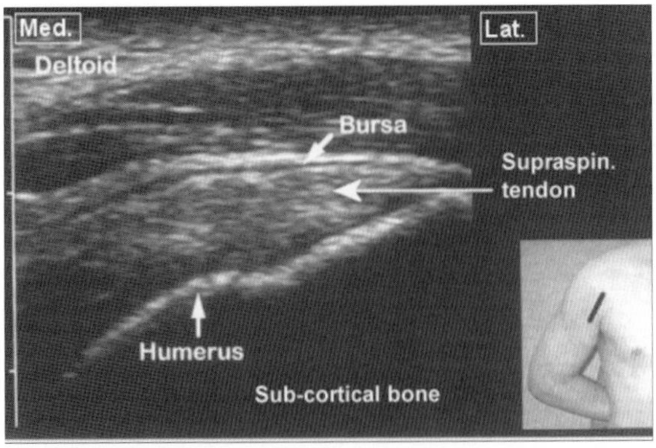

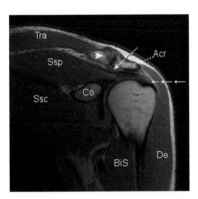

Fig 4.19 Longitudinal ultrasound of the supraspinatus tendon. Note the hypoechoic bursa and the hyperechoic signal from the interface between the deltoid muscle and the bursa. The scanning plane is shown in the inserted photograph (from van Holsbeeck et al 2001, with permission).

Rotator cuff syndrome

The most commonly encountered clinical problems of the shoulder relate to degenerative changes in the rotator cuff: supraspinatus tendinosis and rotator cuff tears. It is now well established that degenerative changes and tears in the rotator cuff are most frequently the result of impingement of the tendons due to, among other factors, aberrant shape or malalignment of the acromion and degenerative changes in the acromio-clavicular joint (Fig 4.20) (Morag et al 2006). MRI has revolutionised the diagnosis of these

degenerative problems and made it possible to visualize the anatomical causes of impingement.

IMAGING OF THE ELBOW

Fractures constitute the most commonly encountered clinical problem at the elbow. Other clinical problems relate to overuse injuries, ligament sprains, and nerve entrapments.

Conventional radiography

The conventional radiographic evaluation consists of an AP view in the anatomical position, lateral view (at 90 degrees of flexion), and oblique views in internal and external rotation. The internal oblique view provides a clear view of the coronoid process, while the external oblique view allows unobstructed view of the radial head, neck and tuberosity.

Conventional radiography of the forearm, frequently performed with radiography of the elbow, most commonly includes the AP forearm view and the lateral view. In the AP forearm view, the forearm is fully supinated; with the entire radius, ulna and wrist visible, as well as the proximal and distal radio-ulnar joints and the wrist. In the lateral view of the forearm, the forearm is seen in profile, with the elbow flexed at 90 degrees.

Advanced imaging

MRI is used for the detection of tendinosis and tendon ruptures, nerve entrapments, bursitis, and subtle fractures (Fig 4.21). Ultrasound has been used for the same

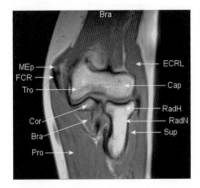

Fig 4.20 Oblique coronal T1 MRI showing impingement of the left supraspinatus tendon. There are substantial degenerative changes (arrowhead) in the acromio-clavicular joint and indentation in the superior surface to the supraspinatus tendon due to intra-articular swelling in the acromio-clavicular joint and hypertrophy of its capsule (arrow). Furthermore, the acromion (Acr) is downsloping laterally. Note the insertion of the supraspinatus tendon on the greater tuberosity (repeating arrows). Trapezius (Tra), supraspinatus muscle (Ssp), subscapularis muscle (Ssc), coracoid process (Co), short head of biceps (BiS), and deltoid muscle (De) (from Kassarjian et al 2006, with permission).

Fig 4.21 Coronal T1 MRI of the left elbow. Note the considerable thickness of the articular cartilage; a light grey shade above the dark outline of the radial head (RadH) and coronoid process (Cor). The image also shows: Brachialis (Bra), medial epicondyle (MEp), tendon of flexor carpi radialis (FCR), trochlea (Tro), pronator teres (Pro), supinator (Sup), radial neck (RadN), capitellum (Cap), and extensor carpi radialis longus (ECRL).

purposes, although not for the evaluation of fractures. Epicondylitis and tears of the collateral ligaments may be best viewed with ultrasound.

Fractures of the elbow

Elbow fractures, which may involve the distal humerus, or proximal ulna, and radial head, are often associated with later functional disturbances (Figs 4.22 & 4.23). This is exemplified by fractures of the proximal ulna. The congruency between the trochlear notch of the ulna and the trochlea of humerus, as well as the tight fit between the olecranon and coronoid processes and their respective fossae in the humerus, may present problems associated with fracture healing, although the tight fit offers excellent medio-lateral stability. Mal-union of fractures in this area can have serious implications for function; fractures of the proximal ulna are associated with loss of ROM in > 50% of cases. Similarly, fractures of the radial head, which may be treated with radial head excision (depending on amount of displacement), result in shortening of the radius. This, in turn, is associated with biomechanical problems at the distal radio-ulnar joint (DRUJ) and wrist.

Fractures of the radial and ulnar shafts are, similarly, associated with functional disturbances at the elbow, wrist, and DRUJ. These fractures most often result from direct trauma, sustained during motor vehicle accidents, blows, or falls. Radial shaft fractures are frequently accompanied by dislocation of the ulno-carpal and distal radio-ulnar joints, as well as avulsion fractures

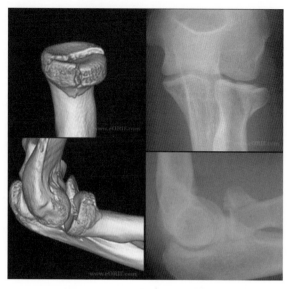

Fig 4.23 Displaced radial head fracture, following a fall on the outstretched hand. AP and lateral radiographs, as well as CT 3D reconstructions show the displacement of the fragment. The patient was treated with open fixation. (Courtesy of eorif.com.)

of the ulnar styloid (Fig 4.24). Ulnar shaft fractures may be accompanied by dislocation of the radio-humeral joint.

IMAGING OF THE HAND AND WRIST

Clinical problems of the wrist and hand are mostly related to instabilities, fractures, and overuse injuries.

Conventional radiography

Radiography of the hand

Unlike other regions of the musculoskeletal system, radiographs are made in the postero-anterior view (PA); not the AP view. An oblique PA view is used to provide an oblique-to-lateral view of the phalanxes and metacarpals, without the superimposition encountered in the lateral view. In the lateral view, most of the structures of the hand, metacarpals and phalanxes are superimposed. However, the lateral view is a true PA view of the thumb.

Radiography of the wrist

The same views apply to the radiographic evaluation of the wrist, with the addition of optional views obtained in radial and ulnar deviation. The lateral view shows the superimposed metacarpals, carpal bones, and the distal radius and ulna. This is a difficult view to evaluate, since

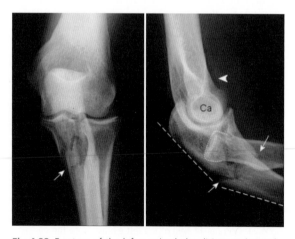

Fig 4.22 Fracture of the left proximal ulna (Monteggia type), with posterior dislocation of the radial head (dotted outline) from the capitellum (Ca). This is a complete (arrows), comminuted fracture, with anterior deviation (dashed lines) and minimal lateral displacement of the ulna. There is displacement of the anterior fat pad of the elbow (arrowhead) (courtesy of Dr. A Gentili).

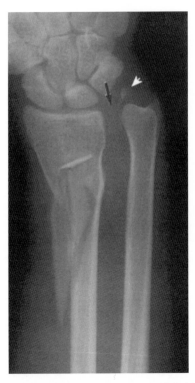

Fig 4.24 Comminuted fracture of the distal third of the radius. The distal-most fragment is laterally displaced and angulated. There is concomitant separation of DRUJ (arrow) and avulsion of the ulnar styloid (arrowhead), indicating injury to the triangular fibrocartilage complex (TFCC) (from Taylor & Resnick 2000, with permission).

a slight change in the angle of the x-ray beam, relative to the hand, can alter the view considerably; carpal bones that previously appeared volarly may now seem to be dorsally situated. Radiographs made with the patient's wrist in ulnar and radial deviation can provide additional information. Ulnar deviation may, for example, 'open up' a scaphoid fracture not visible in the PA view, as well as allowing inferences about the biomechanics of the wrist and ligament ruptures.

Advanced imaging

CT is used to demonstrate the dimensions of the carpal tunnel, since it offers superior presentation of osseous structures. This is the best modality for demonstrating complex fractures, fracture healing, and dislocations.

MRI is widely used in the imaging of pathology and trauma to tendons and ligaments. High field strength in conjunction with surfaces coils is used in order to obtain thin slices and to allow images to be reconstructed in any plane, in order to accommodate for the complex anatomy in this region. Complex ligament injuries in the wrist

can be directly imaged, instead of inferred from the alignment of the osseous structures on conventional radiographs. Faulty alignment can be demonstrated in any plane and diagnosis can be made based on loss of continuity of ligaments, as well as the associated adjacent inflammation.

The carpal tunnel syndrome (CTS) is one of the most common nerve entrapment syndromes. With MRI it has become possible to directly visualize the pathological changes associated with CTS (Fig 4.25). Oedema may be present along the carpal arch, displacing the fat normally adjacent to the osseous structures in this area and there may be flattening of the median nerve. Volar bowing of the transverse carpal ligament may result from increased pressure in the carpal tunnel; all of these changes are well displayed with MRI (White et al 1997).

Ultrasound is used to evaluate tendon pathology: inflammation, fraying, and cavities in the tendons. Tenosynovitis and ganglia, arising from the tendon sheaths, are clearly visualized on ultrasound. CTS is well demonstrated as swelling of the median nerve proximal to the carpal tunnel and flattening of the nerve within the tunnel.

Measurements at the wrist – instability

Many of the biomechanical disturbances resulting from fractures of the ulna and radius relate to changes in ulnar variance. Radiographic measurement and assessment

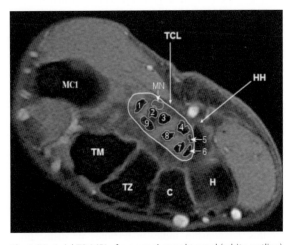

Fig 4.25 Axial T2 MRI of a normal carpal tunnel (white outline) at the level of the hook of the hamate (HH). Transverse carpal ligament (TCL), first metacarpal (MC1), trapezium (TM), trapezoid (TZ), capitate (C), hamate (H), median nerve (M) tendon of flexor pollicis longus (1), tendon TMs of flexor digitorum superficialis (2–5), tendons of flexor digitorum profundus (6–9) (from Bower et al 2006, with permission).

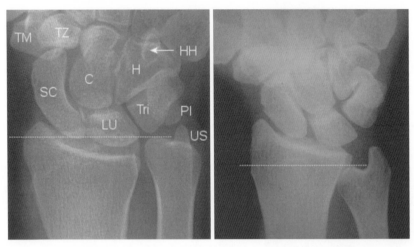

Fig 4.26 Positive ulnar variance (left) and negative ulnar variance (right). Note the different position of the DRUJ. Labels: Trapezium (TM), trapezoid (TZ), capitate (C), hamate (H), hook of the hamate (HH), ulnar styloid (US), pisiform (PI), triquetrum (Tri), lunate (LU), and scaphoid (SC) (from Taylor & Resnick 2000, with permission).

of the alignment of the bones of the forearm are thus very important in the management of wrist and hand problems.

Ulnar variance can be measured in the PA view, in the following manner. When lines are drawn across the articular surfaces of the ulna and radius, there is said to be neutral ulnar variance if these lines overlap. If the radial surface is more distal, there is negative ulnar variance; if the ulnar surface is more distal, there is positive ulnar variance (Fig 4.26). This relationship is frequently altered following fracture of the ulna and/or radius, which may, in turn, lead to functional disturbances of the wrist and altered load on the carpal bones. Negative ulnar variance is associated with Kienbock's disease, avascular necrosis of the lunate, as well as ulnar impingement syndrome; compression of the distal end of the ulna against the medial side of the radius (Cerezal et al 2002). Shortening of the radius, on the other hand, leads to positive ulnar variance. This is associated with ulnar impaction syndrome – degenerative changes associated with excessive load bearing across the ulnar-sided carpal joints and the TFCC. Ligamentous instability and TFCC perforation may result.

In the PA view, the alignment of the bones of the wrist can be checked by drawing three lines: (1) proximal to the distal row, (2) distal to the proximal row, and (3) proximal to the proximal row. These three lines should form arches that are roughly parallel (Fig 4.27). A disturbance in this relationship indicates fractures or dislocations and a gap of more than 3 mm between the lunate and scaphoid is indicative of scapholunate dissociation. Disturbances in normal alignment not only alert us to functional disturbances (such as instabilities), (Fig 4.28) but can help detect fractures missed by simply viewing bones in isolation.

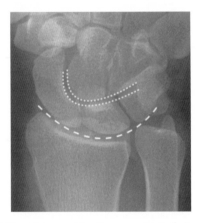

Fig 4.27 Three lines used for the assessment of alignment of the carpal bones. Note the positive ulnar variance. (from Taylor & Resnick 2000, with permission).

In the lateral view, the scapholunate angle can be assessed. The axis of the scaphoid is represented by a line intersecting the midpoints of its proximal and distal poles; the axis of the lunate is formed by a line drawn across its concave distal joint surfaces. The scapholunate angle represents the intersection of the long axis of the scaphoid and a line drawn perpendicular to the long axis of the lunate. This angle should be 30–60 degrees (Fig 4.29). If the angle is increased it could indicate ligamentous disruption (scapholunate dissociation), which frequently results from falls on the hand, or other injury mechanisms that axially load the wrist (Fig 4.30).

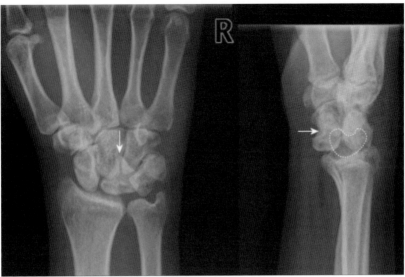

Fig 4.28 The PA radiograph shows disruption of the three lines of the wrist. The lunate (arrow) partly overlaps the capitate and hamate. The lateral radiograph shows that the lunate has dislocated anteriorly (arrow). Its normal position is traced with a dotted outline (from van Kooten et al 2005, with permission).

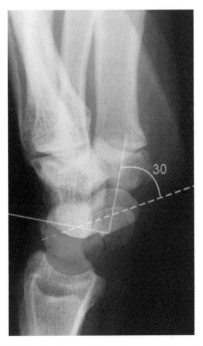

Fig 4.29 A lateral radiograph showing normal scapholunate angle (30°). The lunate is shaded dark and a dashed line represents the long axis of the scaphoid.

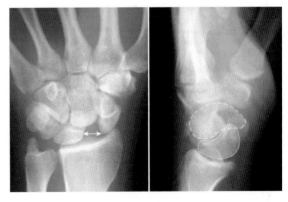

Fig 4.30 PA and lateral radiographs demonstrating scapholunate dissociation. Disruption of the scapholunate ligaments allows the scaphoid (dotted outline) and lunate (dashed outline) to separate and to rotate in opposite directions, increasing the scapholunate angle to 110° (from Manuel & Moran 2007, with permission).

REFERENCES

Agustsson, H., 2005. Radiologic evaluation of the temporomandibular joint. In: McKinnis, L.N. (Ed.), Fundamentals of musculoskeletal imaging. second ed. FA Davis Company, Philadelphia, pp. 183–207.

APTA Education Division, 2004. Coalition for Consensus, A normative model of physical therapist professional education. APTA, Alexandria.

Barr, J.B., 2005. Integration of imaging into physical therapy practice. In: McKinnis, L.N. (Ed.), Fundamentals of musculoskeletal imaging. second ed. FA Davis Company, Philadelphia, pp. 531–548.

Borchgrevink, G., Smevik, O., Haave, I., et al., 1997. MRI of cerebrum and cervical column within two days after whiplash neck sprain injury. Injury 28, 331–335.

Bower, J.A., Stanisz, G.J., Keir, P.J., 2006. An MRI evaluation of carpal tunnel dimensions in healthy wrists: Implications for carpal tunnel syndrome. Clin. Biomech. (Bristol, Avon) 21, 816–825.

Cerezal, L., del Piñal, F., Abascal, F., et al., 2002. Imaging findings in ulnar-sided wrist impaction syndromes. Radiographics 22, 105–121.

Daker-White, G., Carr, A.J., Harvey, I., et al., 1999. A randomised controlled trial. Shifting boundaries of doctors and physiotherapists in orthopaedic outpatient departments. J. Epidemiol. Community Health 53, 643–650.

Deyle, G., 2005. Diagnostic imaging in primary care physical therapy. In: Boissonnault, W.G. (Ed.), Primary care for the physical therapist – examination and triage. WB Saunders, St. Louis, pp. 323–347.

Donato, E.B., DuVall, R.E., Godges, J.J., et al., 2004. Practice analysis: defining the clinical practice of primary contact physical therapy. J. Orthop. Sports Phys. Ther. 34, 284–304.

Graber, M.B., 2005. Diagnostic imaging and differential diagnosis in 2 case reports. J. Orthop. Sports Phys. Ther. 35 (11), 745–754.

Hides, J.A., Stokes, M.J., Saide, M., et al., 1994. Evidence of lumbar multifidus muscle wasting ipsi-lateral to symptoms in patients with acute/subacute low back pain. Spine 19, 165–172.

Hino, H., Abumi, K., Kanayama, M., et al., 1999. Dynamic motion analysis of normal and unstable cervical spines using cineradiography. An in vivo study. Spine 24, 163–168.

Jette, D.U., Ardleigh, K., Chandler, K., et al., 2006. Decision-making ability of physical therapists: physical therapy intervention or medical referral. Phys. Ther. 86, 1619–1629.

Jónsson Jr., H., Bring, G., Rauschning, W., et al., 1991. Hidden cervical injuries in traffic accident victims with skull fractures. J. Spinal Disord. 4, 251–263.

Kassarjian, A., Bencardino, J.T., Palmer, W.E., 2006. MR imaging of the rotator cuff. Radiol. Clin. North Am. 44, 503–523.

Krakenes, J., Kaale, B.R., Nordli, H., et al., 2003. MR analysis of the transverse ligament in the late stage of whiplash injury. Acta Radiol. 44, 637–644.

Kristjánsson, E., Jónsson Jr., H., 2002. Is the sagittal configuration of the cervical spine changed in women with chronic whiplash syndrome? A comparative computer-assisted radiographic assessment. J. Manipulative Physiol. Ther. 25, 550–555.

Magee, D.J., 2006. Orthopedic physical assessment, fourth ed. Elsevier, Philadelphia.

Manuel, J., Moran, S.L., 2007. The diagnosis and treatment of scapholunate instability. Orthop. Clin. North Am. 38, 261–277.

Morag, Y., Jacobson, J.A., Miller, B., et al., 2006. MR imaging of rotator cuff injury: what the clinician needs to know. Radiographics 26, 1045–1065.

Marchiori, D.M., 1999. Skeletal imaging with skeletal, chest, abdominal pattern differentials. Mosby, St. Louis.

Patijn, J., Wilmink, J., van der Linden, F. H., et al., 2001. CT study of craniovertebral rotation in whiplash injury. Euro. Spine J. 10, 38–43.

Pettersson, K., Kjarrholm, J., Toolanen, G., et al., 1995. Decreased width of the spinal canal in patients with chronic symptoms after whiplash injury. Spine 20, 1664–1667.

Steinbach, L.S., Palmer, W.E., Schweitzer, M.E., 2002. Special focus session. MR arthrography. Radiographics 22, 1223–1246.

Stiell, I.G., Wells, G.A., Vandemheen, K. L., et al., 2001. The Canadian C-spine rule for radiography in alert and stable trauma patients. J. Am. Med. Assoc. 286, 1841–1848.

Taylor, J.A.M., Resnick, D., 2000. Skeletal Imaging. Mosby, St. Louis.

Umans, H.R., Pavlov, H., Berkowitz, M., Warren, R.F., 2001. Correlation of radiographic and arthroscopic findings with rotator cuff tears and degenerative joint disease. J. Shoulder Elbow Surg. 10, 428–433.

van Holsbeeck, M.T., Introcaso, J.H., 2001. Musculoskeletal ultrasound. Mosby, St. Louis.

van Kooten, E.O., Coster, E., Segers, M.J., Ritt, M.J., 2005. Early proximal row carpectomy after severe carpal trauma. Injury 36, 1226–1232.

Wang, J.C., Hatch, J.D., Sandhu, H.S., et al., 1999. Cervical flexion and extension radiographs in acutely injured patients. Clin. Orthop. Relat. Res. 365, 111–116.

Watkinson, A., Gargan, M.F., Bannister, G.C., 1991. Prognostic factors in soft tissue injuries of the cervical spine. Injury 22, 307–309.

White, L.M., Schweitzer, M.E., Liu, P.T., 1997. The wrist. In: Deutsch, A.L., Mink, J.H. (Eds.), MRI of the musculoskeletal system: a teaching file. second ed. Lippincott-Raven, Philadelphia, pp. 149–196.

Wong, K.W., Leong, J.C., Chan, M.K., et al., 2004. The flexion-extension profile of lumbar spine in 100 healthy volunteers. Spine 29, 1636–1641.

Chapter | 5 |

Electrodiagnostic studies

Caroline A Quartly

INTRODUCTION

'There are more things in heaven and earth, Horatio, than are dreamt of in your philosophy'

Hamlet to Horatio in Act I, Scene V

an argument against the oversimplification of a doctrine

In the context of neck and arm pain syndromes, there are many diagnostic categories where electrodiagnostic evaluation may be relevant (Box 5.1). However, as with referral for every clinical test in medicine, initiation of referral to an electrodiagnostic service should always be prefaced by clinical reasoning. Will doing the test have a bearing on patient outcome? It behoves us to always remember that just because we have the ability to do a test, this doesn't mean that doing the test serves the patient. When the opportunities for intervention are limited, such as when, for example, spinal MRI studies are done in the absence of clinical signs and/or symptoms of neurological or orthopaedic compromise or of a history suggestive of sinister pathology, we are complicit in the creation/perpetuation of an expensive health care system that does not change patient outcome. Clinical questions that might then be useful in deciding whether to refer for electrodiagnostic testing include:

1. Is the accurate documentation of the presence and severity of this lesion critical to surgical referral for consultation to determine the merits of exploration, decompression, transposition, or nerve graft?
2. Is the accurate documentation of the presence and severity of this condition essential to determining whether specific medication (such as, e.g., prednisone) will change outcome?
3. Is the accurate documentation of the presence and severity of this condition essential to determining whether further investigation will uncover a potentially treatable disorder, such as vitamin B12 deficiency, vasculitis, or diabetes?
4. Is the accurate documentation of the presence and severity of this condition essential to determining whether exercise prescriptions and/or work capacity recommendations will require modification, such as, for example, in the case of severe axonal nerve damage (where potential metabolic exhaustion of recovering or permanently damaged nerve is an issue) or in patients with hereditary sensory-motor neuropathies, entrapment neuropathies, and myopathies?
5. Is the finding of a negative test useful or contextually harmful to patient management?

© 2011 Elsevier Ltd.
DOI: 10.1016/B978-0-7020-3528-9.00005-4

Box 5.1 **Diagnostic categories where nerve conduction studies/EMG evaluation may be relevant to the diagnosis and/or management of upper extremity pain syndromes (source: modified from www.aanem.org)**

Peripheral nerves

1. Suprascapular nerve:
   - Suprascapular motor nerve to the supraspinatus
   - Suprascapular motor nerve to the infraspinatus
2. Long thoracic nerve injury: serratus anterior
3. Thoracodorsal motor nerve to the latissimus dorsi
4. Axillary nerve: isolated deltoid involvement
5. Median nerve:
   - Median motor nerve to the abductor pollicis brevis
   - Median motor nerve, anterior interosseus branch, to the flexor pollicis longus
   - Median motor nerve, anterior interosseus branch, to the pronator quadratus
   - Median motor nerve to the first lumbrical
     Median motor nerve to the second lumbrical
   - Entrapment above the elbow at the ligament of Struthers
   - Entrapments between the two heads of pronator teres
   - Anterior interosseus syndrome (pure motor)
   - Carpal tunnel syndrome
6. Musculocutaneous motor nerve to the biceps brachii
7. Radial nerve:
   - Radial motor nerve to the extensor carpi ulnaris
   - Radial motor nerve to the extensor digitorum communis
   - Radial motor nerve to the extensor indicis proprius
   - Radial motor nerve to the brachioradialis
   - Entrapment at the spiral groove
   - Posterior interosseus syndrome
   - Supinator syndrome
   - Radial tunnel syndrome
   - Superficial sensory branch of the radial nerve
8. Ulnar nerve:
   - Ulnar motor nerve to the abductor digiti minimi
   - Ulnar motor nerve to the palmar interosseus
   - Ulnar motor nerve to the first dorsal interosseus
   - Ulnar motor nerve to the flexor carpi ulnaris
   - Entrapments well above the elbow
   - Tardy ulnar palsy
   - Entrapment in the aponeurosis of the flexor carpi ulnaris
   - Entrapment of the dorsal cutaneous branch of the ulnar nerve
   - Entrapment at Guyon's canal
   - Entrapment of the deep palmar branch

Upper Extremity Sensory and Mixed Nerves

A. Lateral antebrachial cutaneous sensory nerve
B. Medial antebrachial cutaneous sensory nerve
C. Medial brachial cutaneous sensory nerve
D. Median nerve
   1. Median sensory nerve to the 1st digit
   2. Median sensory nerve to the 2nd digit
   3. Median sensory nerve to the 3rd digit
   4. Median sensory nerve to the 4th digit
   5. Median palmar cutaneous sensory nerve
   6. Median palmar mixed nerve
E. Posterior antebrachial cutaneous sensory nerve
F. Radial sensory nerve
   1. Radial sensory nerve to the base of the thumb
   2. Radial sensory nerve to digit 1
G. Ulnar nerve
   1. Ulnar dorsal cutaneous sensory nerve
   2. Ulnar sensory nerve to the 4th digit
   3. Ulnar sensory nerve to the 5th digit
   4. Ulnar palmar mixed nerve

Radiculopathy

Cervical nerve root stimulation
1. Cervical level 5 (C5)
2. Cervical level 6 (C6)
3. Cervical level 7 (C7)
4. Cervical level 8 (C8)

Plexopathy

- Thoracic outlet syndrome
- Brachial neuritis
- Traction palsies (birth trauma)
- Trauma (stretch, laceration, compression)

Myopathy/dystrophy

Proximal versus distal
- Not usually painful unless related to muscle imbalance
- Family history may or may not be relevant
- Pattern of wasting and weakness may be pathognomic

Peripheral neuropathy

- May be sensory, motor, distal, proximal, axonal, and/or demyelinating
- Acquired: e.g., Guillain–Barré syndrome
- Hereditary: e.g., HSMN I or II

As with most clinical tests, when results are taken out of context the value of the test is greatly diminished. By extension, one can infer that utilizing tests out of context carries a higher likelihood of doing more harm than good to the patient (Shekelle et al 2000). It is important to understand that – next to technical issues – perhaps the largest source of error in electrophysiology lies in drawing conclusions from a limited database. The same can of course be said of the hallmarks of the clinical evaluation, history and clinical examination.

There seems to be a growing compulsion to use automated software programs to analyse nerve conduction (Armstrong et al 2008) and even electromyographic data; a compulsion perhaps driven by the erroneous assumption that electrodiagnostic evaluation involves the analysis of a signal as simple and uncomplicated as is elicited by electrocardiogram. The issue, of course, is that either limited or incorrectly interpreted and applied data may lead to an increase in both false negative and false positive findings. Either way, the patient may not be served. To be more specific: if, for example, a limited study is used to identify the presence or absence of carpal tunnel syndrome but the superimposition of other confounding diagnoses is neither considered nor evaluated, surgical decompression may result in poor outcome. Alternatively, the lack of surgical intervention may result in poor outcome if the data set is limited and incorrectly assumes a 'normal' study. A patient who returns with a label of 'normal' after a technical study that is not accompanied by a clinical evaluation may be completely misinterpreted (even to the extent of being called a malingerer) if the referring clinician or the third-party payer does not understand the indications and limitations of the procedure.

Interpretation of the test as 'normal' without the context of the clinical evaluation (history and physical examination) carries with it an enormous burden of responsibility. The responsibility to the patient and to the healthcare system as a whole is in understanding that the results of any given individual clinical test should never be taken out of context. If the clinician making the referral is not fully aware of the symptoms characteristic of a specific peripheral nerve injury, and as such requests only evaluation of a limited and specific diagnosis, it is that clinician who should perhaps bear full responsibility for not only the way in which the test is used technically but also the ultimate medical outcome of the patient.

One has to confront the fact that not all clinicians may be aware that specific presentations may signify an aetiology or even technique of testing outside common knowledge (Seror 2005). On the other hand, it must also be noted that the current literature is replete with a most-welcome focus on removing bias from analysis of specific disorders through more critical and representative studies. For example, comparative analyses of tests such as those used to diagnose entrapment ranging from that as common as carpal tunnel syndrome (Ayyar et al 2001, Bodofsky et al 2005, Chang et al 2006, Dan et al 2006, Aygül et al 2009, Brannagan et al 2009), to the more elusive radial nerve entrapment (Beck et al 1998), and to chronic demyelinating inflammatory and immune-mediated neuropathies (Hattori et al 2005, Latov & Sander 2003) are now even appearing in literature search engines of best evidence. Helpful studies confirming that electrodiagnostic evaluation can be blinded are also starting to emerge (Haig et al 2006).

It is the intent of this chapter that the reader comes to appreciate that the electrodiagnostic evaluation is most appropriately utilized in clinical practice as an extension of the clinical examination. It is not the intent of this chapter to discuss in detail the technical aspects of the ways in which electrodiagnostic studies are performed. Indeed, such information is clearly and extensively covered in numerous texts on the subject; perhaps the most comprehensive of which is *Electrodiagnostic Medicine* (Dumitru et al 2002). More recent publications by acknowledged experts in the field offer invaluable perspective (Aminoff 2005, Buschbacher & Prahlow 2005, Katirji 2007, Daube & Rubin 2009). To facilitate an understanding of the material in this chapter, some basic terminology not otherwise explained in the text is included in Table 5.1.

Table 5.1 A few basic examples of electrodiagnostic terminology		
Configuration of motor unit recorded on EMG	Polyphasic	A potential that crosses the baseline 5 or more times (may be seen in reinnervation/remodelling)
	Serrated	Multiple phases that do not cross the baseline (same inference)
	Long duration	Muscle specific and dependent on innervation ratio of specific muscle May be seen in collateral sprouting / indicative of prior axonal damage
	Large amplitude	Muscle specific and dependent on innervation ratio of specific muscle Recording needle characteristics also influence amplitude, hence normative data are critical
	Small amplitude	Muscle specific and dependent on innervation ratio of specific muscle May indicate myopathy or chronic neuropathy

Continued

Table 5.1 A few basic examples of electrodiagnostic terminology—cont'd

Stigmatic electrode	Recording electrode/cathode The differential signal analysis requires a cathode and an anode	
Terminal latency (motor or sensory)	The time (in milliseconds) it takes for a stimulus to evoke a response from nerve to its nearest recording site (nerve or muscle)	
Spontaneous discharge quoted and explained in text	Fibrillation	Mostly indicative of recent or active denervation.
	Positive sharp wave	May occur as fibrillation or motor unit
	Fasciculation	Spontaneous discharge of motor unit
Recruitment	When used to reflect firing frequency, can be directly correlated with motor unit drop (or axonal loss)	
Interference pattern	Can vary with the presence or absence of superimposed upper motor neuron involvement The firing frequency is not abnormal in the presence of upper motor neuron involvement alone	

EDUCATION AND CERTIFICATION IN ELECTRODIAGNOSTIC MEDICINE

Although not exclusively, two subspecialties of medicine are more likely to perform electrodiagnostic evaluations: neurology and physical medicine and rehabilitation (physiatry). An acknowledged minimal requirement of supervised training in the field of electromyography is six months during residency training. In North America, certification of competency in electrodiagnosis is achieved after successful written and oral examination through organizations such as the American Association of Neuromuscular and Electrodiagnostic Medicine (AANEM) or its Canadian equivalent, the Canadian Society of Clinical Neurophysiologists (CSCN). Basic eligibility to be considered for such examination requires both clinician reference and documentation of a minimum of 200 independent evaluations. During the six-month interval of residency training the focus is primarily on gaining technical skills. The context in which the technical skill is applied is a background of three to four years of medical school and four to five years of specialty residency training (encompassing not only more detailed neuroanatomy and neurophysiology but also in-depth expressions of the influence of disease, trauma, ageing, and genetics upon the neuromuscular system). In rehabilitation medicine, such understanding is also married with knowledge of the myriad presentations of musculoskeletal disorders. In neurology, such understanding may be married with a more extensive background in differential diagnosis of central and peripheral neurological disorders. The above information is inserted not to impress but rather to impress the extent of the art form

upon those who would oversimplify the use and value of electrophysiology.

The easiest part of the electrodiagnostic evaluation is the technical execution of the study (which of course requires a comprehensive understanding of pitfalls in the technical execution of the test). A poorly executed test is just as likely to miss a disease as it is to result in the inference of disease when there is none. Technical competence, as well as understanding which data to collect and how to interpret the findings in context, takes both skill and experience. This becomes the art of the specialty.

While in some jurisdictions (after a year's apprenticeship) a technologist may still become eligible for examination to acquire certification of competency in execution of nerve conduction studies (as an EMG technician), growing recognition of the extent of training required to operate sophisticated electroneurodiagnostic equipment has led to the development of two-year diploma programs in electrophysiology (see, for example, BCIT 2009). Certification of competency within subsets of electroneurophysiology is then acquired by specific examination. Such detailed training should prepare the technologist with the savvy of how to avoid pitfalls and how to problem solve various technical challenges in the acquisition of data.

While technologists have some basic knowledge of instrumentation, they do not usually have the entire medical context to assess the appropriateness of the specifics of the evaluation, nor do they assume the legal responsibility for excluding or including coexisting competing medical, pharmacological, or ageing effects on nerve structure and function. The most comprehensive electrodiagnostic evaluation is, therefore, done either personally by a recognized specialist in the field with the privilege of a comprehensive history and clinical examination or by a certified technologist in partnership with a specialist in the field (who, again, should have access to a comprehensive history and clinical examination, i.e., the context).

PSYCHOMETRIC AND ECONOMIC CONSIDERATIONS

The beauty of the title of this book as 'evidence-informed' as opposed to 'evidence-based' evaluation is that the latter terminology has over time become hackneyed, misunderstood, and misused. The intent of the terminology was indeed originally to raise the culture of awareness of the value of critical appraisal of evidence in clinical decision making. A fundamental tenet of such critical appraisal deals with understanding how bias may pollute clinical decision making. Part of the beauty of how health care decision making has evolved is that the self-regulation of professional competence extends to raising consciousness about the ongoing rigour with which each and every diagnostic test and intervention needs to be examined (Shekelle et al 2000). Each and every test that is used in medicine is limited as to what it tests. It follows that it is important to understand what a test does not test. Sometimes a test is most useful when it is positive; technical and biological variations may make a negative test unreliable. It is always important to bear in mind when assessing the value of a specific clinical tool that the absence of proof is not necessarily the proof of absence. Specific tests may not lend themselves well to rigorous scrutiny because of the rareness of the disorder they reflect.

We know from inter- and intra-rater reliability, that the more explicitly the parameters of normal and/or specific range of disease are described, the higher the likelihood that experts will agree with each other and with themselves. Without such descriptors, inter-rater reliability, specifically in any test that involves perception, is often between 60 and 70%. Intra-rater reliability is known to be higher (at around 80%), as over time we tend to agree with ourselves more consistently.

With regard to the content of the electrodiagnostic evaluation, organizations such as the AANEM and the CSCN are dedicated to assisting in the setting of standards for competent electrodiagnostic evaluation by setting guidelines for the most reasonable number of parameters to include in any given study of a specific diagnosis or constellation of symptoms. These recommendations are based on the strength of evidence after critical appraisal of the literature. Evidence may be robust enough to actually publish guidelines (such as with carpal tunnel syndrome) (Jablecki et al 2002a,b) or less robust (as in the case of chronic idiopathic demyelinating polyneuropathy), forcing us to rely on consensus of expert opinion (Latov & Sander 2003).

When one examines how easily generalized results are, i.e., how closely any given test result represents one's own patient population, one cannot escape consideration of how the business of medicine influences the outcome as well as the practical application and utility of any given test in medicine. What is actually practised in a community may be far different than the standards to which the AANEM and CSCN hold their diplomats. In some jurisdictions, such as British Columbia, payment of service is inherently tied to demonstration of competence by examination. This is not universally the case. Clinics offering electrodiagnostic services may be limited by poor reimbursement of the service, which may in some instances limit the amount of data gathering that can occur. When clinicians assess patients whom they have already seen in consultation, and so have had the privilege of clinical examination, testing may be quite specific, utilizing a selection of the most appropriate electrodiagnostic techniques to diagnose specific conditions in the context of a sound knowledge of the patient's limitations. Reimbursement fees that do not adequately reflect the time needed to gather data or differentiate between the time necessary to rule out a specific disorder, particularly in the presence of confounding disorders that also affect the nervous system (such as diabetes), may contribute to a higher incidence of false negative as well as false positive diagnoses. In either case, neither the patient nor the clinician is well served. Furthermore, as reimbursement schedules frequently reflect neither the expertise of the examiner nor the length of time taken for a test (except in gross terms), there may be no uniformity in what is in actuality gathered or delivered through any given test.

In the United States, reimbursement is directly tied to the time required to execute the test. In order to prevent abuse of the opposite sort (i.e., doing more than is required), the AANEM has culled the opinions of experts to establish an appropriate number of tests to rule in or out a given diagnosis. Such guidelines assist third-party payers in understanding reasonable and customary fees while at the same time addressing inadvertent abuse in an otherwise open-ended system.

In the interest of clarifying the interpretation of reports of electrodiagnostic testing and in order to better serve patient care, caveats may be appended to the conclusions provided at the end of a given test. Such a caveat might read: '... [such and such] nerves only were studied. No abnormality was identified in these specific nerves. Clinical correlation is required...' This caveat might be most applicable in the situation where the patient is referred, for example, to rule out carpal tunnel syndrome, but not for electrodiagnostic consultation, meaning that the tester/interpreter is working in a 'vacuum.'

Other caveats may draw attention to the limitation of the test itself, regardless of how much data is gathered. This will help the referring clinician, third-party payer, and/or legal representative understand the context of an interpretation. For instance, if a referral is made to assess whether there is electrodiagnostic support for a diagnosis of peripheral neuropathy, a disclaimer should perhaps be added to the interpretation of 'normal' that reads: '…a normal nerve conduction velocity does not exclude the presence of either an early dying-back neuropathy or a small-fibre neuropathy. Clinical correlation is recommended…'

Similarly, if the request is to rule out thoracic outlet syndrome, the interpretation of 'normal' should perhaps include a statement such as: '…evidence of either axonal damage or demyelination in thoracic outlet syndrome is rare. A "normal" study does not rule out a symptomatic dynamic compression of the neurovascular bundle within the thoracic inlet or outlet (the result of which may be related to circumstances of compression resulting in temporary nerve ischaemia). Full clinical correlation is suggested…'

ELECTRODIAGNOSTIC FINDINGS AND CLINICAL CORRELATION

Recall that the restoration of homeostasis is the first order of the day for all tissue damage. Any insult or injury to the host will be met with an instantaneous attempt at repair. Sometimes the recovery is complete (such as skin response to a paper cut). Sometimes – if the lesion is deeper – repair will be associated with the development of scar tissue. In milder forms of injury, the scar tissue is sufficient for restoration of normal function. In more severe injury, the repair process (scarring) may interfere with restoration of normal function; the scar tissue will never have the same tensile property of the damaged tissue it replaces. Each tissue in the body has the equivalent of scar formation when damage is repaired. For example, a simple fracture to a bone may heal without eventual radiological evidence of prior trauma. By contrast, the more complicated the fracture, the higher the potential for permanent deformity and impact on functional capacity.

The equivalent of the scar process is not necessarily symptomatic. For example, trauma or loading that exceeds the tensile properties of the vertebral body endplate is thought to cause micro-fracture of the endplate, which in turn will be met with repair that results in bony sclerosis. This repair process is thought to contribute to a decreased ability of the nucleus pulposus to imbibe fluid at night, and hence to eventual dessication of the disc. In the process, the relative instability of the motion segment is met with the development of osteophytes that develop along force lines in an attempt to restore homeostasis and functional capacity (Bogduk & Twomey 1991). Although the radiological expression of this adaptive change frequently carries the misnomer of degenerative disc disease (misnomer because there is no disease), the spondylotic changes noted are frequently asymptomatic. In fact there is no evidence that there is a higher incidence of symptoms in persons with spondylotic changes on X-ray than in persons without such radiological findings (van Tulder et al 1997).

This discourse about the interpretation of radiological changes on X-ray is included to draw attention to a practice in which anatomical changes such as, for example, those that may be identified on X-ray, are frequently labelled as the source of pain generation. By contrast, the absence of anatomical change upon imaging is often interpreted as evidence that a given structure is not a pain generator, somehow ignoring the fact that irritation of the pain fibres that innervate a given structure can in and of themselves be the source of pain. The source of pain does not necessarily have an anatomical correlate on imaging studies. Similarly, for technical reasons, a nerve may be a source of pain but not necessarily show any structural change through electrodiagnostic testing. The converse is also true: a structural change found during the electrodiagnostic examination is not necessarily symptomatic.

Some refer to the presence of motor unit configuration changes, such as serration and/or polyphasicity (Table 5.1), as consistent with stable radiculopathy. In effect, one could think of this label as the equivalent of the presence of scar tissue in the skin or of spondylotic changes reported in spinal X-rays. The changes reflect a repair process and are not necessarily symptomatic or functionally limiting. By contrast, the presence of large, long-duration potentials, as well as decreased recruitment (reflecting axonal damage without recovery or remodelling; Table 5.1), may have much more significant functional consequences. A more limited complement or motor axons trying to supply the same territory of muscle may be more vulnerable to metabolic exhaustion with effort, resulting in decreased endurance and the capacity to act not only as a prime mover but also as a stabilizer. This information may have far more valuable prognostic and management implications if employed thoughtfully toward the clinical presentation. No one experiences such diminished endurance more readily than patients who demonstrate the late effects of polio. Patients that suffer reflex muscle inhibition of the supporting muscles of the suspensory system in post-whiplash-type injuries may also experience a significant functional limitation in their capacity to tolerate dynamic loading of the neck and shoulder girdle, particularly in the presence of coexistent profound single- or multi-nerve axonal damage. Such damage may include injury to the nerve root, plexus, and/or peripheral nerve (such as the suprascapular or long thoracic nerves) (see Box 5.1).

ELECTRODIAGNOSTIC MEDICINE IN NECK AND ARM PAIN SYNDROMES

Electrodiagnosis in the context of neck and arm pain syndromes is taken to encompass nerve conduction studies, electromyography, and somatosensory evoked potentials, all of which are studies that evaluate the integrity of the peripheral nervous system. With the exception of isolated academic laboratories, most practitioners do not routinely utilize electromagnetic stimulation of nerves and motor unit counting. Other electrodiagnostic studies, such as repetitive nerve stimulation, have more relevance to disorders of the neuromuscular junction (such as myasthenia gravis). Single-fibre electromyography is similarly most frequently used in disorders of the neuromuscular junction and not directly in arm pain syndromes. Clearly some arm pain syndromes are central in origin, the evaluation of which is outside the intent of this chapter.

Nerve conduction studies

Electrodiagnostic evaluation concerns itself with the study of sensory, motor, and autonomic nerve fibres. By common parlance, 'EMG' has come to be taken to mean both nerve conduction and EMG studies, even though there is a semantic difference between the two.

Technically, these are two entirely different tests that potentially reveal vastly different information about the nervous system. Nerve conduction studies can only be performed on nerves that are readily accessible for reliable stimulation/recording and, as such, are limited to the testing of a discrete set of peripheral nerves. By contrast, most muscles are accessible to needle EMG evaluation. The EMG, however, only reflects the state of the muscle/innervating nerve supply and is, therefore, limited to reflecting motor nerve/muscle integrity (meaning that conditions in which sensory abnormalities alone are anticipated would not benefit from EMG, but rather sensory nerve conduction alone). Table 5.2 lists potential nerve conduction findings in specific diseases (further reinforcing the fact that interpretation of nerve conduction studies cannot be done out of context, such as the frequent assumption that carpal tunnel syndrome can be comprehensively diagnosed with limited data: 'To a hammer everything looks like a nail').

Table 5.2 Potential findings in confounding (superimposed) medical conditions (Mendell & Sahenk 2003)*

Primary types of painful sensory neuropathy	Electromyography (EMG) and nerve conduction study (NCS)
Idiopathic small-fibre painful sensory neuropathy	Normal
Diabetic peripheral neuropathy	Abnormal EMG and NCS
Inherited neuropathies	Abnormal EMG and NCS
Peripheral neuropathy with connective tissue disease	Abnormal EMG and NCS
Peripheral nerve vasculitis	Abnormal EMG and NCS
MGUS neuropathy	Abnormal EMG and NCS (may be normal)
Paraneoplastic sensory neuropathy	Abnormal EMG and NCS
Familial amyloid polyneuropathy	Abnormal EMG and NCS
Acquired amyloid polyneuropathy	Abnormal EMG and NCS
Neuropathy with renal failure	Abnormal EMG and NCS
Hereditary sensory autonomic neuropathy	Abnormal EMG and NCS
Sarcoid polyneuropathy	Abnormal EMG and NCS
Arsenic neuropathy	Abnormal EMG and NCS
Fabry disease	Normal EMG and NCS
Celiac disease	EMG and NCS may be normal or abnormal
HIV-related neuropathy	EMG and NCS usually abnormal

*When limited studies are done to rule out entrapment neuropathies, the coexistence of these disorders may influence interpretation of abnormal results (MGUS-monoclonal gammopathy of undetermined significance; HIV-human immunodeficiency virus)

Sensory nerves carry information from the external environment towards the spinal cord and brain. When a sensory nerve is stimulated distally and recordings are made from the same nerve proximally, the process is said to reveal orthodromic conduction (conduction in the direction of intent of the impulse; *ortho* meaning straight and *dromic* referring to direction). By contrast, when the same nerve is stimulated proximally and recordings are made distally, the process is said to reveal antidromic conduction (against the direction of conduction; *anti* meaning against).

The cell bodies of the sensory nerve fibres are located in the dorsal root ganglion (DRG). If damage occurs to the sensory nerve proximal to the DRG, stimulation of the nerve in the periphery will fail to elicit an abnormal response. It then follows that an abnormal sensory response reflects structural damage to the sensory nerve distal to the DRG. When easily accessible, a sensory nerve may be stimulated as part of a mixed nerve or as a pure sensory nerve, and recordings can be made either from a sensory nerve or from a mixed nerve. Interpretation of abnormal sensory responses, however, carries with it the obligation of understanding how lack of rigour in technique, in assumptions about instrumentation settings, in temperature control, in anatomical variation, and in pathological processes will influence the quality and integrity of the data collected.

Motor nerves carry information from the spinal cord to muscle, the conduction direction of which is orthodromic for the motor nerves. The cell body of the motor nerve is, of course, the anterior horn cell within the spinal cord. While some nerve fibres carry only motor axons and some are purely sensory, many nerves readily accessible for stimulation to test conduction velocity carry all fibres (motor, sensory, and autonomic). The amplitude of the response recorded from a muscle reflects a compound action potential. The amplitude of the response is a summation of amplitudes evoked by stimulating every motor unit (individual nerve and all of the muscle fibres it supplies). If some axons are demyelinated, the time that the evoked response of those specific axons takes to arrive at the muscle stigmatic/recording electrode will vary, producing a response that is attenuated and of lower amplitude. As long as the area under the curve remains the same, the drop in amplitude does not represent axonal loss. Normative data is electrode dependent (including such factors as size of recording surface area, conductivity, and inter-electrode distance), technique and temperature dependent, and instrumentation (filter setting) dependent.

When any given nerve is stimulated, the propagation of the impulse is bidirectional. A small stimulus (sensory impulse) may travel proximally along a given nerve to stimulate a motor nerve in the anterior horn cell, creating a simple monosynaptic reflex. A motor response generated by such a reflex is referred to as a late response, specifically as an H- or Hoffman reflex. With the exception of the H-reflex that is elicited by stimulating the median nerve and recorded from the flexor carpi radialis (and specific conditions associated with a loss of central inhibition, such as MS), an H-reflex is rarely found in the upper extremity after early childhood. Carefully executed, the H-reflex may be an extremely helpful tool in diagnosing C6 sensory radiculopathy.

A supra-maximal stimulus applied to the nerve may also create a late response. This response is referred to as the F-response (which actually stands for Foot response), a purely motor phenomenon thought to be generated by the bouncing back of a motor-propagated impulse off the axon hillock. The evaluation of F-responses are perhaps most useful in conditions where there is suspected multifocal conduction block, such as Guillain–Barré Syndrome or CRDP (chronic relapsing demyelinating poly-radiculopathy). Because of technical challenges in the execution of the F-responses, controversy continues to exist as to the value of the F-response in conditions of proximal conduction block, such as thoracic outlet syndrome and/or radiculopathy. Some clinicians find the lack of persistence of a volley of F-responses to hold greater significance, correlating with the likelihood of proximal nerve pathology.

In executing a nerve conduction study, usually sensory and/or motor nerves are systematically stimulated to determine patterns of abnormality that may reveal isolated nerve injury or entrapment, radiculopathy, plexopathy, peripheral neuropathy, and/or combinations of these conditions. The process is methodical and the particular pattern of stimulation/results is compared to that of normative data representative of the technique chosen. To calculate motor conduction velocity, a mixed nerve is stimulated at two separate points along the course of the nerve and recordings are made from a muscle. The distance between two points is measured (usually with a tape measure), and the conduction velocity is calculated. The time that it takes for a stimulus to get to the muscle and cause contraction is termed the *terminal motor latency*. Variations in anatomical position during the acquisition of data will greatly influence the results, a fact that is most commonly acknowledged in the elbow flexion angle (the degree of which requires standardization for reproducibility/validity of results when assessing ulnar nerve conduction block/entrapment).

There are a limited number of ways in which a nerve can respond to injury. Within a given nerve a variable number of fibres will be unmyelinated. Of the myelinated fibres, different diameters of nerves will conduct an impulse with variable rates. When a nerve is stimulated, the fastest conducting fibres are reflected in the calculations of conduction velocity. It then follows that the smallest diameter fibres (the unmyelinated nerve fibres, which carry pain sensation) may be damaged, but that the nerve conduction velocity may be recorded as normal. This leads us to consider the following caveats when interpreting nerve conduction velocity study results:

- One may have a small-fibre neuropathy and yet the nerve conduction study may be 'normal.'
- One may have damage to unmyelinated fibres (transmitting pain sensation) and yet the nerve conduction study may be 'normal.' This, of course, is most commonly seen in diabetes.
- One may have damage to the most distal end of a sensory nerve (as in dying-back neuropathies) and yet the nerve conduction may be 'normal.' This is a function of the practical limitations imposed by the location of stimulating and stigmatic electrodes.
- One may have damage to a sensory nerve proximal to the DRG (as in the case of root avulsion) and yet the sensory nerve conduction velocity may be 'normal.'

The number of axons in a given nerve also influences nerve conduction velocity. Indeed, axonal loss can produce a slowing of conduction velocity of about 30% of the baseline normal for a specific nerve. Conduction velocity reduced by more than 30%, however, is more likely to reflect some degree of demyelination. A prolongation of terminal motor latency may reflect either demyelination or more proximal axonal loss. That axonal loss can occur anywhere along the course of the nerve. A prolongation in the terminal motor latency of the median mixed nerve of the thenar muscle may reflect either compression (causing demyelinization) of the median nerve at the level of the carpal tunnel or proximal axonal loss (an entirely different mechanism) within the parent median nerve, lower plexus, or root. The process of compression of the median nerve at the level of the carpal tunnel usually preferentially involves sensory fibres. It thus becomes easy to see that taking prolongation of the terminal motor latency of the median nerve out of context may lead to potential over-diagnosis of carpal tunnel syndrome and under-diagnosis of, for example, a lower plexus lesion.

Different injuries and disease states will affect the pattern of involvement of the peripheral nervous system differently. To facilitate comprehension, two simplistic (but not entirely accurate) models are used to explain nerve function: one referring to a nerve as a cable of wires, the second likening the nerve to a garden hose. It behoves one to never lose sight of how rich in metabolic activity nerves are. Within each axon (or wire or hose) are multiple channels of axoplasm, rich in mitochondria, transporting nutrients at different rates throughout the course of every nerve fibre. Damage to any part of the nerve signals the cell body to initiate repair. The process is a dynamic one. The more extensive the damage and the closer that damage is to the cell body, the less likely the metabolic demands on the cell body will be able to achieve full repair, and the more likely the cell body will die (as in the case of polio). In an attempt to achieve homeostasis and maximally restore function, neighbouring intact nerves will automatically sprout nerve fibres in an attempt to take over the territory of the damaged nerve.

Similarly, damage to the most distal end of the nerve at the neuromuscular junction is met with an immediate response of nerve repair (such as when botulinum toxin type A is incorporated into the terminal nerve twig, interfering with the SNAP 25 receptor and release of acetylcholine across the synaptic cleft). When the cell body produces enough material to repair the SNAP 25 receptor, the sprouted nerve twigs disappear and full restoration of function occurs in the sense of complete reinnervation and remodelling. In other forms of nerve damage, the capacity of the nerve to achieve full repair is dependent upon the number of axons that remain intact and so can receive the regenerating nerve. Crush injury to nerve, by destroying axonal architecture, is likely to produce a far greater functional loss if the recovering nerve cannot find its skeletal framework. As a nerve sprout forms into a tumour-like ending with no pathway of meaningful end, one or multiple neuromas may form. Depending on their location, these may be profoundly disabling. Electrodiagnostic studies are rarely helpful in diagnosing neuromas, except in ruling out other potential sources of entrapment/pain generation. Again, an index of suspicion and careful clinical examination are indicated.

The results of any given nerve conduction study represent a point in time. In isolation and out of context, it may be impossible to know whether an abnormal finding reflects a process that is deteriorating, improving, or remaining static. By gathering sufficient data (through stimulating an adequate number of motor and sensory nerves as well as nerves that receive different peripheral and root innervations), it is possible to categorize nerve response to injury as reflective of damage to an individual peripheral nerve (such as through entrapment), a group of motor and sensory nerves (such as in peripheral neuropathy), predominantly axonal or demyelinating nerves, sensory or motor nerves, and proximal or distal nerves. By categorizing the pattern of involvement it becomes possible to offer a likelihood of diagnosis that is consistent with a specific disease process.

Electromyography

Perhaps no part of the electrodiagnostic examination is as subject to variability in data interpretation as the EMG. Variations in training, technique, and sampling (both time of sampling in relationship to insult and the actual choice of muscles sampled) will profoundly affect interpretation. Technically, the term electromyography refers to the insertion of a microphone in the shape of a pin through muscle fascia and into a muscle belly. The amplified sounds generated by needle/pin (microphone) insertion with the muscle at rest and from muscle contraction are interpreted and compared to normative data. The normative data is injury-stage specific, muscle specific, electrode specific, and age specific.

While electromyographic data may give information about primary disorders of muscle as well as reflecting acute/chronic axonal damage and/or repair of motor nerves, it would be considered of limited use in diagnosing arm pain syndromes, except where weakness is associated with pain or where sensory and motor involvement coexist in the same disease process. In the latter case, the use of electromyography (needle examination) is most helpful by reflecting the severity and acuity of the disorder. A neurosurgeon might be more inclined to perform surgery for radiculopathy in the presence of diffuse fibrillation activity than in a case where there was no evidence of acute or ongoing nerve damage.

Making a decision to undergo surgical intervention in the case of certain entrapment neuropathies on the basis of fibrillation activity alone should arguably be a far more complicated and educated decision-making process. Except when a nerve is incontrovertibly transected, as long as there is clear evidence of some degree of function distal to the lesion, one has to weigh the possibility that nerve grafting will have a worse outcome than the extent of natural recovery (even if incomplete). Exploration and decompression of peripheral nerve injuries other than carpal tunnel syndrome (where the process of damage is most frequently primarily demyelinating), is generally considered to have a more tempered (if not inconsistent) outcome. In practical terms, when damage to a nerve involves demyelination (rather than isolated axonal damage), identification of the point of conduction block is often easy.

The same cannot be said of selective fascicular axonal damage, the localization of which may not be possible (particularly when there are competing hypotheses regarding cause). The thoughtful clinician will carefully examine motor and sensory function of the peripheral nerve in question in an attempt to localize the most likely location of the lesion. In this attempt, the clinician will be guided by the clinical findings on initial examination. When subsequent examination confirms some degree of recovery, there may well be cause to be optimistic. A recovering nerve, however, may become easily metabolically exhausted, particularly if inadvertent abuse/overuse occurs during the recovery process. If at that eventual stage nerve recovery plateaus or appears worse and surgical exploration occurs (out of context of the preceding clinical findings), inaccurate conclusions may be drawn that do not actually reflect the truth or care of the decision-making process.

Fibrillation is the name given to spontaneous activity recorded by a monopolar or concentric needle inserted into a muscle belly while the muscle is at rest. Fasciculation is the name given to a spontaneous firing of an entire motor unit, i.e., a motor axon and all the muscle fibres that it supplies. Fasciculations may be seen in denervated nerves, but are not pathognomonic of that process, as they may also be seen in some central states where there

appears to be a loss of central inhibition. The presence of fibrillation is taken to infer a separation of a nerve twig from an individual muscle fibre. There is a time delay between insult to a nerve and the anticipated time that fibrillation activity will be demonstrable. Examining an extremity too soon after injury may fail to identify the severity of the lesion. Recent or active denervation is quantified by the intensity of fibrillation activity noted, the pattern and significance of which will vary with the innervation ratio of each muscle. As a nerve starts to re-establish connection with muscle (reinnervation), the degree of fibrillation activity decreases. Fibrillation can be categorized by characteristic firing frequency and by configuration. The presence of fibrillation may reflect recent, ongoing, or prior axonal disruption. Disruption refers to separation of the nerve from a muscle fibre. Inflammation of muscle may also cause it to be separated from the nerve fibre, such as in polymyositis where multiple muscle fibres are in essence denervated.

A change in firing frequency of voluntarily recruited motor units may precede the presence of fibrillation and may be the first sign of axonal damage. As soon as the axon is separated from the muscle fibre, however, the body will attempt to repair the process. The cell body becomes quite metabolically active while preparing for the repair process. Initially, nerve sprouts form from proximally intact nerves to reconnect with the muscle. The regenerating nerve seeks an intact endoneurium, eventually re-establishing continuity with the endplate. When substrates are delivered to the nerve terminus, re-establishing viable connection, the sprouts disappear and the process of remodelling and repair begins. If the axon cannot be repatriated, sprouts from neighbouring intact nerves take over the territory of the muscle fibres of the damaged nerve. This will result in fibre grouping, which is observable on muscle biopsy. This process and the obligatory fibre grouping will be evident in the change in duration and/or amplitude as well as firing frequency characteristics of volitional motor units. Clearly, unless motor fibres are involved, the EMG will not be abnormal, and (needle) EMG will not lend any further information to the understanding or management of the process at hand. If, however, there is both pain and weakness, then insertion of an EMG needle into muscle will certainly help estimate how severe the axonal damage is to the mixed nerve. Severe axonal damage may indeed have significant consequences upon the treatment options as well as the anticipated degree of disability/impairment.

When electromyography first became part of clinical testing of nerve and muscle disorders, analogue equipment was used. Learning instrumentation was fundamental to being able to execute a test. The analogue equipment allowed easy manipulation of the signal by changing filter settings. A system of assessment developed. With the advent of digital equipment, the ability to manipulate filter settings became more remote. Variations in filter settings unique to equipment manufacturers reflected company assumptions of how the signal-to-noise ratio could be manipulated to give cleaner data or at least the appearance of cleaner data. The ability to feel confident about whether essential parts of the signal were being lost became challenged, (and hence the possibility of, for example, missing fibrillations on EMG recordings, if present). To the best of my knowledge there is no standardized regulation of filter setting in digital equipment. Regulation of filter settings is at the discretion of the clinician gathering data. The progression of digital equipment has certainly generated more attractive reports (recording nerve conduction values to the hundredth decimal place), giving the appearance of increased accuracy, despite the fact that a low-tech tape measure is still used to measure the inter-stimulation interval. The largest source of error in nerve conduction velocity calculation will occur with variations in the precision with which the inter-stimulus distance is recorded with a tape measure.

Other sources of error in the acquisition of neurophysiological data include failure to adjust results for variation in temperature. A cold extremity may slow down the speed of conduction of impulses, increase the amplitude of sensory nerve responses, and extinguish fibrillation activity. Failure to achieve a supra-maximal stimulus, too short a distance between anode and cathode, filter settings, and lack of skin preparation may all impede accurate recording of data. Lack of appreciation of anatomical variation may lead to confusion and misinterpretation of data. Examples of such variation include the presence of neural anastomosis as common variant, variations in peripheral nerve or in root innervations patterns, pre- or post-fixed plexuses, and angulated courses of spinal nerve roots (associated with ageing). Given the variations in technical examination montages including electrode placement and choice of nerve combinations studied, normative data will vary. Published normative data can be used provided the technique of electrode placement is mirrored exactly. Otherwise only the normative data that is associated with technique choice should be used.

Somatosensory evoked potentials

Somatosensory evoked potentials use a computer averaging technique to sift out a common signal from background noise. Recording electrodes follow a lab-specific standardized montage over the skull. The peripheral sensory nerve pathway up to the somatosensory cortex is evaluated. Somatosensory evoked potentials are commonly used to reflect ongoing nerve integrity during spinal surgery. There may be differences in recording montages from lab to lab, which contributes impediment to reliability and validity testing. Somatosensory responses have been used to evaluate sensory nerves that are not commonly tested such as the lateral femoral cutaneous nerve of the thigh. Unfortunately, technical challenges thwart confidence in the

reliability of data. It is fair to say that one of the great values of this test is achieved when a response is elicited. An absent response unfortunately does not necessarily infer pathology. There are many factors that mitigate accurate elicitation of a response. Perhaps as a result, somatosensory evoked potentials have not been found to be helpful in diagnosing many arm pain syndromes where not done routinely.

Autonomic nerve testing

Autonomic nerves can be easily stimulated and recordings made from the arm or leg. The sympathetic skin response (SSR) is studied. The test is a bit finicky to perform, and the evoked responses can be somewhat frustrating to record. As such, the diagnostic usefulness is good but not great, and its usefulness in prospective and longitudinal studies is yet to be determined (Ravits 1990). This test is also somewhat time consuming, sensitive to a huge number of variables, and may not reflect any consistency despite disease. At the present time the testing does not give more information than can be elicited by standard clinical tests developed to assess autonomic dysfunction.

CONCLUSION

Electrodiagnostic evaluation can be an invaluable tool in establishing pathology as well as the presence or absence of coexisting confounding conditions, in assisting with the determination of the appropriate vigour with which rehabilitation effort is pursued, and in determining prognosis and treatment options. As with all clinical tests, the actual value will depend to a great deal on clarification of the clinical question, the technical execution of the test, and the skills and experience of both the examiner and the interpreter of the data. To best serve the patient, the examination cannot and should not be taken out of context.

There is nothing wrong with doing a limited examination as long as the results are not taken to reflect anything but that fact; (in context) there is nothing wrong with the concept of minimalist evaluation as discussed by Johnson (Pease et al 2007) provided everyone – including the patient – understands that a sometimes limited/focused evaluation was used to exclude a specific pathology, nothing more and nothing less. The important communication to patient and colleague alike must be that other potential causes of the symptoms have not been excluded by this approach. Communication is of paramount importance. Because of the habitual use of the word EMG when only a nerve conduction study is done, clarification of the clinical question will allow the examiner to utilize the tool correctly and with the greatest advantage. The execution of the test must also be properly compensated to ensure that data gathering is comprehensive and appropriate.

The following are recommendations to assist in effective referral for electrodiagnostic testing:

I.   Develop a relationship with the electromyographer.

II. Think about what you want to know from the evaluation and convey that query as succinctly and clearly as possible.

III. Give the electromyographer as much data as possible about potentially confounding insults to the neuromuscular system, the nature of the onset of symptoms (e.g., trauma), coexisting disease, the time frame of the occurrence, and the progression of symptoms, as well as copies of any prior electrodiagnostic data.

IV. Ask for copies of the data sheets and review which nerves were examined to determine if this correlates with your clinical query. If not, pick up the phone, discuss with the specialist, and if necessary re-refer for further testing. Most electromyographers are quick to indicate which tests they have limited comfort in doing accurately (simply from exposure or experience) and know which colleagues may have more advanced experience if the test is deemed necessary.

V.   Maintain an open line of communication; most specialists are happy to explain the limitations of the test and/or confirm the lack of need for further evaluation.

VI. Remember that the test represents a point in time. If the neurological condition deteriorates, further or repeat evaluation may be necessary.

VII. Remember that each lab/electromyographer may use different paradigms when studying the absence or presence of a disorder, that normative data is technique, electrode, temperature, age, and sometimes even equipment specific, and that results of data are not necessarily interchangeable from lab to lab or clinician to clinician (depending on their training).

VIII. Organizations such as the AANEM will direct you to the latest published studies and/or consensus guidelines on specific disorders (Brandstater et al 1999, Jablecki et al 2002a,b).

Additional resources

With a picture as good as a thousand words, the reader is directed to two excellent websites designed to inform the general public on what to expect when referred for electrodiagnostic testing:

- search under emg or nerve conduction at http://www.healthlinkbc.ca/
- patient resources at http://aanem.org/

Under the patient resources icon of the American Association of Neuromuscular and Electrodiagnostic Medicine website is a link to a video clip that clearly demonstrates the application of nerve conduction/EMG testing as a diagnostic tool. Indeed, the AANEM website (www.aanem.org) and the organization itself may be the single most comprehensive international resource of its kind, for patients and clinicians alike.

REFERENCES

Aminoff, M.J., 2005. Electrodiagnosis in clinical neurology, fifth ed. Churchill Livingstone, New York.

Armstrong, T.N., Dale, A.M., Al-Lozi, M.T., Franzblau, A., Evanoff, B.A., 2008. Median and ulnar nerve conduction studies at the wrist: Criterion validity of the NC-stat automated device. J. Occup. Environ. Med. 50, 758–764.

Aygül, R., Demir, R., Kotan, D., Kuyucu, M., Ulvi, H., 2009. Sensitivities of conventional and new electrophysiological techniques in carpal tunnel syndrome and their relationship to body mass index. J. Brachial Plex. Peripher. Nerve Inj. 4, 12.

Ayyar, D.R., Romano, J., Rotta, F., Sharma, K.R., 2001. Early diagnosis of carpal tunnel syndrome: Comparison of digit 1 with wrist and distoproximal ratio. Neurol. Clin. Neurophysiol. 2, 2–10.

BCIT, 2009. Electroneurophysiology. http://www.bcit.ca/study/programs/5750diplt.

Beck, J., Bronson, J., Gillet, J., Kupfer, D.M., Lee, G.W., 1998. Differential latency testing: a more sensitive test for radial tunnel syndrome. J. Hand Surg. 23, 859–864.

Bodofsky, E.B., Campellone, J.V., Greenburg, W.M., Tomaio, A.C., Wu, K.D., 2005. A sensitive new median-ulnar technique for diagnosing mild carpal tunnel syndrome. Electromyogr. Clin. Neurophysiol. 45, 139–144.

Brannagan, T.H., Chin, R.L., De Sousa, E.A., Latov, N., Sander, H.W., 2009. Demyelinating findings in typical and atypical chronic inflammatory demyelinating polyneuropathy: sensitivity and specificity. J. Clin. Neuromuscul. Dis. 10, 163–169.

Brandstater, M.E., Busis, N.A., Carroll, D. J., Chokroverty, S., Chiou-Tan, F.Y., Cockrell, J.L., 1999. Practice parameter for needle electromyographic evaluation of patients with suspected cervical radiculopathy. Muscle Nerve 22, S225–S229.

Bogduk, N., Twomey, L.T., 1991. Clinical anatomy of the lumbar spine. Churchill Livingstone, Melbourne.

Buschbacher, R.M., Prahlow, N.D., 2005. Manual of nerve conduction studies, second ed. Demos Medical Publishing, New York.

Chang, M.H., Chiang, H.L., Hsieh, P.F., Lee, Y.C., Liu, L.H., Wei, S.J., 2006.

Comparison of sensitivity of transcarpal median motor conduction velocity and conventional conduction techniques in electrodiagnosis of carpal tunnel syndrome. Clin. Neurophysiol. 117, 984–991.

Dan, Y.F., Fook-Chong, S., Leoh, T.H., Lo, Y.L., Nurjannah, S., Prakash, K.M., 2006. Sensitivities of sensory nerve conduction study parameters in carpal tunnel syndrome. J. Clin. Neurophysiol. 23, 565–567.

Daube, J.R., Rubin, D.I., 2009. Clinical neurophysiology. Oxford University Press, New York.

Dumitru, D., Amato, A.A., Zwarts, M.J., 2002. Electrodiagnostic medicine, second ed. Hanley & Belfus, St. Louis.

Haig, A.J., Harris, M., Kendall, R., Miner, J., Parres, C.M., 2006. Assessment of the validity of masking in electrodiagnostic research. Am. J. Phys. Med. Rehabil. 85, 475–481.

Hattori, T., Kuwabara, S., Misawa, S., Mori, M., Nakata, M., Tamura, N., 2005. Superficial radial sensory nerve potentials in immune-mediated and diabetic neuropathies. Clin. Neurophysiol. 116, 2330–2333.

Jablecki, C.K., Andary, M.T., Floeter, M.K., Miller, R.G., Quartly, C.A., Vennix, M.J., et al., 2002a. Practice parameter: Electrodiagnostic studies in carpal tunnel syndrome: Report of the American Association of Electrodiagnostic Medicine, American Academy of Neurology, and the American Academy of Physical Medicine and Rehabilitation. Neurology 58, 1589–1592.

Jablecki, C.K., Andary, M.T., Floeter, M.K., Miller, R.G., Quartly, C.A., Vennix, M.J., Wilson, J.R., 2002b. Practice parameter for electrodiagnostic studies in carpal tunnel syndrome: Summary statement. Muscle Nerve 25, 918–922.

Katirji, B., 2007. Electromyography in clinical practice: A case study approach, second ed. Mosby, Philadelphia.

Latov, N., Sander, H.W., 2003. Research criteria for defining patients with CIDP. Neurology 60, S8–S15.

Mendell, J.R., Sahenk, Z., 2003. Painful sensory neuropathy. N. Engl. J. Med. 348, 1243–1255.

Pease, W., Lew, H., Johnson, E.W., 2007. Johnson's practical electromyography, fourth ed. Lippincott Williams and Wilkins, Baltimore.

Ravits, J., 1990. Autonomic nervous system testing: An AAEM Workshop. AAEM, Milwaukee, pp. 1–8.

Shekelle, P.G., Kravitz, R.L., Beart, J., Marger, M., Wang, M., Lee, M., 2000. Are nonspecific practice guidelines potentially harmful? A randomized comparison of the effect of nonspecific versus specific guidelines on physician decision making. Health Serv. Res. 34, 1429–1448.

Seror, P., 2005. Frequency of neurogenic thoracic outlet syndrome in patients with definite carpal tunnel syndrome: An electrophysiological evaluation in 100 women. Clin. Neurophysiol. 116, 259–263.

Van Tulder, M.W., Assendelft, W.J., Koes, B.W., Bouter, L.M., 1997. Spinal radiographic findings and non-specific low back pain: A systematic review of observational studies. Spine 22, 427–434.

Chapter | 6 |

Myofascial trigger points in the workplace

Jo L M Franssen, Carel Bron, Jan Dommerholt

INTRODUCTION

Complaints in the neck, shoulder and arm are frequently related to work and the work environment, which has led to the recent use of symptom based descriptions of upper limb disorders such as repetitive strain injury (RSI), computer related disorders, mouse arm, overuse syndrome, cumulative trauma disorder, upper extremity cumulative trauma disorders, occupational overuse syndrome, restrictive immobilization syndrome, and work related musculoskeletal disorder (Melhorn 1998, Ireland 1998). These descriptions refer to the alleged cause of the complaint, respectively: injuries caused by repetitive overloading, computer use, mouse use, overuse, including cumulative use of the upper extremities, occupational activity, lack of exercise, and work.

A Dutch agency proposed a new term to reduce confusion under the motto 'curing the disease by killing its definition'. The agency suggested referring to these complaints as 'Complaints of the arm, neck and/or shoulder region' (CANS). CANS is defined as symptoms of disorders of the locomotor system in the arm, neck and/or shoulder, which are not based on acute trauma or underlying systemic diseases. A disorder is called specific, if it has distinctive features and the diagnosis can be made reproducibly. Specific CANS are a distinct group of 23 disorders, differentiated on the basis of physical abnormalities and include cervical hernia, suprascapular compression, tears of the glenoid labrum, rotator cuff tears, sub-acromial impingement syndrome (rotator cuff syndrome, tendinosis and bursitis in the shoulder region), instability of the shoulder, frozen shoulder, biceps tendinosis, bursitis in the elbow region, instability of the elbow, cubital tunnel syndrome, lateral epicondylitis, medial epicondylitis, radial tunnel syndrome, Guyon canal syndrome, carpal tunnel syndrome, Oarsman's wrist, De Quervain's disease, Dupuytren's disease, trigger finger, local arthritis of one joint of the upper extremity, complex regional pain syndrome, and Raynaud's phenomena. Several of these entities are discussed in more detail in other chapters of this textbook.

Complaints that are not specific within the concept of CANS are referred to as non-specific CANS. The objective of redefining the terminology was to be able to differentiate

© 2011 Elsevier Ltd.
DOI: 10.1016/B978-0-7020-3528-9.00006-6

diagnosable disorders from non-specific CANS. The group of non-specific CANS is still a large collection of unexplained symptoms, which may be reduced to so-called garbage diagnoses, whereby the symptoms become the disease. This is in contrast to the traditional disease model of clinical conditions, which is based on objectively demonstrable patho-physiological substrates. The relationship between the symptom-based model and the traditional disease model is displayed in a model presented by Nathan & Meadows (2000). Nathan maintains that 'the exclusive use of subjective diagnostic criteria creates a greatly expanded prevalence of symptom-based conditions elevated to the level of 'pathology'. Under this model there is no defined pathway to treatment, since specific tissue pathology usually is not identified. Symptoms essentially become the disease, creating a circumstance in which the goal of treatment is to palliate symptoms rather than cure pathology (Nathan & Meadows 2000).

In Figure 6.1 the circle represents the symptoms and the oval represents objective pathology. The part of the oval that falls within the circle shows the area where diagnostic criteria from the two models overlap. This represents the group of clinical conditions, which are the focus of the traditional disease model. The part of the oval that falls outside the circle represents objective asymptomatic pathology, which can be demonstrated, but is not yet clinically relevant. The focus of the symptom-based model includes the entire circle, which in this context is referred as CANS. Symptoms that are confirmed by objective pathology are called 'specific CANS', symptoms that are not confirmed by pathophysiological substrates are referred to as 'non-specific CANS'. There is contradictory and limited evidence for interventions to reduce symptoms by improving working conditions in the workplace, such as speech recognition software, breaks, work rest, ergonomic tools, measures to reduce the workload, organizational measures, education, corporate exercise programmes and cognitive training

(Cherniack & Warren 1999, Nathan & Meadows 2000, Verhagen et al 2007, 2009).

SYMPTOMS AND PREVALENCE OF NON-SPECIFIC CANS

A 2003 Dutch study showed that more than one in five workers (23.4%) presented with complaints in the arm–neck–shoulder region. A study of 15 European countries came to the same conclusion with 22.8%. Recent research has demonstrated that the incidence does not appear to decrease (Eltayeb et al 2008). The symptoms include pain, stiffness, loss of muscle strength, paraesthesias, clumsiness, loss of coordination, skin discoloration, temperature differences, and fatigue.

A study of 354 factory workers identified 'non-specific discomfort' in addition to carpal tunnel syndrome, epicondylitis, radiculopathy, bursitis, arthritis, ganglion, and mononeuropathy (Strasser et al 1999). This 'non-specific discomfort' was found in 16.7% of the workers in their elbows and forearms, 30.2% in the fingers, wrists and hands, and 34% in the neck, shoulder, and upper arm, which suggests that 80.9% of the complaints were considered non-specific. Other studies showed that poorly defined concepts like RSI account for only 20% of diagnosable disorders (specific CANS) with a residual group of 80% described as 'localized non-specific musculoskeletal symptoms' (Grieco et al 1998) or 'vague soft-tissue complaints' (Vender & Kasdan 1999). Another Dutch agency reported an even lower percentage (10%) of specific diseases and came to the conclusion that 90% of the presented RSI symptoms could not be diagnosed. As a result the estimated prevalence of non-specific CANS is 80–90%.

RISK FACTORS OF NON-SPECIFIC CANS

What are the work-related risk factors of non-specific CANS? A wide variety of work activities and occupations in relation to disorders are described: video display unit work (Dembe 1999), industrial work (Muggleton et al 1999), machine milking (Stal et al 1999), urological endoscopic examinations (Luttmann et al 1998), musicians (Markison et al 1998, Pascarelli 1999, Davies 2002), interpreters for the hearing impaired (Scheuerle et al 2000), and ultrasonographers (Schoenfeld 1998). It is clear that certain work-related activities are associated with occupational risks. The likelihood of symptoms increases with static work, increased force demands, increased precision requirements, suboptimal joint positions, increased time of exertion, decreased numbers of breaks, increased operation speed, adverse environmental factors (e.g. noise, temperature), increased time pressure, stress, and poor work organization (Spekle et al 2005).

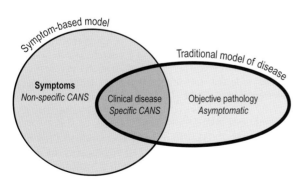

Fig 6.1 CANS as a symptom-based model.

CAUSE–EFFECT RELATIONSHIP BETWEEN WORK AND NON-SPECIFIC CANS

The diagnosis of a clinical disease, which based on its distinctive diagnostic features is reproducible, would give greater clarity about cause–effect relationship between non-specific CANS and work-related ailments. A distinct medical diagnosis will provide more insights into a possible relationship, considering the epidemiology, etiology, symptoms and pathogenesis. The evaluation of cause-and-effect relationships is one of the most difficult challenges in biomedical research. There are six criteria used to establish causation (Hill 1965, Feinstein 1985, Lobbezoo & Lavigne 1997, Vender & Kasdan 1999):

1) In the case of non-specific CANS, there should be a strong relationship between work and the condition without any preconceived notions (i.e. using suggestive terms as 'mouse-arm' and 'computer-related disorders'), by coincidences (i.e. simultaneous developed diseases with a different aetiology), or disturbing influences (musculoskeletal overloading with certain hobbies or other activities).
2) This relationship should be consistent among different people (a significant number of employees should have similar complaints from performing the same tasks), in different places (a significant number of employees performing the same task should have similar complaint irrespective of location), circumstances (complaints will be present under the same circumstances, such as ergonomic conditions, work stressors, etc.), and duration (the complaints will appear after exposure to a certain amount of work).
3) The cause should precede the effect, meaning that the complaints are triggered by a certain workload and worsen with continued exposure.
4) The relationship of work and illness should be specific. In other words, the effect would not occur without the presumed cause.
5) A relationship should exist between the magnitude of the noxious stimulus (dose) and magnitude of the effect (response).
6) There should be a biological plausibility between the work and the complaint.

Once the clinician takes a symptom-based model as non-specific CANS for granted, by definition none of the six criteria are being met. Indeed, the collective term already implies a particular kind of relationship, which yet remains to be proven. The subjective symptom complex can not be diagnosed consistently, because the symptoms are defined without any evidence of a patho-physiological substrate.

MYOFASCIAL TRIGGER POINTS AS NON-SPECIFIC CANS

The question arises whether there is an ubiquitous clinical musculoskeletal disease, with comparable symptoms and risk factors, and a prevalence of 80%, which could be considered a non-specific CANS. Ninety-three percent of 96 patients in a pain management centre presented with myofascial trigger points (TrPs), which played a significant role in the complaints. In 74% of patients, the primary cause of the pain was attributed to TrPs (Gerwin 1997, 1999, 2001). In another pain centre, the cause of pain was attributed to TrPs in 85% of the cases (n = 283) (Fishbain et al 1986). In the clinic for neck, shoulder, and arm complaints in Groningen, the Netherlands, approximately 80% of the patients referred with non-specific CANS presented with TrPs during physical examination. Patients reported pain with palpation of clinically relevant TrPs and they were diagnosed with myofascial pain and dysfunction (Fishbain et al 1986, Gerwin 1997, 1999).

Myofascial pain syndrome (MPS) is based on the presence of TrPs and accepted as a clinical disease (Mense & Simons 2001). TrPs are described in the life work of Janet G. Travell and David G. Simons 'Myofascial Pain and Dysfunction – The Trigger Point Manual: Volume 1–2' (Travell & Simons 1992, Simons et al 1999). A TrP is defined as a sensitive spot in a skeletal muscle associated with a palpable taut band. The motor symptoms of active TrPs, which produce a clinical complaint, include stiffness, restricted range of motion, fatigue, and disordered coordination. The sensory symptoms include pain, hyper- and hypoaesthesia, peripheral and central sensitization and referred pain. Autonomic symptoms include lacrimation, vasodilatation, vasoconstriction, and piloerection, among others. A latent TrP does not produce spontaneous pain, but it may produce other symptoms, including increased muscle tension, muscle shortening, and altered muscle activation patterns. A detailed clinical history, examination of movement patterns, and consideration of muscle referred pain patterns assist clinicians in determining which muscles may harbour clinically relevant TrPs. The diagnosis of a TrP starts with the identification of the taut band by palpating perpendicular to the fibre direction. A TrP is identified as a discrete area of intense pain and hardness. There is a good overall inter-rater reliability reported for identifying taut bands, TrP, and referred pain (Bron et al 2007, Lucas et al 2009).

TrPs are characterized by pathophysiological changes, e.g. multiple contraction knots (Simons & Stolov 1976, Mense et al 2003), pathological alterations of the mitochondria (Windisch et al 1999), significantly increased concentrations of H^+ and cytokines (calcitonin-gene-related-peptide, bradykinin, substance P, tumour necrosis factor-α, interleukin-1β, serotonin, and norepinephrine) in the biochemical milieu of an active TrP (Shah et al 2008), and characteristic electrical activity in the endplate zone referred to as endplate noise (EPN) (Hubbard & Berkoff 1993, Simons 2001, Simons et al 2002). The expanded integrated TrP hypothesis provides a detailed explanation of TrP phenomena (Gerwin et al 2004).

Besides mechanical overload as a cause of the development of TrPs, many predisposing factors, direct and indirect precipitating factors, and perpetuating factors are described. Predisposing factors may include lack of exercise, poor diet, smoking, sleep disorders, poor posture, joint problems, and hypermobility. Direct precipitating factors are acute overload, unusual exercise, chronic overload, exhaustion, entrapment, and immobilization. Indirect precipitating factors are visceral diseases, other TrPs, joint dysfunction, stress, and tension. Perpetuating factors include mechanical and postural overload (short leg, small hemi pelvis), vitamin or mineral insufficiencies, depression, inadequate pain behaviour, chronic infections, and allergies. In addition to inactivating TrPs, clinicians must eliminate all predisposing, precipitating, and perpetuating factors, and educate patients regarding generic and muscle-specific issues.

That TrPs are frequently overlooked by practitioners may be related to the fact that no medical specialty has claimed muscle as its focus organ, thereby reducing muscle to an 'orphan organ'. Although skeletal muscle occupies nearly half of our body weight, muscles remain an overlooked source of musculoskeletal pain and dysfunction (Simons 2007). Referred pain phenomena further contribute to an under-appreciation of TrPs, since usually the TrP causing the symptoms is proximal from the region of the complaint. Phenomena of referred pain and the pathophysiology of TrPs are discussed in Chapter 32.

THERAPEUTIC APPROACH OF NON-SPECIFIC CANS

The symptoms, prevalence, and risk factors of non-specific CANS largely match those of myofascial pain and dysfunction. In this section, common treatment methods of non-specific CANS will be reviewed. The management of non-specific CANS focuses first on eliminating risk factors to create the conditions to allow overloaded structures the opportunity to recover from the overload situation. It has been shown that reduction of the load quantity can be effective (Battevi et al 1998). It is assumed that the broader the approach is, the more successful the intervention will be (Peper et al 2003, 2005). Peper & Gibney (1999) emphasized seven components: work style, ergonomics, somatic awareness, stress management, regeneration, vision care, and fitness. Surface EMG plays an important role by 'taking the guesswork out of assessment, monitoring and training'. Because the influence of

muscle behaviour is paramount, surface EMG is an important tool. Surface EMG is ideally suited to evaluate five muscle-specific properties: muscle strength (Hof 1984, Hermens et al 1984, Anders et al 2005, Kallenberg & Hermens 2006), muscle endurance (Hagberg 1981a,b, Hagberg & Kvarnstrom 1984, Mesin et al 2009), coordination (Graven-Nielsen et al 1997, Lucas et al 2004, Falla et al 2007), the ability to lengthen muscle (McGlynn et al 1979, Neblett et al 2003a,b), and muscle relaxation (Pollard & Katkin 1984, Hagg et al 2000).

Although surface EMG may provide additional and more precise information, in the context of myofascial pain, the ability to detect and measure even the slightest muscle activity is essential in assessing and correcting excessive muscle use. The insertion of micro-breaks, during which the muscle has to relax completely every minute for a few seconds, can be taught with EMG-feedback or myofeedback. The EMG-signal can be displayed visually or auditory (Peper et al 2005). In summary, the activity of superficial muscles can be directly, accurately, and quantitatively related to muscular activity, by demonstrating the EMG signal to the patient or subject, which makes myofeedback didactically an indispensable and powerful tool (Fig 6.2) (Franssen 1995, Donaldson et al 2003). A possible treatment approach of non-specific CANS integrating Peper's work and the management of TrPs will be reviewed in the next section.

WORK STYLE

The work style determines whether an individual is likely to manage daily tasks without increased risk of fatigue and injury. A good work style is characterized by frequent breaks, including macro-breaks and micro-breaks. In particular, sustained static muscle contractions have negative

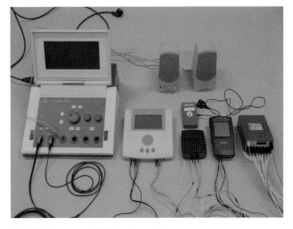

Fig 6.2 Common EMG equipment.

consequences for the blood and lymphatic circulation (Peper, personal communication). Whether a workplace features micro-breaks appears to be more predictive of the occurrence of symptoms in stereotypical work in factory workers than the degree of muscle contractions (Veiersted et al 1990). There are two probable explanatory models.

Damage caused by prolonged static contraction is best explained by the so-called 'Cinderella hypothesis' (Sjogaard et al 2000, Hagg 2000, Westerblad et al 2000, Hermens & Hutten 2002, Andersen et al 2008), which is based on the 'size principle of Henneman' (Henneman et al 1965, Henneman & Olson 1965).

When muscle contractions gradually get stronger, especially smaller motor units of type I red muscle fibres are recruited. During prolonged contractions, as is required during many professional activities, such as typing or playing musical instruments, the Cinderella motor units with primarily red muscle fibres are more likely to get damaged. Structural changes in type I muscle fibres have been confirmed (Simons 1984, Gissel 2000, Zennaro et al 2003, 2004, Andersen et al 2008). The lack of relaxation is significantly more important than the absolute levels of muscle contractions. Psychosocial factors need to be taken into account when low threshold motor units are more and longer active during physical activity leading to damage and symptoms (McNulty et al 1994).

The second model suggests that intramuscular pressures, which occur during a muscle contraction, may deteriorate the blood circulation within the muscle. In this model the architecture of a pinnate muscle is presented with muscle fibres running from one tendinous sheet to another tendinous sheet (Fig 6.3A). During the muscle contraction, the tendinous sheets are displaced by shortening fibres (Fig 6.3B). By further shortening of the muscle, the total available space for the muscle fibres diminishes and needed space can only be achieved through curving of the tendinous sheets (Fig 6.3C). The curving from the tendinous sheets has implications for the pressure conditions in the muscle (Fig 6.3D). In the mathematical calculations, the pressures increased to more than 100 Kilopascal, which is equivalent to 750 mmHg or 1 atmosphere. Results of an experiment as measured during tetanic contractions of the gastrocnemius muscle of a toad confirm the mathematical calculations (Fig 6.3E). Since the pressure in the capillaries are only 5.3–9.3 Kilopascal, which is equivalent to 40–70 mmHg or 0.05–0.09 atmosphere, even during light contractions the circulation around the origin and the attachment of a muscle would significantly decrease. This model applies to prolonged static contraction of a muscle and will have adverse effects on the microcirculation (Otten 1988). Mathematical calculations of intramuscular pressures using muscle models reveal areas in the muscle with extremely high pressures exceeding the vascular pressure. These high pressure areas are experimentally confirmed

by actual measurements of the gastrocnemius muscle of a toad. At relatively low level activities, this may have important implications for the blood and lymph circulation. Damage by overloading a muscle is not equally divided throughout the muscle, but is expected primarily in the high pressure zones of the muscle. These areas agree remarkably well with the preferred sites of enthesopathies (Otten 1988, Palmerud et al 2000).

A work style without micro-breaks, or with excessive and unnecessary muscle activity will contribute to the development or persistence of TrPs (Treaster et al 2005, Hoyle et al 2010). Sufficient oxygen and adenosine triphosphate (ATP) supplies are essential for the proper functioning of muscle and for restoring TrPs, which have been shown to feature very low oxygen saturations (Brüeckle et al 1990). Training patients in the use of micro-breaks is an essential part of the treatment in addition to inactivating muscle TrPs. Surface EMG is the only non-invasive method to achieve total relaxation of multiple muscles, and to learn how to create micro-breaks. For instance, with a nearly perfect ergonomic set up (Fig 6.4), it should be possible to minimize muscle contractions of the muscles in the neck and shoulder region to maintain optimal posture. The endodontist's shoulders are hanging down, the upper arms are in a vertical position, the forearms are supported, and the wrists are held in slight extension. Because of the precise nature of the work tasks, the endodontist maintains a continuous contraction of most of the cervical and shoulder muscles as measured by the EMG-registration (Fig 6.5). The EMG-recording of 12 muscles during a 1-minute period in the 19th minute of 71 minutes of continuous recordings was typical of the entire registration period and shows continuous muscle activity. Occasionally, there was some relaxation of a few muscles, including the left infraspinatus, deltoid, and biceps muscles. The endodontist would benefit from utilizing frequent mini-breaks each minute for all involved muscles with each mini-break lasting a few seconds.

In addition, muscle retraining remains guesswork without myofeedback. Figure 6.6 shows a 1-minute EMG-registration of 12 muscles revealing that during a short break of 30 seconds most muscles relaxed properly with the exception of the left trapezius muscle. Activity in the left and right extensor digitorum muscles reflects the subject lifting the hands. The recording was made during the 67th minute.

SOMATIC AWARENESS

The ability to sense muscle tension is generally poorly developed and often, it is difficult to respond appropriately and let go physically, mentally and emotionally. Simultaneous EMG-registrations and measurements of

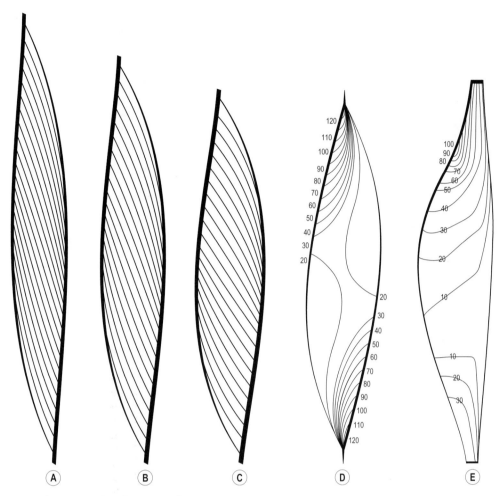

Fig 6.3 Pressure in a contracting pinnate muscle.

subjective muscle awareness are poorly correlated, which may lead to excessive and unnecessary tightening of muscles and dysponesis (Franssen 1995, Peper & Gibney 1999). Dysponesis is defined as a condition to describe misdirected physical reactions to various stimuli (i.e. emotions, bodily sensations, environmental events, and thoughts) and the effects of these reactions throughout the body (Jonas 2005). In painful muscles, changes in contraction patterns are even more pronounced (Middaugh & Kee 1987, Graven-Nielsen et al 1997, Fry et al 1998, Madeleine et al 1999, Falla et al 2007, Oostrom et al 2007, Falla & Farina 2008). Training with myofeedback can significantly improve muscle awareness and is an important aspect of the treatment of persons with non-specific CANS. For instance, a hairdresser using a blow-dryer was not able to take any micro-breaks (Fig 6.7). Considering the relative rest of other muscles, it would be prudent to alternate the hand that holds the

blow dryer. Both upper trapezius muscles are contracted during right-handed blow drying and left handed combing with the right side contracting more, then the left. Noteworthy is the activity in the right lower trapezius muscle which fixates the scapula while raising the arm (Fig 6.8).

Persons with TrPs in certain muscles may display poor coordination, reflected for example as problems with handwriting due to TrPs in the lower arm muscles (Simons et al 1999) or poor muscle awareness (Moussawi et al 2008). Sixty-five percent of 2341 patients with neck–shoulder–arm complaints and TrPs in the trapezius muscle presented with increased EMG activity in the descending part of the trapezius muscle when assessed in standing with the arms hanging down (Franssen 1995). In the treatment of patients with clinically relevant TrPs, it is critical to use myofeedback applied to relevant muscles and treat TrPs with manual or dry needle techniques.

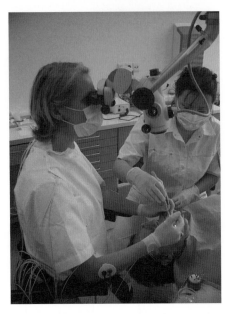

Fig 6.4 An endodontist with a nearly perfect ergonomic set up.

reflected in increased EMG-activity of one or multiple muscles. As such, EMG recordings can be used to objectively assess whether ergonomic adjustments, such as modifying the height of a seat or desk, a new type of keyboard, mouse, or trackball actually reduce muscle activity.

Familiarity with the approximately 150 referred pain areas of TrPs described by Travell and Simons adds a new dimension to assessing and modifying the workplace of a patient with pain. The location of the pain will point clinicians familiar with typical referred pain patterns to relevant muscles with TrPs. Palpation of taut bands and TrPs may trigger the patient's recognizable pain. By combining the assessment of TrPs with surface EMG, an optimal approach to ergonomics can be developed. Clinicians will be able to accurately assess those muscles with clinically relevant TrPs and offer the most appropriate resolution to the patient's unique circumstances (Donaldson et al 2003). Figure 6.9 shows two 1-minute EMG recordings of a 45-minute recording of 12 muscles (6 left and 6 right) during a computer task (responding to e-mail correspondence). Figure 6.9B shows that few muscles relax shortly: a continuous contraction is visible in the left upper trapezius muscle, whereas Figure 6.9C shows that after myofeedback training the same work is conducted with significantly more micro-breaks.

ERGONOMICS

Under optimal ergonomic conditions, working with minimal muscle tension would be the norm. Ergonomic recommendations can be made much more specific by including EMG-recordings of multiple muscles (Bullock 1990, Jonsson 1991, Hagg et al 2000, Clasby et al 2003, Peper et al 2003, 2005). Less than optimal ergonomic conditions are

REGENERATION

Regeneration is important for organ systems to find an optimal balance between ergotropic and trophotropic situations. These terms are introduced by W.R. Hess to denote those mechanisms and the functional status of the nervous system that favour the organism's capacity

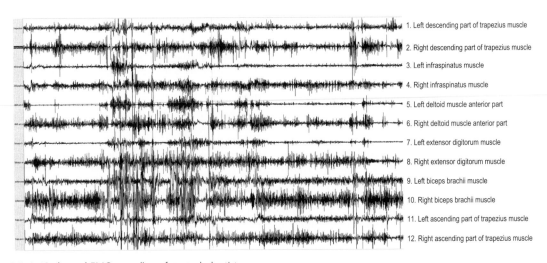

1. Left descending part of trapezius muscle
2. Right descending part of trapezius muscle
3. Left infraspinatus muscle
4. Right infraspinatus muscle
5. Left deltoid muscle anterior part
6. Right deltoid muscle anterior part
7. Left extensor digitorum muscle
8. Right extensor digitorum muscle
9. Left biceps brachii muscle
10. Right biceps brachii muscle
11. Left ascending part of trapezius muscle
12. Right ascending part of trapezius muscle

Fig 6.5 A 12-channel EMG-recording of an endodontist.

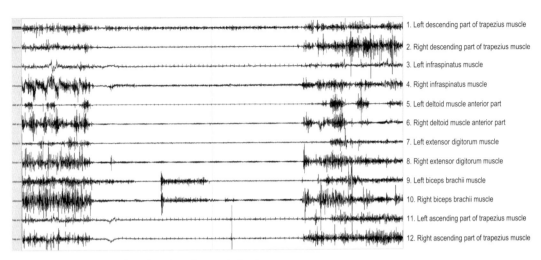

1. Left descending part of trapezius muscle
2. Right descending part of trapezius muscle
3. Left infraspinatus muscle
4. Right infraspinatus muscle
5. Left deltoid muscle anterior part
6. Right deltoid muscle anterior part
7. Left extensor digitorum muscle
8. Right extensor digitorum muscle
9. Left biceps brachii muscle
10. Right biceps brachii muscle
11. Left ascending part of trapezius muscle
12. Right ascending part of trapezius muscle

Fig 6.6 Myofeedback training for relaxation of an endodontist.

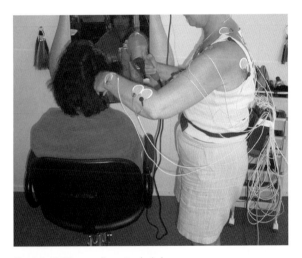

Fig 6.7 EMG-recording at a hairdresser.

to expend energy, as distinguished from trophotropic mechanisms promoting rest and reconstitution of energy stores. In general, the balance between ergotropic and trophotropic nervous mechanisms corresponds in large part to that between the sympathetic and parasympathetic subdivisions of the autonomic nervous system. Timely recognition of signs of fatigue and subsequent corrective actions will assure that catabolic processes will not dominate anabolic processes. Good habits, such as regular work–rest rotations, may help staying healthy and energetic. Physical and mental activities are considered ergotropic conditions which mean that regular macro-breaks should be implemented. TrPs, which are indicative of a local energy crisis in the vicinity of dysfunctional endplates, occur in all occupational groups during low level prolonged muscle activity (Andersen & Gaardboe 1993, Rosen 1993, Kaergaard et al 2000, Fallentin et al 2001). Therefore, the impact of TrPs may decrease by creating a finely tuned balance between ergotropic and trophotropic conditions in the workplace. TrPs can be activated and maintained by both physical and mental stressors, which in turn would challenge the balance between ergotropic and trophotropic conditions.

VISION CARE

Another aspect of ergonomic measures and smart work practices involves reducing eye strain. It is important to prevent drying of the eyes and to avoid excessive efforts of the eye muscles, which can be achieved by taking regular breaks, by staring into the distance, by preventing glare on the screen, and by avoiding extreme difference between the luminance of the screen and any background light, such as when working in front of the bright window. Rather than facing the window, the line of sight should be parallel to the window to avoid sharp contrasts. Sitting directly in front of the monitor or source documents will also reduce eye strain.

The development of TrPs was correlated with visual stress in the trapezius muscle during continuous computer work for 30 min (Treaster et al 2006). Interestingly, in those situations where visual stress existed without postural stress, an increase in the development of TrPs was observed. According to the researchers, TrPs provide a

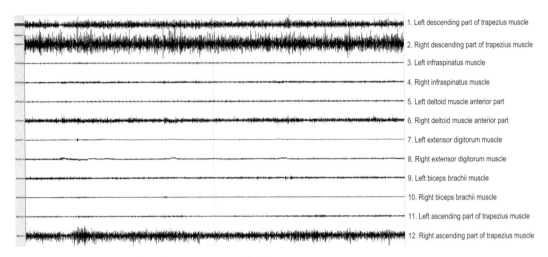

1. Left descending part of trapezius muscle
2. Right descending part of trapezius muscle
3. Left infraspinatus muscle
4. Right infraspinatus muscle
5. Left deltoid muscle anterior part
6. Right deltoid muscle anterior part
7. Left extensor digitorum muscle
8. Right extensor digitorum muscle
9. Left biceps brachii muscle
10. Right biceps brachii muscle
11. Left ascending part of trapezius muscle
12. Right ascending part of trapezius muscle

Fig 6.8 A 12-channel EMG-recording for 94 minutes at a hairdresser.

good explanatory model for the development of muscle pain and other non-specific symptoms, which may occur as the result of static low-level exertions (Treaster et al 2006, Hoyle et al 2010).

FITNESS

Fitness is included as a preventive measure for non-specific CANS. Possible recommended instructions include gentle stretching exercises, muscle strengthening, and regular movements. Even for relatively light work a good overall condition is required (computer athlete). In muscle TrPs, stretching exercises are also recommended, but stretching may be painful and therefore, compliance can be poor. A combination of brief cold applications and stretching, as described by the so-called 'spray and stretch' technique, has been proven to be very effective to inactivate TrPs and diminish any restrictions of the involved muscles (Simons et al 1999). Although the presence of TrPs has a negative impact on muscle strength and coordination, it is not recommended to strengthen painful muscles, because this may actually activate TrPs not only in the involved muscles but also in agonist and antagonist muscles, leading to more widespread weakness, loss of coordination, and pain. Inactivating TrPs is effective to restore muscle strength and range of motion (Simons et al 1999, Moussawi et al 2008).

STRESS MANAGEMENT

Stress management consists of learning to recognize and handle stressors, stress responses and also stress. A stressor is any chemical, physical, psychological, or social stimulus which disturbs the homeostasis of the organism. A stress response is the response of the organism to a stressor to counteract the disturbance of the homeostasis or to restore the disturbed balance. Stress is the altered condition of the organism with changes in the autonomic, endocrine, immune, and movement system and motor behaviour. Learning to recognize stressors, stress symptoms and also stress, with their management are part of the treatment of non-specific CANS. By increasing awareness of the effects of stressors on muscle behaviour, surface EMG is an excellent method to demonstrate changes in work style during various stressful situations as illustrated in Figure 6.10 (Peper & Gibney 2006).

Other biofeedback modalities are also used in stress management, including feedback of the galvanic skin response or heart coherence training (HCT). HCT is a biofeedback method, where feedback of the natural heart rate variability is provided by a sensor on the index finger. With a fluent or coherent pattern a good balance between parasympathetic and sympathetic activity is assumed, in which mental and physical recovery can occur.

In painful TrPs, specific electrical discharges are described during needle EMG, which are described as 'end-plate noise' (EPN). This electrical noise from the motor endplate is probably due to an abnormal excessive release of acetylcholine, which also points to dysfunctional endplates (Mense et al 2003). There is a positive correlation between the prevalence of EPN in a TrP and the pain intensity of that TrP (Kuan et al 2007). Mental tasks, such as counting backwards, show an increased EPN in a TrP when monitored with needle EMG (Hubbard & Berkoff 1993, McNulty et al 1994). To the contrary, autogenic relaxation shows a reduction of electrical activity (Dommerholt et al 2006, Banks et al 1998). The presence of alpha en beta adrenergic

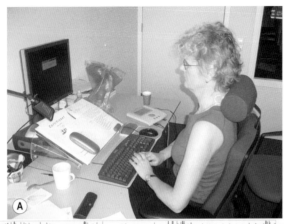

(A)

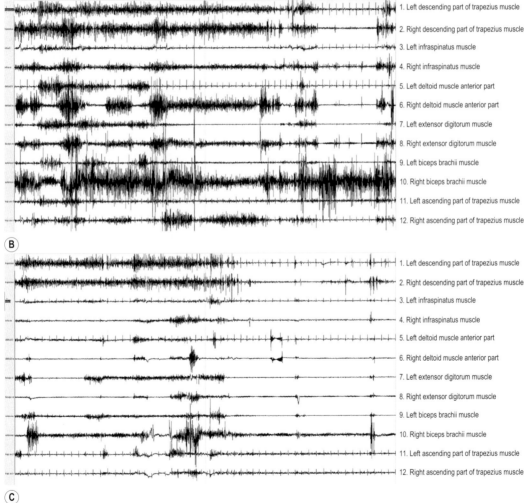

1. Left descending part of trapezius muscle
2. Right descending part of trapezius muscle
3. Left infraspinatus muscle
4. Right infraspinatus muscle
5. Left deltoid muscle anterior part
6. Right deltoid muscle anterior part
7. Left extensor digitorum muscle
8. Right extensor digitorum muscle
9. Left biceps brachii muscle
10. Right biceps brachii muscle
11. Left ascending part of trapezius muscle
12. Right ascending part of trapezius muscle

(B)

1. Left descending part of trapezius muscle
2. Right descending part of trapezius muscle
3. Left infraspinatus muscle
4. Right infraspinatus muscle
5. Left deltoid muscle anterior part
6. Right deltoid muscle anterior part
7. Left extensor digitorum muscle
8. Right extensor digitorum muscle
9. Left biceps brachii muscle
10. Right biceps brachii muscle
11. Left ascending part of trapezius muscle
12. Right ascending part of trapezius muscle

(C)

Fig 6.9 (A) The computer task being assessed. (B) A 12-channel EMG-recording and myofeedback during a computer task. (C) A 12-channel EMG-recording during the same computer task as seen in (B) with significant more micro-breaks after the myofeedback training.

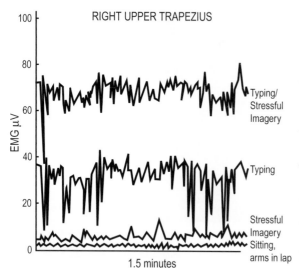

Fig 6.10 Influence of stress on muscle activity measured in the descending part of the trapezius muscle. In sitting with hands in the lap, the impact of fantasy-induced stress, is shown (on bottom) in two EMG-recordings of the descending part of the trapezius muscle. There is a small visible difference between rest and stressful imagery. During fantasy induced stress a person thinks, feels, imagines, visualizes an angry, resentful, and frustrating job-related or personal experience and indicates when these angry, resentful feelings and thoughts are present. During typing the impact of fantasy-induced stress is significantly increased. While during 90 seconds of relaxed typing, a number of microbreaks were measured, it is noteworthy that no micro-breaks were measured during the stressful situation, in which the EMG-activity also increased significantly again. *Reprinted with permission from E. Peper.*

receptors on the motor endplate suggests a possible involvement of the autonomic nervous system in TrPs (Gerwin et al 2004).

THERAPEUTIC APPROACH OF TRIGGER POINTS (TrPs)

Therapeutic measures for non-specific CANS, in which surface EMG may play a relevant role, are designed to eliminate any predisposing, precipitating and perpetuating factors of TrPs. Interventions such as learning microbreaks, increasing muscle awareness, stress management, have a preventive and corrective influence on the development or inactivation of TrPs. Combining myofascial pain concepts and surface EMG offers both diagnostic and therapeutic value. The knowledge and recognition of referred pain, the skill of identifying TrPs in taut bands of muscles, and the principles and practical applications of surface EMG are skills within the scope of physiotherapy practice.

If symptoms are attributed at least partially to TrPs, treatment should start with inactivating those TrPs, which yield much quicker results than waiting for the indirect and long-term results of a wide range of preventive measures (Rosen 1993, 1994, Davies 2002). As Travell & Simons stated: 'Fortunately most authors approached resolution of occupational myalgias by reducing the overload and/or overuse whenever possible. This way, the mechanical perpetuating factors that could have been aggravating TrPs were ameliorated or eliminated, allowing the muscle to partially, or occasionally completely, recover normal function. However, if the source of pain and dysfunction of occupational myalgias were specifically related to TrPs in the muscle being overused, local TrP management of that muscle would expedite return to normal function. The employees or patients could be trained to recognize activities that abused the involved muscles and to tailor routine activities and stretching exercises to maintain normal function of those muscles, which would greatly reduce the likelihood of reactivation' (Simons et al 1999).

CAUSE–EFFECT RELATIONSHIP BETWEEN WORK AND TRIGGER POINTS (TrPs)

It is obvious that myofascial pain and dysfunction with its known aetiology, symptomatology, and pathogenesis, provide more research opportunities on the cause–effect relationship between work and complaints, than the symptom based non-specific CANS. The six criteria listed in the introduction will be reviewed again, but now in the context of TrPs as a clinical disease (Fig 6.11). First, overloaded muscles with TrPs can be identified easier by applying knowledge of referred pain areas, which can assist in establishing the relationship between a client's complaints and muscle behaviour. Whether these muscles are electromyographically active can easily be determined with surface EMG in the workplace and also during work. An assumed relationship can be confirmed or rejected by the EMG-recording. This does not only apply to work conditions, but can also be applied to spontaneous symptoms, hobbies, general stressors, or other underlying pathology. Second, surface EMG allows for comparisons between individuals, places and circumstances, and also assist in establishing patterns of the relationship between complaints and muscle behaviour. Thirdly, the time relationship that exists between the activation of a TrP and the pain caused by the TrP is present but is not necessarily linear. The multifactorial pathogenesis and activation of

Fig 6.11 Myofascial pain syndrome included within the traditional disease model. If Myofascial Pain Syndrome would be recognized as a clinical disease, i.e. as specific CANS is defined, it would provide significantly more clues for explaining and treating work related disorders in the neck, shoulder, and arm regions. The non-specific CANS-group would be remarkably reduced by this inclusion and possibly even be eliminated.

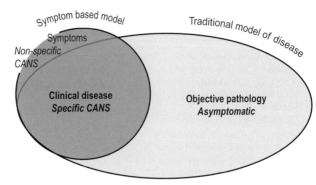

TrPs provide further insights into the complexity of the development of complaints in the workplace.

The same applies to the fourth criterion which states that the relationship between work and disease has to be specific and that the effect does not occur without the preceding cause. Yet, a TrP does not get activated until a certain load has been applied for certain duration, and therefore, muscle overuse is not necessarily always the only direct cause of dysfunction. The work load can be better estimated with EMG-recordings of those muscles with activated TrPs. The fifth criterion states that a quantitative relationship should exist between the noxious stimulus (dose) and the effect (response). The sixth requirement, that the relationship between work and pain complaint should be biologically plausible, can also be determined in the workplace using surface EMG of muscles with TrPs. Given the similarities between the prevalence of non-specific CANS and the prevalence of TrPs (Fishbain et al 1989, Gerwin & Shannon 2000, Dommerholt et al 2006), it seems reasonable to perform an assessment with multi-channel surface EMG of muscles with TrPs.

Finally, we can conclude that once clinicians incorporate TrPs management in a work condition, the six criteria can be appreciated better compared to non-specific CANS. After all, myofascial pain syndrome is a clinical disease, which can be reliably diagnosed, and which is characterized by pathophysiological mechanisms.

CONCLUSION

The management of arm, neck, shoulder complaints in the workplace consists first of careful mapping of the problem. The history must include the genesis, location, frequency, provocation, and intensity of the symptoms. Next, a multi-dimensional analysis of the health problem must be completed, which may include an assessment of lifestyle and co-morbidity, among others. An analysis of workplace factors, including ergonomic features, regeneration opportunities, and work organization, in addition to an analysis of psychosocial factors in which work stress, work pressure and work experience are estimated, gives an impression of the risk factors at work. By using surface EMG, an impression of work style and somatic awareness can be obtained. An assessment of movement anxiety or kinesiophobia, or activities which exceed an individual's pain threshold may direct the clinician to certain behaviours or patterns, which may hinder recovery. Based on the patient's pain complaints, pathophysiological changes in bone, tendons, connective tissue, joints, neurological and muscular system are examined. Particular attention should be paid to muscles with their specific referred pain patterns and TrPs, since TrPs play an important role with nearly all non-specific pain problems.

Pain management strategies must include the inactivation of relevant muscle TrPs combined with the elimination of all recorded predisposing, direct and indirect precipitating, and perpetuating factors. Myofeedback on the workplace provides the opportunity to train muscle awareness, learn micro-breaks, correct dysponesis, optimize work posture, and align optimal ergonomics. Furthermore attention is paid to vision care, regeneration, general fitness and stress management with or without other biofeedback procedures. Regular screening using surface EMG is a powerful way to prevent relapses.

REFERENCES

Anders, C., Bretschneider, S., Bernsdorf, A., Schneider, W., 2005. Activation characteristics of shoulder muscles during maximal and sub-maximal efforts. Eur. J. Appl. Physiol. 93, 540–546.

Andersen, J.H., Gaardboe, O., 1993. Musculoskeletal disorders of the neck and upper limb among sewing machine operators: a clinical investigation. Am. J. Ind. Med. 24, 689–700.

Andersen, L.L., Suetta, C., Andersen, J.L., Kjaer, M., Sjogaard, G., 2008. Increased proportion of megafibers in chronically painful muscles. Pain 139, 588–593.

Banks, S.L., Jacobs, D.W., Gevirtz, R., Hubbard, D.R., 1998. Effects of autogenic relaxation training on electromyographic activity in active myofascial trigger points. J. Musculoskeletal Pain 6 (4), 23–32.

Battevi, N., Bergamasco, R., Girola, C., 1998. Criteria for the reintegration in the workforce of workers with musculoskeletal disorders of the upper limbs, based on preliminary practical experience. Ergonomics 41, 1384–1397.

Bron, C., Franssen, J.L.M., Wensing, M., Oostendorp, R.A.B., 2007. Interrater Reliability of Myofascial Trigger Points in Three Shoulder Muscles. J. Man. Manip. Ther. 15, 203–215.

Brückle, W., Suckfüll, M., Fleckenstein, W., Müller, W., 1990. Gewebe-pO2-Messung in der verspannten Rueckenmuskulatur (m. erector spinae). Z. Rheumatol. 49, 208–216.

Bullock, M.I., 1990. Ergonomics – The Physiotherapist in the Workplace – International perspectives in Physical therapy. vol. 6, Churchill Livingstone, Edinburgh, London, Melbourne and New York.

Cherniack, M., Warren, N., 1999. Ambiguities in office-related injury: the poverty of present approaches. Occup. Med. 14, 1–16.

Clasby, R.G., Derro, D.J., Snelling, L., Donaldson, S., 2003. The use of surface electromyographic techniques in assessing musculoskeletal disorders in production operations.

Appl. Psychophysiol. Biofeedback 28, 161–165.

Davies, C., 2002. Musculoskeletal Pain from Repetitive Strain in Musicians. Med. Probl. Perform. Art. 42–49.

Dembe, A.E., 1999. The changing nature of office work: effects on repetitive strain injuries. Occup. Med. 14, 61–72.

Dommerholt, J., Bron, C., Franssen, J.L.M., 2006. Myofascial Trigger Points: An Evidence-Informed Review. J. Man. Manip. Ther. 14, 203–221.

Donaldson, S., Donaldson, M., Snelling, L., 2003. SEMG evaluations: an overview. Appl. Psychophysiol. Biofeedback 28, 121–127.

Eltayeb, S.M., Staal, J.B., Hassan, A.A., Awad, S.S., de Bie, R.A., 2008. Complaints of the arm, neck and shoulder among computer office workers in Sudan: a prevalence study with validation of an Arabic risk factors questionnaire. Environ. Health 7, 33.

Falla, D., Farina, D., 2008. Neuromuscular adaptation in experimental and clinical neck pain. J. Electromyogr. Kinesiol. 18, 255–261.

Falla, D., Farina, D., Graven-Nielsen, T., 2007. Experimental muscle pain results in reorganization of coordination among trapezius muscle subdivisions during repetitive shoulder flexion. Exp. Brain Res. 178, 385–393.

Fallentin, N., Juul-Kristensen, B., Mikkelsen, S., et al., 2001. Physical exposure assessment in monotonous repetitive work: the PRIM study. Scand. J. Work Environ. Health 27, 21–29.

Feinstein, A.R., 1985. The Architecture of Clinical Research. Saunders, Philadelphia: PA.

Fishbain, D.A., Goldberg, M., Meagher, B.R., 1986. Male and female chronic pain patients categorized by DSM–III psychiatric diagnostic criteria. Pain 26, 181–197.

Fishbain, D.A., Goldberg, M., Steele, R., Rosomoff, H., 1989. DSM–III diagnoses of patients with myofascial

pain syndrome (fibrositis). Arch. Phys. Med. Rehabil. 70, 433–438.

Franssen, J., 1995. Handboek oppervlakte-elektromyografie. De Tijdstroom, Utrecht.

Fry, H.J., Hallett, M., Mastroianni, T., Dang, N., Dambrosia, J., 1998. Incoordination in pianists with overuse syndrome. Neurology 51, 512–519.

Gerwin, R., Shannon, S., 2000. Inter-examiner reliability and myofascial trigger points. Arch. Phys. Med. Rehabil. 81, 1257–1258.

Gerwin, R.D., 1997. Myofascial pain syndromes in the upper extremity. J. Hand Ther. 10, 130–136.

Gerwin, R.D., 1999. Myofascial Pain syndromes from Trigger Points. Current Revalidation and Pain 3, 153–159.

Gerwin, R.D., 2001. Classification, epidemiology, and natural history of myofascial pain syndrome. Curr. Pain Headache Rep. 5, 412–420.

Gerwin, R.D., Dommerholt, J., Shah, J.P., 2004. An expansion of Simons' integrated hypothesis of trigger point formation. Curr. Pain Headache Rep. 8, 468–475.

Gissel, H., 2000. Ca^{2+} accumulation and cell damage in skeletal muscle during low frequency stimulation. Eur. J. Appl. Physiol. 83, 175–180.

Graven-Nielsen, T., Svensson, P., Arendt-Nielsen, L., 1997. Effects of experimental muscle pain on muscle activity and co-ordination during static and dynamic motor function. Electroencephalogr. Clin. Neurophysiol. 105, 156–164.

Grieco, A., Molteni, G., De Vito, G., Sias, N., 1998. Epidemiology of musculoskeletal disorders due to biomechanical overload. Ergonomics 41, 1253–1260.

Hagberg, M., 1981a. Electromyographic signs of shoulder muscular fatigue in two elevated arm positions. Am. J. Phys. Med. 60, 111–121.

Hagberg, M., 1981b. Muscular endurance and surface electromyogram in isometric and dynamic exercise. J. Appl. Physiol. 51, 1–7.

Hagberg, M., Kvarnstrom, S., 1984. Muscular endurance and electromyographic fatigue in myofascial shoulder pain. Arch. Phys. Med. Rehabil. 65, 522–525.

Hagg, G.M., 2000. Human muscle fibre abnormalities related to occupational load. Eur. J. Appl. Physiol. 83, 159–165.

Hagg, G.M., Luttmann, A., Jager, M., 2000. Methodologies for evaluating electromyographic field data in ergonomics. J. Electromyogr. Kinesiol. 10, 301–312.

Henneman, E., Olson, C.B., 1965. Relations between structure and function in the design of skeletal muscles. J. Neurophysiol. 28, 581–598.

Henneman, E., Somjen, G., Carpenter, D.O., 1965. Excitability and inhabitability of motorneurons of different sizes. J. Neurophysiol. 28, 599–620.

Hermens, H.J., Hutten, M.M.R., 2002. Muscle activation in chronic pain: its treatment using a new approach of myofeedback. Int. J. Ind. Ergon. 30, 325–336.

Hermens, H.J., Boon, K.L., Zilvold, G., 1984. The clinical use of surface EMG. Electromyogr. Clin. Neurophysiol. 24, 243–265.

Hill, A., 1965. The environment and disease: Association or causation. Proc. R. Soc. Med. 8, 295–300.

Hof, A.L., 1984. EMG and muscle force: an introduction. Hum. Mov. Sci. 3, 119–153.

Hoyle, J.A., Marras, W.S., Sheedy, J.E., Hart, D.E., 2010. Effects of postural and visual stressors on myofascial trigger point development and motor unit rotation during computer work. Journal of Electromyography and Kinesiology, in press.

Hubbard, D.R., Berkoff, G.M., 1993. Myofascial trigger points show spontaneous needle EMG activity. Spine 18, 1803–1807.

Ireland, D.C., 1998. Australian repetition strain injury phenomenon. Clin. Orthop. Relat. Res. 351, 63–73.

Jonas, W.B., 2005. Dictionary of Complementary and Alternative Medicine. .

Jonsson, B., 1991. Electromyography in ergonomics. In: Anderson, P.A., Hobart, D.J., Danoff, J.V. (Eds.), Electromyographical kinesiology. Excerpta Medica, Oxford, pp. 133–136.

Kaergaard, A., Andersen, J.H., Rasmussen, K., Mikkelsen, S., 2000. Identification of neck-shoulder disorders in a 1 year follow-up study. Validation of a questionnaire-based method. Pain 86, 305–310.

Kallenberg, L.A., Hermens, H.J., 2006. Behaviour of motor unit action potential rate, estimated from surface EMG, as a measure of muscle activation level. J. Neuroeng. Rehabil. 3, 15.

Kuan, T.S., Hsieh, Y.L., Chen, S.M., et al., 2007. The myofascial trigger point region: correlation between the degree of irritability and the prevalence of endplate noise. Am. J. Phys. Med. Rehabil. 86, 183–189.

Lobbezoo, F., Lavigne, G.L., 1997. Do bruxism and temporomandibular disorders have a cause-and-effect relationship? J. Orofac. Pain 11, 15–23.

Lucas, K.R., Polus, B.I., Rich, P.A., 2004. Latent myofascial trigger points: their effects on muscle activation and movement efficiency. J. Bodyw. Mov. Ther. 2004, 160–166.

Lucas, N., Macaskill, P., Irwig, L., Moran, R., Bogduk, N., 2009. Reliability of physical examination for diagnosis of myofascial trigger points: a systematic review of the literature. Clin. J. Pain 25, 80–89.

Luttmann, A., Sokeland, J., Laurig, W., 1998. Muscular strain and fatigue among urologists during transurethral resections using direct and monitor endoscopy. Eur. Urol. 34, 6–13.

Madeleine, P., Lundager, B., Voigt, M., Arendt-Nielsen, L., 1999. Shoulder muscle co-ordination during chronic and acute experimental neck–shoulder pain: An occupational pain study. Eur. J. Appl. Physiol. 79, 127–140.

Markison, R.E., Johnson, A.L., Kasdan, M.L., 1998. Comprehensive care of musical hands. Occup. Med. 13, 505–511.

McGlynn, G.H., Laughlin, N.T., Rowe, V., 1979. Effect of electromyographic feedback and static stretching on artificially induced muscle soreness. Am. J. Phys. Med. 58, 139–148.

McNulty, W.H., Gevirtz, R., Hubbard, D., Berkoff, G., 1994. Needle electromyographic evaluation of trigger point response to a psychological stressor. Psychophysiology 31, 313–316.

Melhorn, J.M., 1998. Cumulative trauma disorders and repetitive strain injuries. The future. Clin. Orthop. 351, 107–126.

Mense, S., Simons, D.G., 2001. Muscle pain. Lippincott Williams & Wilkins, Baltimore.

Mense, S., Simons, D.G., Hoheisel, U., Quenzer, B., 2003. Lesions of rat skeletal muscle after local block of acetylcholinesterase and neuromuscular stimulation. J. Appl. Physiol. 94, 2494–2501.

Mesin, L., Cescon, C., Gazzoni, M., Merletti, R., Rainoldi, A., 2009. A bi-dimensional index for the selective assessment of myoelectric manifestations of peripheral and central muscle fatigue. J. Electromyogr. Kinesiol. 19, 851–863.

Middaugh, S.J., Kee, W.G., 1987. Advances in electromyographic monitoring and biofeedback in the treatment of chronic cervical and low back pain. Adv. Clin. Rehabil. 1, 137–172.

Moussawi, Z.K., Cooper, J.E., Shwedijk, E., 2008. The effect of treatment for myofascial trigger points on the EMG fatigue parameters of shoulder muscles, vol. 97. Oct 30; Chicago, IL, USA, pp. 1082–1085.

Muggleton, J.M., Allen, R., Chappell, P. H., 1999. Hand and arm injuries associated with repetitive manual work in industry: a review of disorders, risk factors and preventive measures. Ergonomics 42, 714–739.

Nathan, P.A., Meadows, K.D., 2000. Neuromusculoskeletal conditions of the upper extremity: are they due to repetitive occupational trauma? Occup. Med. 15, 677–693.

Neblett, R., Gatchel, R.J., Mayer, T.G., 2003a. A clinical guide to surface-EMG-assisted stretching as an adjunct to chronic musculoskeletal pain rehabilitation. Appl. Psychophysiol. Biofeedback 28, 147–160.

Neblett, R., Mayer, T.G., Gatchel, R.J., 2003b. Theory and rationale for surface EMG-assisted stretching as an adjunct to chronic musculoskeletal pain rehabilitation. Appl. Psychophysiol. Biofeedback 28, 139–146.

Oostrom, S.Hv., Huysmans, M.A., Hoozemans, M.J.M., Dieen, J.Hv., 2007. Verminderde propriocepsie bij RSI. Nederlands Tijdschrift voor Fysiotherapie 117, 49–53.

Otten, E., 1988. Concepts and models of functional architecture in skeletal muscle. Exerc. Sport. Sci. Rev. 16, 89–137.

Palmerud, G., Forsman, M., Sporrong, H., Herberts, P., Kadefors, R., 2000. Intramuscular pressure of the infra- and supraspinatus muscles in relation to hand load and arm posture. Eur. J. Appl. Physiol. 83, 223–230.

Pascarelli, E.F., 1999. Training and retraining of office workers and musicians. Occup. Med. 14, 163–172.

Peper, E., Gibney, K.H., 1999. Healthy Computing with Muscle Biofeedback – Taking the guesswork out of assessment, monitoring and training. Woerden (The Netherlands).

Peper, E., Gibney, K.H., 2006. Muscle Biofeedback at the Computer – A Manual to prevent RSI by taking the Guesswork out of Assessment, Monitoring and training, second ed. The Biofeedback Foundation of Europe.

Peper, E., Wilson, V.S., Gibney, K.H., et al., 2003. The integration of electromyography (SEMG) at the workstation: assessment, treatment, and prevention of repetitive strain injury (RSI). Appl. Psychophysiol. Biofeedback 28, 167–182.

Peper, E., Gibney, K.H., Wilson, V., 2005. Integrated group training with sEMG feedback to reduce discomfort at the computer: A controlled outcome study with a nine month follow-up [abstract]. In: Integrated group training with sEMG feedback to reduce discomfort at the computer: A controlled outcome study with a nine month follow-up.

Pollard Jr., R.Q., Katkin, E., 1984. Placebo effects in biofeedback and self-perception of muscle tension. Psychophysiology 21, 47–53.

Rosen, N., 1994. Physical medicine and rehabilitation approaches to the management of myofascial pain and fibromyalgia syndromes. Bailliéres Clin. Rheumatol. 8, 881–916.

Rosen, N.B., 1993. Myofascial pain: the great mimicker and potentiator of other diseases in the performing artist. Md. Med. J. 42, 261–266.

Scheuerle, J., Guilford, A.M., Habal, M. B., 2000. Work-related cumulative trauma disorders and interpreters for the deaf. Appl. Occup. Environ. Hyg. 15, 429–434.

Schoenfeld, A., 1998. Ultrasonographer's wrist – an occupational hazard. Ultrasound Obstet. Gynecol. 11, 313–316.

Shah, J.P., Danoff, J.V., Desai, M.J., et al., 2008. Biochemicals associated with pain and inflammation are elevated in sites near to and remote from active myofascial trigger points. Arch. Phys. Med. Rehabil. 89, 16–23.

Simons, D.G., 1984. Myofascial pain syndromes. Arch. Phys. Med. Rehabil. 65, 561.

Simons, D.G., 2001. Do endplate noise and spikes arise from normal motor endplates? Am. J. Phys. Med. Rehabil. 80, 134–140.

Simons, D.G., 2007. Orphan organ. Journal of Musculoskeletal Pain 15 (2), 7–9.

Simons, D.G., Stolov, W.C., 1976. Microscopic features and transient contraction of palpable bands in canine muscle. Am. J. Phys. Med. 55, 65–88.

Simons, D.G., Travell, J., Simons, L.S., 1999. Myofascial Pain and Dysfunction – The Trigger Point Manual – Volume 1. Upper Half of Body, Second ed. Baltimore.

Simons, D.G., Hong, C.Z., Simons, L.S., 2002. Endplate potentials are common to midfiber myofascial trigger points. Am. J. Phys. Med. Rehabil. 81, 212–222.

Sjogaard, G., Lundberg, U., Kadefors, R., 2000. The role of muscle activity and mental load in the development of pain and degenerative processes at the muscle cell level during computer work. Eur. J. Appl. Physiol. 83, 99–105.

Spekle, E.M., Hoozemans, M.J.M., Beek, A.vd., et al., 2005. Validation of a questionnaire to assess risk factors and complaints related to upper extremity disorders [abstract]. In: Validation of a questionnaire to assess risk factors and complaints related to upper extremity disorders, 18th International symposium on epidemiology in occupational health.

Stal, M., Hansson, G.A., Moritz, U., 1999. Wrist positions and movements as possible risk factors during machine milking. Appl. Ergon. 30, 527–533.

Strasser, P.B., Lusk, S.L., Franzblau, A., Armstrong, T.J., 1999. Perceived psychological stress and upper extremity cumulative trauma disorders. AAOHN J. 47, 22–30.

Travell, J.G., Simons, D.G., 1992. Myofascial pain and dysfunction: the trigger point manual – Vol. 2: The lower extremities. Williams & Wilkins, Baltimore.

Treaster, D., Marras, W.S., Burr, D., Sheedy, J.E., Hart, D., 2006. Myofascial trigger point development from visual and postural stressors during computer work. J. Electromyogr. Kinesiol. 16, 115–124.

Veiersted, K.B., Westgaard, R.H., Andersen, P., 1990. Pattern of muscle activity during stereotyped work and its relation to muscle pain. Int. Arch. Occup. Environ. Health 62, 31–41.

Vender, M., Kasdan, M.L., 1999. Work-related upper extremity complaints. J. Am. Acad. Orthop. Surg. Instructional Course Lectures 48, 693–697.

Verhagen, A.P., Karels, C., Bierma-Zeinstra, S.M., et al., 2007. Exercise proves effective in a systematic review of work-related complaints of the arm, neck, or shoulder. J. Clin. Epidemiol. 60, 110–117.

Verhagen, A.P., Karels, C.C., Bierma-Zeinstra, S.M., et al., 2009. Ergonomic and physiotherapeutic interventions for treating work-related complaints of the arm, neck or shoulder in adults. Cochrane Database Systematic Reviews (3) CD003471.

Westerblad, H., Bruton, J.D., Allen, D.G., Lannergren, J., 2000. Functional significance of Ca^{2+} in long-lasting fatigue of skeletal muscle. Eur. J. Appl. Physiol. 83, 166–174.

Windisch, A., Reitinger, A., Traxler, H., et al., 1999. Morphology and histochemistry of myogelosis. Clin. Anat. 12, 266–271.

Zennaro, D., Laubli, T., Krebs, D., Klipstein, A., Krueger, H., 2003. Continuous, intermitted and sporadic motor unit activity in the trapezius muscle during prolonged computer work. J. Electromyogr. Kinesiol. 13, 113–124.

Zennaro, D., Laubli, T., Krebs, D., Krueger, H., Klipstein, A., 2004. Trapezius muscle motor unit activity in symptomatic participants during finger tapping using properly and improperly adjusted desks. Hum. Factors 46, 252–266.

Chapter | 7 |

Mechanical neck pain

Bryan S Dennison, Michael H Leal

MECHANICAL NECK PAIN DEFINITION

Neck pain is a common problem affecting individuals worldwide. Prevalence data suggests that neck pain can span the ages, affecting children and the elderly alike, without gender discrimination. Similar to low back pain, neck pain is episodic in nature (Hogg-Johnson et al 2009) with complete resolution of symptoms evading the majority of neck pain sufferers (Carroll et al 2009) resulting in quality of life and economic impacts (Borghouts et al 1999, Wright et al 1999).

Despite its common presence, there is wide variability in defining neck pain (Fejer et al 2006). This is due, in part, to the presence of both physical and psychosocial contributors to cervical spine pain. As a result of the multifactorial presentation of neck pain and the inability to identify the exact source of presenting cervical spine symptoms (Borghouts et al 1998), the label non-specific neck pain has been assigned to any un-diagnosable symptomatic disorder of the cervical spine. The vagueness of this descriptive term has resulted in further variance of what compromises non-specific neck pain. As such, terms like occupational cervico-brachial disorder, tension neck

© 2011 Elsevier Ltd.
DOI: 10.1016/B978-0-7020-3528-9.00007-8

syndrome, cervical spondylosis, thoracic outlet syndrome, cervical osteoarthritis and mechanical neck pain have been synonymously applied to non-specific neck pain (Koes & Hoving 2002). Contributing to this terminology confusion is the reality that specific, valid and reproducible diagnostic criteria are absent (Buchbinder et al 1996a; Buchbinder et al 1996b).

In an effort to standardize a working definition of neck pain, steps have been taken to identify the symptomatic boundaries that comprise the neck pain experience. The following definition for neck pain or cervical spinal pain was proposed (Fig 7.1):

'Pain perceived as arising from anywhere within the region bounded superiorly by the superior nuchal line, inferiorly by an imaginary transverse line through the tip of the first thoracic spinous process, and laterally by the sagittal planes tangential to the lateral borders of the neck.'

(Merskey & Bogduk 1994)

In 2009, The Neck Pain Task Force put forth its working definition for neck symptoms covering non-descript terms such as non-specific, soft tissue and mechanical neck pain. The Task Force excluded neck pain associated with systemic or pathologic disease or neck pain as a result of 'skin lesions, throat disorders, tumour, infections, fractures and dislocations' (Guzman et al 2009). They defined neck pain as symptoms 'located in the anatomic region of the neck as outlined (Fig 7.2), with or without radiation to the head, trunk and upper limbs' (Guzman et al 2009).

The definitions above are intended to provide a uniform definition for neck pain. However, the following operational definitions have been used in research to define

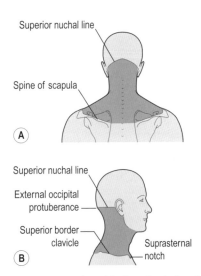

Fig 7.2 A new conceptual model of mechanical neck pain (based on Guzman et al 2009, with permission).

mechanical neck pain. Cleland et al (2005) defined mechanical neck pain as 'non-specific pain in the area of the cervico–thoracic junction that is exacerbated by neck movements'. Others (Martinez-Segura et al 2006, Fernandez-de-las-Peñas et al 2007b, Gonzalez-Iglesias et al 2009a,b, Mansilla-Ferragut et al 2009) have used the following definition of mechanical neck pain by Fernandez-de-las-Penas et al (2007a), or a slight variation thereof: 'generalized neck and/or shoulder pain with mechanical characteristics including: symptoms provoked by maintained neck postures or by movement, or by palpation of the cervical muscles'. Still others have grouped symptoms like headache of cervical origin, mechanical neck disorder with radicular signs and symptoms, neck disorder associated with whiplash and neck disorder associated with degenerative changes as subsets of mechanical neck disorders (Gross et al 2002). Kanlayanaphotporn et al (2009) used the following definition of neck pain: 'pain primarily confined in the area on the posterior aspect of the neck that can be exacerbated by neck movements or by sustained postures.' These operational definitions of neck pain denote the location of and potential provocative manoeuvres for the patient's symptoms but do not infer causation of the patient's perceived symptoms. This dilemma has led to efforts being made in current research to explain the neck pain experience and guide effective interventions.

PREVALENCE OF MECHANICAL NECK PAIN

Neck pain presents a global healthcare challenge to the medical profession with personal and economic impact. Prevalence estimates are of interest to researchers in order

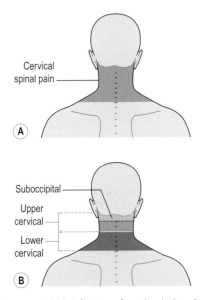

Fig 7.1 Topographical definition of mechanical neck pain.

to help assess the population impact of neck pain and direct future investigations into the etiology and management of this phenomenon. This ability to accurately analyse the worldwide impact of neck pain is challenged by the immense variation in the results and quality of the research to date.

A recent systematic review by Fejer et al (2006) investigated the worldwide prevalence of neck pain as reported in the literature from 1980–2002. Their search resulted in 56 papers meeting their inclusion criteria from Scandinavia (46%), the rest of Europe (23%), Asia (16%) and North America (11%). Australia (two papers) and Israel (one paper) also made contributions investigating the prevalence of neck pain in their respective countries. Variation in the investigated studies was obvious. Various sample sizes were seen ranging from 300 to 51,050 subjects. Variation as to what constituted neck pain, both in terms of anatomical location and an operational definition, was present as well. However, in 79% of the studies investigated, unbiased and randomized population samples were used. Over half of the studies critiqued had sample sizes of over 1000 subjects. The most common categories of prevalence periods investigated and their collective results are shared below.

The point prevalence of neck pain was investigated in 8 studies (13%) ranging from 5.9–38.7%. This data was further broken down by age categories resulting in prevalence ranges of 5.9–22.2% for individuals age 15–74 years, and 38.7% for individuals specifically over the age of 65.

One-week prevalence data was investigated in six studies (10%) with a range of 1.4–36%. However, one study used a unique definition of neck pain not used anywhere else. Excluding this study resulted in five remaining studies with a range of 1.4% to 19.5% of individuals 15–90 years of age reporting a one-week prevalence of neck pain.

One-month prevalence statistics were investigated in six studies (10%) resulting in a range of 15.4% to 41.1% for individuals between 16–79 years of age. One study by Wedderkopp et al (2001) investigated children (ages 8–10) and adolescents (ages 14–16) and reported a one-month prevalence rate of neck pain at 6.9%.

Seven studies (11%) reported 6-month prevalence data for adults 18–80 years of age ranging from 6.9% to 54.2%. Three of these studies reported ranges from 6% to 45% for 12-year-old males and 18-year-old females respectively.

The largest reported prevalence rate was in the one-year category. Twenty-two studies (39%) reported ranges of 16.7% to 75.1% for individuals aged 17–70 years old. Two studies reported ranges for adolescents. Niemi et al (1997) reported a one-year prevalence rate of 15.8% for 714 (408 girls, 306 boys – age ranges not specified) high school students. A second study by Holmen et al (2000) reported one-year prevalence data for 4279 junior high and high school students aged 13–18 years. In this population, adolescents reported a 22.1% one-year prevalence of neck and shoulder pain. In addition, the systematic critical review by Fejer et al (2006) goes on to delineate a range of 8.8–11.6% one-year prevalence as reported by three studies (Woo et al 1994, Isacsson et al 1995, Brochet et al 1998) of the elderly population (age > 65, 68 years of age, and age > 70 respectively).

Life-time prevalence rates were reported in eight studies (13%), two of which were gathered from the Tokelau Islands in the South Pacific Ocean. There, lifetime prevalence rates ranged from 0.2–2.1%. The remaining six studies reported prevalence rates of 14.2–71% for individuals 18–84 years of age. One study (Aoyagi et al 1999) focused on 860 women ages 60–79 years living in Japan or Hawaii. The results of this study reported 14.8% lifetime prevalence ('which of your joints have ever been painful...') of neck joint pain in the combined populations. However, in the systematic critical review by Fejer et al (2006), one of their inclusion criteria was to look at populations that were representative of the general population. In light of this, the Hawaiian–Japanese cohort was not considered representative of the Hawaiian population. Therefore, only the Japanese data was included, resulting in a lifetime prevalence for this group (n = 222) of 17.1%.

In summary, the literature has revealed varying descriptors of neck pain which can affect the quality of the studies. Interestingly, Fejer et al (2006) did not find a correlation between the variation in the studies they reviewed and prevalence estimates. This suggests that the quality of the studies (presence of heterogeneity) reviewed may not be a factor in neck pain prevalence estimates. In addition, the longer duration of the prevalence period the higher the reported prevalence estimates (i.e. one-year prevalence estimates where higher than one-month prevalence estimates). Gender differences were also seen. Women consistently reported neck pain 83% more than men (25 out of 30 studies; see Table 7.1).

Financial impact of mechanical neck pain

In addition to disability, neck pain carries significant economic impact as well. In the Netherlands, total costs of neck pain were estimated to be $686.2 million comprising about 1% of the 1996 total health care expenditures in the Netherlands. Health service costs for patients with neck pain, denoted as 'direct (medical) costs', comprised $159.6 million of the $686.2 million total cost. The remaining $526.5 million represented 'wealth lost to society' or 'indirect (non-medical) costs' (Koopmanschap & Rutten 1996) as a result of neck pain (Borghouts et al 1999). In the US, cervical spine disorders present challenges to the health care system, accounting for billions of dollars spent on indemnity and medical costs in the

Table 7.1 Prevalence of mechanical neck pain

Neck pain	Age (years)	World population (%)
Point Prevalence	15–74	5.9–22.2
	65+	38.7
One-Week Prevalence	15–90	1.4–19.5
One-Month Prevalence	16–79	15.4–41.1
	8–10 & 14–16	6.9
Six-Month Prevalence	18–80	6.9–54.2
	18 (female population)	45
	12 (male population)	6
One-Year Prevalence	17–70	16.7–75.1
	high school & 13–18	15.8–22.1
	65+	8.8–11.6
Lifetime Prevalence	18–84	14.2–71
	60–79	17.1

worker's compensation system, which are second only to worker's compensation costs associated with lumbar spine disorders (Wright et al 1999).

Risk factors and prognosis in mechanical neck pain

In light of current evidence, neck pain cannot be looked at in isolation. Rather this phenomenon is generally non-traumatic and multifactorial with evidence supporting the dual interaction of the physical and psychosocial arenas (Ariens et al 2001, Croft et al 2001, Guzman et al 2009, Cote et al 2009, Jull & Sterling 2009, Sterling 2009) as contributors to the pain experience. Identifying risk factors for, or predictors of, neck pain is useful at helping direct measures to prevent initial neck injury (primary prevention) or interventions for addressing factors that contribute to persistent symptoms and/or recurrent neck pain (secondary prevention) (Hill et al 2004).

Historically, risk factors for neck pain have been broken down into categories. These categories have been identified as work-related or non-work-related risk factors. These categories can further be broken down into three basic sub-groups: (1) physical risk factors, (2) psychosocial risk factors and (3) individual risk factors (i.e. coping behaviour) (Ariens et al 2000, 2001).

Early research (1966–1997) into risk factors (Ariens et al 2000, 2001), both physical and psychological, has consisted primarily of methodology using cross-sectional study designs. However, this style of research inquiry limits the ability to establish cause and affect relationships (Croft et al 2001, Carroll et al 2009). Research has evolved in the last 10 years, improving upon this methodological dilemma, by contributing larger numbers of prospective studies (Cote et al 2009). Prospective study designs allow a more confident establishment of relationships and, thus, contribute more deeply to the systematic review process.

Prevalence of neck pain in working individuals

A recent systematic review (Cote et al 2009) sought to investigate the prevalence of neck pain risk factors for working individuals. They found frequent or persistent neck disorders can develop in at least 5% of the work force with 10%, of those that develop neck pain, succumbing to activity limitation (due to neck pain) at least one time. Over half of those workers (50%) who develop neck pain will go on to report neck pain one year later (Carroll et al 2009). Identifying the contributors of neck pain has pointed researchers away from single risk factors and towards complex relationships involving interactions among individual, cultural and work-related variables. Furthermore, age, previous musculoskeletal pain, quantitative job demands, social support at work, job insecurity, low physical capacity, poor computer workstation design and work posture, sedentary work position, repetitive work, and precision work suggest an episode of neck pain. Contributors to the development of neck pain included variables of gender, a history of headache, emotional problems, smoking, awkward work postures, physical work environment and ethnicity (Box 7.1).

Prognostic factors of neck pain in working individuals

Prognostic factors for workers with neck pain have also been investigated (Carroll et al 2009) revealing 60% of workers noting persistent or recurrent neck pain one year later after an onset of symptoms. Gender also played a role in neck pain with women more likely than men to report persistent or recurrent pain. Outcomes such as prior musculoskeletal pain, prior sick leave and occupational type (blue-collar versus white-collar) were associated with poor neck pain prognostics. The only psychosocial variable that demonstrated a prognostic role was a report of having little self-perceived influence over one's own work situation. This was associated with another report of neck pain 4 years later. A challenge after identification of these poor prognosticators is the

Box 7.1 **Risk factors for mechanical neck pain in the working population**

Risk factors: an episode of neck pain	Risk factors: developing neck pain
Age	Gender
Previous musculoskeletal pain	History of headache
Quantitative job demands	Emotional problems
Social support at work	Smoking
Job insecurity	Awkward work
Low physical capacity	postures
Poor computer workstation	Physical work
design and work posture	environment and
Sedentary work position	ethnicity
Repetitive work	
Precision work	

Box 7.1 **Risk factors for mechanical neck pain in the working population**

Risk factors: an episode of neck pain	Risk factors: developing neck pain
Age	Gender
Previous musculoskeletal pain	History of headache
Quantitative job demands	Emotional problems
Social support at work	Smoking
Job insecurity	Awkward work
Low physical capacity	postures
Poor computer workstation	Physical work
design and work posture	environment and
Sedentary work position	ethnicity
Repetitive work	
Precision work	

Box 7.3 **Risk factors for mechanical neck pain in the general population**

Unfavourable risk factors	Favourable risk factors
Middle age, additional health complaints, psychological factors	Younger age

assumptions in medicine, cervical spine disc degeneration failed to be a risk factor for neck pain. In addition to physical risk factors, psychological factors predicted and presented with neck pain complaints (Box 7.3).

Prognostic factors of neck pain in the general population

Carroll et al (2008) investigated prognostic factors in the general population. Neck pain affects each sex with higher reports among women than men. However, gender only weakly predicted neck pain recovery. Younger age is associated with a more favourable prognosis. In contrast, old age is a predictor of poorer prognosis and a weak predictor of recovery. But, middle age individuals (45–59 years of age) were the highest risk and carried the poorest prognosis for neck pain.

In studies of neck pain, physical activity and exercise are assessed by self-reported questionnaires. This poses challenges to the conclusions that are able to be drawn from this data. Regular physical activity is favourable for a number of musculoskeletal issues from a prophylactic perspective, including being a component of neck pain management. However, prognostic studies evaluating its effect provided no relationships between the persistence or recurrence of neck pain when compared at the start and end of the studies.

Psychosocial health plays a factor in the prognosis of neck pain. For individuals that utilize a passive coping mechanism, their outcomes were worse than those with greater social support and better psychological health. In contrast, neck pain is associated with poorer psychological health which was also a risk factor for a new episode of neck pain (Box 7.4).

realization of the limited ability to modify these variables. But, improved outcomes were noted with changing jobs (for sewing machine operators) and exercise (Box 7.2).

Prevalence of neck pain in the general population

Hogg-Johnson et al (2009) reviewed the literature for risk factors in the general population. Their review revealed equivocal findings regarding age as a risk factor. The incidence of neck pain occurs across all ages, increasing in its prevalence as the years pass. There appears to be a peak in the prevalence of neck pain in the middle years and less prevalent in the later years of life.

Evidence has suggested a multifactorial presentation of neck pain. This includes additional health complaints (i.e. headache, low back pain, poorer self-rated health) that accompany neck pain complaints. Contrary to popular

Box 7.2 **Prognostic variables for mechanical neck pain in the working population**

Poor prognostic variables	Favourable prognostic variables
Prior neck pain	Changing jobs (for
Musculoskeletal pain	sewing machine
Prior sick leave and	operators)
occupational type (blue-collar	Exercise
versus white-collar, etc.)	
Having little self-perceived	
influence over one's own	
work situation	

Box 7.4 **Prognostic variables for mechanical neck pain in the general population**

Poor prognostic variables	Favourable prognostic variables
Middle age,	Younger age
Passive coping	Greater social support
mechanism	Better psychological health

REVIEW OF ANATOMY SPECIFIC TO MECHANICAL NECK PAIN

Any innervated structure in the cervical spine can be a pain generator, e.g. the posterior musculature, cervical zyga-pophyseal joints, lateral atlanto-occipital joint, atlanto-occipital joint, median atlanto-axial joint, dura mater of the spinal cord, pre-vertebral and lateral muscles of the neck, inter-vertebral discs, vertebral artery, synovial joints, anterior and posterior longitudinal ligaments, atlanto-axial ligaments, and internal carotid artery (Bogduk 2003). The reader is referred elsewhere for more detailed discussions of the cervical spine anatomy and its associated innervations (Bogduk 2002, 2003, Bogduk & McGuirk 2006). It is important to note that while these innervated structures can certainly be credited with the pain experience, the presence of innervation alone does not confirm the structure as the source of symptoms (Bogduk 2003).

CAUSES OF MECHANICAL NECK PAIN

Similar to low back pain, identifying exact sources of neck pain is challenging, if not impossible. The ability of any innervated structure in the cervical spine to act as a pain generator makes identification of the source of neck pain a challenge (Bogduk 2002). Further, pathological conditions (i.e. malignancy, cervical myelopathy, fracture, systemic disease and arterial dysfunction) can also cause neck pain.

Current spine research, both in low back and cervical spine regions, is encouraging a shift in clinical decision making away from previously emphasized tissue-based models of pain towards multifactorial causes (Ariens et al 2000, Guzman et al 2009). The biomedical model is repeatedly found to account for only part of the pain experience in certain spinal conditions. The International Association for the Study of Pain (IASP) has encouraged a broader clinical reasoning framework when working with patients in pain. Specifically, they have encouraged clinicians to consider possible hypotheses beyond tissue-based sources. Assisting clinicians to move beyond simple tissue-based sources, the IASP provided the following definition of pain: 'An unpleasant sensory and emotional experience associated with actual or potential tissue damage, or described in terms of such damage' (Merskey & Bogduk 1994). Based on current evidence suggesting the failure of tissue-based models to accurately explain all types of neck pain, today's clinician must be aware of both 'actual' and 'potential' sources of neck pain. Thus, a bio-psychosocial model is now being looked to as a more comprehensive model of spine pain. This model provides a combination of biomedical, psychological and social contributors to neck pain. It has been introduced in an attempt to more accurately account for the multidimensional aspect of neck pain (Jull & Sterling 2009, Sterling 2009).

Neck pain and cervical radicular pain are two categories that have been indentified for spinal related pain of the cervical region. Cervical radicular pain, pain that is perceived in the upper limb (Slipman et al 1998, Bogduk 2003) emanates from the cervical spine. Due to the ability of the cervical spine to create pain locally in the neck as well as distally in the upper extremity, the terms 'cervical radicular pain' and 'neck pain' are used interchangeably. This association, however, is incorrect. Despite the commonality of the cervical anatomic region responsible for creating symptoms, neck pain and cervical radicular pain are not interchangeable terms. Adding to this confusion is the use of the term 'cervical radiculopathy' as a synonym for cervical radicular pain. Briefly, cervical radiculopathy is a 'neurologic condition, characterized by objective signs of loss of neurologic function, that is, some combination of sensory loss, motor loss, or impaired reflexes in a segmental distribution' (Bogduk 2003). This is a result of pathology involving compression or compromise of the spinal nerve roots or the spinal nerve itself. This is objectively assessed as a loss of function and not pain. If pain is involved in a compressive condition in the cervical spine, it is due to compression of the dorsal root ganglion (see Chapter 8). Compression of nerve roots does not cause illicit nociceptive activity (Howe et al 1977). Compression of the dorsal root ganglion evokes activity in the $A\beta$ and C fibers (Howe et al 1977). This neural behaviour is more than nociceptive activity (which is predominantly $A\Delta$ and C fiber transmission). Because of the involvement of the $A\beta$ fibres with dorsal root ganglion compression, this establishes a distinction between radiculopathy (a reflection of a loss nerve function and not necessarily pain) and radicular pain (a reflection of dorsal root ganglion involvement beyond simple nociceptive function). Paraesthesia is associated with radicular pain which reflects involvement of $A\beta$ fibres (Bogduk 2003). From this perspective, the seemingly intuitive thought that pain results from 'pinched' or 'compressed' nerves does not hold true unless the dorsal root ganglion is involved in that compression.

CLINICAL PRESENTATION OF NECK PAIN

Within a sound clinical reasoning framework, it is still important for physical therapists to have an appreciation for potential tissue-based sources of neck pain. Epidemiological studies have provided support for prevalence rates of neck pain from around the world. This information is useful for helping clinicians and prognosticate direct research and prognosticates about this subgroup of patients. However, these studies are not useful in providing insight into the sources

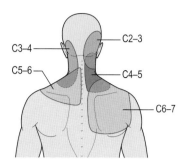

Fig 7.3 Referral patterns from spine zygapophyseal joints and inter-vertebral discs (from Bogduk 2002, with permission).

of neck pain (Yin & Bogduk 2008). Having an appreciation for possible causes of neck pain can assist the clinician in identifying pre-test probabilities for neck conditions, which then allows the clinician to prioritize their evaluation and match the patient to interventions that are associated with a higher level of success (Yin & Bogduk 2008).

The patient with neck pain creates a clinical reasoning challenge due to the vast possible causes behind the patient's chief complaint. Clinicians commonly evaluate their patients looking for a familiar pattern of symptoms that will then lead the clinician to hypothesize about a particular tissue-based source of the patient's chief complaint. In this regard, research on normal and symptomatic patients has provided identifiable referral patterns for the cervical spine zygapophyseal joints (Fig 7.3 and Fig 7.4) and intervertebral discs (Fig 7.3), spinal nerves (Fig 7.5) and soft tissue (Fig 7.6). Nociceptive stimulation of the cervical spine, without involvement of cervical nerves or nerve

roots, can refer symptoms to the upper limb, anterior chest wall, interscapular region and head (Bogduk 2002, 2003, 2006, Grubb & Kelly 2000) (Fig 7.7).

PROPOSED MANAGEMENT OF MECHANICAL NECK PAIN

Current best evidence has advocated a treatment-based classification approach for the management of patients with neck pain. Emphasis has been placed on matching the patient to optimal interventions based on the identification of signs and symptoms collected during the patient interview and physical examination (Childs et al 2004, Cleland et al 2006, Fritz & Brennan 2007, Childs et al 2008). The clinical decision-making process involved in applying this treatment-based classification strategy consists of two distinct levels (Cleland et al 2006). The first level requires that the therapist determine if the patient is appropriate for physical therapy services through a comprehensive medical screen including red and yellow flag assessments. The second level of the classification schema involves directing the patient to their matched intervention (s) or subgroup based on presenting signs and symptoms as well as their respective physical examination findings (Cleland et al 2006, Fritz & Brennan 2007).

First level of classification

Step one of this classification approach begins with a comprehensive review of the patient's medical history and a medical screen encompassing both a review of

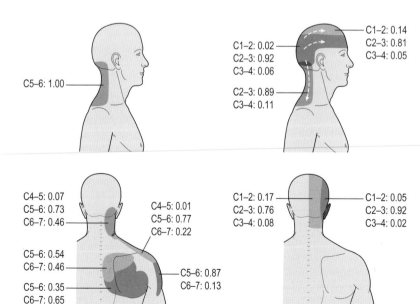

Fig 7.4 Referral patterns from spine zygapophyseal joints and inter-vertebral discs (data taken from Cooper & Bogduk 2005).

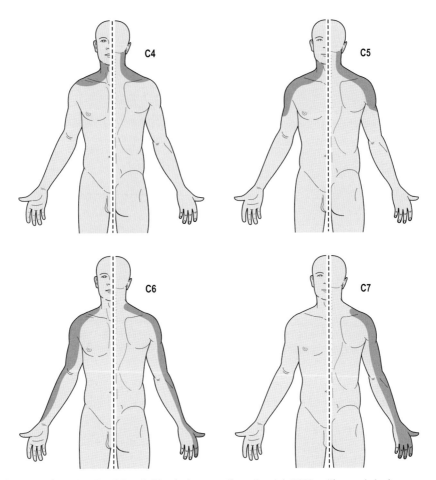

Fig 7.5 Referral patterns from C4, C5, C6 and C7 spinal nerves (from Bogduk 2002, with permission).

general health and specific systems (Boissonnault 2005). General health questions should be asked of all patients inquiring about the following: (1) fatigue, (2) malaise, (3) weakness, (4) unexplained weight loss/gain, (5) nausea, (6) paraesthesia or numbness, (7) dizziness or light-headedness, (8) change in mentation or cognition, and (9) chills, sweats, or fever.

Patient self-administered questionnaires can assist with this data collection. They have been shown to be accurate for reporting important health history information and in assisting the clinician in deciding whether or not to proceed further to the second level of classification (Pecoraro et al 1979, Boissonnault 2005).

A specific system screen (Cardiovascular, Pulmonary, Gastrointestinal, Urogenital Endocrine, Nervous system, Integumentary) follows based on the initial information gathered from the general health questions review including the body chart and self-administered questionnaires. The patient interview is a key component in attempting to recognize serious spinal pathology that may warrant

additional concern including appropriate medical follow-up with a primary care practitioner (Greene 2001, Greenhalgh & Selfe 2009).

Red flag screening

A screen for possible red flags (signs or symptoms that may suggest a more serious underlying pathology) is the first step in the classification process for determining if the patient is appropriate for physical therapy services (Nordin et al 2009). It has been suggested that the clinician needs to determine one of three potential courses of action after the initial medical screening is complete: treat the individual and proceed to the second level of classification; treat the patient and proceed to the second level of classification with notification to the individual's physician regarding signs or symptoms that may warrant concern; or refer to a physician, without any form of treatment during the initial visit, for further diagnostic work-up due to patient interview/examination findings (Boissonnault 2005). There is a small

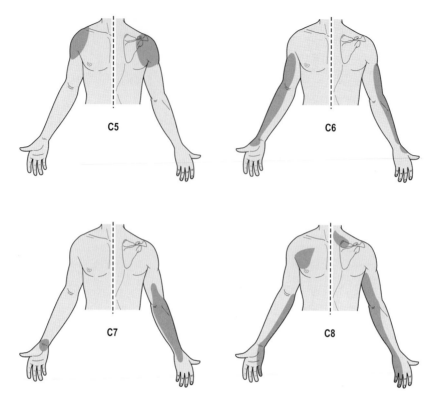

Fig 7.6 Referral patterns from inter-spinous muscles (from Bogduk & McGuirk 2006, with permission).

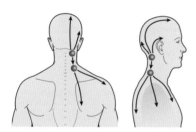

Fig 7.7 Referral patterns from nociceptive stimulation of the cervical spine.

prevalence of more serious related sources such as spinal fractures, spinal or central cord compression, neoplastic conditions, vascular compromise, system or inflammatory disease, as well as upper cervical spine ligamentous instability that the practicing clinician should be aware of. The medical screening process, combined with a thorough red flag screen, alert the clinician to the possibility of a more serious underlying condition (Cleland et al 2006).

Spinal fractures

Spinal fractures usually occur with some type of mechanical trauma or injury. Typically fractures occur from a fall, blunt trauma, the application of compressive or axial load force, or the result of a motor vehicle collision. It has been shown that risk factors such as a patient's age, as well as the height of the fall (> 3 m), are risk factors that increase the risk of cervical spine fractures. Incidents involving axial loads, diving incidents, and collisions all raise the risk of potential cervical spine fracture. The highest occurrences take place with motor vehicle collisions at speeds >100 km/hr (Thompson et al 2009). The Canadian Cervical Spine Rule is a clinical prediction rule used to determine if cervical spine radiography is needed for an alert and stable individual who has suffered a cervical spine injury (Stiell et al 2001, 2003). The rule is based on various high and low risk criteria as well as the ability of the patient to rotate their neck. If the rule is positive and the patient has not had any radiographs performed, the therapist should ensure that the appropriate radiographic evaluation be undertaken prior to the initiation of formal physical therapy services (see Chapter 2 for the Canadian C-Spine Rule).

Cervical myelopathy

Cervical myelopathy is a disorder that involves compression of the spinal cord canal resulting in neurological compromise. Canal obstruction can be caused by a variety of factors including: degenerative changes of the intervertebral discs, hypertrophy of the ligamentum flavum, or osteophyte formation due to the degenerative processes occurring at the intervertebral disc level. Cervical myelopathy is reported as the most common form of spinal cord dysfunction in individuals over the age of 55, affecting 90% of individuals as they approach their seventies (Cook et al 2009). Common symptoms include sensory disturbances of the hands, gait disturbances or balance unsteadiness, decreased motor strength with associated muscle wasting in the upper extremities, as well as bowel and bladder disturbances. Current research reported only moderate to substantial reliability for the clinical tests for cervical spine myelopathy. Furthermore performing a cluster of commonly used tests for this disorder did not improve the diagnostic accuracy greater than the Babinski test alone (Cook et al 2009). Readers are referred to Chapter 8 for further information on cervical myelopathy.

Primary neoplastic conditions

Primary neoplastic conditions are rare in the cervical spine representing 0.4% of all tumours and accounting for less than 5% of tumours that occur above the sacrum (Abdu & Provencher 1998). A more common clinical presentation may be from a Pancoast tumour, which is a malignant tumour of the upper apices of the lungs or within the superior pulmonary sulcus of the lung. It has been estimated that Pancoast tumours account for 2–5% of all cancers of the lung (Kovach & Huslig 1984). A common clinical presentation will include shoulder pain that radiates into the arm and/or hand with or without the presence of neck pain. These individuals may or may not have pulmonary signs or symptoms. Often a patient may exhibit a clinical presentation similar to Horner's syndrome or an ulnar nerve dermatomal pattern due to the close proximity of the tumour to the lower trunk of the brachial plexus (C8–T1). Pancoast tumours affect men more than women and typically show an increased incidence rate over the age of 50, especially with a history of tobacco usage. In the low back literature a systematic review looking at malignancy found a combination of age > 50, a previous history of cancer, unexplained weight loss (more than 5–10% of your body weight within a month), and failure to improve after 1 month, was 100% sensitive in diagnosing a primary metastasis (Henschke et al 2007). Given the fact that lung cancer leads the cause of death among active cancers and is the second most common cancer in men and women in the United States (Centers for Disease Control Resource page), it is important that clinicians screen for the disease appropriately.

Cervical arterial dysfunction

Cervical arterial dysfunction (CAD) is a recent term that describes the arterial events that can occur in both the anterior and posterior arterial systems of the cervical spine. The anterior system is composed of the internal carotid arteries (ICA) and provides blood flow to the eyes as well as the cerebral hemispheres. The posterior system is composed of the vertebro-basilar arteries (VBA) and provides blood flow to the hind-brain (Kerry & Taylor 2009). These pathologies can mimic cervico-cranial pain. The clinician must be able to differentially diagnosis a likely arterial presentation versus symptoms due to a musculoskeletal source based on physical examination findings encountered during a comprehensive screen and subsequent physical examination. The exact prevalence rate of spontaneous vertebral dissections and vertebro-basilar insufficiency is unknown. Therefore the clinician should have a high suspicion of CAD, especially in cases involving cervical spine trauma. Although the prevalence rate for these conditions is quite low, the clinician should be aware of the limitations surrounding the current objective examination for CAD. This awareness should lead to decreased clinical reasoning errors that occur when these tests are used in isolation during the differential diagnosis process.

This paradigm shift encourages the patient interview to include a thorough review of vascular risk factors such as hypertension, hypercholesterolaemia diabetes mellitus, a history of smoking, infection, coagulation abnormalities and direct vessel trauma. During the objective component of the evaluation, additional tests such as a cranial nerve and eye examination can be used to assist the clinician in a comprehensive perspective of the patient's current haemodynamic status (Kerry & Taylor 2009). This comprehensive evaluation is extremely important as current literature is supporting the hypothesis that neck movements are not valid screening tools in determining who is at risk for a vertebro-basilar artery dissection (Haldeman et al 1999). The concept of pre-manipulative testing has also been discouraged when there is a strong suspicion of a vertebro-basilar artery dissection. It has also been suggested that pre-manipulative testing adds little clinical information needed for decision making. In light of this, clinicians should question whether or not provocation tests add any benefit to the patient screening process with a realization that a comprehensive approach to screening for cervical arterial disorders is the key to early identification (Thiel et al 2005).

Clinical cervical spine instability (CCSI)

CCSI can occur from a variety of traumatic and non-traumatic events. CCSI has been difficult to diagnose due to the subtle clinical features that are associated with this condition (Cook et al 2005), the relative low prevalence rate, and the lack of clinical tests that have been shown to be reliable and valid in assisting the clinician in their clinical decision making process (Mintken et al 2008). The clinician should undertake a screening process that looks at ruling out ligamentous instability after any injury to the cervical spine, especially after a fall, blunt trauma, or a motor vehicle accident. There are a variety of non-traumatic diagnoses clinicians should be aware of that carry the potential for ligamentous instability such as rheumatoid arthritis, Down syndrome, ankylosing spondylitis, as well as prolonged oral contraceptive or corticosteroid use (Boissonnault 2005). A combination of the application of the Canadian Cervical-Spine rules, and a thorough history and physical examination aimed at identifying ligamentous structures, are key components of the clinician's examination process when attempting to rule out ligamentous instability. Despite the absence of strong empirical data for testing the integrity of the alar and transverse ligaments, they are considered essential components of the evaluation process, often performed due to potential medicolegal ramifications (Cleland et al 2006). From a clinical reasoning perspective, it is helpful to understand that due to the weak empirical evidence behind these tests, one must use caution when obtaining a negative result on either of these tests in terms of ruling out the diagnosis.

In addition to the physical examination findings, the patient interview may reveal statements that increase the probability of CCSI. A large Delphi study reported common subjective identifiers as noted by expert physical therapists (Board Certified Orthopaedic Clinical Specialists (OCS) and Fellows of the American Academy of Orthopaedic Manual Physical Therapists (FAAOMPT)). A consensus of common patient complaints were noted as follows: 'intolerance to prolonged static postures', 'fatigue and inability to hold head up', 'better with external support, including hands or collar', 'frequent need for self-manipulation', 'feeling of instability, shaking, or lack of control', 'frequent episodes of acute attacks', and 'sharp pain, possibly with sudden movements' (Cook et al 2005). These patient reports may assist the clinician in identifying patients with CCSI.

Yellow flag screening

After clinicians have completed the first level of classification and concluded that there are no red flags or systemic issues present, the next step in the evaluation process is to perform a yellow flags assessment. Yellow flags are defined as patient indicators that require further investigation by the clinician regarding the cognitive and behavioural aspects of the patient presentation (Pincus et al 2002). These psychosocial variables have been demonstrated in the research literature as a link between neck pain in both the acute and sub-acute tissue healing phases (Linton 2000, Bot et al 2005, Carroll et al 2008). Epidemiological studies have demonstrated that 47% of all individuals who experienced a neck pain episode had either continued persistent pain or a worsening of symptoms at an annual follow-up (Cote et al 2004).

Fear of movement has been identified in the research literature as a psychosocial indicator that can assist in predicting disability in the neck pain population. It may be a key variable in explaining why individuals continue to have pain up to a year after their initial episode. The Fear-avoidance Beliefs Questionnaire is a tool the clinician can use to objectify the patient's fear of movement. Although primarily studied in the low back pain population there is data to suggest similar prognostic capabilities, although with weaker statistical associations, for functional outcomes using this tool in the cervical spine population (George et al 2001). Once the clinician determines the presence of any yellow flags, they can adjust the treatment plan accordingly (Fear-Avoidance based model) including notification of the patient's primary care physician or referring individual regarding the clinical findings which may affect the patient's future prognosis. Once the red flag and yellow flag assessment has been completed the clinician can then move on to the second level of classification involving matching the patient to the most appropriate interventions for their clinical findings.

Second level of classification

Once the patient has been evaluated for any potential red and yellow flags and the decision is made that the individual is appropriate for physical therapy services, the clinician can then move to the second level of classification (Fig 7.8). Here the clinician can start to classify the patient in terms of key impairments, appropriately matching them to selected interventions. This current treatment-based classification system is based on presenting signs and symptoms obtained from the history and physical examination with subsequent decision-making using a clinical algorithm (Fritz & Brennan 2007). The individual is then matched accordingly to the most appropriate interventions most likely to benefit their current clinical presentation (Childs et al 2004, Fritz & Brennan 2007). Preliminary studies of this treatment-based classification have shown that individuals receiving matched interventions were found to have strong associations with greater improvements in neck disability scores (NDI), as well as pain ratings, than individuals receiving non-matched interventions (Fritz & Brennan 2007).

Mechanical neck pain classification

Mechanical neck pain is often managed with a conservative, non-surgical approach, which has traditionally been the mainstay of treatment interventions for this population. Historically physical therapists have used a variety of different interventions including modalities, joint mobilization and/or manipulation, therapeutic exercise, and cervical spine mechanical traction (Cleland et al 2007).

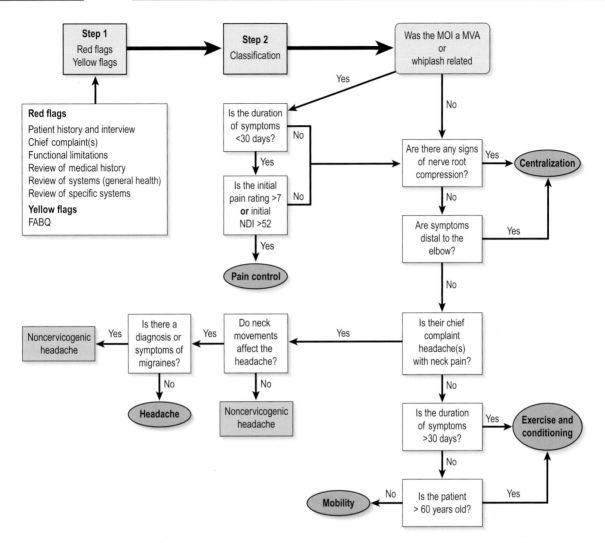

Fig 7.8 Treatment-based classification algorithm. MOI = mechanism of injury; MVA = motor vehicle accident; NDI = Neck Disability Index. (based on Fritz & Brennan 2007, with permission).

These interventions have largely been accepted as the standard practice of care although high-quality evidence describing their usage is often absent or inconclusive (Childs et al 2004, Fritz & Brennan 2007). This individualized and personalized clinical decision-making approach to patient care has been described as professional uncertainty or Wennberg's hypothesis. Wennberg's hypothesis states that when a clinician is faced with diagnostic uncertainty, treatment options are based on idiosyncratic factors. This outcome can lead to differences amongst providers in terms of the evaluative methods of their patients as well as subsequent treatment options (Wennberg et al 1982, Jette & Jette 1997). A previous critical appraisal revealed a scarcity of evidence for the treatment of individuals with neck pain. They concluded more decisive research was needed to support conclusions regarding the efficacy of physical therapy interventions for patients with neck pain (Hoving et al 2001).

A series of reviews from the Cochrane Library reported exercise, mobilization, manipulation, and electrotherapy had limited evidence of efficacy, and it was unclear if there were any potential benefit of their usage. Suggestions for improving the validity and statistical strength of future trials included obtaining larger patient sample sizes as well as establishing a model for the standardization for treatment for this population (Gross et al 2004, Kroeling et al 2005). Variability in practice and the absence of uniform professional decision-making has been reported as key potential causes for the lack of high quality studies within the neck pain population. Smaller effect sizes leading to a fair to moderate quality of evidence rating, combined with reported subsequent data with only moderate success in patient outcomes, could potentially be a result of this lack of standardization of care (Fritz & Brennan 2007).

Treatment based classification

Due to the lack of high quality evidence for the management of this population, a treatment-based classification system (TBC) was proposed that can assist the practitioner in their clinical decision-making process (Wang et al 2003, Childs et al 2004, Fritz & Brennan 2007). This is different from a patho-anatomical approach to patient care, which is influenced by the search for the correct 'diagnosis' or tissue source. The patho-anatomical approach has been shown to be a large failure based on the inadequacies of the medical model for low back pain (Fritz & Brennan 2007). Previous studies have shown that diagnostic uncertainty at the primary care level is as high as 85% in the low back population. One can therefore infer that this would be a similar statistic for the cervical spine population (Jarvik 2003). In the absence of using a treatment-based classification system, physical therapy interventions are applied to individuals with the perception that the patient has an equal chance of failure or success, which is largely based on a patho-anatomical model. The classification approach uses a clinical reasoning process that focuses on classifying clinical data into certain categories for the purpose of making clinical decisions regarding therapeutic management. This current treatment-based classification model therefore assists the clinician in sub-grouping larger groups of patients into smaller, similar homogeneous entities. The focus is less on the identification of a patho-anatomical source and more on recognizing key impairments gained from the patient history, self-report measures, and the results of the physical examination, to guide the treatment approach (Childs et al 2004, Fritz & Brennan 2007).

Classification categories

Although high quality evidence is absent, there have been a series of studies that help guide intervention strategies once the patient has been classified into a sub-group. These interventions are the product of current, best, available evidence. They are supplemented with expert opinion and common practice when necessary. The current treatment-based classification system for patients with neck pain is composed of five classification categories (Fritz & Brennan 2007). The classification categories are: mobility, centralization, exercise and conditioning, pain control, and headache. An algorithm is used to aid the clinician in determining which appropriate classification their

patient should be assigned to (see Fig 7.1). Interventions are applied according to best current evidence and standard practice of care.

Patients in the mobility classification will often present with a recent onset of symptoms, rarely have upper quarter symptoms (active range of motion does not peripheralize symptoms and no signs of nerve root compression) and usually demonstrate active range of motion discrepancies. In the mobility classification, matched interventions will include mobilization/manipulation directed at the cervical or thoracic spine. Neuromuscular re-education and strengthening of the deep neck flexors are also included as interventions within this subgroup (Cleland et al 2005, 2007).

The centralization classification typically consists of patients presenting with a referral pattern of pain into the upper extremity and/or hands with or without concomitant neck pain. They may have pain in a radicular pattern, as well as peripheralization of symptoms with active range of motion. A test item cluster has been developed to assist the practitioner in determining if the patient's presentation is cervical radiculopathy. The four items of this cluster are: ipsilateral cervical spine rotation < 60°, a positive upper limb median nerve neurodynamic test, manual distraction relieves their current symptoms and a positive Spurling's test (Wainner et al 2003). Typical interventions may include: manual mechanical cervical traction and cervical retraction exercises based on the centralization phenomenon. Current research has also proposed a manual therapy approach including mobilization and manipulation techniques directed at the cervical and thoracic spine (Cleland et al 2007, Young et al 2009). Symptom response is then recorded for possible centralization or peripheralization of symptoms. This has been shown to assist in the clinician's prognostic reasoning (Werneke et al 2003, 2008).

Within the exercise and conditioning classification patients will have lower pain and disability scores, a longer duration of symptoms (> 30 days), no signs of nerve root compression, and no signs of peripheralization or centralization. Common interventions will include both general strengthening for the upper quarter as well as motor control exercises focused on the deep neck flexor muscle area (Bronfort et al 2001). Individuals often begin in one specific classification and then move into this category as they start to improve.

The pain control classification includes individuals who have higher initial pain and disability scores, a recent onset of symptoms, which is usually due to trauma, concomitant cervicogenic headaches, referred pain into the upper quarter, as well as poor tolerance to participation in the physical examination. Interventions include pain relieving modalities and cervical spine range of motion exercises.

Finally, the headache classification has patients who present with a one-sided or unilateral headache pattern with certain cervical spine motions exacerbating symptoms. The following interventions have been recommended for this population: cervical spine manipulation or mobilization, motor control exercises for the deep neck flexor muscles, and strengthening of the upper quarter musculature (Jull et al 2002).

CERVICAL SPINE SELF-REPORT MEASURES OF PAIN AND FUNCTION

The administration and collection of self-report measures is gaining increased awareness in physical therapy clinical practice and published research. These health status questionnaires look at a variety of variables such as general health, functional limitations and current levels of the individual's self perceived disability. It has been advocated that the use of these measures can assist the practitioner in their clinical performance as well as their overall professional accountability to the patient in providing the best care possible (Delitto 2006).

Common measures in the cervical spine population include the Numeric Pain Rating Scale (NPRS), Neck Disability Index (NDI), Patient Specific Functional Scale (PSFS), Fear-avoidance Belief Questionnaire (FABQ), and the Global Rating of Change scale (GRC). When applying these measures to a specific patient population it is helpful to know the tool's psychometric properties, especially the minimum detectable change (MDC) and the minimum clinically important difference (MCID). It is helpful to define MDC and MCID as their value is related to the clinical relevance of the measure used as well as determining if a clinical meaningful change had occurred based upon a certain treatment approach. The MDC is defined as the least amount of change that falls outside of the normal measurement error (Kovacs et al 2008). MCID is the smallest amount of change, or difference that the patient perceives as being beneficial (Jaeschke et al 1989).

Currently there is a lack of published evidence that suggests an optimal timeframe for an appropriate follow up when using self-report measures. The authors recommend that a numeric pain rating (NPRS) and change between sessions (GRC) be measured at each visit. Tools that look at perceived functional limitations (PSFS) should be measured weekly. Fear avoidance behaviour (FABQ) and self reported disability (NDI) should be evaluated at the initial evaluation and at time of discharge (Table 7.2). One may administer these tools more often based on the patient's specific case presentation. These are general guidelines to assist the clinician in their preliminary usage of these tools in the clinical setting.

Numerical pain rating scale

The Numerical Pain Rating Scale (NPRS) is a subjective measure in which individuals rate their pain on an eleven-point numerical scale. The scale is composed of 0 (no pain at all) to 10 (worst imaginable pain). It has been shown that a composite scoring system including best, worse, and current level of pain over the last 24 hours was sufficient to pick up changes in pain intensity with maximal reliability (Jensen et al 1999). The MCID has been found to be a change in score of 1.3 points or higher in the mechanical neck pain population (Cleland et al 2008).

Neck disability index

The Neck Disability Index (NDI) is the most common region specific tool in use for measuring neck related disability. It has been shown to be a reliable and valid tool. In a recent study there was no difference in NDI scores in patients with or without unilateral arm pain suggesting that the NDI adequately accounts for UE symptoms in conjunction with neck pain (Young et al 2009). There are 10 questions each scored with a possible 0–5 value with the larger number indicating a higher self-reported disability status. The score on this questionnaire can range from 0–50. In order to calculate a percentage, simply multiply the final value by two. In a recent study the MCID was found to be 7.5 points and an MDC of 10 points.

Table 7.2 Self reported measures for the cervical spine population

Measure	Score	MCID / MDC	Frequency
Numeric Pain Rating Scale (NPRS)	0–10	1.3	Every session
Patient Specific Functional Scale (PSFS)	0–10	2	Weekly
Neck Disability Index (NDI)	0–50	7.5 / 10.2	Initial & Discharge
Global Rate of Change (GROC)	−5 to +5	+2	Every session
Fear Avoidance Belief Questionnaire (FABQ)	0–24 (PA)*	>19 (PA)*	Initial & Discharge
*PA: Physical activity subscale			

It is recommended that the MDC be used as this exceeds the standard error of measurement that one would find with this tool if accepting the current MCID value (7.5 points) (Young et al 2009).

Patient specific functional scale

The Patient Specific Functional Scale (PSFS) is an outcome measure that asks the patient to identify and rate limited functional activities. It is based on a 0–10 scale with score of 10 establishing their ability to perform the activity prior to injury and zero representing their current inability to perform the activity at all. The PSFS has been shown to be highly reliable in the neck pain population (Westaway et al 1998). Currently there is a lack of evidence that supports an actual MCID for this tool in the mechanical neck pain population, but a study looking at individuals with suspected cervical spine radiculopathy established an MCID of 2 points (Cleland et al 2006).

Fear avoidance belief questionnaire

The Fear Avoidance Belief Questionnaire (FABQ) was originally developed in 1993 and was used to measure subjects' beliefs and fears about how their physical activity or work activity may contribute to their current pain state (Waddell et al 1993). The FABQ has a total of 66 points and consists of a total of 16 questions which can be scored from 0–6. Outlier questions are present resulting in the work subscale (FABQW) containing a total of 42 points (questions 6, 7, 9, 10, 11, 12, 15), while the physical activity subscale (FABQPA) has a total of 24 points (questions 2, 3, 4, 5). A recent study used this tool in the development of a clinical prediction rule for those individuals with neck pain that may benefit from thoracic spine manipulation, exercise, and patient education. They found that a score of < 12 on the FABQPA was one of the predictors of a successful outcome (Cleland et al 2007). An additional study in 2007 showed that a chronic neck pain sub-sample total score of 41 for the FABQ (T), 19 for the FABQ (PA) and 19 for the FABQ (W) could identify prolonged disability 6 months later (Landers et al 2008). There is no published data at this time that describes an MDC or MCID for this tool.

Global rating of change scale

The Global Rating of Change scale (GRC) is used to look at the patient's self perceived progress during the course of their treatment. This tool adds objectivity to the frequently asked clinical question, 'How are you feeling today – better, worse, or the same as compared to when you first started physical therapy?'. The GRC asks the patient to rate their progress from a previous point in their care (often the initial evaluation) to their current state. The most common version of this scale used in the physical therapy literature is a 15-point scale that has data points ranging from −7 (A great deal worse) to +7 (A great deal better). The original literature that had described this tool was based on a patient population that was diagnosed with chronic lung or heart disease (Jaeschke et al 1989). The authors used the 15-point scale in defining treatment success using an arbitrary cut-off system. A recent review of the GRC found using an 11-point scale ranging from −5 (very much worse) to +5 (completely recovered) or a 15-point scale, as previously mentioned, yielded the same results in terms of responsiveness. Given the lack of empirical evidence for the arbitrary cut off points used in the 15-point scale, it is the author's opinion that the 11-point scale be used with a corresponding MCID of 2 points (Kamper et al 2009).

CONCLUSION

Neck pain is a common occurrence affecting individuals around the world. Similar to low back pain, it is difficult to identify exact sources of neck pain, strengthening the likelihood of a multifactorial presentation to this pain phenomenon. Epidemiologic studies provide data to guide future research with the goal of optimizing management strategies. Physical therapists must be aware of current best practice standards regarding neck pain. This includes screening patients for the appropriateness of physical therapy services prior to initiating treatment. Once the decision is made to proceed with physical therapy care, a treatment-based classification system is proposed as an ideal starting point for managing this population. Outcome measures provide objective data to support the clinical decision making process for individuals with cervical spine pain. Future research is needed to provide further insight into the management of patients with neck pain.

REFERENCES

Abdu, W.A., Provencher, M., 1998. Primary bone and metastatic tumors of the cervical spine. Spine 23, 2767–2777.

Aoyagi, K., Ross, P.D., Huang, C., et al., 1999. Prevalence of joint pain is higher among women in rural Japan than urban Japanese-American women in Hawaii. Ann. Rheum. Dis. 58, 315–319.

Ariëns, G.A., van Mechelen, W., Bongers, P.M., et al., 2000. Physical risk factors for neck pain. Scand. J. Work. Environ. Health 26, 7–19.

Ariëns, G.A., van Mechelen, W., Bongers, P.M., et al., 2001. Psychosocial risk factors for neck pain: a systematic review. Am. J. Ind. Med. 39, 180–193.

Bogduk, N., 2002. Innervation and Pain Patterns of the Cervical Spine. In: Grant, R. (Ed.), Physical Therapy of the Cervical and Thoracic Spine. third ed. Churchill Livingstone, Edinburgh, pp. 399–412.

Bogduk, N., 2003. The anatomy and pathophysiology of neck pain. Phys. Med. Rehabil. Clin. N. Am. 14, 455–472.

Bogduk, N., McGuirk, B., 2006. Management of Acute and Chronic Neck Pain: An Evidence-Based Approach. Elsevier, Edinburgh.

Boissonnault, W.G., 2005. Primary Care for the Physical Therapist Examination and Triage. Elsevier Saunders, St. Louis, pp. 53–104.

Borghouts, J.A., Koes, B.W., Bouter, L.M., 1998. The clinical course and prognostic factors of non-specific neck pain: a systematic review. Pain 77, 1–13.

Borghouts, J.A., Koes, B.W., Vondeling, H., et al., 1999. Cost-of-illness of neck pain in The Netherlands in 1996. Pain 80, 629–636.

Bot, S.D.M., van der Waal, J.M., Terwee, C.B., et al., 2005. Predictors of outcome in neck and shoulder symptoms: a cohort study in general practice. Spine 30, E459–E470.

Brochet, B., Michel, P., Barberger-Gateau, P., et al., 1998. Population-based study of pain in elderly people: a descriptive survey. Age Ageing 27, 279–284.

Bronfort, G., Evans, R., Nelson, B., 2001. A randomized clinical trial of exercise and spinal manipulation for patients with chronic neck pain. Spine 26, 788–797.

Buchbinder, R., Goel, V., Bombardier, C., 1996a. Lack of concordance between the ICD-9 classification of soft tissue disorders of the neck and upper limb and chart review diagnosis: one steel mill's experience. Am. J. Ind. Med. 29, 171–182.

Buchbinder, R., Goel, V., Bombardier, C., et al., 1996b. Classification systems of soft tissue disorders of the neck and upper limb: do they satisfy methodological guidelines? J. Clin. Epidemiol. 49, 141–149.

Carroll, L.J., Hogg-Johnson, S., van der Velde, G., et al., 2008. Course and prognostic factors for neck pain in the general population: results of the Bone and Joint Decade 2000–2010 Task Force on Neck Pain and Its Associated Disorders. Spine 33 (Suppl. 4), S75–S82.

Carroll, L.J., Hogg-Johnson, S., Côté, P., et al., 2009. Course and prognostic factors for neck pain in workers: results of the Bone and Joint Decade 2000–2010 Task Force on Neck Pain and Its Associated Disorders. J. Manipulative Physiol. Ther. 32 (Suppl. 2), S108–S116.

Centers for Disease Control, http://www.cdc.gov/cancer/lung/statistics/index.htm. Website accessed 2009.

Childs, J.D., Fritz, J.M., Piva, S.R., et al., 2004. Proposal of a classification system for patients with neck pain. J. Orthop. Sports Phys. Ther. 34, 686–700.

Childs, J.D., Cleland, J.A., Elliott, J.M., et al., 2008. Neck pain: Clinical practice guidelines linked to the International Classification of Functioning, Disability, and Health from the Orthopedic Section of the American Physical Therapy Association. J. Orthop. Sports Phys. Ther. 38, A1–A34.

Cleland, J.A., Childs, J.D., McRae, M., et al., 2005. Immediate effects of thoracic manipulation in patients with neck pain: a randomized clinical trial. Man. Ther. 10, 127–135.

Cleland, J.A., Fritz, J.M., Whitman, J.M., et al., 2006. The reliability and construct validity of the Neck Disability Index and patient specific functional scale in patients with cervical radiculopathy. Spine 31, 598–602.

Cleland, J.A., Childs, J.D., Fritz, J.M., et al., 2007. Development of a clinical prediction rule for guiding treatment of a subgroup of patients with neck pain: use of thoracic spine manipulation, exercise, and patient education. Phys. Ther. 87, 9–23.

Cleland, J.A., Childs, J.D., Whitman, J.M., 2008. Psychometric properties of the Neck Disability Index and Numeric Pain Rating Scale in patients with mechanical neck pain. Arch. Phys. Med. Rehabil. 89, 69–74.

Cook, C., Brismée, J., Fleming, R., et al., 2005. Identifiers suggestive of clinical cervical spine instability: a Delphi study of physical therapists. Phys. Ther. 85, 895–906.

Cook, C., Roman, M., Stewart, K.M., et al., 2009. Reliability and diagnostic accuracy of clinical special tests for myelopathy in patients seen for cervical dysfunction. J. Orthop. Sports Phys. Ther. 39, 172–178.

Cooper, G., Bogduk, N., 2005. Cervical zygapophyseal joint pain maps (Poster 97). Arch. Phys. Med. Rehabil. 86 (9), e22–e23.

Côté, P., Cassidy, J.D., Carroll, L.J., et al., 2004. The annual incidence and course of neck pain in the general population: a population-based cohort study. Pain 112, 267–273.

Côté, P., van der Velde, G., Cassidy, J.D., et al., 2009. The burden and determinants of neck pain in workers: results of the Bone and Joint Decade 2000–2010 Task Force on Neck Pain and Its Associated Disorders. J. Manipulative Physiol. Ther. 32 (Suppl. 2), S70–S86.

Croft, P.R., Lewis, M., Papageorgiou, A.C., et al., 2001. Risk factors for neck pain: a longitudinal study in the general population. Pain 93, 317–325.

Delitto, A., 2006. Patient outcomes and clinical performance: Parallel paths or inextricable links?. J Orthop Sports Phys Ther. 36, 548–549.

Fejer, R., Kyvik, K.O., Hartvigsen, J., 2006. The prevalence of neck pain in the world population: a systematic critical review of the literature. Eur. Spine J. 15, 834–848.

Fernández-de-Las-Peñas,, C., Alonso-Blanco,, C., Miangolarra,, J. C., 2007a. Myofascial trigger points in subjects presenting with mechanical neck pain: A blinded, controlled study. Man. Ther. 12, 29–33.

Fernández-de-las-Peñas, C., Palomeque-del-Cerro, L., Rodríguez-Blanco, C., 2007b. Changes in neck pain and active range of motion after a single thoracic spine manipulation in subjects presenting with mechanical neck pain: a case series. J. Manipulative Physiol. Ther. 30, 312–320.

Fritz, J.M., Brennan, G.P., 2007. Preliminary examination of a proposed treatment-based classification system for patients receiving physical therapy interventions for neck pain. Phys. Ther. 87, 513–524.

George, S.Z., Fritz, J.M., Erhard, R.E., 2001. A comparison of fear-avoidance beliefs in patients with lumbar spine pain and cervical spine pain. Spine 26, 2139–2145.

González-Iglesias, J., Fernández-de-las-Peñas, C., Cleland, J.A., et al., 2009a. Inclusion of thoracic spine thrust manipulation into an electro-therapy/thermal program for the management of patients with acute mechanical neck pain: a randomized clinical trial. Man. Ther. 14, 306–313.

González-Iglesias, J., Fernández-de-las-Peñas, C., Cleland, J.A., et al., 2009b. Thoracic spine manipulation for the management of patients with neck pain: a randomized clinical trial. J. Orthop. Sports Phys. Ther. 39, 20–27.

Greene, G., 2001. Red Flags': essential factors in recognizing serious spinal pathology. Man. Ther. 6, 253–255.

Greenhalgh, S., Selfe, J., 2009. A qualitative investigation of Red Flags for serious spinal pathology. Physiotherapy 95, 224–227.

Gross, A.R., Kay, T., Hondras, M., et al., 2002. Manual therapy for mechanical neck disorders: a systematic review. Man. Ther. 7, 131–149.

Gross, A.R., Hoving, J.L., Haines, T.A., et al., 2004. A Cochrane review of manipulation and mobilization for mechanical neck disorders. Spine 29, 1541–1548.

Grubb, S.A., Kelly, C.K., 2000. Cervical discography: clinical implications from 12 years of experience. Spine 25, 1382–1389.

Guzman, J., Hurwitz, E.L., Carroll, L.J., et al., 2009. A new conceptual model of neck pain: linking onset, course, and care: the Bone and Joint Decade 2000–2010 Task Force on Neck Pain and Its Associated Disorders. J. Manipulative Physiol. Ther. 32 (Suppl. 2), S17–S28.

Haldeman, S., Kohlbeck, F.J., McGregor, M., 1999. Risk factors and precipitating neck movements causing vertebrobasilar artery dissection after cervical trauma and spinal manipulation. Spine 24, 785–794.

Henschke, N., Maher, C.G., Refshauge, K.M., 2007. Screening for malignancy in low back pain patients: a systematic review. Eur. Spine J. 16, 1673–1679.

Hill, J., Lewis, M., Papageorgiou, A.C., et al., 2004. Predicting persistent neck pain: a 1-year follow-up of a population cohort. Spine 29, 1648–1654.

Hogg-Johnson, S., van der Velde, G., Carroll, L.J., et al., 2009. The burden and determinants of neck pain in the general population: results of the Bone and Joint Decade 2000–2010 Task Force on Neck Pain and Its Associated Disorders. J. Manipulative Physiol. Ther. 32 (Suppl. 2), S46–S60.

Holmen, T.L., Barrett-Connor, E., Holmen, J., et al., 2000. Health problems in teenage daily smokers versus nonsmokers, Norway, 1995–1997: the Nord-Trøndelag Health Study. Am. J. Epidemiol. 151, 148–155.

Hoving, J.L., Gross, A.R., Gasner, A.R., et al., 2001. A critical appraisal of review articles on the effectiveness of conservative treatment for neck pain. Spine 26, 196–205.

Howe, J.F., Loeser, J.D., Calvin, W.H., 1977. Mechanosensitivity of dorsal root ganglia and chronically injured axons: a physiological basis for the radicular pain of nerve root compression. Pain 3, 25–41.

Isacsson, A., Hanson, B.S., Ranstam, J., 1995. Social network, social support and the prevalence of neck and low back pain after retirement. A population study of men born in 1914 in Malmö, Sweden. Scand. J. Soc. Med. 23, 17–22.

Jaeschke, R., Singer, J., Guyatt, G.H., 1989. Measurement of health status. Ascertaining the minimal clinically important difference. Control. Clin. Trials. 10, 407–415.

Jarvik, J.G., 2003. Imaging of adults with low back pain in the primary care setting. Neuroimaging Clin. N. Am. 13, 293–305.

Jensen, M.P., Turner, J.A., Romano, J.M., et al., 1999. Comparative reliability and validity of chronic pain intensity measures. Pain 83, 157–162.

Jette, D.U., Jette, A.M., 1997. Professional uncertainty and treatment choices by physical therapists. Arch. Phys. Med. Rehabil. 78, 1346–1351.

Jull, G., Sterling, M., 2009. Bring back the biopsychosocial model for neck pain disorders. Man. Ther. 14, 117–118.

Jull, G., Trott, P., Potter, H., et al., 2002. A randomized controlled trial of exercise and manipulative therapy for cervicogenic headache. Spine 27, 1835–1843; discussion 1843.

Kamper, S.J., Maher, C.G., Mackay, C., 2009. Global Rating of Change Scales: A Review of Strengths and Weaknesses and Considerations for Design. J. Man. Manip. Ther. 17, 163–170.

Kanlayanaphotporn, R., Chiradejnant, A., Vachalathiti, R., 2009. The immediate effects of mobilization technique on pain and range of motion in patients presenting with unilateral neck pain: a randomized controlled trial. Arch. Phys. Med. Rehabil. 90, 187–192.

Kerry, R., Taylor, A.J., 2009. Cervical arterial dysfunction: knowledge and reasoning for manual physical therapists. J. Orthop. Sports Phys. Ther. 39, 378–387.

Koes, B.W., Hoving, J.L., 2002. Efficacy of Manual Therapy in the Treatment of Neck Pain. In: Grant, R. (Ed.), Physical Therapy of the Cervical and Thoracic Spine. third ed. Churchill Livingstone, Edinburgh, pp. 399–412.

Koopmanschap, M.A., Rutten, F.F., 1996. A practical guide for calculating indirect costs of disease. Pharmacoeconomics 10, 460–466.

Kovach, S.G., Huslig, E.L., 1984. Shoulder pain and Pancoast tumor: a diagnostic dilemma. J. Manipulative Physiol. Ther. 7, 25–31.

Kovacs, F.M., Abraira, V., Royuela, A., et al., 2008. Minimum detectable and minimal clinically important changes for pain in patients with nonspecific neck pain. BMC Musculoskelet. Disord. 9, 43.

Kroeling, P., Gross, A.R., Goldsmith, C.H., 2005. A Cochrane review of electrotherapy for mechanical neck disorders. Spine 30, E641–E648.

Landers, M.R., Creger, R.V., Baker, C.V., et al., 2008. The use of fear-avoidance beliefs and nonorganic signs in predicting prolonged disability in patients with neck pain. Man Ther. 13, 239–248.

Linton, S.J., 2000. A review of psychological risk factors in back and neck pain. Spine 25, 1148–1156.

Mansilla-Ferragut, P., Fernández-de-Las Peñas, C., Alburquerque-Sendín, F., et al., 2009. Immediate effects of atlanto-occipital joint manipulation on active mouth opening and pressure pain sensitivity in women with mechanical neck pain. J. Manipulative Physiol. Ther. 32, 101–106.

Martínez-Segura, R., Fernández-de-las-Peñas, C., Ruiz-Sáez, M., et al., 2006. Immediate effects on neck pain and active range of motion after a single cervical high-velocity low-amplitude manipulation in subjects presenting with mechanical neck pain: a randomized controlled trial. J. Manipulative Physiol. Ther. 29, 511–517.

Merskey, H., Bogduk, N., 1994. Classification of Chronic Pain. Description of Chronic Pain Syndromes and Definitions of Pain Terms, second ed. IASP Press, Seattle.

Mintken, P.E., Metrick, L., Flynn, T.W., 2008. Upper cervical ligament testing in a patient with os odontoideum presenting with headaches. J. Orthop. Sports Phys. Ther. 38, 465–475.

Niemi, S.M., Levoska, S., Rekola, K.E., et al., 1997. Neck and shoulder symptoms of high school students and associated psychosocial factors. J. Adolesc. Health 20, 238–242.

Nordin, M., Carragee, E.J., Hogg-Johnson, S., et al., 2009. Assessment of neck pain and its associated disorders: results of the Bone and Joint Decade 2000–2010 Task Force on Neck Pain and Its Associated Disorders. J. Manipulative Physiol. Ther. 32 (Suppl. 2), S117–S140.

Pecoraro, R.E., Inui, T.S., Chen, M.S., et al., 1979. Validity and reliability of a self-administered health history questionnaire. Public Health Rep. 94, 231–238.

Pincus, T., Vlaeyen, J.W.S., Kendall, N.A.S., et al., 2002. Cognitive-behavioral therapy and psychosocial factors in low back pain: directions for the future. Spine 27, E133–E138.

Slipman, C.W., Plastaras, C.T., Palmitier, R.A., et al., 1998. Symptom provocation of fluoroscopically guided cervical nerve root stimulation. Are dynatomal maps identical to dermatomal maps? Spine 23, 2235–2242.

Sterling, M., 2009. Neck pain: much more than a psychosocial condition. J. Orthop. Sports Phys. Ther. 39, 309–311.

Stiell, I.G., Wells, G.A., Vandemheen, K.L., et al., 2001. The Canadian C-spine rule for radiography in alert and stable trauma patients. J. Am. Med. Assoc. 286, 1841–1848.

Stiell, I.G., Clement, C.M., McKnight, R.D., et al., 2003. The Canadian C-spine rule versus the NEXUS low-risk criteria in patients with trauma. N. Engl. J. Med. 349, 2510–2518.

Thiel, H., Rix, G., 2005. Is it time to stop functional pre-manipulation testing of the cervical spine? Man Ther. 10, 154–158.

Thompson, W.L., Stiell, I.G., Clement, C.M., Brison, R.J., et al., 2009. Association of injury mechanism with the risk of cervical spine fractures. CJEM 11, 14–22.

Waddell, G., Newton, M., Henderson, I., et al., 1993. A Fear-Avoidance Beliefs Questionnaire (FABQ) and the role of fear-avoidance beliefs in chronic low back pain and disability. Pain 52, 157–168.

Wainner, R.S., Fritz, J.M., Irrgang, J.J., et al., 2003. Reliability and diagnostic accuracy of the clinical examination and patient self-report measures for cervical radiculopathy. Spine 28, 52–62.

Wang, W.T.J., Olson, S.L., Campbell, A.H., et al., 2003. Effectiveness of physical therapy for patients with neck pain: an individualized approach using a clinical decision-making algorithm. Am. J. Phys. Med. Rehabil. 82, 203–218.

Wedderkopp, N., Leboeuf-Yde, C., Andersen, L.B., et al., 2001. Back pain reporting pattern in a Danish population-based sample of children and adolescents. Spine 26, 1879–1883.

Wennberg, J.E., Barnes, B.A., Zubkoff, M., 1982. Professional uncertainty and the problem of supplier-induced demand. Soc. Sci. Med. 16, 811–824.

Werneke, M., Hart, D.L., 2003. Discriminant validity and relative precision for classifying patients with nonspecific neck and back pain by anatomic pain patterns. Spine 28, 161–166.

Werneke, M.W., Hart, D.L., Resnik, L., et al., 2008. Centralization: prevalence and effect on treatment outcomes using a standardized operational definition and measurement method. J Orthop Sports Phys Ther. 38, 116–125.

Westaway, M.D., Stratford, P.W., Binkley, J.M., 1998. The patient-specific functional scale: validation of its use in persons with neck dysfunction. J. Orthop. Sports Phys. Ther. 27, 331–338.

Woo, J., Ho, S.C., Lau, J., Leung, P.C., 1994. Musculoskeletal complaints and associated consequences in elderly Chinese aged 70 years and over. J. Rheumatol. 21, 1927–1931.

Wright, A., Mayer, T.G., Gatchel, R.J., 1999. Outcomes of disabling cervical spine disorders in compensation injuries. A prospective comparison to tertiary rehabilitation response for chronic lumbar spinal disorders. Spine 24, 178–183.

Yin, W., Bogduk, N., 2008. The nature of neck pain in a private pain clinic in the United States. Pain Med. 9, 196–203.

Young, I.A., Michener, L.A., Cleland, J.A., et al., 2009. Manual therapy, exercise, and traction for patients with cervical radiculopathy: a randomized clinical trial. Phys. Ther. 89, 632–642.

Chapter | 8 |

Whiplash associated disorders

Michele Sterling

INTRODUCTION

Whiplash associated disorders are common, disabling, and costly conditions that occur as a consequence of a motor vehicle crash (MVC). Recent data indicate that rapid improvement in levels of pain and disability occur in the first three months post injury with little if any change after this period and that the majority of injured people will not fully recover (Kamper et al 2008). The associated cost secondary to whiplash injury, including medical care, disability, lost work productivity, as well as personal costs is substantial (Crouch et al 2006, MAIC 2004).

Whiplash is a recalcitrant condition for some individuals. Management options for both the acute and chronic stages of whiplash are not straightforward and whilst offering some improvements in pain and disability are far from being a panacea. Trials of treatment for acute whiplash have not demonstrated efficacy in terms of decreasing the incidence of those who develop persistent symptoms (Provinciali et al 1996, Borchgrevink et al 1998, Rosenfeld et al 2000, 2003). Whilst these trials have provided evidence to show that maintenance of activity is superior to rest and prescription of a collar for most whiplash injured people (Scholten-Peeters et al 2002), significant numbers of patients still transition to chronicity. Further, trials of treatment for the chronic stage of the condition, including various exercise forms have offered only modest effects with only 10–20% of patients having a completely successful outcome, that is minimal or no disability at the 12-month follow-up (Jull et al 2007, Stewart et al 2007).

Recent research findings show that whiplash is a remarkably complex and heterogeneous condition and this heterogeneity may explain the modest effects of treatment strategies investigated to date. Most trials have previously investigated relatively non-specific approaches to treatment without targeting interventions toward specific physical or psychological characteristics of the condition. However recent investigations have begun to provide insight into the characteristics of the whiplash condition – both physical and psychological – that allows speculation on the potential underlying mechanisms.

This chapter will outline the whiplash condition and classification before discussing the burgeoning knowledge

© 2011 Elsevier Ltd.
DOI: 10.1016/B978-0-7020-3528-9.00008-X

of physical and psychological manifestations of the condition and the implications for clinical practice.

THE WHIPLASH CONDITION

A motor vehicle crash can lead to bony or soft-tissue damage, which in turn may result in a variety of clinical manifestations called whiplash-associated disorders (WAD). The primary symptom is neck pain, although headache, arm pain, paraesthesia, dizziness and cognitive difficulties are also frequently reported (Spitzer et al 1995).

It is conceivable that virtually any cervical spine structure may sustain injury following whiplash. Bioengineering studies where cadavers were subjected to simulated rear end crashes have demonstrated perturbations in segmental movement including inter-segmental hyperextension, S-curve formation and differential acceleration of the upper cervical spine (Cusick et al 2001). This together with evidence from autopsy (Taylor & Taylor 1996) and animal studies (Winkelstein et al 2000) indicates that lesions may occur to cervical structures including bony elements, intervertebral discs and zygapophyseal joints, ligaments, muscles and nerve tissues. Unfortunately, in vivo identification of structural pathology has proved difficult probably due to the insensitivity of current radiological diagnostic imaging (Davis et al 1991, Uhrenholt et al 2002), although recent studies begin to provide hope that this situation may change in the future for at least some structures (Krakenes & Kaale 2006). It is also generally accepted that in some persons with chronic whiplash, the zygapophyseal joint is a symptomatic structure, demonstrated by placebo controlled nerve blocks to these joints (Lord et al 1996).

Whilst it could be argued to be beneficial if specific structural lesion(s) could be identified in whiplash injured persons, it has more recently been promoted that the identification of the patho-anatomical source of symptoms provides little basis for appropriate management of musculoskeletal pain disorders and emphasis should instead be placed on treatment approaches directed toward mechanisms and processes underlying the painful condition (Jensen & Baron 2003). With respect to WAD, there is evidence that a variety of physical and psychological impairments characterize the condition.

CLASSIFICATION OF WHIPLASH INJURY

Classification systems have been proposed in order to assist in the early assessment, prognosis and management of whiplash. The most commonly used classification system is the Quebec Task Force (QTF) system (Spitzer et al 1995). It broadly defines the condition into four groups

as WAD I (neck complaint, without musculoskeletal signs); WAD II (with musculoskeletal signs); WAD III (with neurological deficits) and WAD IV (with a fracture or dislocation). While this system provides some necessary information related to condition classification, a major systematic flaw exists as the majority of whiplash injured people are grouped within one classification (WAD II), which falsely assumes homogeneity of the most common complaints within this group (Sterling 2004). The QTF Classification system has received some criticism in the past for the lack of scientific validation (Hartling et al 2001), failure to accommodate the heterogeneity of the WAD presentation (Sterling 2004) and its lack of prognostic capacity (Kivioja et al 2008).

To date, neither the QTF classification system for WAD nor trials investigating various management approaches for this condition have considered both the physical (biological) and psychological factors that are emerging as playing a role in the pain and disability of whiplash. It is becoming apparent that whiplash is a heterogeneous condition and more complex than previously assumed. Furthermore, it is emerging that whiplash is in some ways different from neck pain conditions of a non-traumatic nature. In particular chronic whiplash shows marked sensory features indicative of central nervous system hyperexcitability that have now consistently been shown not to be a feature of chronic non-traumatic neck pain (Chien et al 2010, Elliott et al 2008, Scott et al 2005).

PHYSICAL AND PSYCHOLOGICAL CHARACTERISTICS OF THE WHIPLASH CONDITION

Historically much past research and certainly the clinical assessment of spinal pain conditions, including whiplash has aimed to identify the patho-anatomical source(s) of the patient's reported symptoms. This approach has had limited success as a patho-anatomical diagnosis is not possible in the vast majority of patients with common musculoskeletal pain conditions nor does such a diagnosis necessarily shed light on the most optimal intervention for a specific condition or patient. As a consequence, the focus has shifted in recent years more towards attempting to identify the underlying mechanisms or processes of the patient's pain syndrome (Max 2000). The purpose of this more specific diagnosis and classification of musculoskeletal pain syndromes is to help tailor interventions toward identifiable underlying processes to try to improve treatment success, particularly in some of the more recalcitrant conditions. Of all neck and upper quadrant conditions, there is arguably the most data for motor, sensory and psychological characteristics available for whiplash. One reason for this may be due to the easily defined onset of injury (MVC) versus a more insidious onset that often occurs with other conditions.

Motor and sensori-motor control dysfunction

One of the most common clinical characteristics of patients with WAD is that of movement loss or decreased cervical range of movement (Heikkila & Wenngren 1998, Dall'Alba et al 2001). Most prospective studies have shown that all whiplash injured subjects have a loss of cervical active range of movement from soon after injury (Radanov et al 1995, Kasch et al 2001b, Sterling et al 2004). Kasch et al (2001b) reported that restoration of movement loss occurred in all individuals by three months post-injury, irrespective of recovery or non-recovery. However if whiplash subjects are classified more precisely, it can be seen that those with persistent moderate/severe levels of pain and disability (measured with NDI) continue to display active movement loss several years post injury (Sterling et al 2006). In contrast, participants who had recovered or reported lesser (but still significant) pain and disability showed restoration of movement loss within 2–3 months of injury (Sterling et al 2003b), similar to that seen by Kasch et al (2001b). This demonstrates the importance of differentiating individuals with whiplash based on pain and disability levels.

Altered patterns of muscle recruitment in both the cervical spine and shoulder girdle regions have been clearly shown to be features of chronic WAD (Nederhand et al 2002, Jull et al 2004). Longitudinal data demonstrate that these changes are apparent from very soon after injury (Nederhand et al 2002, Sterling et al 2003b) with greater deficits in those reporting higher levels of pain and disability (Sterling et al 2003b). Sterling et al (2003b, 2006) observed that the disturbed motor patterns persisted, not only in those with ongoing chronic symptoms, but also in those with milder pain and disability and those who reported full recovery with this phenomena occurring at significant time periods post-injury – up to 2 years. These persisting deficits in muscle control may leave recovered individuals more vulnerable to future episodes of neck pain but this proposal needs to be substantiated with further investigation (Sterling et al 2006). Altered patterns of muscle recruitment are not unique to whiplash and identical changes have also been observed in neck pain of insidious onset (idiopathic neck pain) (Nederhand et al 2002, Jull et al 2004, Woodhouse & Vasseljen 2008). These findings suggest that the driver of such motor changes may be more due to the nociceptive input rather than the injury mechanism itself.

Recent investigation, using MRI, has shown marked morphological changes to cervical spine muscles in people with chronic whiplash. Elliott et al (2006, 2010) demonstrated the presence of fatty infiltrate in both deep and superficial cervical extensor and flexor muscles in WAD patients compared to an asymptomatic control group. Although the fatty infiltrate was generally higher in all muscles investigated for the patient group, it was highest in the deeper muscles, the rectus capitis minor/major and multifidi (Elliott et al 2006). In contrast to muscle recruitment changes, preliminary data indicate that similar morphological changes are not apparent in individuals with chronic idiopathic neck pain (Elliott et al 2008). The relevance of these findings in terms of pain, disability or functional recovery and the cause of the muscle changes are not yet known but the findings illustrate the profound disturbances in motor function present in people with chronic WAD.

Dysfunction of sensori-motor control is also a feature of both acute and chronic WAD. Greater joint re-positioning errors have been found in patients with chronic WAD and also in those within weeks of their injury, and with moderate/severe pain and disability (Sterling et al 2003b, Treleaven et al 2003). Loss of balance and disturbed neck influenced eye movement control are present in chronic WAD (Treleaven et al 2005a,b) but their presence in the acute stage of the injury are yet to be determined. It is important to note that sensori-motor disturbances seem to be greater in patients who also report dizziness in association with their neck pain (Treleaven et al 2005a,b).

Most of the documented motor deficits (movement loss, altered muscle recruitment patterns) seem to be present in whiplash injured individuals irrespective of reported pain and disability levels and rate or level of recovery (Sterling et al 2003b). Additionally, apart from cervical movement loss, motor deficits do not appear to have predictive capacity (Sterling et al 2005). Further, treatment directed at rehabilitating motor dysfunction and improving general movement shows only modest effects on reported pain and disability levels (Jull et al 2007, Stewart et al 2007). Together these findings suggest that motor deficits, although present, may not play a key role in the development and maintenance of chronic or persistent symptoms following whiplash injury. However, this is not to say that management approaches directed at improving motor dysfunction should not be provided to patients with whiplash. Rather the identification of motor deficits alone may not equip the clinician with useful information to either gauge prognosis or potential responsiveness to physical interventions.

Augmented pain processing mechanisms in whiplash

There is now considerable and consistent evidence of sensory disturbances in WAD which indicate the presence of augmented central pain processing mechanisms. Changes include both sensory hypersensitivity (or decreased pain thresholds) to numerous stimuli such as pressure, thermal, electrical stimulation and light touch in both acute and chronic WAD (Curatolo et al 2001, Sterling et al 2003a, Raak & Wallin 2006). Sensory hypersensitivity is found not only over the cervical spine (area of injury) but also at remote uninjured areas such as the upper and lower limbs (Koelbaek-Johansen et al 1999, Sterling et al 2003a). The absence of tissue damage at the site of testing suggests that central sensitization of nociceptive pathways is the cause of the pain hypersensitivity. Recently the presence of widespread hypoaesthesia (that is, elevated detection thresholds) occurring concurrently with hypersensitivity has also been found in WAD and suggests disturbances in central inhibitory processes as well (Chien et al 2008a,b).

Hypersensitivity has been shown not only to be present in testing involving a cognitive response from the participant. Facilitated flexor withdrawal reflexes in the lower limbs of participants with chronic WAD have been demonstrated following electrical stimulation of the sural nerve (Banic et al 2004, Sterling et al 2008). In this test, reflex activity of the biceps femoris was measured and evidence of spinal cord hyper-excitability (central sensitization) was provided without relying on the subject's self reported response to the stimuli, as is required with pain threshold testing. It has also been shown that the heightened reflex responses are not associated with psychological factors such as catastrophization and distress (Sterling et al 2008).

In contrast to the apparently uniform presence of motor dysfunction, sensory disturbances seem to differentiate whiplash from less severe neck pain conditions and whiplash sub-groupings with higher or lower levels of self-reported pain and disability. Individuals with chronic WAD manifest a more complex presentation involving lowered pain thresholds to pressure, heat and cold stimuli

in areas remote to the cervical spine which are not present in those with idiopathic (non-traumatic) neck pain (Scott et al 2005, Elliott et al 2008, Chien et al 2010). Similarly widespread hypoaesthesia to vibration, thermal and electrical stimulation, whilst present in WAD is not a feature of idiopathic neck pain (Chien et al 2010). However the presence of central hyper-excitability is not unique to whiplash with other painful musculoskeletal conditions such as fibromyalgia, tension-type headache and migraine also manifesting such signs (Yunus 2007). With respect to the cervical spine and upper quadrant, widespread sensory hypersensitivity is a feature of cervical radiculopathy with this condition and whiplash reporting similar pain and disability levels (Chien et al 2008b) (Figs 8.1 & 8.2). This suggests that chronic whiplash and chronic cervical radiculopathy share similar underlying mechanisms but differ from idiopathic neck pain illustrating the diversity of processes involved in various neck pain conditions.

The reason as to why some whiplash injured people develop a hypersensitive state is not clear but appears to be related to levels of pain and disability (Sterling et al 2003a). Numerous cervical spine structures are implicated as possible sources of nociception following whiplash injury. It is possible that injuries to deep cervical structures do not rapidly heal and thus become a nociceptive 'driver' of central nervous system hyper-excitability. Whilst this proposal may meet opposition from those who believe injured soft tissues are healed within several weeks, it is gaining support as a possible contributor to the development of chronic musculoskeletal pain including whiplash (Curatolo et al 2006, Vierck 2006). There is also evidence from cadaver studies that certain lesions

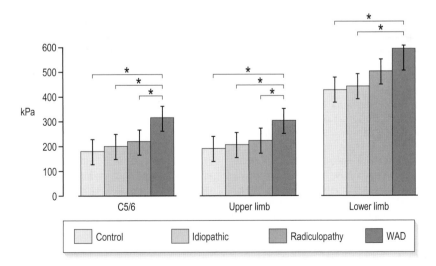

Fig 8.1 Pressure pain thresholds (PPTs) (mean and standard deviation) at C5/6, upper and lower limbs of patients with idiopathic (non-traumatic) neck pain, whiplash associated disorders (WAD) and cervical radiculopathy compared to asymptomatic controls. The three neck pain groups showed decreased PPTs at the neck (C5/6) and upper limbs. The WAD and radiculopathy groups also showed widespread decreased PPTs in the lower limb (*p < 0.05).

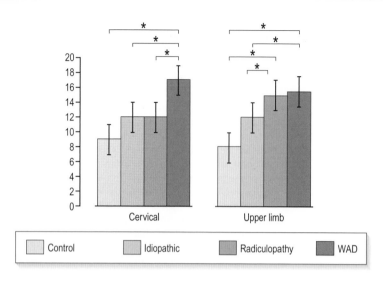

Fig 8.2 Cold pain thresholds (mean and standard deviation) measured over the cervical spine and upper limb of patients with idiopathic (non-traumatic) neck pain, whiplash associated disorders (WAD) and cervical radiculopathy compared to asymptomatic controls. The WAD and radiculopathy groups showed cold hyperalgesia over the cervical spine compared to the idiopathic neck pain group and controls. Only the WAD group showed cold hyperalgesia in the upper limb (*$p < 0.05$).

can persist unresolved in MVC survivors who die of unrelated causes some years later (Taylor & Finch 1993). Additionally, the sensory hypersensitivity seen in whiplash is often also associated with other disturbances such as impaired sympathetic vasoconstriction (Sterling 2006) and stress related factors (Sterling & Kenardy 2006). The co-occurrence of these factors suggests that a complex interplay between various mechanisms may lead to this almost systemic response in some following whiplash injury. Research is now focusing on investigating such complex models which may in the future shed light on this intriguing issue (McLean et al 2005, Passatore & Roatta 2006, Sterling & Kenardy 2006).

Psychological factors in whiplash associated disorders

There is no doubt that chronic whiplash is associated with psychological distress including affective disturbances, anxiety, depression and behavioural abnormalities such as fear of movement (Williamson et al 2008). Psychological distress is also present in the acute post-injury stage with most people showing some distress regardless of symptom levels (Sterling et al 2003c). Data from some studies indicate that the ongoing psychological distress is associated with non-resolving pain and disability. A large cross-sectional study showed an association between anxiety, depression and pain and disability in people whose accidents occurred over two years previously, but not in those with acute injury, suggesting that symptom persistence is the trigger for psychological distress (Wenzel et al 2002). Longitudinal data indicate that initially elevated levels of distress decrease in those who recover, closely paralleling decreasing levels of pain and disability (Sterling et al 2003c).

Unique psychological factors may be involved in the etiology and development of chronic whiplash (Sterling et al 2003c) when compared to other painful musculoskeletal conditions. For example, the role of fear of movement beliefs seems to be a less important factor in whiplash (Sterling et al 2005) than in low back pain (Vlaeyen et al 1995). The role of coping styles or strategies in whiplash is unclear. Some data indicate that a palliative reaction (e.g. seeking palliative relief of symptoms such as distraction, smoking or drinking) was associated with longer symptom duration (Buitenhuis et al 2003, Carroll et al 2006). In contrast Kivioja et al (2005) found no evidence that different coping styles in the early stage of injury influenced the outcome at one year post-accident. The different cohort inception times of these studies may account for the differences in findings indicating that coping strategies may vary depending on the stage of the condition and this requires further investigation.

One factor that is likely unique to WAD (when compared to other common musculoskeletal conditions), due to the mode of onset being a traumatic event, is that of post-traumatic stress. Symptoms of post-traumatic stress have been shown to be present in a proportion of people following a whiplash injury due to a MVC (Drottning et al 1995, Sterling et al 2003c, Kongsted et al 2008) and these symptoms have shown prognostic capacity for poor functional recovery at six months and two years post-MVC (Sterling et al 2005, Buitenhuis et al 2006, Sterling et al 2006). These studies mostly utilized the Impact of Events Scale (IES) (Horowitz et al 1979), an instrument that measures distress associated with a specific event (in the case of whiplash a MVC). It should be noted that a diagnosis of post-traumatic stress disorder cannot be made from IES scores. However recent data utilizing a more robust tool, The Post-traumatic Stress Diagnostic Scale (Foa et al 1997) demonstrated that 22% of a prospective sample of 155 whiplash injured people had a probable diagnosis of PTSD at three months post-MVC with this figure dropping slightly to 17% by 12 months post-injury (Sterling et al 2009). These findings indicate the need for further psychological evaluation of these patients (Forbes et al 2007) and clinicians should be aware of this factor in their assessment of whiplash injured people.

THE PREDICTION OF OUTCOME FOLLOWING WHIPLASH INJURY

The capacity to predict those at risk of poor recovery following whiplash injury is important because it may allow the institution of appropriate early interventions targeted at modifiable risk factors. This could potentially reduce the transition to chronicity in those individuals deemed at risk. Numerous factors have been investigated for their prognostic capability including: sociodemographic status; crash related variables; compensation and/or litigation, psychosocial and physical factors (Radanov et al 1995, Cassidy et al 2000, Kasch et al 2001a). However, recent systematic reviews of prospective cohort studies on whiplash found that only greater initial pain intensity and greater initial disability were the most consistent predictors of delayed functional recovery (Carroll et al 2008, Kamper et al 2008, Walton 2010). Other factors reported by individual systematic reviews include post-injury psychological factors such as coping strategies (Carroll et al 2008), less than post-secondary education, female gender, history of previous neck pain (Walton 2010) and symptoms of post-traumatic stress and poor self-efficacy (Williamson et al 2008). Whilst some of these factors such as pain intensity, psychological distress may be modifiable many of the others (age, education) are not. Furthermore when potentially modifiable factors of initial pain and disability levels are considered alone, whilst having high specificity had relatively low sensitivity to predict those with ongoing moderate to severe symptoms at six months post-accident (Sterling et al 2005). Furthermore measurement of pain and disability levels alone is unlikely to assist in the direction of secondary and tertiary management stages of this condition. Nonetheless it will be important for clinicians to obtain a measure of reported pain and disability (e.g. Neck Disability Index) in the assessment of the whiplash injured.

Additional prognostic factors have emerged but require replication and validation in further studies before they are included in systematic reviews. These include physical factors of decreased range of neck movement, cold hyperalgesia or cold intolerance and impaired sympathetic vasoconstriction (Kasch et al 2005, Sterling et al 2005, 2006). The psychological domain of post-traumatic stress symptoms is emerging as a dominant factor in poor outcome following whiplash injury (Buitenhuis et al 2006, Sterling et al 2006) with the latter study demonstrating a superior predictive capacity of this variable when compared to other psychological domains. Additional psychological factors such as high catastrophising, low self efficacy and palliative coping strategies have also been identified, in some studies, as potentially influencing recovery (Buitenhuis et al 2003, Hendricks et al 2005).

The role of the controversial issue of compensation related factors is inconclusive with some studies showing it has predictive capacity (Carroll et al 2008) and others reporting no predictive capacity of this factor (Scholten-Peeters et al 2003). A recent systematic meta-review outlined the limitations of research of the influence of injury compensation on health outcomes including the low quality of primary research papers in this area, the heterogeneous nature of compensation schemes studies and the lack of use of validated health outcome measures (Spearing & Connelly 2010). These authors could find only one systematic review that could be considered both internally and externally valid and based on this, their findings were: 'that there is evidence of no association between fault-based injury compensation and poor health outcomes among people with whiplash' (Spearing & Connelly 2010).

IMPLICATIONS FOR ASSESSMENT OF WHIPLASH

It is clear that the whiplash condition involves complexities between physiological and psychological factors. Whilst the presence of high initial levels of pain and/or disability are consistent predictors of poor outcome (Scholten-Peeters et al 2003), the additional presence of sensory hypersensitivity (particularly cold hyperalgesia) and also post-traumatic stress symptoms have been shown to substantially improve predictive capacity (Sterling et al 2005). These factors have also been shown to be associated with non-responsiveness to physical interventions (Jull et al 2007). The long-term functional status following whiplash may be established within a few months of injury with little further improvement after this time (Kamper et al 2008). This reiterates the important role clinicians play in the early post-injury stage and even towards the prevention of chronicity.

The patient assessment will need to include an adequate history such as previous history of neck pain and headache as well as the possible mechanism of injury. The patient should be screened for the presence of any 'red flag' condition (WAD IV – fracture or dislocation). Whilst accident related features have not been shown to be consistent prognostic indicators of outcome (Scholten-Peeters et al 2003), they have shown some predictive capacity in certain studies (Sturzenegger et al 1995). Since pain and disability levels have been repeatedly shown to be a consistent indicator of prolonged recovery (Hendricks et al 2005), it is essential that a validated questionnaire, such as the NDI, is used in the initial assessment. Certain physical factors, such as loss of neck movement, cold hyperalgesia, are predictive of poor recovery and must also be carefully assessed for. With respect to whiplash injury the psychological factor of post-traumatic stress appears to be involved in the transition from the acute to chronic stages of the condition and clinicians may want to include a measure of post-traumatic stress symptoms (e.g. Impact of Events Scale) in their assessment of the whiplash injured patient.

Recent calls have been made to direct clinical examination toward the recognition and identification of mechanisms involved in the patient's pain syndrome (Max 2000, Treede et al 2002). At present sensory examination such as that required to detect the variety of sensory disturbances outlined above is rarely performed and if it is performed, is usually limited to rudimentary assessment of muscle power, deep tendon reflexes and light touch sensation. More detailed assessment of sensory changes in neck pain patients is necessary. The first stage of this assessment would be thorough recording of the patient's symptoms including the nature of pain. Although the usefulness of symptom classification as a way of clarifying pain mechanisms is debatable, it is a necessary part of the patient's assessment (Jensen & Baron, 2003). In recent times questionnaires have been developed that aim to specifically identify neuropathic like pain (Bennett et al 2007). Using the S-LANSS questionnaire (Bennett et al 2005), it has been shown that 20% of an acute whiplash cohort likely have a predominantly neuropathic pain condition with certain items being particularly associated with higher levels of pain and disability (Sterling & Pedler 2009). These were 'electric shock' type pain that comes in bursts, burning pain in the neck and hyperalgesia to manual pressure. Inclusion of this questionnaire with particular attention to these items may be a useful addition to the clinical assessment of acute WAD.

Quantitative sensory testing can also be used. This could include the measurement of mechanical pain thresholds with pressure algometry (Fig. 8.3) and determination of the presence of allodynia with light tactile stimulation. Cold hyperalgesia is emerging as an important factor in both the prediction of outcome (Sterling et al 2005) and for gauging treatment responsiveness (Jull et al 2007). It is more difficult to measure clinically but options may include the use of thermorollers set at predetermined temperatures (Sterling 2008) or the time taken to reach pain threshold following the application of ice (Cathcart & Pritchard 2006). However, it has been shown that there is little relationship between S-LANSS items and cold pain threshold indicating that physical measures of sensory hyper-sensitivity will also need to be included

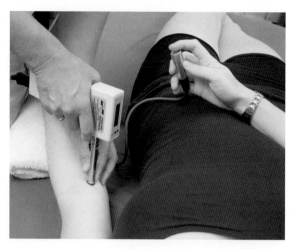

Fig 8.3 Measurement of pressure pain thresholds (PPT) (Somedic AB, Sweden) over the median nerve trunk. Decreased pressure pain thresholds in areas remote to the cervical spine may reflect augmented central pain processing mechanisms.

in the assessment of acute whiplash (Sterling & Pedler 2009).

However it should be noted that whilst such sensory assessments can provide useful information, at present there is no consensus about the most appropriate method to use and what to compare findings with (Jensen & Baron 2003). The development of the most appropriate sensory examination of whiplash injured patients is at an early stage and moves toward further development into clinically valid and useful measures is of vital importance.

Physiotherapists routinely assess cervical range of movement and this will remain a mainstay of assessment of whiplash due to the prognostic capacity of this measure. Assessment will also need to include muscle recruitment patterns of the cervical and shoulder girdle regions. Further, the assessment of sensori-motor control is relatively simple to undertake in the clinical situation and will be particularly important in whiplash injured patients who report dizziness associated with their neck pain. Readers are referred to Jull et al (2008) for a detailed account of how to undertake these assessments.

IMPLICATIONS FOR MANAGEMENT OF WHIPLASH ASSOCIATED DISORDERS

Clinical guidelines for the management of acute and chronic WAD promote education, assurance to the patient, the maintenance of activity levels, general and specific exercises, simple analgesics and encouragement of coping strategies (Scholten-Peeters et al 2002, MAA 2007, TRACsa 2008). Some recent clinical guidelines have become more cognizant of the complex presentation of some individuals with whiplash and have attempted to include recommendations for the identification of factors such as sensory disturbance and psychological distress (MAA 2007).

Whilst the resumption of activity is almost universally recommended, the case for the avoidance of pain provocation may be an important aim of any physical intervention for patients demonstrating features of sensory hypersensitivity. The application of non-judicious physical mechanically stimulating treatments may serve to maintain and prolong this hypersensitivity and have a deleterious effect on the patient's long-term outcome (Sterling & Kenardy 2008). It is not suggested that these patients avoid activity, as the maintenance of activity levels opposed to rest and use of a collar has been shown to be important in the management of acute whiplash (Rosenfeld et al 2003). Certainly studies investigating fibromyalgia syndrome, a condition also proposed to have disturbed central pain processing mechanisms, have shown that sensory hypersensitivity increases following some forms of exercise including isometric and sub-maximal aerobic exercise (Vierck 2006).

Possible treatment modalities for central hyperexcitability in pain of musculoskeletal origin are largely unexplored. Pharmacological management approaches have been suggested (Curatolo et al 2006) but effectiveness of this form of treatment is yet to be investigated in WAD. Furthermore the side-effects of some drug therapy approaches are daunting (Vierck 2006). A predominantly medication-based approach to management, particularly in the acute stage may not be feasible. An important unanswered question is whether specific physiotherapy interventions have the capacity to modulate central hyperexcitability in WAD.

Theoretically physical interventions such as TENS and acupuncture may be useful in modulating sensory hypersensitivity and these have not been specifically investigated in WAD. Few studies have investigated the effects of psychologically based interventions in this condition. However Blanchard et al (2003) found that psychological intervention directed toward post-traumatic stress disorder in chronic whiplash, whilst influencing post-traumatic stress symptoms, did not have an effect of pain levels in this group.

This is not to suggest that exercise and movement approaches are not indicated for those with a more 'complicated' whiplash presentation. A combined specific exercise and manual therapy approach has demonstrated efficacy in the management cervicogenic headache (idiopathic neck pain) (Jull et al 2002) and this treatment approach has shown to decrease pain and disability in patients with chronic whiplash *without* the presence of mechanical and cold hyperalgesia (Jull et al 2007). It may be that such an approach has a greater role in these subgroups of neck pain. However it is apparent that it will be important to identify those patients with the presence of sensory hypersensitivity (and psychological distress, particularly post-traumatic stress) such that additional management can be provided.

CONCLUSIONS

Whiplash is a complex, heterogeneous intriguing condition involving both physical (motor and sensory) disturbances and psychological distress. It is also one of the most frustrating conditions for clinicians to manage. It would appear that the quest to better understand WAD has only just begun and the results from recent research efforts have paved the way for further directions for research. As new knowledge emerges, the clinical assessment of the condition will become more informed and this will translate to improved outcome for injured people.

REFERENCES

Banic, B., Petersen-Felix, S., Andersen, O., Radanov, B., Villiger, P., Arendt-Nielsen, L., et al., 2004. Evidence for spinal cord hypersensitivity in chronic pain after whiplash injury and in fibromyalgia. Pain 107, 7–15.

Bennett, M., Smith, B., Torrance, N., Potter, J., 2005. The S-LANSS score for identifying pain of predominantly neuropathic origin: validation for use in clinical and postal research. J. Pain 6, 149–158.

Bennett, M., Attal, N., Backonja, M., Baron, R., Bouhassira, D., Freynhagen, R., et al., 2007. Using screening tools to identify neuropathic pain. Pain 127, 199–203.

Blanchard, E., Hickling, E., Devineni, T., Veazey, C., Galovski, T., Mundy, E., et al., 2003. A controlled evaluation of cognitive behaviour therapy for posttraumatic stress in motor vehicle accident survivors. Behav. Res. Ther. 41, 79–96.

Borchgrevink, G., Kaasa, A., McDonagh, D., Stiles, T., Haraldseth, O., Lereim, I., 1998. Acute treatment of whiplash neck sprain injuries. A randomized trial of treatment during the first 14 days after a car accident. Spine 23, 25–31 *LHM: Herston Medical, Biological Sciences *LHC: RD768.S67.

Buitenhuis, J., Spanjer, J., Fidler, V., 2003. Recovery from acute whiplash – the role of coping styles. Spine 28, 896–901.

Buitenhuis, J., DeJong, J., Jaspers, J., Groothoff, J., 2006. Relationship between posttraumatic stress disorder symptoms and the course of whiplash complaints. J. Psychosom. Res. 61, 681–689.

Carroll, L., Cassidy, D., Cote, P., 2006. The role of pain coping strategies in prognosis after whiplash injury: passive coping predicts slowed recovery. Pain 124, 18–26.

Carroll, L., Holm, L., Hogg-Johnson, S., Cote, P., Cassidy, D., Haldeman, S., et al., 2008. Course and Prognostic Factors for Neck Pain in Whiplash-Associated Disorders (WAD). Results of the Bone and Joint Decade 2000–2010 Task Force on Neck Pain and Its Associated Disorders. Spine 33, 583–592.

Cassidy, J.D., Carroll, L.J., Cote, P., Lemstra, M., Berglund, A., Nygren, A., 2000. Effect of eliminating compensation for pain and suffering on the outcome of insurance claims for whiplash injury. N. Engl. J. Med. 20, 1179–1213.

Cathcart, S., Pritchard, D., 2006. Reliability of pain threshold measurement in young adults. J. Headache Pain 7, 21–26.

Chien, A., Eliav, E., Sterling, M., 2008a. Hypoaesthesia occurs in acute whiplash irrespective of pain and disability levels and the presence of sensory hyper-sensitivity. Clin. J. Pain 24, 759–766.

Chien, A., Eliav, E., Sterling, M., 2008b. Whiplash (Grade II) and cervical radiculopathy share a similar sensory presentation: An investigation using quantitative sensory testing. Clin. J. Pain 24, 595–603.

Chien, A., Eliav, E., Sterling, M., 2010. Sensory hypoaesthesia is a feature of chronic whiplash but not chronic idiopathic neck pain. Man. Ther. 15, 48–53.

Crouch, R., Whitewick, R., Clancy, M., Wright, P., Thomas, P., 2006. Whiplash associated disorder: incidence and natural history over the first month for patients presenting to a UK emergency department. Emerg. Med. J. 23, 114–118.

Curatolo, M., Petersen-Felix, S., Arendt-Nielsen, L., Giani, C., Zbinden, A., Radanov, B., 2001. Central hypersensitivity in chronic pain after whiplash injury. Clin. J. Pain 17, 306–315.

Curatolo, M., Arendt-Nielsen, L., Petersen-Felix, S., 2006. Central hypersensitivity in chronic pain: mechanisms and clinical implications. Phys. Med. Rehabil. Clin. N. Am. 17, 287–302.

Cusick, J., Pintar, F., Yoganandan, N., 2001. Whiplash syndrome: kinematic factors influencing pain patterns. Spine 26, 1252–1258.

Dall'Alba, P., Sterling, M., Trealeven, J., Edwards, S., Jull, G., 2001. Cervical range of motion discriminates between asymptomatic and whiplash subjects. Spine 26, 2090–2094.

Davis, S., Teresi, L., Bradley, W., Ziemba, M., Bloze, A., 1991. Cervical spine hyperextension injuries: MR findings. Radiology 180, 245–251.

Drottning, M., Staff, P., Levin, L., Malt, U., 1995. Acute emotional response to common whiplash predicts subsequent pain complaints: a prospective study of 107 subjects sustaining whiplash injury. Nord. J. Psychiatry. 49, 293–299.

Elliott, J., Jull, G., Noteboom, T., Darnell, R., Galloway, G., Gibbon, W., 2006. Fatty infiltration in the cervical extensor muscles in persistent whiplash associated disorders: an MRI analysis. Spine 31, E847–E851.

Elliott, J., Jull, G., Sterling, M., Noteboom, T., Darnell, R., Galloway, G., 2008. Fatty infiltrate in the cervical extensor muscles is not a feature of chronic insidious onset neck pain. Clin. Radiol. 63, 681–687.

Elliott, J., O'Leary, S., Sterling, M., Hendrikz, J., Pedler, A., Jull, G., 2010. MRI findings of fatty infiltrate in the cervical flexors in chronic whiplash. Spine 35, 948–954.

Foa, E., Cashman, L., Jaycox, L., Perry, K., 1997. The validation of a self-report measure of posttraumatic stress disorder: the posttraumatic diagnostic scale. Psychol. Assess. 9, 445–451.

Forbes, D., Creamer, M., Phelps, A., Bryant, R., McFarlane, A., Devilly, G., et al., 2007. Australian guidelines for the treatment of adults with acute stress disorder and posttraumatic stress disorder. Aust. N. Z. J. Psychiatry 41, 637–648.

Hartling, L., Brison, R., Ardern, C., Pickett, W., 2001. Prognostic value of the Quebec classification of whiplash associated disorders. Spine 26, 36–41.

Heikkila, H., Wenngren, B., 1998. Cervicocephalic kinesthetic sensibility, active range of cervical motion and oculomotor function in patients with whiplash injury. Arch. Phys. Med. Rehabil. 79, 1089–1094.

Hendricks, E., Scholten-Peeters, G., van der Windt, D., Neeleman-van der Steen, C., Oostendorp, R., Verhagen, A., 2005. Prognostic factors for poor recovery in acute whiplash patients. Pain 114, 408–416.

Horowitz, M., Wilner, N., Alvarez, W., 1979. Impact of Event Scale: a measure of subjective stress. Psychosometric Medicine 41, 209–218.

Jensen, T., Baron, R., 2003. Translation of symptoms and signs into mechanisms in neuropathic pain. Pain 102, 1–8.

Jull, G., Trott, P., Potter, H., Zito, G., Niere, K., Emberson, J., et al., 2002. A randomized controlled trial of physiotherapy management for cervicogenic headache. Spine 27, 1835–1843.

Jull, G., Kristjansson, E., Dall'Alba, P., 2004. Impairment in the cervical flexors: a comparison of whiplash and insidious onset neck pain patients. Man. Ther. 9, 89–94.

Jull, G., Sterling, M., Kenardy, J., Beller, E., 2007. Does the presence of sensory hypersensitivity influence outcomes of physical rehabilitation for chronic whiplash? A preliminary RCT. Pain 129, 28–34.

Jull, G., Sterling, M., Falla, D., Treleaven, J., O'Leary, S., 2008. Whiplash, headache and neck pain: research based directions for physical therapies. Elsevier, Edinburgh.

Kamper, S., Rebbeck, T., Maher, C., McAuley, J., Sterling, M., 2008. Course and prognostic factors of whiplash: a systematic review and meta-analysis. Pain 138, 617–629.

Kasch, H., Flemming, W., Jensen, T., 2001a. Handicap after acute whiplash injury. Neurology 56, 1637–1643.

Kasch, H., Stengaard-Pedersen, K., Arendt-Nielsen, L., Jensen, T., 2001b. Headache, neck pain and neck mobility after acute whiplash injury. Spine 26, 1246–1251.

Kasch, H., Qerama, E., Bach, F., Jensen, T., 2005. Reduced cold pressor pain tolerance in non-recovered whiplash patients: a 1 year prospective study. Eur. J. Pain 9, 561–569.

Kivioja, J., Jensen, I., Lindgren, U., 2005. Early coping strategies do not influence the prognosis after whiplash injuries. Injury 36, 935–940.

Kivioja, J., Jensen, I., Lindgren, U., 2008. Neither the WAD-classification nor the Quebec Task Force follow-up regimen seems to be important for the outcome after a whiplash injury. A prospective study on 186 consecutive patients. Eur. Spine J. 17, 930–935.

Koelbaek-Johansen, M., Graven-Nielsen, T., Schou-Olesen, A., Arendt-Nielsen, L., 1999. Muscular hyperalgesia and referred pain in chronic whiplash syndrome. Pain 83, 229–234.

Kongsted, A., Bendix, T., Qerama, E., Kasch, H., Bach, F., Korsholm, L., et al., 2008. Acute stress response and recovery after whiplash injuries. A one year prospective study. Eur. J. Pain 12, 455–463.

Krakenes, J., Kaale, B., 2006. Magnetic resonance imaging assessment of cranio-vertebral ligaments and membranes after whiplash trauma. Spine 31, 2820–2826.

Lord, S., Barnsley, L., Wallis, B., Bogduk, N., 1996. Chronic cervical zygapophyseal joint pain after whiplash: a placebo-controlled prevalence study... including commentary by Derby R Jr. Spine 21, 1737–1745.

MAA, 2007. Guidelines for the management of whiplash associated disorders. Motor Accident Authority (NSW), Sydney.www.maa.nsw.gov.au.

MAIC, 2004. Annual Report 2004. Motor Accident Insurance Commission, Brisbane.

Max, M., 2000. Is mechanism-based pain treatment attainable? Clinical trial issues. J. Pain 1, 2–9.

McLean, S., Clauw, D., Abelson, J., Liberzon, I., 2005. The development of persistent pain and psychological morbidity after motor vehicle collision: integrating the potential role of stress response systems into a biopsychosocial model. Psychosom. Med. 67, 783–790.

Nederhand, M., Hermens, H., Ijzerman, M., Turk, D., Zilvold, G., 2002. Cervical muscle dysfunction in chronic whiplash associated disorder

grade 2. The relevance of trauma. Spine 27, 1056–1061.

Passatore, M., Roatta, S., 2006. Influence of sympathetic nervous system on sensorimotor function: whiplash associated disorders (WAD) as a model. Eur. J. Appl. Physiol. 98, 423–449.

Provinciali, L., Baroni, M., Illuminati, L., Ceravolo, M., 1996. Multimodal treatment to prevent the late whiplash syndrome. Scand. J. Rehabil. Med. 28, 105–111.

Raak, R., Wallin, M., 2006. Thermal thresholds and catastrophising in individuals with chronic pain after whiplash injury. Biology Research Nursing 8, 138–146.

Radanov, B., Sturzenegger, M., Di Stefano, G., 1995. Long-term outcome after whiplash injury. A 2-year follow-up considering features of injury mechanism and somatic, radiologic, and psychological findings. Medicine 74, 281–297.

Rosenfeld, M., Gunnarsson, R., Borenstein, P., 2000. Early intervention in whiplash-associated disorders. A comparison of two protocols. Spine 25, 1782–1787.

Rosenfeld, M., Seferiadis, A., Carllson, J., Gunnarsson, R., 2003. Active intervention in patients with whiplash associated disorders improves long-term prognosis: a randomised controlled clinical trial. Spine 28, 2491–2498.

Scholten-Peeters, G., Bekkering, G., Verhagen, A., van der Windt, D., Lanser, K., Hendriks, E., et al., 2002. Clinical practice guideline for the physiotherapy of patients with whiplash associated disorders. Spine 27, 412–422.

Scholten-Peeters, G., Verhagen, A., Bekkering, G., van der Windt, D., Barnsley, L., Oostendorp, R., et al., 2003. Prognostic factors of Whiplash Associated Disorders: a systematic review of prospective cohort studies. Pain 104, 303–322.

Scott, D., Jull, G., Sterling, M., 2005. Sensory hypersensitivity is a feature of chronic whiplash associated disorders but not chronic idiopathic neck pain. Clin. J. Pain 21, 175–181.

Spearing, N., Connelly, L., 2010. Is compensation "bad for health"? A sytematic meta-review. Injury Jan 7 [Epub ahead of print].

Spitzer, W., Skovron, M., Salmi, L., Cassidy, J., Duranceau, J., Suissa, S., et al., 1995. Scientific Monograph of Quebec Task Force on Whiplash associated Disorders: redefining "Whiplash" and its management. Spine 20, 1–73.

Sterling, M., 2004. A proposed new classification system for whiplash associate disorders – implications for assessment and management. Man. Ther. 9, 60–70.

Sterling, M., 2006. Sensory hypersensitivity and psychological distress following whiplash injury: Is there a relationship?, Australian Pain Society Annual Scientific Meeting. Melbourne.

Sterling, M., 2008. Testing for sensory hypersensitivity or central hyperexcitability associated with cervical spine pain. J. Manipulative Physiol. Ther. 31, 534–539.

Sterling, M., Kenardy, J., 2006. The relationship between sensory and sympathetic nervous system changes and acute posttraumatic stress following whiplash injury – a prospective study. J. Psychosom. Res. 60, 387–393.

Sterling, M., Kenardy, J., 2008. Physical and psychological aspects of whiplash: important considerations for primary care assessment. Man. Ther. 13, 93–102.

Sterling, M., Pedler, A., 2009. A neuropathic pain component is common in acute whiplash and associated with a more complex clinical presentation. Man. Ther. 14, 173–179.

Sterling, M., Jull, G., Vicenzino, B., Kenardy, J., 2003a. Sensory hypersensitivity occurs soon after whiplash injury and is associated with poor recovery. Pain 104, 509–517.

Sterling, M., Jull, G., Vicenzino, B., Kenardy, J., Darnell, R., 2003b. Development of motor system dysfunction following whiplash injury. Pain 103, 65–73.

Sterling, M., Kenardy, J., Jull, G., Vicenzino, B., 2003c. The development of psychological changes following whiplash injury. Pain 106, 481–489.

Sterling, M., Jull, G., Vicenzino, B., Kenardy, J., 2004. Characterization of acute whiplash associated disorders. Spine 29, 182–188.

Sterling, M., Jull, G., Vicenzino, B., Kenardy, J., Darnell, R., 2005. Physical and psychological factors predict outcome following whiplash injury. Pain 114, 141–148.

Sterling, M., Jull, G., Kenardy, J., 2006. Physical and psychological predictors of outcome following whiplash injury maintain predictive capacity at long term follow-up. Pain 122, 102–108.

Sterling, M., Pettiford, C., Hodkinson, E., Curatolo, M., 2008. Psychological factors are related to some sensory pain thresholds but not nociceptive flexion reflex threshold in chronic whiplash. Clin. J. Pain 24, 124–130.

Sterling, M., Hendrikz, J., Kenardy, J., 2009. Developmental trajectories of pain/disability and PTSD symptoms following whiplash injury, Australian Spine Society Annual Conference. Brisbane.

Stewart, M., Maher, C., Refshauge, K., Herbert, R., Bogduk, N., Nicholas, M., 2007. Randomised controlled trial of exercise for chronic whiplash associated disorders. Pain 128, 59–68.

Sturzenegger, M., Radanov, B., Stefano, G.D., 1995. The effect of accident mechanisms and initial findings on the long-term course of whiplash injury. J. Neurol. 242, 443–449.

Taylor, J., Finch, P., 1993. Acute injury of the neck: anatomical and pathological basis of pain. Ann. Acad. Med. Singapore 22, 187–192.

Taylor, J., Taylor, M., 1996. Cervical spinal injuries: an autopsy study of 109 blunt injuries. Journal of Musculoskeletal Pain 4, 61–79.

TRACsa, 2008. A clinical pathway for best practice management of acute and chronic whiplash-associated disorders. South Australian Centre for Trauma and Injury Recovery, Adelaide.

Treede, R.D., Rolke, R., Andrews, K., Magerl, W., 2002. Pain elicited by blunt pressure: neurobiological basis and clinical relevance. Pain 98, 235–240.

Treleaven, J., Jull, G., Sterling, M., 2003. Dizziness and unsteadiness following whiplash injury – characteristic features and relationship with cervical joint position error. J. Rehabil. 34, 1–8.

Treleaven, J., Jull, G., Low Choy, N., 2005a. Standing balance in persistent whiplash: a comparison between subjects with and without dizziness. J. Rehabil. Med. 37, 224–229.

Treleaven, J., Jull, G., Low Choy, N., 2005b. Smooth pursuit neck torsion test in whiplash associated disorders: relationship to self-report of neck pain and disability, dizziness and anxiety. J. Rehabil. Med. 37, 219–223.

Uhrenholt, L., Grunnet-Nilsson, N., Hartvigsen, J., 2002. Cervical spine lesions after road traffic accidents. A systematic review. Spine 27, 1934–1941.

Vierck, C., 2006. Mechanisms underlying development of spatially distributed chronic pain (fibromyalgia). Pain 124, 242–263.

Vlaeyen, J., Kole-Snijders, A., Boeren, R., 1995. Fear of movement/re-injury in chronic low back pain patients and its relation to behavioural performance. Pain 62, 363–372.

Walton, D., 2010. Prognosis for chronic pain and disability following whiplash: A meta-analysis. J. Orthop. Sports Phys. Ther. (in press).

Wenzel, H., Haug, T., Mykletun, A., Dahl, A., 2002. A population study of anxiety and depression among persons who report whiplash traumas. J. Psychosom. Res. 53, 831–835.

Williamson, E., Williams, M., Gates, S., Lamb, S., 2008. A systematic review of psychological factors and the development of late whiplash syndrome. Pain 135, 20–30.

Winkelstein, B.A., Nightingale, R.W., Richardson, W.J., Myers, B.S., 2000. The cervical facet capsule and its role in whiplash injury. Spine 25, 1238–1246.

Woodhouse, A., Vasseljen, O., 2008. Altered motor control patterns in whiplash and chronic neck pain. BMC Musculoskelet. Disord. 9, 90.

Yunus, M., 2007. Fibromyalgia and overlapping disorders: the unifying concept of central sensitivity syndromes. Semin. Arthritis Rheum. 36, 339–356.

Chapter | 9 |

Cervical myelopathy and radiculopathy

Chad E Cook, Amy E Cook

INTRODUCTION

Cervical/neck pain is a common musculoskeletal complaint affecting 66–70% of individuals within their lifetime (Anderson et al 1993) with 54% having experienced symptoms within the previous 6 months (Cote et al 1998). Cervical pain can significantly affect both physical and social functions (Bovim et al 1994, Brown et al 2009), with correspondingly high levels of healthcare use and costs (Brattberg et al 1989) and up to 5%

© 2011 Elsevier Ltd.
DOI: 10.1016/B978-0-7020-3528-9.00009-1

of individuals indicating high disability (Cote et al 1998). Cervical spine pain is more prevalent in individuals who are educated, who have a history of injury or trauma, and who suffer from consistent headaches (Brown et al 2009).

Cervical pain can originate from a tumour, injurious event, infection, inflammatory disorder, metabolic condition, and/or degeneration (Ahn et al 2007, Binder 2007). The most common cause is degeneration (called cervical spondylosis). Cervical spondylosis is caused by degeneration of tissues such as the cervical disc and cartilaginous end plates, osteophytes along the vertebral body, facets, and unco-vertebral joints, and ossification or thickening of the ligamentum flavum or posterior longitudinal ligament (Rao & Fehlings 1999, McCormick et al 2003).

Two specific diagnoses associated with degenerative changes in the cervical area are cervical myelopathy and cervical radiculopathy. Both conditions involve debilitating neurological symptoms that may progress toward disability if inadequately treated (Muller & Dvorak 2001, McCormick et al 2003). In severe cases, radiculopathic and myelopathic changes can occur simultaneously resulting in myeloradiculopathy. Cervical myeloradiculopathy is a major management challenge and often leads to significant movement disorders (Wong et al 2004).

It has been purported that myelopathy is present in 90% of individuals by the seventh decade of life (Dvorak 1998) and is recognized as the most common form of spinal cord dysfunction in an individual over the age of 55 (Brown et al 2009). Cervical myelopathy most commonly affects males (Montgomery & Brower 1992) and those of Asian descent (Jayakumar et al 1996). It is believed that a large percentage of elderly patients have mild cervical myelopathy that often goes unnoticed, as signs and symptoms are frequently attributed to a normal ageing process (Brown et al 1991, 2009).

Cervical radiculopathy is defined simply as an abnormality of a nerve root, which originates in the cervical spine (Polston 2007). Cervical radiculopathy has a purported prevalence of 3.3 cases per 1000 people (Wainner et al 2003) to 83.2 per 100,000 (Polston 2007), affecting men more frequently than women (Radhakrishnan et al 1994). The condition has a peak annual incidence of 2.1 cases per 1000, and occurs most commonly in the fourth and fifth decades of life (Wainner & Gill 2000). The seventh (60%) and the sixth (25%) cervical nerve roots are the most common regions affected (Malanga 1997).

The natural history of myeloradiculopathy is unclear, the signs and symptoms are inconsistent, and the patho-physiological mechanisms are multifactorial in nature. The prevalence of myeloradiculopathy is unknown, although patients with movement disorders, e.g. cerebral palsy, torticollis and Tourette syndrome, demonstrate accelerated propensity for either spondylosis or myeloradiculopathy (Wong et al 2004). Infectious conditions such as schistosomiasis are the most investigated disease processes associated with myeloradiculopathy in the literature. Schistosomal myeloradiculopathy is a japonicum infection with trematodes of the spinal cord and is usually associated with acute transverse myelitis involving the lower portions of the spinal cord (Lambertucci et al 2008).

Cervical myelopathy, cervical radiculopathy, and cervical myeloradiculopathy may cause significant pain and debilitation and are the focus of this chapter. In particular, we plan to focus on correct diagnosis, prognosis, and treatment of each condition.

REVIEW OF ANATOMY SPECIFIC TO THE PATHOLOGY

Anatomical knowledge of the cervical spinal is necessary for an understanding of the patho-biomechanics of cervical myelopathy, radiculopathy, and myeloradiculopathy. A single spinal segment is identified by two contiguous vertebral units (e.g. C4 and C5). There are five primary articulations between adjacent vertebrae. The first is the intervertebral disc which cushions and controls movement between two vertebral bodies. Two uncinate processes articulate laterally and provide control of side flexion-based movements, and two zygapophyseal joints guide movements such as rotation. The intervertebral discs allow movement in all three planes, plus torsion. The zygapophyseal joints are considered translational joints and allow sliding motions that depend on the orientation of the joint plane. The uncinate processes allow sliding movements as well but are thought to be limited to those associated with convex and concave movements such as side flexion and sagittal movements (Cook 2006).

Within this boundary are two foramens, the spinal canal, which houses the spinal cord and the intervertebral foramen, in which the cervical spine roots exit. For the spinal canal, the lateral and posterior aspects are bordered by the superior and inferior lamina. The ligamentum flavum provides a dorsal boundary and is attached to two-thirds of the undersurface of the superior lamina. Inferiorly the ligamentum flavum is attached to the superior edge of the lower lamina (Cook 2006). Anteriorly, the spinal canal is bordered by the intervertebral disc and anterior-laterally by the unco-vertebral joints.

Each nerve root exits above the correspondingly numbered vertebral body from C2 to C7 in regions identified as intervertebral foramen. Nerve roots in the cervical spine are identified by the caudal segment of the intervertebral foramen. For example, the C3 nerve root exits above C3 vertebral body, as does the C5 nerve root above the C5 body. The intervertebral foramen is bordered superiorly and inferiorly by the pedicle, posteriorly by the facet joint, posterior-medially by the ligamentum flavum, anteriorly by the unco-vertebral joint, and anterior-medially by the intervertebral disc and posterior longitudinal ligament (Cook 2006).

REVIEW OF PROPOSED PATHOLOGY AND PATHO-BIOMECHANICS

Myelopathy, radiculopathy, and myeloradiculopathy involve both structural and movement-related abnormalities. Structurally, progressive degenerative changes result in disc height losses and reduction of space in the spinal canal and intervertebral foramina. Structural changes to the inter-vertebral discs, ligaments, and capsule lead to visco-elastic losses and movement abnormalities (Pope 2001). In particular, flexion-extension movements may cause a variety of neurological symptoms in severe degenerated conditions (Wilson et al 1991). During extension, the spinal canal shortens and narrows because of infolding of ligaments. The ligamentous infolding causes dorsilateral encroachment in the canal. In addition, the disc may bulge posteriorly in selected situations, further reducing space dorsilaterally. These structural changes may lead to kinetic changes such as decreased movement, compression on dorsilateral nerve roots or nerve root ganglia, compression on the spinal cord, and pain (Pope 2001).

Cervical myelopathy is hallmarked by the stenotic encroachment of the cervical spinal cord and subsequent neurological changes (Brown et al 2009). The encroachment may lead to structural and vascular changes and originates from sagittal narrowing of the canal. The narrowing may cause compression of the spinal cord and often originated from (1) osteophytes secondary to degeneration of intervertebral joints, (2) stiffening of connective tissues such as the ligamentum flavum at the dorsal aspect of the spinal canal which can impinge on the cord by buckling when the spine is extended, (3) degeneration of intervertebral disc together with subsequent bony changes, and (4) other degenerative connective tissue changes (Wong et al 2004). Non-degenerative, structural-based conditions may be associated with syringomyelia, an arachnoid cyst, a tumour, or epidural lipomatosis (Durrant & True 2002).

Dynamic movements of the spinal cord are regulated by the spinal column and the anchoring elements of the spinal cord. The primary anchoring elements are the dentate ligaments and the filum terminale (Durrant & True 2002). In normal subjects, length changes of the spinal cord are from 4.5 to 7.5 cm, with flexion increasing tension in the spinal cord and with extension decreasing tension (Breig 1978). Spinal cord compression occurs from a number of mechanisms, most notably from the friction that is present from degenerative changes during movements of extension and flexion. Ventral osteophytes can prevent upward and downward movement of the spinal cord during physiological motions (Bartels et al 2007).

Furthermore, thickening of tissues and bony changes called a spondylitic bar increases the friction placed upon the spinal cord during movements and causes permanent damage (Bartels et al 2007).

Cervical radiculopathy is caused by a cascade of events that lead to nerve root distortion, intraneural edema, impaired circulation and focal nerve ischaemia, a localized inflammatory response and altered nerve conduction (Truumees & Herkowitz 2000). The localized inflammatory response is stimulated by chemical mediators within the disc, which may incite the production of inflammatory cytokines, substance P, bradykinin, tumour necrosis factor α, and prostaglandins (Albert & Murrell 1999, Rhee et al 2007). These chemical pain mediators are not typically present in chronic disc lesions (Durrant & True 2002). Along with the production of chemicals, the membrane surrounding the dorsal root ganglion, which is more permeable allowing a local inflammatory response, may contribute to cervical radiculopathy (Rao & Fehlings 1999).

The most common compressive causes of cervical radiculopathy are disc herniation and degenerative spine components, e.g. osteophytes, facet joint hypertrophy, and ligament hypertrophy (Truumees & Herkowitz 2000). Disc herniation occurs when nuclear material from the acute soft disc herniation impinges on a nerve root either posterolaterally or intraforaminally (Rhee et al 2007). The degenerative causes are associated with a loss of disc height and a 'hard disc' bulging with resultant compressive elements such as the ligaments (Albert & Murrell 1999) and osteophytes (Rhee et al 2007). Location-wise, anterior causes (soft or hard disc herniation and osteophytes from the uncinate processes) are the most common cause of radicular symptoms (Rhee et al 2007). Other causes include ischaemia, trauma, neoplastic infiltration, spinal infections, post-radiation, immune-mediated diseases, lipoma, and congenital disorders (Truumees & Herkowitz 2000).

Cervical myeloradiculopathy is believed to occur during chronic spondylosis and repetitive compressive damage to the cervical spinal cord and roots, but may also occur acutely upon a flexion/extension injury (Ito et al 2004, Lewis et al 2008). Compression may result from anterior spondylotic spurs, posterior infolding of ligaments, or both (Frank 1993). Changes involve demyelination, vascular compromise and inflammation of the nerve roots.

CLINICAL SIGNS AND SYMPTOMS

Myelopathy

Myelopathy is characterized by a variable distribution pattern (Brown et al 2009) and may involve clinical findings in the lower extremities first, with subsequent gait related changes, weaknesses of the legs and spasticity (Bartels et al 2007, Harrop et al 2007). Gait disturbances are associated with upper motor neuron changes involving corticospinal tracts and spinocerebellar tracts dysfunction. Later, lower motor neuron findings in the upper extremities such as loss of strength, atrophy, and difficulty in fine finger movements may present (Cook et al 2007, Harrop et al 2007, Cook et al 2009).

Additional signs and symptoms of cervical myelopathy manifest as pain in the cervical, upper quarter region or shoulder, widespread numbness, paraesthesia and sensory and ataxic changes of the lower extremities (Polston 2007). Findings may include tetraspasticity (Dvorak 1998), gait-related clumsiness (Dvorak 1998), spasticity, hyper-reflexia (Crandall & Batzdorf 1966), and the presence of primitive reflexes (Hawkes 2002). Other clinical findings indicative of progressive decline include acquired spastic paraparesis (Hawkes 2002), tetraparesis, or paraparesis (Montgomery & Brower 1992). Because the signs and symptoms are often sequential, weakness and stiffness of the legs (Adams & Victor 1999) typically precedes pain and the occasional findings of bowel and bladder changes (Thongtrangan et al 2004).

There is a distinct possibility of mixed presentation of signs and symptoms with myelopathy. Reflexes and sensibility changes may actually be depressed at the level of compression (C5–C8) with hyper-reflexia at the levels below the lesion (Brown et al 2009). Since myelopathy can involve a number of cervical levels, most commonly, C5–C8, changes below the affected level may manifest as hyper-reflexia, whereas problems above the level are generally hyporeflexic (Brown et al 2009). In addition, uncommon symptoms may be present with myelopathic conditions, including restless legs secondary to loss of descending inhibition of the corticospinal tract, nausea, dizziness and dysphagia which can occur from compression of vertebral artery (Brown et al 2009).

Radiculopathy

For cervical radiculopathy, neurological symptoms may lead to pain, motor weakness or sensory deficits along the affected nerve root (Rao & Fehlings 1999, Polston 2007, Rhee et al 2007). Depending on the nerve root affected, symptoms may exist concurrently in the neck, shoulder, upper arm or forearm (Polston 2007). Often, pain and sensibility changes are not consistent and may result in a dull ache to a severe burning pain in the neck and arm. Pain is typically noted in the medial border of the scapula and shoulder, which can progress down the ipsilateral arm and hand along the sensory distribution of the involved nerve root (Wolff & Levine 2002). The pain may not be localized because multiple nerve roots can cause similar distribution patterns (Ellenberg et al 1994).

Motor weakness associated with radiculopathy may provide a variety of clinical scenarios and is associated with specific nerve root levels (Polston 2007, Rao & Fehlings 1999). Specific nerve root weakness typically presents in the following patterns: scapular weakness with C4; shoulder abduction or forearm flexion weakness with C5; wrist extension/supination with C6; triceps, wrist flexion/pronation with C7; and finger flexors/interossei with C8 (Tsao et al 2003). Others have noted (Tsao et al 2003) that motor weakness often with fasciculations is present in 61–68% of patients. Advanced cervical radiculopathy cases may present with muscle wasting and fasciculations (Polston 2007). In a study of 846 patients, Henderson et al (1983) noted triceps weakness due to C7 radiculopathy was present in 37% of the subjects and biceps weakness was present in 28%.

Sensibility changes (sensation variations) of the affected nerve roots may help localize the level of the lesion. C4 nerve root distribution tends to affect the shoulder and upper arm, C5 nerve root distribution the lateral aspect of the arm, C6 nerve root affects the lateral aspect of the forearm, hand, and thumb, the C7 nerve root the dorsal lateral forearm and 3rd digit, and the C8 nerve root the medial forearm, hand and 4th and 5th digits (Chien et al 2008).

Cervical radiculopathy typically presents with diminished deep tendon reflexes (muscle stretch reflex). Deep tendon reflexes are an involuntary response which offers an objective assessment for neurological impairment (Durrant & True 2002). Loss of deep tendon reflexes is usually said to be the most reliable clinical finding (Marshall & Little 2002) and is noted in 70% of the cases (Tsao et al 2003). Generally, the decline in reflexes follows a predictable radicular pattern.

Myeloradiculopathy

The combination of signs and symptoms of cervical myeloradiculopathy lead to a complex clinical presentation (Baba et al 1998). In most cases, the presentation of myeloradiculopathy involves both the cardinal signs and symptoms of the two separate diseases. For example, a common presentation is radicular symptoms in the arm (pain and weakness) and myelopathic symptoms in the legs (gait disturbances, loss of position and vibratory sense and spasticity) (Frank 1993). The challenges occur when clinical signs and symptoms overlap. In these selected cases, which typically involved highly affected, chronic spondylitic changes, differentiation of the condition is less probable and recognition of the need for decompressive surgery is the key clinical finding.

CURRENT BEST EVIDENCE WITH REGARD TO DIAGNOSIS

Cervical myelopathy

Patient history

In most cases, myelopathic changes are slow and progressive (Masdeu et al 1997). The duration of symptoms often spans a number of years and is present with concomitant conditions associated with spondylosis such as stiffness and pain. Initial symptoms are typically vague and are often mistaken as changes associated with 'old age'. Often, patients will indicate problems after or period of rest or inactivity (Masdeu et al 1997, Bednarik et al 2004). Gait problems are the first symptoms associated with myelopathy but it's often motor changes such as spasticity, weakness, and clumsiness of the arms and hands that warrants the pursuance of work up (Masdeu et al 1997, Bednarik et al 2004).

Myelopathic changes either occur after a prolonged bout of spondylitic changes or after trauma in those patients with relatively recent degenerative changes. Most patients are older, have experienced range of motion limitations, pain with selected positions such as end range rotation and extension, and routinely have had bouts of radiculopathy in the past (Bednarik et al 2004). In fact, the strongest predictor of future myelopathy is a history of radiculopathy (Bednarik et al 2004).

Sensory changes are inconsistent and generally occur later more so than early, and in the upper extremities more than the lower extremities (Masdeu et al 1997). Initial symptoms in milder cases can start with hand clumsiness or numbness, which may be unilateral at first, before gait abnormalities are noted (Masdeu et al 1997, Polston 2007). Hand clumsiness or numbness involves less sensory loss than motor dysfunction and is, in essence, an apraxia of the distal upper extremities and hands (Good et al 1984). Diminished vibration sense is often seen in the lower extremities (Masdeu et al 1997).

Other symptoms may include decreased appreciation of pain, hot, or cold (Brown et al 2009), decreased response to sharp or dull, and restless legs (Brown et al 2009). Long-term cases may involve wasting or fasciculations of the biceps (Harrop et al 2007). In very rare cases, bowel and bladder disturbances may occur. Presence of urinary retention, dribbling incontinence or faecal incontinence should raise concern of a condition outside of myelopathy such as cauda equina syndrome (Masdeu et al 1997).

Outcomes measures

There are a number of clinician-scored outcomes for myelopathy represented in the literature. The oldest is the Nurick-score consisting of five definitive explanations of the effects of the condition, and is scored from 0 to 5 (0 representing root involvement but no evidence of spinal cord disease, 5 representing chair bound or bedridden status). The Nurick-score suffers from a lack of responsiveness as each grade reflects substantial jumps in clinical condition (Nurick 1972).

The most used appears to be the Japanese Orthopaedic Association Score (JOA), which is effective at measuring changes in patients' conditions (Vitzhum & Dalitz 2007). The JOA is a disease-specific, physician-oriented

scale designed to assess the neurological status of a patient and allows surgeons to measure pre- and post-intervention changes (Dalitz & Vitzhum 2008). The scale involves a number of constructs including scoring of feeding, upper extremity shoulder and elbow function, lower extremity gait capabilities, sensory involvements, and bowel and bladder control (Dalitz & Vitzhum 2008).

The European Myelopathy Score (EMS) is a disease-specific, physician oriented scale that involves a number of constructs including gait function, walking dysfunction, climbing stairs, bladder and bowel function, handwriting, eating, and dressing, and activities associated with sensory losses and proprioception (Vitzhum & Dalitz 2007). The scale is more sensitive to change than the JOA and the Nurick but is not routinely used in clinical practice.

Physical examination

a) *Observation*: Diagnosis of myelopathy is challenging, particularly in the early stages of the condition, as symptoms may present as hyper-reflexia (MacFadyen 1984, Polston 2007), clumsiness in gait (Matsuda et al 1991, Bednarik et al 2004), neck stiffness (Montgomery & Brower 1992, Chiles et al 1999), shoulder pain (Lev et al 2001), paraesthesia in 1 or both arms or hands (Good et al 1984), or radiculopathic signs (Nurick 1972, Montgomery & Brower 1992).

b) *Active and passive movements*: Both active and passive neck movements are often limited, specifically rotation, side flexion, and extension. Range of motion loss in the upper extremity is inconsistently found. Symptoms may or may not be reproduced during movements. In some cases, extension triggers neurological symptoms down the thoracic spine but this condition typically only occurs in patients with chronic spondylar changes.

c) *Gait symptoms* associated with myelopathy are slow and progressive. Symptoms may involve difficulty in initiating movements, walking briskly, and tendencies to trip (Masdeu et al 1997). Other gait changes include development of paraparesis described as heaviness of legs, trembling and cramping of thigh and calf muscles, and difficulty negotiating steps, curbs, and getting in and out of vehicles (Masdeu et al 1997).

d) *Clinical tests* such as single leg stance, tandem walking, and basic coordination exercises will be challenges to patients with myelopathy. A test referred to as the head shake and gait involves having the patient attempt to walk a straight line while moving one's head up and down (as if shaking one's head in agreement). In patients with spondylitic bars, the friction of the cord during the movements often facilitates the challenges in normal gait and coordination.

In some occasions, symptoms may include hyper-reflexia, which in severe cases may involve bilateral clonus and extensor plantar reflexes. Pathological reflexes are generally only present in long standing, chronic degenerative conditions (Brown et al 2009). Upper extremity reflex changes are less consistent and are often dependent on the site of structural impairment (Masdeu et al 1997). Higher level cervical involvement can cause hyper-reflexia throughout the upper and lower extremities. Mid or lower levels of cervical involvement may result in hyporeflexia (radicular symptoms) at the levels above the site of the injury and hyper-reflexia below the levels.

Coordination testing such as nose to hand tests, braiding, Frenkel's, and arm rolling are often poorly performed in patients with late-stage myelopathy. Patients may overshoot targets and demonstrate poor dexterity during activities and struggle with fine motor tasks.

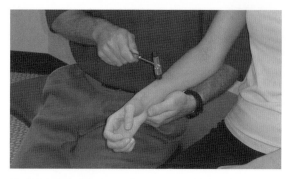

Fig 9.2 Inverted supinator sign.

Confirmation tests

The clinical examination for myelopathy includes the use of Hoffmann's test (Emery et al 1998, Cook et al 2007, 2009), deep tendon reflex testing (Denno & Meadows 1991, Cook et al 2007, 2009), inverted supinator sign (Estanol & Marin 1976), suprapatellar quadriceps reflex testing (de Freitas & Andre 2005), hand withdrawal reflex testing (Denno & Meadows 1991), Babinski sign (Ghosh & Pradhan 1998), and clonus (Young 2000). Nearly all of these tests are specific, versus sensitive, and are useful to rule in a suspected condition versus ruling out the condition. Despite the fact that most of these tests are routinely used to screen for myelopathy, the inherent diagnostic accuracy of each test limits the effectiveness as screens.

a) *Hoffmann's Sign* (Fig. 9.1). Hoffmann's sign consists of involuntary flexion of a varied combination of the neighbouring fingers and/or thumb, and is commonly used to detect an upper motor neuron dysfunction (Emery et al 1998). The test is performed by stabilizing the middle finger proximal to the distal interphalangeal joint and striking the fingernail of the middle finger with the opposite hand. A number of studies have analysed the sensitivity and specificity of the tests and have demonstrated that the Hoffmann's sign is

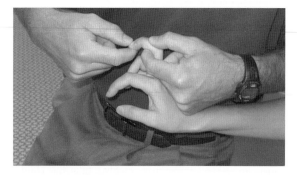

Fig 9.1 Hoffman's sign.

generally a specific test having yielded sensitivity values of 25–68% (Glaser et al 2001, Houten & Noce 2008, Cook et al 2009).

b) *Inverted Supinator Sign* (Fig. 9.2). The inverted supinator sign is a C7 response during a deep tendon reflex assessment of C6 (brachioradialis). The test is performed in the same fashion as a brachioradialis deep tendon reflex test and the response for a pathological finding involves finger flexion and/or elbow extension, versus a normal response of wrist pronation and/or elbow flexion. To our knowledge, the test has been investigated only once and demonstrated a sensitivity of 61% and a specificity of 78% (Cook et al 2009).

c) *Suprapatellar Reflex Test*. The suprapatellar reflex test involves a tapping of the quadriceps tendon just superior to the patella. A normal response involves slight knee extension, whereas an abnormal response associated with upper motor neuron problems involves an exaggerated knee extension response, a possible hip flexion response, and in some occasions internal rotation and adduction of the hip joint. The test has been investigated only once and demonstrated a sensitivity of 56%; but only a specificity of 33% (Cook et al 2009).

d) *Babinski Test*. The Babinski test involves the elicitation of an extensor toe sign during stroking of the plantar aspect of the foot. The test is more specific than sensitive, demonstrating a sensitivity of 33% (Houten & Noce 2008) and 24% in two recent studies (Cook et al 2009). Cook et al (2009) found the Babinski sign to have the best diagnostic value of all tests for confirmation providing a positive likelihood ratio of 4.0 (95% CI 1.1–16.6).

e) *Clonus Test*. Repetitive beats of 3 or more upon striking the anterior aspect of the patient's foot during sitting is associated with a positive finding of clonus. Clonus has been investigated in two studies, both of which have demonstrated poor sensitivity, 10% in Houten & Noce (2008) and 14% in Cook et al (2009).

Combinations of testing

Only one study has combined values to determine if clusters of clinical findings improve the diagnostic accuracy of the tests. Cook et al (2009) reported no improvement in post-test probability adjustments after clustering patient history factors such as clumsiness in the hands or gait problems with clinical tests such as clonus, Babinski, Hoffmanns, and others.

Cervical radiculopathy

Patient history

It is important to determine the main complaint (numbness, weakness, location of symptoms) of the subject (Wolff & Levine 2002). If pain is a complaint, a pain drawing is beneficial to establish a pattern and location of the pain. A pain drawing allows one to determine if the pain radiates and if so, the distribution of the symptoms (Honet & Puri 1976). In addition to identifying the main complaint it is important to isolate activities or head movements that trigger the concordant symptoms. One must also check for presence of concomitant symptoms such as gait changes, bowel or bladder or lower extremity conditions which are suggestive of myelopathy, and address if there were any similar episodes in the past and if any treatment was provided for the present and/or past episodes. Identifying demographic and social history such as age, sex, stress, occupation, recreational activities, and nicotine use is suggested (Honet & Puri 1976).

Outcomes measures

There are no specific outcomes measures for cervical radiculopathy. The Neck Disability Index (NDI) is the most frequently used functional outcome tool for cervical related disabilities. This outcome assessment tool was created by modifying the Oswestry Disability Index and is extremely reliable. The NDI determines the extent of disability and is designed to measure activity limitations due to neck pain and disability (Pietrobon et al 2002). The NDI has been used regularly in previous studies that have investigated functional status (Smith 1979).

Visual Analogue Scale (VAS) or a Numeric Analogue Scale is a common scale used to quantify pain and has historically been used as an outcome tool (Downie et al 1978, Langley & Sheppeard 1985). The VAS for pain in the cervical spine has a test-retest reliability of 0.95 to 0.97 (McCormick et al 2003) and MCID of 12 ± 3 mm (Kelly et al 2005). The VAS involves quantification of pain on a numbered line (0–100, the level of pain he/she is currently experiencing: 0 indicates no pain and 100 indicates the worst pain imaginable). The scale is easy to administer but lacks any dimensions other than intensity (Szpalski & Gunzburg 2001).

Physical examination

a) *Observation*: Patients with cervical radiculopathy will often hold their head away from the injurious side avoiding rotation to the offending side (Wolff & Levine 2002). In some cases, the patients may cradle their affected arm or place the arm behind or on top of their head to reduce the tension on the nerve root (Davidson et al 1981).

b) *Active and Passive Movements*: All planes of motion of the cervical spine should be assessed with active and passive movements. Active range of motion is typically decreased, specifically rotation to the offending side (Wainner et al 2003) and extension. Range of motion assessment is typically reliable and is considered a useful clinical measure (Fletcher & Bandy 2008). Responses to look for are any movements that are associated with the pain/symptoms noted during the history portion of the exam.

c) *Dermatome Testing*: Dermatome testing involves examination of motor function, sensibility changes, and deep tendon reflex modifications along a nerve root distribution. Cervical nerve roots exit above their correspondingly numbered pedicles (e.g. C6 exits between C5 and C6 vertebra), with the exception of the C8 nerve root which exits above T1. With infrequent exceptions, disc herniation or some other space offending structure at a specific site (e.g. C4–5) will affect the nerve root from that site (Rhee et al 2007).

For two primary reasons, it is important to note that absence of radiating symptoms in a dermatomal distribution does not rule out the presence of nerve root compression (Rhee et al 2007). Firstly, the presence of upper trapezius or interscapular pain may be the extent of the symptoms for that patient (Rhee et al 2007). As the condition progresses, symptoms may or may not migrate to the upper arm. Secondly, the clinical tests associated with motor testing, sensibility testing, and deep tendon reflex testing have routinely demonstrated very low sensitivity values suggesting that the clinical findings may be below the threshold of these particular tests (Cook & Hegedus 2008). The most common nerve roots affected are C5, C6, C7, C8, and T1. Specific nerve roots may demonstrate predictable patterns of motor functional losses, sensory changes, or reflex changes.

A manual muscle test is performed to identify minimal weakness along a myotome distribution to determine a local nerve root involvement. According to Yoss et al (1958), a manual muscle test offers greater specificity than either the reflex or sensory testing and single root level involvement can be diagnosed clinically 75–80% of the time. The manual muscle tests may best be initiated in a gravity induced position, testing the uninvolved limb first for a comparison of both sides. The clinician should look for subtle changes and apply the force proximal to the next distal joint (Ellenberg et al 1994, Malanga 1997). Grading of 0 to 5 is recommended as follows: 0/5 no movement; 3/5 antigravity; 5/5 normal (Honet & Puri 1976).

The grading of deep tendon reflexes (DTR) are from 0 (absent) to 4 (clonus, very brisk). Reflex abnormality is found primarily from nerve root involvement of C5 through C8 (Polston 2007, Chien et al 2008). The DTR is tested with the muscle of the tendon relaxed and the clinician applying a slight stretch to the tendon followed by tapping the tendon with a reflex hammer. Reflex abnormality of deltoid, biceps, brachioradialis is noted from C5 and C6 involvement, triceps from C7, and finger flexors from C8 (Honet & Puri 1976).

Confirmation tests

There are a few provocation tests that are typically performed when assessing for cervical radiculopathy. *Spurling's sign* combines the motions of cervical lateral bending and compression which reduces space within the foraminal area (Tsao et al 2003). The test is considered positive if symptoms of radicular pain are reproduced or worsen. According to Honet & Puri (1976) the Spurling's sign demonstrates high specificity and low sensitivity for cervical radiculopathy (Cook & Hegedus 2008) (Fig. 9.3).

The *cervical distraction test* is another test offered for cervical radiculopathy assessment. The test is performed with the patient supine and the clinician supporting the head with a chin cradle grip. The clinician applies a traction force to the cervical area (Fig. 9.4). If symptoms are reduced with this test, it is considered positive. Viikari-Junatura et al (2000) noted a specificity of 100 with a QUADAS score of 11 for ruling in cervical radiculopathy.

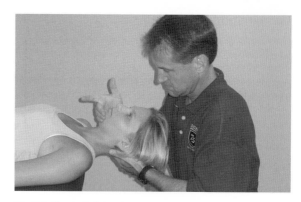

Fig 9.4 Cervical distraction test.

Another test to consider is the *Upper Limb Tension Sign* (ULTT). According to Cook & Hegedus (2008) this test is excellent as a screening test for ruling out cervical radiculopathy. The test is performed with the patient supine, forearm supinated, wrist and fingers extended. Ulnar deviation is applied. If no symptoms are reproduced the clinician then extends the elbow (Fig. 9.5). If symptoms are still not reproduced lateral flexion of the neck is performed. Reproduction of concordant, asymmetric symptoms in the distal area denotes a positive test.

Combinations of tests

Wainner et al (2003) developed a clinical prediction rule for ruling in cervical radiculopathy: the combined tests include Spurling's, ROM < 60 degrees, the cervical distraction test and ULTT. When all 4 tests are positive the specificity was 99% with a LR+ of 30.0 (QUADAS = 10).

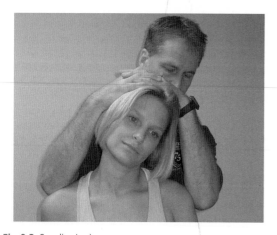

Fig 9.3 Spurling's sign.

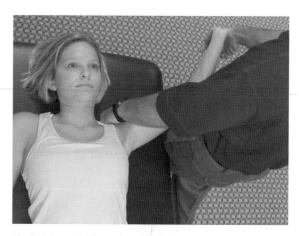

Fig 9.5 Upper limb tension sign.

Cervical myeloradiculopathy

Patient history

The most common report of symptoms include subtle neck pain, radiculitis and radicular pain in the arms and trouble with gait or coordination of the lower extremities. In chronic conditions, patients may indicate difficulty with upper extremity coordination activities as well. Most of the reported signs and symptoms are analogous to concomitant myelopathy and radiculopathy. Outside of infectious condition most myeloradiculopathic symptoms are insidious, progressive, and have a chronic presentation.

Physical examination

Positive findings may occur with stenotic movements of rotation, side flexion and extension. Most patients will exhibit problems with gait examination but typically only during higher level gait changes such as single legged stance, tandem walking and Rhomberg positions. Coordination losses may be prevalent in the lower and potentially, upper extremities, with sensation changes most common in the upper extremities.

Outcomes measures

There are no exclusive outcomes measures for myeloradiculopathy, thus the same tools used for measurement of myelopathy (e.g. Nurick scale, JOA, and European Myelopathy Scale) and radiculopathy (NDI and VAS) are used to evaluate changes in patients' conditions.

Confirmation tests

There are no dedicated clinical tests designed to identify myeloradiculopathy. Typically, the same tests used to confirm myelopathy (Hoffmann, Inverted supinator sign, suprapatellar reflex) and radiculopathy (Spurling's sign, cervical distraction test) are used in the clinical confirmation phase.

Imaging

Plain film radiograph

Plain film radiography is useful in identifying stenosis and the extensiveness of degenerative joint disease (Brown et al 2009). In addition, radiography is used to determine canal stenosis and at present, 13 millimetres of anterior-posterior (sagittal diameter) width or less is considered a risk factor in the development of myelopathy (Brown et al 2009). Nonetheless, smaller patients may have decreased diameters and this value may not be as useful as a ratio measure (Brown et al 2009).

Magnetic resonance imaging (MRI) and computed tomography (CT) scan

MRI is considered the best imaging method for myelopathy because it expresses the amount of compression placed on the spinal cord (Fukushima et al 1991), and demonstrates relatively high levels of sensitivity (79–95%) and specificity (82–88%) (LR+ = 4.39–7.92; LR− = 0.06–0.27) in identifying selected abnormalities such as space occupying tumours (Fujiwara et al 1989), disc herniation (Yousem et al 1992), and ligamentous ossification (Mizuno et al 2001). The MRI provides the ability to rule out a tumour or syrinx (fluid-filled cavity that develops in the spinal cord), and provides detailed views of the spinal cord, intervertebral disc, vertebral osteophytes and ligaments, all structures that potentially compress the spinal cord (Gross & Benzel 1999). Furthermore, MRI findings have been shown to correlate with preoperative severity of cervical compressive myelopathy and prognosis after surgery (Ono 1977, Yousem et al 1992). Patients with advanced cord changes often demonstrate poor outcomes after surgery and those with only minor compression tend to demonstrate fair recovery or retardation of progression of symptoms (Yoshimatsu et al 2001).

Changes associated with myelopathy may lead to anterior-posterior width reduction of the spinal cord, cross sectional evidence of cord compression, or obliteration of the sub-arachnoid space (Fukushima et al 1991). At present, there are no definitive objective findings on MRI consistently described by radiologists that are reflective of myelopathy with the exception of myelomalacia (identified through signal intensity changes to the cord). Signal intensity changes have been described as the most appropriate 'gold standard' for confirmation of a spinal cord compression myelopathy (Fukushima et al 1991), but are also only present in advanced chronic cases (Fig. 9.6).

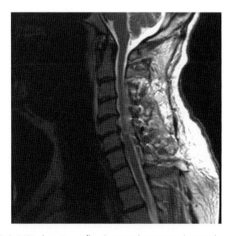

Fig 9.6 MRI changes reflecting cord compression and myelomalacia.

MRI findings are not conclusively indicative of cervical myelopathy (Bednarik et al 2004). Cord related changes and subsequent symptoms from cervical myelopathy overlap other types of intrinsic myelopathy, e.g. multiple sclerosis, syrinx or amyotrophic lateral sclerosis. Careful screening of the MRI, including the presence of T2 weighted changes, is crucial to show clear, relevant, spinal cord compression (Jeffreys 2007). False positives are common as cord compression alone does not directly equate to clinical signs and symptoms (Estanol & Marin 1976). Diagnosis is usually made from a detailed history of progressive patient symptoms, weakness and hyper-reflexia on examination, and clear compression of the spinal cord at an appropriate symptomatic level on the MRI scan, with or without T2 changes. Since T2 MRI changes usually do not abate with surgery (Wada et al 1999), these changes are more indicative of damage rather than reversible ischemia. A dedicated criterion standard, such as the singular use of an MRI scan used to determine myelopathy does not exist (Sung & Wang 2001).

The MRI has demonstrated superiority in identification of a herniated nucleus pulposis (Wilmink 2001) and structural changes from spondylosis (Wilmink 2001). The MRI has demonstrated comparable findings with myelography and cervical radiculopathy-myelography (Larsson et al 1989) but may exhibit limitations in identifying the extent of root compression (Barlett et al 1996).

It is difficult to differentiate a soft and a hard disc herniation through imaging methods (Rhee et al 2007). Specificity of the MRI for nerve root compression is suspect, identifying abnormal findings in 10% of subjects who were asymptomatic (Boden et al 1990). Sensitivity of an MRI is very good (Birchall et al 2003). Significant compression can occur before one sees changes clinically (Birchall et al 2003).

As a whole, the most compelling findings are associated with complete occlusion of the entrance to the intervertebral foreman by a laterally migrated mass on MRI followed by narrowing of a foramen by osteophytes (may only cause nerve root swelling). Poorest association includes disc herniation because the nerve root can often move out of the way of the offending intruder (Birchall et al 2003).

Computed tomography (CT) is less commonly used in assessment of the extent of degenerative of the cervical spine. Although CT is less costly and is faster and more reliable, it does have significant limitations in detection of both cervical radiculopathy and myelopathy. The inherent low-contrast resolution during assessment of soft tissue obviates the need for a CT myelography, which is troublesome when dealing with small disc herniations or limited intrusion into the intervertebral foramina (Maigne & Deligne 1994).

Nerve condition responses

Aside from MRI, a neuromuscular test, such as an electromyogram/electroneurogram (EMG/ENG), is often used to differentiate cervical myelopathy from carpal tunnel syndrome, or other peripheral nerve problems. Since cervical myelopathy is an upper motor neuron syndrome, the EMG is expected to display a normal finding unless there are intervening root or peripheral nerve problems. Kang & Fan (1995) reported normal results for EMG in 100% of patients diagnosed with cervical myelopathy. Evoked potentials have demonstrated the greatest assistance with the diagnosis of cervical myelopathy. Motor evoked potentials have a reported 70% sensitivity in the upper extremity muscles and 95% sensitivity for muscles of the lower extremity for the diagnosis of cervical myelopathy (De Mattei et al 1993). From an electrodiagnostic standpoint, the use of sensory evoked potentials (SEP) have demonstrated superior diagnostic ability as Kang & Fan (1995) reported abnormal SEP in 19/20 patients diagnosed with cervical myelopathy.

Tests of nerve condition responses such as electromyography (EMG) and nerve conduction studies (often abbreviated to NCV, V for velocity) tests are occasionally used to differentiate radiculopathy for peripheral entrapment disorders (Rhee et al 2007). Because of limitations in nerve condition testing, the MRI has supplanted nerve condition responses as the tool of choice (Polston 2007). For example, of the cervical spinal nerves, only C4–C8 has limb representation that allows differentiation (Truumees & Herkowitz 2000). In addition, results of the tests may vary considerably depending on the age of the lesion, the segmental level analysed, and the diagnostic application of the test (Polston 2007).

EMG is an electrical recording of muscle activity and involves insertion of a fine needle into the tested muscle. In order to diagnose with an EMG the reading must be abnormal for two or more different muscles and peripheral nerves from the same nerve root (Durrant & True 2002). The EMG is considered a useful diagnostic tool for cervical radiculopathy (Durrant & True 2002). Two recordings are taken, one at rest and one during a contraction. A normal response involves only brief EMG activity during needle insertion, then no activity when the muscle is at rest. During contraction, motor unit action potentials that reflect electrical activity within the muscle appears on the recording screen with corresponding increases as more muscle fibres are solicited.

Abnormal responses exhibit electrical activity at rest, alterations in the pattern of firing activity and decreases in amplitude and duration of the spikes on the recording screen. The findings may demonstrate contractions of other muscles (compensatory) and poor recruitment in nerve related disorders such as radiculopathy. Concentric needle EMG testing has demonstrated sensitivities of 50–93% and appears to be the best and most widely accepted method of electrodiagnostic testing (Prahlow & Buschbacher 2003).

A NCV consists of stimulation of the nerve and recording of the evoked potential, either from the muscles, or from the nerve (to study the sensory response). NCV assesses the extent of axonal loss of large myelinated nerve fibre (Cook et al 2009). The test involves measurement of the time delay between stimulation and response at two stimulation sites with a calculation of the distance of the sites (Smith 1979).

The two late responses most commonly analysed include the H-reflex and the F-wave. The H-reflex (Hoffmann's reflex) assesses an afferent 1a sensory nerve and an efferent alpha motor nerve. The F-wave analyses motor nerves only and is often normal in patients who have suspected radiculopathy. Because of a propensity for poor sensitivity, NCV tests should never be used in isolation (Rhee et al 2007).

Selective diagnostic nerve root block (SNRB) is a test to identify if a specific nerve root is causing the patient's pain. The test is considered sensitive and specific for radiculopathy (Malanga 1997).

ESSENTIAL ASPECTS OF DIFFERENTIAL DIAGNOSIS

Two definitive elements of differential diagnosis are necessary. Firstly, one must rule out the presence of red flags such as fever, chills, history of cancer, intravenous drug use, and other sinister conditions. Secondly, infectious conditions such as schistosomiasis will have a rapid onset (uncharacteristic of spondylotic causes) and may progress toward quicker debilitation. Cervical myelopathy requires differentiation from a number of other conditions including amyotrophic lateral sclerosis, multiple sclerosis, spinal cord tumours, and cerebrovascular disease (Brown et al 2009). In some cases, viral diseases can cause spinal cord degeneration. The most difficult differential diagnosis is when both radicular and myelopathic changes are present (Table 9.1).

Table 9.1 Differentiation of referred pain characteristics

Characteristic	Radiculopathy	Myelopathy	Somatic referred pain	Visceral pain
Axial Distribution	+	+	+	+
Upper Extremity Muscle Weakness	+	+	−	−
Lower Extremity Muscle Weakness	+	+	−	−
Upper Extremity Sensory Disturbance	+	+	−	−
Lower Extremity Sensory Disturbance	+	+	−	−
Clumsiness	−	+	−	−
Gait Disturbance	+ or −	+	−	−
Spurling's Sign	+	−	+ or −	−
Sensory Deficit	+ or −	+ or −	−	−
Loss of Vibratory Sense	−	Yes (LE)	−	−
Tendon Reflex Changes	Diminished + or −	Increased	−	−
Muscle Wasting	Unilateral + or −	Bilateral	−	−
Babinski Sign	−	+	−	−
Hoffman's Sign	−	+	−	−
Muscle Tone	Normal	Increased	Normal	Normal
Limb Tension Test	+	+ or −	−	−

CURRENT BEST EVIDENCE WITH REGARD TO PROGNOSIS

Prognosis for myelopathy and myeloradiculopathy without surgical intervention is mixed. Generally, it is assumed that the condition, which is a progressive degenerative process, will result in continuing worse outcomes over time. However, a number of subjects with mild cases of cord compression who do not receive prophylactic surgery do not decline and maintain their current level of function (Matsumoto et al 2000).

There is limited research on the prognosis of cervical radiculopathy. Most authors indicate that about two-thirds of conditions of cervical radiculopathy resolve with conservative care (Lees & Turner 1963). Some authors note that due to the benign course of cervical radiculopathy, with up to 75% rate of natural recovery, conservative care is the recommended treatment initially (Polston 2007). A long-term follow up study of 51 subjects with cervical radiculopathy who were treated conservatively showed that 45% had one episode of pain and 30% had mild symptoms (Lees & Turner 1963).

CURRENT BEST EVIDENCE WITH REGARD TO TREATMENT

Conservative approaches

Myelopathy

Conservative management including treatment of pain, limb mobility, treatment of gait impairments and reduction of risk of falls may be appropriate for a number of patients because myelopathy may exhibit only minor impairment with no progression (Matsumoto et al 2000). Initially, immobilization of the cervical spine with a collar is used to stabilize the spine in neutral or slight flexion. While some evidence exists for the effective treatment of early myelopathic changes via conservative physical therapy interventions (traction and thoracic manipulation) (Browder et al 2004, Murphy et al 2006), conclusive evidence for the effectiveness of surgical intervention for myelopathy suggests that surgery should be pursued when symptoms are progressive and destructive (Fujiwara et al 1989). Conservative care has been shown beneficial in 30–50% of patients (McCormick et al 2003).

Treatment after surgical intervention may include strengthening weakened areas, gait training, and proprioceptive exercises. At present, there is no literature that supports or refutes the use of conservative rehabilitation after surgical management of myelopathy.

Radiculopathy

A stepwise approach addressing predominant signs and symptoms of cervical radiculopathy is usually used. Typically, during the acute stage of cervical radiculopathy the treatment should aim at reducing inflammation and pain, patient education, and avoidance of increasing any neurological deficits. Treatment for inflammation and pain may include ice, heat, NSAIDS, analgesics, rest, possible immobilization, and traction.

A recent derivation clinical prediction rule was developed that outlined patients with neck pain who were most likely to benefit from a concomitant program of cervical traction and exercise (Raney et al 2009). The study identified: (1) a positive abduction test, (2) peripheralization of symptoms, (3) a positive upper limb tension test, (4) a positive neck distraction test, and (5) age $\geqq$ 55 years. Although the authors reported an increase in post-test probability of improvement to 94.8% when four of five variables were present, one must use caution as the findings demonstrated very wide confidence intervals (2.5–227.9).

There is no evidence that immobilization via a cervical collar/brace will reduce the duration or severity of cervical radiculopathy (Naylor 1979). If immobilization is administered, the timeframe should be limited to 1–2 weeks due to the negative effects from long-term immobilization. Limited evidence is available to support traction as an early intervention. A recent randomized clinical trial by Young et al (2009) reported no significant differences between two patient groups classified with cervical radiculopathy when evaluating the effectiveness of mechanical cervical traction. Jensen & Harms-Ringdahl (2007) found that when comparing acute and chronic neck pain interventions, range of motion had the strongest evidence in reducing pain in the acute phase, and combined physical agents for acute and chronic pain reduction.

Patient education should address the cause of the pain, activity modification to improve or reduce further progression of the symptoms. Patients showed reduction in pain and increased patient satisfaction when instructed on an individual home exercise program compared to written information (Jensen & Harms-Ringdahl 2007). Patients should have a home programme of stretching and strengthening once the radiculopathy symptoms have resolved.

During subacute management physical therapy is typically prescribed. Modalities such as heat, ice, massage, ultrasound, and electrical stimulation are not verified in the literature for long-term benefits but have shown some benefit in uncontrolled studies (Rhee et al 2007). These modalities are typically administered to address muscle pain and spasm. Once the patient's pain and inflammation are reduced, a progression by physical therapy to address ROM, flexibility, and strength is initiated. Strengthening exercises include isometrics of the cervical muscles and isotonics for stabilization of the scapular region, which includes the trapezius, rhomboids, serratus anterior, and latissimus dorsi (Malanga 1997). Progression to resistive exercises is appropriate as long as the patient's symptoms are not aggravated. The literature also encourages continued aerobic exercise throughout the course of rehabilitation to reduce overall de-conditioning (Malanga 1997, Tsao et al 2003).

Steroid injection is a common intervention in patients with cervical radiculopathy for reduction of inflammation despite only a few randomized clinical trials to support the efficacy of the approach (Polston 2007). The injections are often offered when a patient is not responding to a course of conservative treatment including meds, rest, and physical therapy. Studies that have been performed show a positive outcome of up to 60% for long-term relief (Malanga 1997).

Myeloradiculopathy

At present, conservative treatment for myeloradiculopathy includes palliative care, gait training by physical therapists, and range of motion and strengthening exercises to retard the progression of the degenerative changes. There is a dearth of evidence to support conservative care for this condition as most patients receive surgical intervention.

Surgical approaches

Surgical approaches are aimed at removing the offending compressive disorders from the nerve and decompressing the cord to allow the cord to move without friction and further damage (Frank 1993). In order to decide which surgical approach to use, surgeons must consider lesion location (Witwer & Trost 2007), the number of levels involved (Witwer & Trost 2007), the specific pathology (Witwer & Trost 2007), patient age, neurological function and cervical alignment (Heller et al 2001), radiographic imaging (Witwer & Trost 2007) as well as an individual surgeon's familiarity with technique (Heller et al 2001).

Surgical treatment has been shown to retard the effects of cervical myelopathy when caught in an expeditious manner (Fujiwara et al 1989). A number of factors can influence the outcome of surgery, most notably, chronicity of symptoms (Matsumoto et al 2000), whether radiculopathy is also present with myelopathy (Shamji et al 2009), and age and integrity of the spine (Fujiwara et al 1989). In addition, the type of surgical approach is often selected based on the symptoms at hand. All surgeries involve some element of decompression of the spinal canal and may involve an anterior or posterior approach (McCormick et al 2003). At present, a series of trials has failed to prove the superiority of one versus the other although short-term complications are higher in patients who receive posterior approaches (Cybulski & D'Angelo 1988).

It is important to note that in some occasions, continued neurological deterioration can occur after surgery secondary to ischaemia (Smith-Hammond et al 2004). This condition is a diagnosis of exclusion (once hematoma and dislocation is ruled out) and has a gradual but damaging progression.

Anterior approaches

Anterior surgery is performed for unilateral/bilateral radiculopathy or myelopathy when there is a single dominant cervical level or in the face of kyphosis. Anterior fusion is considerably more common but is associated with increased operative time and use of instrumentation (Iwasaki et al 2007).

Generally, anterior decompression and fusion is performed when one or two levels of cervical myelopathy are present (Cybulski & D'Angelo 1988). The approach generally involves an anterior osteophysectomy and removal of the vertebral bodies. One significant benefit of this approach is that further formation of anterior and posterior bony spurs should no longer occur, spurs present may actually regress, and since the segment is distracted during the surgery, the buckling of the ligamentum flavum is improved (Masaki et al 2007).

The procedure involves a transverse (1 or 2 levels) or vertical (multiple levels) anterior approach following the anterior border of the sternocleidomastoid muscle. The discs are removed and replaced typically, with a bone intradisc transplant. In most cases, anterior plating is provided to reduce the risk of nonunion. The approach is considered useful when addressing the vascular elements associated with myelopathy and may reduce scar formations associated with a posterior approach (Masaki et al 2007).

The success rate for anterior decompression and fusion is very high (90%) (Masaki et al 2007) and complications are generally low (Cybulski & D'Angelo 1988). Many have promoted the use of anterior fusion versus laminectomy or laminoplasty indicating it results in fewer complications, vascular damage, and less osteophyte growth (Masaki et al 2007). Furthermore, an anterior approach may be preferred over a posterior approach such as laminoplasty when ossification of the posterior longitudinal ligament is prevalent (Glaser et al 2001). However, physician preference and skill-set likely dictates the selection of the surgical method to a greater extent than patient presentation and published outcomes.

Posterior approaches

Posterior surgery is preferred for deformity, multi-segmental and dorsal pathology (Witwer & Trost 2007) and in cases of severe myelopathy as it decompresses the entire relevant cervical spine, but is not preferred when there is a single dominant level or for kyphosis (Iwasaki et al 2007). When multiple levels are involved, partial removal of two or more vertebral bodies, removal of the posterior longitudinal ligament, and any remaining spurs may be necessary. Anterior approaches are not warranted when radicular symptoms are predominant.

There are two primary posterior approaches to myelopathy: laminectomy with fusion, and laminoplasty. Posterior laminectomy and fusion is indicated when cervical stenosis causes lower extremity and/or upper extremity losses of function. Complications have included nerve damage, lack of fusion, high levels of blood loss during surgery, insufficient decompression, and infection (Epstein 2003). A laminoplasty is indicated in cases of cervical stenosis, which has originated from posterior longitudinal ligament ossification, buckling of the ligamentum flavum, or structural changes within the spinal canal. The most common complications reported have included loss of range of motion, inadequate decompression, and loss of sagittal alignment (Epstein 2002). The surgical approach involves decompression of the spinal cord posteriorly by enlarging the spinal canal but retaining the laminae. A laminoplasty is not considered superior to an anterior or posterior approach because it decompresses less space.

A laminoplasty involves one of two methods, the most common an open door laminoplasty. A cervical open door laminoplasty expands the diameter of the spinal canal decompressing the nerves and spinal cord. This surgery is typically performed in about two hours. During a cervical laminoplasty, an incision is performed in the back of the neck. The posterior portion of the bony spinal canal or lamina will be elevated. A portion of the thickened ligament is also removed. The spinal canal diameter will be widened, decompressing the spinal cord and nerves. The lamina will then be held in the open position using titanium miniplates.

A laminectomy and fusion approach generally involves posterior unilateral or bilateral removal of the lamina and a partial facetectomy. Candidates are patients who have adequate preservation of the cervical lordosis (minimum of 10 degrees) (Epstein 2002). Often, the decompression represents two segments above and below and is much more extensive than an anterior decompression. The procedure typically involves a posterior midline incision and dissection of the para-cervical muscles from the spinous processes between C2 and T1 (Heller et al 2001). The laminectomy requires removal of either moderate or large amounts of the facets, furthering the likelihood of instability after surgery, unless fusion is concurrently employed.

To our knowledge, there is only one study (Kaminsky et al 2004) that has retrospectively analysed outcomes for patients with myelopathy and radiculopathy and one study (Herkowitz 1988) that retrospectively compared anterior cervical fusion, posterior fusion and laminectomy, and laminoplasty. Another study (Nakano et al 1988) analysed outcomes for patients with myeloradiculopathy. At present, no studies have prospectively randomly assigned comparable patients with myelopathy for a comparison of outcomes after laminoplasty or laminectomy and fusion.

CONCLUSIONS

The diagnoses of cervical radiculopathy, myelopathy, and myeloradiculopathy are clinical and involve both clinical and imaging findings. Conservative treatment outcomes for radiculopathy are mixed, whereas conservative outcomes for myelopathy and myeloradiculopathy are currently unknown. Outcomes associated with surgery are mixed in all three diagnoses and should involve careful reflection prior to selection.

REFERENCES

Adams, R., Victor, M., 1999. Diseases of the spinal cord, peripheral nerve and muscle. In: Adam, R.D., Victor, M. (Eds.), Principles of Neurology. fifth ed. McGraw Hill Book, New York, pp. 1100–1101.

Ahn, N.U., Ahn, U.M., Ipsen, B., et al., 2007. Mechanical neck pain and cervicogenic headache. Neurosurgery 60 (Supp1. 1), S21–S27.

Albert, T.J., Murrell, S.E., 1999. Surgical management of cervical radiculopathy. J. Am. Acad. Orthop. Surg. 7 (6), 368–376.

Anderson, H.I., Ejlertsson, G., Leden, I., et al., 1993. Chronic pain in a geographically defined population: studies of differences in age, gender, social class and pain localisation. Clin. J. Pain 9 (3), 174–182.

Baba, H., Maezawa, Y., Uchida, K., et al., 1998. Cervical myeloradiculopathy with entrapment neuropathy: a study based on the double crush. Spinal Cord 36 (6), 399–404.

Barlett, R.J., Hill, C.A., Devlin, R., et al., 1996. Two-dimensional MRI at 1.5 and 0.5 T versus CT myelography in the diagnosis of cervical radiculopathy. Neuroradiology 38 (2), 142–147.

Bartels, R.H., Verbeek, A.L.M., Grotenhuis, J.A., 2007. Design of Lamifuse: a randomized, multi-centre controlled trial comparing laminectomy without or with doral fusion for cervical myeloradiculopathy. BMC Musculoskelet. Disord. 8, 111.

Bednarik, J., Kadanak, Z., Dusek, L., et al., 2004. Presymptomatic spondylotic cervical cord compression. Spine 29 (20), 2260–2269.

Binder, A.I., 2007. Cervical spondylosis and neck pain. Br. Med. J. 334 (7592), 527–531.

Birchall, D., Connelly, D., Walker, L., et al., 2003. Evaluation of magnetic resonance myelography in the investigation of cervical spondylotic radiculopathy. Br. J. Radiol. 76 (908), 525–531.

Boden, S.D., McCowin, P.R., Davis, D. O., et al., 1990. Abnormal magnetic-resonance scans of the cervical spine in asymptomatic subjects: a prospective investigation. J. Bone Joint Surg. Am. 72 (8), 1178–1184.

Bovim, G., Schrader, H., Sand, T., 1994. Neck pain in the general population. Spine 19 (12), 1307–1309.

Brattberg, G., Thorslund, M., Wikman, A., 1989. The prevalence of pain in a general population: the results of a postal survey in a county of Sweden. Pain 37 (2), 215–222.

Breig, A., 1978. Adverse mechanical tension in the central nervous system: an analysis of cause and effect, relief by functional neurosurgery. John Wiley, Stockholm.

Browder, D.A., Erhard, R.E., Piva, S.R., 2004. Intermittent cervical traction and thoracic manipulation for management of mild cervical compressive myelopathy attributed to cervical herniated disc: a case series. J. Orthop. Sports Phys. Ther. 34 (11), 701–712.

Brown, S., Guthmann, R., Hitchcock, K., et al., 2009. Clinical inquiries: which treatments are effective for cervical radiculopathy? J. Fam. Pract. 58 (2), 97–99.

Brown, P.J., Marino, R.J., Herbison, G.J., et al., 1991. The 72-hour examination as a predictor of recovery in motor complete quadriplegia. Arch. Phys. Med. Rehabil. 72, 546–548.

Chiles 3rd, B.W., Leonard, M.A., Choudhri, H.F., et al., 1999. Cervical spondylotic myelopathy: patterns of neurological deficit and recovery after anterior cervical decompression. Neurosurgery 44 (4), 762–770.

Chien, A., Eliav, E., Sterling, M., 2008. Whiplash (grade II) and cervical radiculopathy share a similar sensory presentation: an investigation using quantitative sensory testing. Clin. J. Pain 24 (7), 595–603.

Cook, C., 2006. Orthopedic manual therapy: an evidence based approach. Prentice Hall, Upper Saddle River, NJ.

Cook, C., Hegedus, E., 2008. Orthopedic physical examination tests: an evidence based approach. Prentice Hall, Upper Saddle River, NJ.

Cook, C.E., Hegedus, E., Pietrobon, R., et al., 2007. A pragmatic neurological screen for patients with suspected cord compressive myelopathy. Phys. Ther. 87 (9), 1233–1242.

Cook, C., Roman, M., Stewart, K., et al., 2009. Reliability and diagnostic accuracy of clinical special tests for myelopathy in patients seen for cervical dysfunction. J. Orthop. Sports Phys. Ther. 39 (3), 172–178.

Cote, P., Cassidy, L., Carroll, L., 1998. The Saskatchewan Health and Back Pain Survey: the prevalence of neck pain and related disability in Saskatchewan adults. Spine 23 (15), 1689–1698.

Crandall, P.H., Batzdorf, U., 1966. Cervical spondylotic myelopathy. J. Neurosurg. 25 (1), 57–66.

Cybulski, G.R., D'Angelo, C.M., 1988. Neurological deterioration after laminectomy for spondylotic cervical myeloradiculopathy: the putative role of spinal cord ischaemia. J. Neurol. Neurosurg. Psychiatry 51 (5), 717–718.

Dalitz, K., Vitzhum, H.E., 2008. Evaluation of five scoring systems for cervical spondylogenic myelopathy. Spine J. Sep 5 [Epub ahead of print].

Davidson, R., Dunn, E., Metzmaker, J., 1981. The shoulder abduction test in the diagnosis of radicular pain in cervical extradural compression monoradiculopathies. Spine 6 (5), 441–445.

de Freitas, G.R., Andre, C., 2005. Absence of the Babinski sign in brain death: a prospective study of 144 cases. J. Neurol. 252 (1), 106–107.

De Mattei, M., Paschero, B., Sciarretta, A., et al., 1993. Usefulness of motor evoked potentials in compressive myelopathy. Electromyogr. Clin. Neurophysiol. 33 (4), 205–216.

Denno, J.J., Meadows, G.R., 1991. Early diagnosis of cervical spondylotic myelopathy: a useful clinical sign. Spine 16 (12), 1353–1355.

Downie, W.W., Leatham, P.A., Rhind, V. M., et al., 1978. Studies with pain rating scales. Ann. Rheum. Dis. 37 (4), 378–381.

Durrant, D.H., True, J.M., 2002. Myelopathy, radiculopathy, and peripheral entrapment syndromes. CRC, London.

Dvorak, J., 1998. Epidemiology, physical examination, and neurodiagnostics. Spine 23 (24), 2663–2673.

Ellenberg, M.R., Honet, J.C., Treanor, W. J., 1994. Cervical radiculopathy. Arch. Phys. Med. Rehabil. 75 (3), 342–352.

Emery, S.E., Bohlman, H.H., Bolesta, M. J., 1998. Anterior cervical decompression and arthrodesis for the treatment of cervical spondylotic myelopathy: two to seventeen-year follow-up. J. Bone Joint Surg. 80A (7), 941–951.

Epstein, N., 2003. Laminectomy for cervical myelopathy. Spinal Cord 41 (6), 317–327.

Epstein, N., 2002. Posterior approaches in the management of cervical spondylosis and ossification of the posterior longitudinal ligament. Surg. Neurol. 58 (3–4), 194–208.

Estanol, B.V., Marin, O.S., 1976. Mechanism of the inverted supinator reflex: a clinical and neurophysiological study. J. Neurol. Neurosurg. Psychiatry 39, 905–908.

Fletcher, J.P., Bandy, W.D., 2008. Intrarater reliability of CROM measurement of cervical spine active range of motion in persons with and without neck pain. J. Orthop. Sports Phys. Ther. 38 (10), 640–645.

Frank, E., 1993. Approaches to myeloradiculopathy. West. J. Med. 158 (1), 71–72.

Fujiwara, K., Yonenobu, K., Ebara, S., et al., 1989. The prognosis of surgery for cervical compression myelopathy – an analysis of the factors involved. J. Bone Joint Surg. Br. 71 (3), 393–398.

Fukushima, T., Ikata, T., Taoka, Y., et al., 1991. Magnetic resonance imaging study on spinal cord plasticity in patients with cervical compression myelopathy. Spine 16 (Suppl. 10), S534–S538.

Ghosh, D., Pradhan, S., 1998. 'Extensor toe sign' by various methods in spastic children with cerebral palsy. J. Child Neurol. 13 (5), 216–220.

Glaser, J.A., Cure, J.K., Bailey, K.L., et al., 2001. Cervical spinal cord compression and the Hoffmann sign. Iowa Orthop. J. 21, 49–52.

Good, D.C., Couch, J.R., Wacaser, L., 1984. Numb, clumsy hands' and high cervical spondylosis. Surg. Neurol. 22 (3), 285–291.

Gross, J., Benzel, E., 1999. Camins, M.D. (Ed.), Techniques in neurosurgery. Lippincott Williams & Wilkins, Philadelphia, pp. 162–176.

Harrop, J.S., Hanna, A., Silva, M.T., et al., 2007. Neurological manifestations of cervical spondylosis: an overview of signs, symptoms and pathophysiology. Neurosurgery 60 (1 Suppl. 1), S14–S20.

Hawkes, C., 2002. Smart handles and red flags in neurological diagnosis. Hosp. Med. 63 (12), 732–742.

Heller, J.G., Edwards, C., Murakami, H., et al., 2001. Laminoplasty versus laminectomy and fusion for multilevel cervical myelopathy. Spine 26 (12), 1330–1336.

Henderson, C.M., Hennessy, R.G., Shuey, H.M., et al., 1983. Posterior-lateral foraminotomy as an exclusive operative technique for cervical radiculopathy: a review of 846 consecutively operated cases. Neurosurgery 13 (5), 504–512.

Herkowitz, H.N., 1988. A comparison of anterior cervical fusion, cervical laminectomy, and cervical laminoplasty for the surgical management of multiple level spondylotic radiculopathy. Spine 13 (7), 774–780.

Honet, J.C., Puri, K., 1976. Cervical radiculitis: treatment and results in 82 patients. Arch. Phys. Med. Rehabil. 57 (1), 12–16.

Houten, J.K., Noce, L.A., 2008. Clinical signs of cervical myelopathy and the Hoffmann sign. J. Neurosurg. Spine 9 (3), 237–242.

Ito, S., Panjabi, M.M., Ivancic, P.C., et al., 2004. Spinal canal narrowing during simulated whiplash. Spine 29 (12), 1330–1339.

Iwasaki, M., Okuda, S., Miyauchi, A., et al., 2007. Surgical strategy for cervical myelopathy due to ossification of the posterior longitudinal ligament. Part 2: advantages of anterior decompression and fusion over laminoplasty. Spine 32 (6), 654–660.

Jayakumar, P.N., Kolluri, V.R., Vasudev, M.K., et al., 1996. Ossification of the posterior longitudinal ligament of the cervical spine in Asian Indians: a multiracial comparison. Clin. Neurol. Neurosurg. 98 (2), 142–148.

Jeffreys, E., 2007. Disorders of the cervical spine. Butterworth, London.

Jensen, I., Harms-Ringdahl, K., 2007. Strategies for prevention and management of musculoskeletal conditions: neck pain. Best Pract. Res. Clin. Rheumatol. 21 (1), 93–108.

Kaminsky, S.B., Clark, C.R., Traynelis, V. C., 2004. Operative treatment of cervical spondylotic myelopathy and radiculopathy: a comparison of laminectomy and laminoplasty at five year average follow up. Iowa Orthop. J. 24, 95–105.

Kang, D.X., Fan, D.S., 1995. The electrophysiological study of differential diagnosis between amyotrophic lateral sclerosis and cervical spondylotic myelopathy. Electromyogr. Clin. Neurophysiol. 35 (4), 231–238.

Kelly, K.G., Cook, T., Backonja, M.M., 2005. Pain ratings at the thresholds are necessary for interpretation of quantitative sensory testing. Muscle Nerve 32 (2), 179–184.

Lambertucci, J.R., Voieta, I., Silveira Idos, S., 2008. Cerebral schistosomiasis mansoni. Rev. Soc. Bras. Med. Trop. 41 (6), 693–694.

Langley, G.B., Sheppeard, H., 1985. The visual analogue scale: its use in pain measurement. Rheumatol. Int. 5 (4), 145–148.

Larsson, E.M., Holtås, S., Cronqvist, S., et al., 1989. Comparison of myelography, CT myelography and magnetic resonance imaging in cervical spondylosis and disk herniation: pre- and postoperative findings. Acta Radiol. 30 (3), 233–239.

Lees, F., Turner, J.W., 1963. Natural history and prognosis of cervical spondylosis. Br. Med. J. 2 (5373), 1607–1610.

Lev, N., Maimon, S., Rappaport, Z.H., et al., 2001. Spinal dural arteriovenous fistulae: a diagnostic challenge. Isr. Med. Assoc. J. 3 (7), 492–496.

Lewis, P.B., Rue, J.P., Byrne, R., et al., 2008. Cervical syrinx as a cause of shoulder pain in 2 athletes. Am. J. Sports Med. 36 (1), 169–172.

MacFadyen, D.J., 1984. Posterior column dysfunction in cervical spondylotic myelopathy. Can. J. Neurol. Sci. 11 (3), 365–370.

Maigne, J.Y., Deligne, L., 1994. Computed tomographic follow-up study of 21 cases of nonoperatively treated cervical intervertebral soft disc herniation. Spine 19 (2), 189–191.

Malanga, G.A., 1997. The diagnosis and treatment of cervical radiculopathy. Med. Sci. Sports Exerc. 29 (Suppl. 7), S236–S245.

Marshall, G.L., Little, J.W., 2002. Deep tendon reflexes: a study of quantitative methods. J. Spinal Cord Med. 25 (2), 94–99.

Masaki, T., Yamazaki, M., Okawa, A., et al., 2007. An analysis of factors causing poor surgical outcome in patients with cervical myelopathy due to ossification of the posterior longitudinal ligament: anterior decompression with spinal fusion versus laminoplasty. J. Spinal Disord. Tech. 20 (1), 7–13.

Masdeu, J.C., Sudarsky, L., Wolfson, L., 1997. Gait disorders of aging: falls and therapeutic strategies. Lippincott-Raven, Philadelphia.

Matsuda, Y., Miyazaki, K., Tada, K., et al., 1991. Increased MR signal intensity due to cervical myelopathy: analysis of 29 surgical cases. J. Neurosurg. 74 (6), 887–892.

Matsumoto, M., Toyama, Y., Ishikawa, M., et al., 2000. Increased signal intensity of the spinal cord on magnetic resonance images in cervical compressive myelopathy: does it predict the outcome of conservative treatment? Spine 25 (6), 677–682.

McCormick, W.E., Steinmetz, M.P., Benzel, E.C., 2003. Cervical spondylotic myelopathy: make the difficult diagnosis, then refer for surgery. Cleve. Clin. J. Med. 70 (10), 899–904.

Mizuno, J., Nakagawa, H., Hashizume, Y., 2001. Analysis of hypertrophy of the posterior longitudinal ligament of the cervical spine, on the basis of clinical and experimental studies. Neurosurgery 49 (5), 1091–1098.

Montgomery, D.M., Brower, R.S., 1992. Cervical spondylotic myelopathy: clinical syndrome and natural history. Orthop. Clin. North Am. 23 (3), 487–493.

Muller, A., Dvorak, J., 2001. Neurological symptoms. In: Szpalski, M., Gunzburg, R. (Eds.), The degenerative cervical spine. Lippincott-Williams & Wilkins, Philadelphia.

Murphy, D.R., Hurwitz, E.L., Gregory, A. A., 2006. Manipulation in the presence of cervical spinal cord compression: a case series. J. Manipulative Physiol. Ther. 29 (3), 236–244.

Nakano, N., Nakano, T., Nakano, K., 1988. Comparison of the results of laminectomy and open-door laminoplasty for cervical spondylotic myeloradiculopathy and ossification of the posterior longitudinal ligament. Spine 13 (7), 792–794.

Naylor, A., 1979. Factors in the development of the spinal stenosis syndrome. J. Bone Joint Surg. Br. 61-B (3), 306–309.

Nurick, S., 1972. The natural history and the results of surgical treatment of the spinal cord disorder associated with cervical spondylosis. Brain 95 (1), 101–108.

Ono, K., 1977. Cervical myelopathy secondary to multiple spondylotic protrusions: a clinicopathologic study. Spine 2 (2), 125.

Pietrobon, R., Coeytaux, R.R., Carey, T. S., et al., 2002. Standard scales for measurement of functional outcome for cervical pain or dysfunction: a systematic review. Spine 7 (5), 515–522.

Polston, D.W., 2007. Cervical radiculopathy. Neurol. Clin. 25 (2), 373–385.

Pope, M.H., 2001. Cervical spine biomechanics. In: Szpalski, M., Gunzburg, R. (Eds.), The degenerative cervical spine. Lippincott-Williams & Wilkins, Philadelphia.

Prahlow, N.D., Buschbacher, R.M., 2003. An introduction to electromyography: an invited review. J. Long Term Eff. Med. Implants 13 (4), 289–307.

Radhakrishnan, K., Litchy, W.J., O'Fallon, W.M., et al., 1994. Epidemiology of cervical radiculopathy: a population-based study from Rochester, Minnesota, 1976 through 1990. Brain 117 (part 2), 325–335.

Raney, N.H., Petersen, E.J., Smith, T., et al., 2009. Development of a clinical prediction rule to identify patients with neck pain likely to benefit from cervical traction and exercise. Eur. J. Spine 18 (3), 382–391.

Rao, S., Fehlings, M.G., 1999. The optimal radiologic method of assessing spinal cord compromise and cord compression in patients with cervical spinal cord injury: Part 1: an evidence based analysis of the published literature. Spine 24 (6), 598–604.

Rhee, J.M., Yoon, T., Riew, K.D., 2007. Cervical radiculopathy. J. Am. Acad. Orthop. Surg. 15 (8), 486–494.

Shamji, M.F., Cook, C., Pietrobon, R., et al., 2009. Impact of surgical approach on complication and resource utilization of cervical spine fusion: a nationwide perspective to the surgical treatment of diffuse cervical spondylosis. Spine J. 9 (1), 31–38.

Smith, M.S., 1979. Babinski Sign – Abduction also Counts. J. Am. Med. Assoc. 242 (17), 1849–1850.

Smith-Hammond, C.A., New, K.C., Pietrobon, R., et al., 2004. Prospective analysis of incidence and risk factors of dysphagia in spine surgery patients: comparison of anterior cervical, posterior cervical, and lumbar procedures. Spine 29 (13), 1441–1446.

Sung, R.D., Wang, J.C., 2001. Correlation between a positive Hoffmann's reflex and cervical pathology in asymptomatic individuals. Spine 26 (1), 67–70.

Szpalski, M., Gunzburg, R., 2001. The degenerative cervical spine. Lippincott-Williams and Wilkins, Philadelphia.

Thongtrangan, I., Le, H., Park, J., et al., 2004. Cauda equina syndrome in patients with low lumbar fractures. Neurosurg. Focus 16 (6), e6.

Tsao, B.E., Levin, K.H., Bodner, R.A., 2003. Comparison of surgical and electrodiagnostic findings in single root lumbosacral radiculopathies. Muscle Nerve 27 (1), 60–64.

Truumees, E., Herkowitz, H.N., 2000. Cervical spondylotic myelopathy and radiculopathy. Instr. Course Lect. 49, 339–360.

Viikari Junatura, E., Takala, E., Riihimaki, H., et al., 2000. Predictive validity of signs and symptoms in the neck and shoulders. J. Clin. Epidemiol. 53 (8), 800–808.

Vitzhum, H.E., Dalitz, K., 2007. Analysis of five specific scores for cervical spondylogenic myelopathy. Eur. Spine J. 16 (12), 2096–2103.

Wada, E., Yonenobu, K., Suzuki, S., et al., 1999. Can intramedullary signal change on magnetic resonance imaging predict surgical outcome in cervical spondylotic myelopathy? Spine 24 (5), 455–462.

Wainner, R.S., Fritz, J.M., Irrgang, J., et al., 2003. Reliability and diagnostic accuracy of the clinical examination and patient self-report measures for cervical radiculopathy. Spine 28 (1), 52–62.

Wainner, R.S., Gill, H., 2000. Diagnosis and nonoperative management of cervical radiculopathy. J. Orthop. Sports Phys. Ther. 30 (12), 728–744.

Wilmink, J.T., 2001. Cervical imaging: dynamic aspects and clinical significance. In: Szpalski, M., Gunzburg, R. (Eds.), The degenerative cervical spine. Lippincott-Williams and Wilkins, Philadelphia.

Wilson, D.W., Pezzuti, R.T., Place, J.N., 1991. Magnetic resonance imaging in the preoperative evaluation of cervical radiculopathy. Neurosurgery 28 (2), 175–179.

Witwer, B.P., Trost, G.R., 2007. Cervical spondylosis: ventral or dorsal surgery. Neurosurgery 60 (1 Suppl. 1), S130–S136.

Wolff, M.W., Levine, L.A., 2002. Cervical radiculopathies: conservative approaches to management. Phys. Med. Rehabil. Clin. N. Am. 13 (3), 589–608.

Wong, T.M., Leung, H.B., Wong, W.C., 2004. Correlation between magnetic resonance imaging and radiographic measurement of cervical spine in cervical myelopathic patients. J. Orthop. Surg. (Hong Kong) 12 (2), 239–242.

Yoshimatsu, H., Nagata, K., Goto, H., et al., 2001. Conservative treatment for cervical spondylotic myelopathy: prediction of treatment effects by multivariate analysis. Spine J. 1 (4), 269–273.

Yoss, R.E., Corbin, K.B., MacCarty, C.S., et al., 1958. Significance of symptoms and signs in localization of involved root in cervical disk protrusion. Neurology 7 (10), 673–685.

Young, I.A., Michener, L.A., Cleland, J.A., et al., 2009. Manual therapy, exercise, and traction for patients with cervical radiculopathy: a randomized clinical trial. Phys. Ther. 89 (7), 632–642.

Young, W.F., 2000. Cervical spondylotic myelopathy: a common cause of spinal cord dysfunction in older persons. Am. Fam. Physician 62 (5), 1064–1073.

Yousem, D.M., Atlas, S.W., Hackney, D.B., et al., 1992. Cervical spine disc herniation: comparison of CT and 3DFT gradient echo MR scans. J. Comput. Assist. Tomogr. 16 (3), 345–351.

Chapter | **10** |

Thoracic outlet syndrome

Susan W Stralka

OVERVIEW AND HISTORY OF THORACIC OUTLET SYNDROME

Thoracic outlet syndrome (TOS) is a broad term used to describe upper extremity symptoms. These symptoms are related to compression or tension of the brachial plexus, the sub-clavian artery and vein in an area located above the first rib and behind the clavicle. Often, one patient may be seen by numerous specialists before this syndrome is identified. The anterior scalene muscle, the middle scalene muscle and the first rib, border the thoracic outlet. Pathological or dysfunction related to these structures as well as the clavicle bone, pectoralis minor, omohyoid, subclavius, scalene minimus, cervical rib or transverse process of C7 have been associated with TOS (Mackinnon 1996). These neurovascular structures in their course from the inter-scalene triangle to the axilla are covered with a fascial sheath that is part of the deep cervical fascia, which can become problematic (Atasoy 2004). Fibrous bands, both congenital and acquired, also restrict movements of the clavicle and first rib. The term TOS does not specify the compressing agent and does not identify the structure being compressed. This syndrome should be differentiated by using the term arterial TOS (ATOS), venous TOS (VTOS) or neurogenic TOS (NTOS).

Peet first used the term thoracic outlet syndrome in 1956 and indicated that compression of neurovascular

DOI: 10.1016/B978-0-7020-3528-9.00010-8

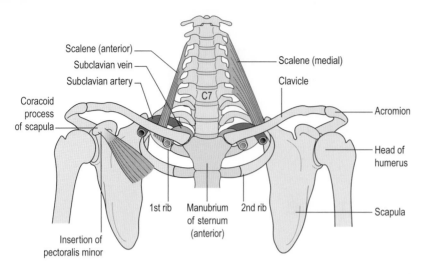

Fig 10.1 Anatomy of the thoracic outlet area.

Scalene (anterior)
Subclavian vein
Subclavian artery
Coracoid process of scapula
Scalene (medial)
Clavicle
C7
Acromion
Head of humerus
1st rib
Manubrium of sternum (anterior)
2nd rib
Scapula
Insertion of pectoralis minor

structures occur in the inter-scalene triangle causing cervical-brachial pain, numbness and other disorders of the upper extremity. He used this term to group them under only one name representing a single common element of neurovascular structures (Samarasam et al 2004). It was not until 1958, that Robb proposed the term thoracic outlet compression syndrome. The clinical signs are variable due to the variety of tissue that can be involved as well as the compression or entrapment area (Fig 10.1). Today TOS is classified into three sections: brachial plexopathy (NTOS) which occurs 90% or greater, the sub-clavian vein (VTOS) which occurs 6–7% and the sub-clavian artery (ATOS) at 3–4% (Sanders et al 2008).

Compression of the vascular system is easier to identify and presents more urgently with arterial or venous thrombosis than the symptoms with NTOS (Fugate et al 2009). The main controversy in patients with this syndrome (NTOS) relates to diagnosis. Neurological type complaints such as paraesthesia, numbness and pain must be based on interpretation of the history, symptoms or clinical examination. These symptoms make the NTOS syndrome somewhat of an enigma as some healthcare professionals tend to overdiagnose it and others underdiagnose it with or without correlating the clinical signs and symptoms.

PATHO-ANATOMICAL CAUSES OF THORACIC OUTLET SYNDROME

The thoracic outlet region includes three major areas in which compression can occur: inter-scalene space or triangle, costo-clavicular space, and sub-pectoralis minor space. Other causes are congenital bony structures, fibro-muscular anomalies, postural deviations and muscle imbalances. It has been reported that subjects who have congenital bony or fibro-muscular variations in the

thoracic outlet region and experience some type of trauma are at risk to develop TOS. Trauma can result in muscle spasm, inflammation and fibrosis, which further narrows the spaces and results in compression of the neurovascular structure (Atasoy 2004).

The incidence of a cervical rib is less than 1% and may be bilateral. The cervical rib size varies from a bony exostosis to a full grown cervical rib with ligamentous cartilaginous or bony attachment to the first rib. The female: male ratio is 2:1 (Atasoy 2004). A cervical rib or other rib anomalies cause the brachial plexus to be pulled against the fascial bands and C8–T1 symptoms can develop. A cervical rib, along with forward shoulders and poor posture, can cause pressure on the plexus and the vessels. Following a fracture of the first rib, excess callous formation can occur creating a narrow space leading to pressure on the brachial plexus and sub-clavian vessels.

Functional causes of thoracic outlet syndrome (MediFocus Guide 2009)

Poor posture, abnormal breathing patterns, cervical or thoracic dysfunctions, muscle imbalances and shoulder pathologies are commonly seen in TOS. Abnormal posture in which the head and shoulders are held in a forward position along with arm elevation greater than 90° may cause neurovascular consequences. Over time, shortening of various neck musculatures may occur which, in turn, causes posterior shoulder girdle weakness. The longus and longissimus cervicis, upper and middle rhomboids and lower trapezius become weakened. To compensate for the forward orientation of the glenoid fossa of the humerus, the serratus anterior muscle becomes shortened by abduction of the scapula. This scenario causes lengthening of the lower and middle trapezius in supporting the scapula causing a mechanical disadvantage and early fatigue. These alterations result in the upper trapezius, rhomboids major and minor muscles, along with the levator scapulae having to function as accessory muscles to elevate the shoulder and arm.

The entire cycle continues to cause weakness in some muscles and shortening of other muscles. Other functional causes, such as abduction over 110°, put tension on the median nerve causing the ancillary artery to be compressed in the bicipital groove. In the axilla, compression can be caused by a fibrous extension of the latissimus dorsi and pectoralis major muscle as they insert in the bicipital groove. With arm abduction or external rotation, the neurovascular bundle is compressed under the arch producing symptoms. There are histopathological changes that occur to a nerve undergoing chronic compression, which takes place in TOS. A thorough history, comprehensive physical examination and specific provocation test can identify the structure causing compromise as well as to help determine muscle weakness and tightness.

Entrapment sites

Inter-scalene space triangle

The neurovascular bundle which includes the brachial plexus trunks and sub-clavian vessels runs from the base of the neck towards the axilla and the arm. The first narrowing area is the most proximal and is named inter-scalene triangle. This triangle is bordered by the anterior scalene muscle anteriorly, the middle scalene muscle posteriorly, and inferiorly along with the base is the medial surface of the first rib (Atasoy 2004) (Fig 10.2).

The scalene minimus muscle, which is found in only 30–50% of TOS cases, is located between the sub-clavian artery and the T1 root of the brachial plexus which can be a source of compression. The anterior and middle scalene muscles

are respiratory muscles, which elevate the first rib as well as slightly flex and rotate the neck. The insertion of these muscles in the first rib overlaps and causes a V formation. This overlapping creates a narrow space, which causes the sub-clavian artery and the brachial plexus to be in a high position. It has been noted in some cases the middle scalene muscle inserts along the full length of the first rib creating a narrow space through which the neurovascular structures must pass. When there is overlapping of the scalene muscle, there is also a prominent transverse process of the C7 process and the cervical rib. This has often been described as a U or sling formation by these muscles. This may cause elevation and pressure from the structures below. At the proximal portion of the triangle, the scalene muscles may overlap which again causes a decrease in the opening thus causing pressure from the brachial plexus above. It has been noted that at times a thick fibrous coverage of the plexus extending from the scalene sheathe can cause adhesions and pressure on the plexus. The scalene muscles can scar or hypertrophy with trauma or repetitive motion that further contributes to compression. Some researchers have found atrophy of type II muscle fibres, predominance of type I fibres and a 25% increase in connective tissue in the scalene muscles (Sanders 1990) following injury.

Costo-clavicular space (Talu 2005)

The costo-clavicular space is a triangular area bordered anteriorly by the middle third of the clavicle, postero-medially by the first rib, and postero-laterally by the upper border of the scapula. The sub-clavian artery, vein and brachial plexus all pass through the costo-clavicular space (see Fig 10.2). Compression of the brachial plexus and the sub-clavian artery and vein can occur as the result

Fig 10.2 Three potential spaces in the thoracic outlet area that can be responsible for TOS.

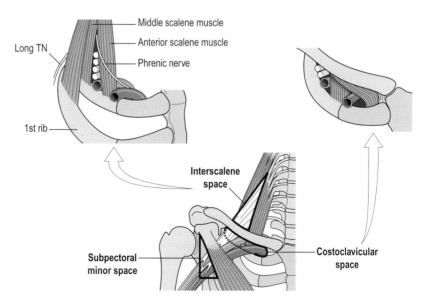

Long TN
Middle scalene muscle
Anterior scalene muscle
Phrenic nerve
1st rib
Interscalene space
Subpectoral minor space
Costoclavicular space

of congenital abnormalities, trauma to the first rib or clavicle, and structural changes in the sub-clavian muscle or the costo-coracoid ligament.

Compression can occur if the clavicle or first rib is fractured following by a hematoma occurring at the fracture site resulting in excessive scar tissue and callus build-up. As mentioned earlier, persons with forward shoulders which represents poor posture or a disabling illness, may develop narrowing of the costo-clavicular space, which has been shown to lead to TOS symptoms. With shoulder abduction, the scapula and coracoid move downward which causes traction on the subclavius muscle and costo-coracoid ligament adding additional pressure on the neurovascular structures. The clavicle, during shoulder abduction, moves backward and upward 30–35° at the sternoclavicular joint, which may add narrowing to the costo-clavicular space.

Sub-pectoralis minor space

The sub-pectoralis minor space is located just below the coracoid process and under the pectoralis minor muscle insertion to this process (see Fig. 10.2). The pectoralis minor runs from the 3rd to the 5th ribs over the thorax and ends at coracoid process. This muscle is completely covered by the pectoralis major muscle. With shortening, the pectoralis minor can lead to a narrowing in the sub-pectoralis minor space increasing pressure on the blood vessels and brachial plexus. The tight pectoralis minor muscle may also compress the neurovascular structures during hyper-abduction. Wright termed this syndrome as *hyper-abduction syndrome* which closes down the costo-clavicular space due to the up and down motion of the clavicle (Beyer & Wright 1951).

AETIOLOGY OF THORACIC OUTLET SYNDROME

TOS is 3–4 times as frequent in women as in men between the ages of 20–50 years of age (Brismee et al 2004). It is speculated that females have less developed muscles, a greater tendency for drooping shoulders due to additional breast tissue, a narrowed thoracic outlet and an anatomical lower sternum all changing the angle between scalene muscles. This may be a reason females are more prone to develop this syndrome (Hursh & Thanki 1985). Another rationale, why females are more prone to develop TOS, could be an increase in hormones that cause laxity thus resulting in superior subluxation of the first rib due to hormonal influence (Brismee et al 2004) (Table 10.1). Common symptoms collected from 17 reports are listed in Table 10.2 (Sanders & Haug 1991).

Table 10.1 Conditions causing nerve trauma (modified from Sanders & Haug 1991)

Aetiology	%
Neck trauma	86
Rear end auto accident	32
Side or front end auto accident	24
Work injury, including RSI	22
Other neck trauma	8
Cervical or anomalous first rib	2
Unknown or spontaneous	12
	100

Table 10.2 Symptoms from nerve irritation (modified from Sanders & Haug 1991)

Symptoms	%
Neck pain	92
Shoulder pain	70
Arm pain	80
Paraesthesia	95
All 5 fingers	46
Fingers 1–3	30
Fingers 4–5	14
No paraesthesia	10

CLINICAL SYMPTOMS OF THORACIC OUTLET SYNDROME (SANDERS ET AL 2008)

The term vascular TOS is non-specific and it does not imply neurogenic, arterial or venous compression, and not address what structure is involved. Historically, symptoms and physical findings are more specific. Patient typically complains of pain in the sub-scapular, scapular, cervical, cervical thoracic regions and occipital headaches. Paraesthesia and numbness may be present in the entire hand region or parts of it. Often using the arms in an elevated position exacerbates the symptoms and complaints are a heavy, tired, aching sensation along with numbness or paraesthesia.

Common clinical presentation of TOS includes:

- Numbness/tingling in ring and small finger but can encompass entire hand
- Paraesthesia occur at night and/or during daily activities
- Vague pain in the uninvolved extremity can occur in hand, elbow, shoulder and/or cervical spine
- Subjective complaints of hand/arm weakness, especially with arms raised overhead
- Subjective complaints of swelling in the absence of true swelling
- The common symptoms collected from 17 reports are listed in Table 10.2.

Neurological symptoms

TOS symptoms may develop spontaneously or following injury in the neck and/or shoulder region. A list of conditions causing nerve trauma are found in Table 10.1. Basic concepts of TOS are a mechanical predisposition (Brantigan & Roos 2004). Symptoms are primarily neurologic structural anomalies causing the problem. Trauma may precipitate the neurologic type of TOS in certain susceptible individuals. The upper plexus includes symptoms involving the C5, C6 and C7 while the lower plexus principally involves the C8–T1 levels.

When the upper plexus is involved, there is pain in the side of the neck and this pain may radiate to the ear and face. Headaches are not uncommon when the upper plexus is involved. Some patients state that on the affected side, there is a 'stuffy ear'. Often the pain radiates from the ear posteriorly to the rhomboids and anteriorly over the clavicle and pectoralis regions. The pain may move laterally to the trapezius, deltoid muscle and down the C5–C6 radial nerve area. Lower plexus patients have symptoms that present in the anterior or posterior shoulder region radiating down the ulnar side of the forearm into the hand, the ring and small finger, as well as muscle tenderness with trigger points which can be located in the supra-clavicular and infra-clavicular area. Headaches may be disabling and can increase with arm activity. At times, the pain with lower plexus involvement mimics the pain associated with cardiac angina.

Injury or repetitive stresses causing chronic muscle spasm may precipitate the syndrome. A common problem is hyperextension-flexion or whiplash injury of the neck. The TOS symptom may show up immediately or may be delayed for weeks or months. Usually cervical and shoulder sprain symptoms occur immediately after the whiplash with persisting symptoms of neck and shoulder pain and stiffness before being diagnosed as TOS (Brantigan & Roos 2004). As the whiplash symptoms

gradually improve over time, the post-traumatic TOS involving the brachial plexus worsens.

Arterial symptoms

Symptoms of ATOS usually develop spontaneously unrelated to trauma or work. These patients often have true claudication of the arm particularly when the arm is elevated. These arterial symptoms occur from compression of the sub-clavian artery in the area of the first rib. Arterial symptoms differ from the whole arm numbness and heaviness that persists when the arm is elevated in patients with neurologic TOS as well as presenting with very little shoulder or neck symptoms. Patients with arterial symptoms may have a cervical rib or an enlarged transverse process of C7 causing the problem.

Physical findings are those of arterial occlusion: loss of pulses at rest, perhaps colour changes and ischemic finger tips as well as coldness, paraesthesia and fatigue. Arterial symptoms include digital and hand ischemia symptoms (coldness, pallor, paraesthesia and fatigue of the arm). In the supra-clavicular area, there is sometimes a tender lump, bony prominence or even pulsation of the sub-clavian artery. Arterial TOS accounts for less than 5% of TOS and typically results from long-term intermittent vascular compression. A cervical x-ray is used as a screening test to rule out ATOS (Brantigan & Roos 2004).

Venous symptoms

The VTOS comprises 2–3% of all TOS patients. Venous symptoms may be preceded by excessive activity with the upper extremity. The precipitating factor that leads to thrombosis is excessive activity of the arm such as throwing a baseball, swimming, weight lifting or working with arms elevated. Swelling, oedema, cyanosis and arm discomfort, which is aggravated with exercise along with distended superficial veins, shoulder and chest wall, are results of venous symptoms.

It is not uncommon to have a sub-clavian vein thrombosis at the first rib level. When this occurs, there is a sudden onset of dusky cyanosis, edema and extreme limb discomfort. It is important to diagnose this immediately and surgical decompression is necessary so that the symptoms do not become chronic. Physicians who diagnose only the vascular forms of TOS are misdiagnosing the vast majority of patients who have nonvascular TOS (Brantigan & Roos 2004).

SYMPATHETIC MEDIATED PAIN IN THORACIC OUTLET SYNDROME

Some of the painful symptoms in individuals with NTOS may be due to overlapping signs and symptoms of complex regional pain syndrome (CRPS) (Kaymak & Ozcakar

2004). In NTOS, the coldness and colour changes may not be caused by ischemia due to obstruction of the sub-clavian vessels, but due to an overactive sympathetic nervous system (SNS). Allodynia, hyperalgesia, prolonged periods of red or blue hand, persistent edema, excessive warmth and sweating changes are often present.

Sympathetic mediated pain may be related to a direct injury to the sympathetic axons in the cords or trunks of the brachial plexus as well as an activation of the somato-sympathetic reflex in which a somatic root injury will activate the sympathetic system over several ascending and descending dermatomes (Schwartzman 1987, Casey et al 2003). Anatomically, the SNS fibers run on the circumference of the nerve root of C8, T1 and lower trunk of the brachial plexus. When the nerves are compressed the sympathetic fibres are activated producing Raynaud's phenomenon. This may explain how the coldness and colour changes are frequently seen with both NTOS and ATOS.

Often, clinicians use the term compressor or releaser to categorize symptoms. The term, compressor, is used to evaluate patients who complain of symptoms when performing overhead activities. These patients have not paraesthesia at night unless the arm is overhead and whose occupation requires overhead work for long periods. This compression occurs when the arm is raised overhead which then causes the brachial plexus to turn over the first rib then under the clavicle at the costo-clavicular space. When the patient lowers their arm, the compression on the blood supply to the nerve is off and the symptoms decrease.

Women often report release phenomenon more often than men due to the weight of the breasts pulling on their bra straps and/or kyphotic posture. The bra straps are capable of creating compression of the brachial plexus while the kyphotic posture in which there is an increase of the shoulder girdle causes increased tension of the brachial plexus and closes down the thoracic outlet. Brismee et al (2004) showed that women were found to report symptoms associated with the release phenomenon about twice as often as men. The Roos Test is often positive when a patient has what is commonly called compressor TOS.

The term 'releaser' is used to identify patients that experience symptoms primarily at night who work in more sedentary jobs and these patients may have poor posture along with large or heavy upper extremities. The term 'release phenomenon' means the brachial plexus is being pulled down then venous pooling occurs around the nerve, which inhibits blood flow to the peripheral nerve. Gravity has an effect when sitting and standing which places tension on the nerve. When the patient lies down, the tension is gradually released and the blood flow returns to the nerves. As reported by Liu, it takes 4–6 hours after the removal of compression for the blood flow to return to the nerve. This may explain why a patient

aches at the same time every night with paraesthesia or pain. Lundborg (1970) believes this happening at night is due to the axons firing and patients experience paraesthesia.

DIAGNOSING THORACIC OUTLET SYNDROME

The diagnosis of TOS is essentially based on history and clinical examination. In order to diagnose accurately, clinical presentation must be evaluated as either neurogenic or vascular. Neurogenic is linked to compression of the brachial plexus and vascular is compression of the sub-clavian vessels. TOS manifestations are varied and there is no single definitive test. Common symptoms experienced with TOS include paraesthesia, numbness, pain and burning. Advanced symptoms include muscle weakness especially in the ulnar nerve distribution.

Diagnosis is based on a total clinical picture that is comprised of a careful meticulous history, review of medical records and clinical examination. For NTOS, the examination also includes tenderness over the scalene muscles, trapezius muscle and anterior chest wall, a positive Tinel sign over the brachial plexus in the neck, reduced sensation to very light touch in the fingers and a positive response to several provocative manoeuvres that put stress on the plexus to elicit symptoms. A list of these manoeuvres and incidence of positive responses is seen in the symptoms in Table 10.2.

Differential diagnosis (Brantigan & Roos 2004)

To have a precise diagnosis, it must be made by history, physical examination, provocative tests, and if needed, ultrasound, radiologic evaluation and/or electrodiagnostic evaluation (Brantigan & Roos 2004). There are multiple diagnoses to consider in the differential diagnosis of TOS. Consideration must be given to musculoskeletal pathology that could mimic a TOS presentation. Cervical radiculopathy as well as ulnar neuropathy may present with similar symptoms as TOS including hypothenar and/or intrinsic wasting (Box 10.1).

Provocative test – used in diagnosis of thoracic outlet syndrome

The physical examination as well as the other tests must be done as to not exacerbate the symptom. Clinicians rely on clinical tests for alteration of radial pulse. A few of these tests are listed below (For all tests, the patient is in a seated position and the examiner palpates the radial pulse):

Box 10.1 Differential diagnosis of thoracic outlet syndrome (TOS)

- Cervical disc disease
- Cervical facet disease, spondylosis
- Malignancies (Pancoast tumour, local tumours; e.g. nerve sheath tumours, spinal cord tumours)
- Peripheral nerve entrapments (ulnar and/or median nerve entrapment)
- Brachial plexitis
- Shoulder pathology
- Muscular spasms, fibromyalgia
- Neurologic disorders (multiple sclerosis)
- Chest pain, angina
- Vasculitis
- Vasospastic disorder (Raynaud disease)
- Neuropathic syndromes of upper extremity (CRPS I, II)
- Thoracic 4 Syndrome (T4)
- Sympathetic mediated pain
- Dull pain, discomfort, aching with tightness in mid-thoracic area

(A) *Adson Test*: The patient is asked to rotate the head and elevate his chin toward the affected side. If the radial pulse on that side is absent or decreased, the test is positive showing that vascular component of the neurovascular bundle is compressed by the scalene anterior muscle or cervical rib. This test has shown a sensitivity of 79% and specificity of 76% (Gillard et al 2001).

(B) *Wright's Test*: The patient's arm is hyper-abducted. If there is a decrease or absence of a pulse on one side, the test is positive showing that the axillary artery is compressed by the pectoralis minor muscle or coracoid process due to stretching of the neurovascular bundle. Gillard et al (2001) found a sensitivity of 70% and specificity of 53% for pulse abolition.

Patients with intermittent symptoms that are associated with specific movements or positions of the upper quadrant, which increases or decreases the compression and tension of neuro structures, will need to utilize these tests below:

(A) *Roos Test*: the patient has arms at 90° abduction and the therapist puts downward pressure on the scapula as the patient opens and closes the fingers. If the TOS symptoms are reproduced within 90 seconds, the test is positive.

(B) *Cyriax Release Test*: the patient can be sitting or standing with arms supported or resting on a pillow with forearm at neutral for a period of at least 3 minutes since symptoms, such as paraesthesia and numbness may not occur instantly. This position passively elevates the shoulder girdle bilaterally with the patient's trunk positioned posteriorly to assure shoulder girdle end range. A positive test is when a release phenomenon occurs including reproduction of symptoms. One theory suggests that paraesthesia is the most common symptom for those individuals with a release phenomenon followed by numbness and occasionally, pain. According to Cyriax (1978), paraesthesia and numbness appear when a nerve trunk or cord is first compressed, followed by a return of normal sensation. After pressure is released from the plexus, these symptoms reoccur latently. This outcome is different from the phenomenon associated with nerve root compression, which produces persistent symptoms until the root pressure is released (Cyriax 1978, Brismee et al 2004). Brismee et al (2004) showed that a one-minute modified Cyriax Release Test is the optimal time limit to maximize the specificity of the test (specificity of 97%).

(C) *Costo-clavicular Test*: This test may be used for both neurological and vascular compromise. The patient brings his shoulders posteriorly and hyper-flexes his chin. A decrease in symptoms means that the test is positive and that the neurogenic component of the neurovascular bundle is compressed. This test has shown a specificity ranging from 53% to 100% depending on the assessment of vascular changes or pain, respectively (Ryan & Jensen 1995, Nord et al 2008).

(D) *Elevated First Rib Test*: For right first rib elevation, patients will demonstrate a significant loss of right lateral flexion with hard end-fill in the position of left rotation indicating an elevated hypo-mobile first rib on the involved side. The second phase of the test consists of passively rotating the neck to the symptomatic side (example: right) to end range then followed by lateral flexion of the neck to the left. This test is considered positive when there is a decrease of lateral flexion and a hard end-fill on the effected side as compared to the contralateral side.

(E) *Upper Limb Neurodynamics Testing*: This test is used to rule out neurogenic pain and to provoke symptoms. Neural tissue assessment can be assessed by active movement dysfunction, passive movement dysfunction, adverse response to neural tissue provocation test, hyperalgesic response to palpation of nerve trunks, hyperalgesic responses to palpation of related cutaneous tissue and evidence of related local pathology (Hall & Elvey 1999). For this topic see Chapter 38.

The study by Sanders et al (2008) reported on 50 patients with positive provocative testing (Table 10.3). Gillard et al (2001) showed that a cluster of two provocative tests displayed the highest sensitivity (90%), whereas a cluster of five provocative tests increased the specificity to 84%.

Table 10.3 Positive physical findings (modified from Sanders et al 2008)

Positive physical findings – 50 patients	%
Upper limb tension test (ULTT)	98
90° abduction in external rotation	100
Scalene muscle tenderness	94
Scalene pressure yields radiating symptoms	92
Neck rotation to opposite side	90
Head tilt to opposite side	90
Sensation to light touch	68

Imaging assessment of thoracic outlet syndrome

TOS presents a challenge to diagnosticians and controversy exists regarding what test and imaging assessment should be used for diagnosis. Unfortunately, many physicians doubt the diagnosis of the pathology because it cannot be radiographically or electro-physiologically determined. One school of thought suggests that patients must demonstrate true neurological signs to be diagnosed with TOS and be confirmed by electromyography or nerve conduction velocity for brachial plexus compression and/or Doppler studies for vascular compromise as well as radiography to rule out cervical rib.

Another school of thought would diagnose TOS by the interpretation of the history, symptoms and clinical examination. Clinical testing of TOS has been highly debated in literature and no single test or questionnaire is universally accepted for the diagnosis of TOS (Mackinnon & Novak 2002).

Clinical diagnosis can be assisted by the use of imaging to demonstrate the nature and location of the structure undergoing compression and the structure producing compression but this is not always necessary. The first radiographic procedure should be a cervical plain radiography to assess for bone abnormalities as well as to differentiate the diagnosis. Computed tomography and angiography or magnetic resonance imaging (MRI) should be performed with postural manoeuvres in order to dynamically show the compression (Demondion et al 2006).

CLINICAL TREATMENT AND MANAGEMENT OF THORACIC OUTLET SYNDROME

Conservative treatment is indicated in patients unless there is significant neural loss or vascular compromise (Leffert 1991). The focus for conservative treatment is to decrease extrinsic pressure reducing intrinsic irritation. The goal is to decrease pressure on the neurovascular bundle and give the patient the tools to manage their TOS. Conservative management of TOS consists of (not in any particular order): restore normal breathing patterns, reduce inflammation, decrease muscle tension, elongate tight muscles, strengthen weak musculature, maintain neural excursion, maintain mobile joints, improve posture and body mechanics, and to restore muscle balance (Watson et al 2009).

Therapy evaluation of thoracic outlet syndrome

The subjective history examination is most helpful to understand patients' perception of the symptoms and duration of time or chronicity of the symptoms. The diagnosis and effective treatment of patients presenting with TOS is challenging due to a syndrome involving many pain sources. Provocation and specific functional tests provide information to design an orthopedic manual therapy management programme as well as addressing other dysfunctions. TOS can cause pain in the cervical and thoracic area, in specific muscle groups and paraesthesia and numbness in the upper extremity. It is important to identify the structure causing the symptoms and identifying areas of hypo-mobility or hyper-mobility. The provocation tests are important to assist in isolating the pain generators and the mobility testing determines areas of segmental dysfunction. It is this author's experience that identifying the abnormalities in the following areas and designing a treatment programme around these abnormalities will assist in successful outcomes.

Breathing patterns

Analysing the patient's breathing pattern cannot be understated. Patients with TOS tend to breath with their upper thorax without any abdominal movement. When this occurs the accessory muscles, particularly the scalene, elevate the first rib thus causing narrowing of the thoracic outlet. When examining a patient who uses the accessory respiratory muscle, as opposed to diaphragmatic breathing, it is not uncommon to find a decrease in hand temperature and decrease in blood flow because of abnormal sympathetic tone or vascular compromise. The sympathetic nervous system uses this normal protective response of vasal restriction that alters blood flow. It is important to change the breathing pattern to a more relaxed diaphragmatic breathing that allows for opening in the thoracic outlet and reduces muscle tension. The abnormal breathing pattern of not using the diaphragm perpetuates a vicious cycle of pain, spasm and congestion. The key to teaching is to ask the patient to lie supine with both hands placed on the upper abdomen and lower rib cage. The abdomen lifts with respiration and lowers with expiration. Observing hand movement will determine if breathing is done correctly. The scalene, in abnormal breathing, tends to contract through the full inspiratory phase. This maintains the elevation of the first rib, which in turn, will compromise the space for the sub-clavian vein to not be compressed.

By performing relaxed repeated breathing patterns, there is a decrease in muscle tension. Imbalances in the pressure gradients with TOS cause an increase in tunnel pressure causing venous stasis and hypoxia. If this hypoxia continues the oedema around the nerve as well as fibroblastic changes can cause scarring. Edgelow (2004) uses an analogy to describe this situation as a river flowing into a lake and a river flowing out of the lake, in which the inflow equals the outflow. In this state, the volume of the lake is constant, the oxygen content is high, and the pollution content is low. Should there be an obstruction affecting the outflow, then the volume of the lake would increase, the oxygen content would decrease and the pollution would increase

Muscle imbalance

Muscle imbalance is a major source of symptoms in patients with TOS. Abnormal posture, such as forward head, rounded shoulders and protracted shoulders are damaging posture for the scapular and neck muscles and should be addressed immediately. It is important to make sure that the scalene muscles, which elevate the first rib, are not tense. If the scapula muscles are weak, then an abnormal scapular movement pattern will result in weakness in the middle and lower trapezius and serratus anterior muscles. The scalene can overwork thus causing more entrapment. A posture evaluation should include evaluating multiple joint and scapula movements. It is important to assist the scapula position at rest and see if the scapula is depressed and downwardly rotated which can be contributing factors to TOS. With the above example, the scapula would be lower than T2–T7 and the slope of the shoulders would be increased which would make the neck appear longer. With scapula depression during overhead reaching, there are changes occurring at the acromio-clavicular joint (AC) especially with large and heavy arms. The AC joint, usually at the end range, will show creases that increase in overhead activities. Scapula, downwardly rotated, can be identified because the inferior angle of the scapula is closer to the spine than the superior angle. Another way to assess downwardly scapula rotation is evaluating movement into flexion and abduction. This movement normally causes signs of pulling or pain located in the teres major and latissimus dorsi region (Sahrmann 2002).

Joint stiffness

The brachial plexus can be compressed with joint stiffness or capsular tightness. Several authors have proposed mobilization of the cervical, thoracic, sternoclavicular, acromio-clavicular and costo-transverse joints to improve joint stiffness or hypo-mobility, range of motion and capsular tightness in upper quadrant conditions (Brismée et al 2005, Vanti et al 2007). Manual therapy techniques aimed at the joints, soft tissue and neural structure of the upper quadrant including the cervical and thoracic spine have been successful in treatment. Research has shown that thoracic mobilization, especially at the T4 area, is helpful to provide an inhibitory influence on the sympathetic nervous system and causes immediate post treatment pain relief (Yip-Menck et al 2000). Thoracic mobilization has proven effective in improving posture, hand and skin temperature as well as pain in TOS (see Chapter 11). The study by Stralka (2010), using grade III oscillation movement PA at T4 level, showed similarities in increased hand and skin temperature. Taskaynatan et al (2007) reported that inclusion of mechanical cervical traction reduced complaints of numbness in patients with TOS.

Evidence exists that thoracic joint mobilization decreases pain (Colachis et al 1966, Saal et al 1966, Browder et al 2004) and it has been theorized that biomechanical disturbances of the thoracic spine can contribute to cervical disorders (Greenman 1996, Norlander et al 1997, Browder et al 2004, Gross et al 2004). When the sympathetic nervous system (SNS) responds there is a normal protective response of vasoconstriction that alters blood flow. Automatic improper breathing patterns along with pain, stress and anxiety can cause SNS activity that maintains a cycle of pain, tension and dysfunction. The involvement of SNS by researchers is controversial but my experience has shown that by changing the sympathetic activity, there can be a positive influence on the patients' symptoms.

Neurogenic pain

It is the author's experience that upper limb nerve tension testing provocative manoeuvres along with clinical examination are extremely helpful in identifying NTOS. Neural mobility is an important part of a successful outcome. The provocation testing will reveal if the patient is a releaser or a compressor and this is useful in educating the patient to which positions of comfort will decrease symptoms. This upper limb nerve tension testing is useful to identify the area of specific entrapments of the brachial plexus. With TOS, the lower trunk/medial cord (C7–T1) is most commonly involved. The upper limb nerve tension testing and Tinels often locate the neurogenic irritability both proximal and distal, which is commonly referred to as a double crush syndrome (Plewa & Delinger 1998). These tests should not aggravate the symptoms (see Chapter 38).

Reproduction of radiating neurogenic arm pain with paraesthesia is a positive response. When this test is positive, it is an indicator of compression against the nerve roots or brachial plexus.

Intervention for thoracic outlet syndrome

There are many schools of thought contributing to the therapy management of TOS. Peter Edgelow, a physiotherapist, utilizes three concepts that are the guiding principles for effective treatment of neurovascular entrapment, which are built on the fundamental idea that this entrapment occurs as a consequence of trauma affecting the nerve or vascular system (Edgelow 2004). His first concept is patient empowerment, which means the patient must be responsible and in control of his own care in order for treatment to be long lasting. The importance of treating the whole person cannot be underestimated and is supported by this author. The most successful outcomes are a multi-factorial approach starting with patient empowered to take care of their own problems by understanding their TOS dilemma as well as understanding the treatment solution. In treating, it is important to gain the patient's trust, stay in contact with them and make sure they understand their problem. The impact of having this long pain syndrome without correctly being diagnosed as TOS allows individuals to feel their life is out of control. Restoring the feeling of being in control has a positive impact on the individual. It has been my experience that there is no quick fix in treating patients with thoracic outlet syndrome. That is why patients must understand the length of the programme and being diligent with the exercise programmes. It is also important for the patient to understand the risks and rewards in paying close attention to symptoms. By understanding the problem and the solution, it adds control in the patient's life. Edgelow also suggests that individual risk factors, health habits, daily living demands and belief systems that can be controlled are important for the treatment of TOS.

The second concept is that neurovascular entrapment is a problem of stenosis. Stenosis should not be thought of as a rigid narrowing of an anatomic part, rather a series of events and circumstances. These events may result in irreversible narrowing. The stenosis caused by the presence of a cervical rib or dysfunction of the scalene may be irreversible but the stenosis due to abnormal breathing patterns and abnormal posture can be reversible (Edgelow 2004).

The third concept that Edgelow stresses is the concept of fluid dynamics. As structural and fluid changes cause restriction in the size of the thoracic outlet they also cause changes in the pressure gradient, which also effects the local neural circulation and the venous and lymphatic return to the whole upper extremity.

CONCLUSION

Communication between the referring physician and physical therapist is a necessity to assure positive outcomes. Many authors combined treatment of soft tissues and joints with neural tissue treatment (Edgelow 2004). This management includes posture correction, treatment of affected structures including nerve excursions, muscular, articular, as well as addressing the emotional component, which is necessary for successful outcomes.

The goal of treatment is to teach the patient to open up the space between the clavicle and first rib by stretching tight muscles, strengthening weak musculature, decrease nerve tension in the upper quadrant, improve temperature differences in the hand, improve diaphragmatic breathing and increase spinal mobility in the cervical-thoracic area. A clear understanding and interpretation of the provocative test are necessary for successful outcomes. The patient must realize that a period of 6 months or longer may be necessary to make a lasting effect on their symptoms.

As we manage patients, I have found that patients perform stretching exercises without using proper techniques. Most patients do not understand that lateral flexion, without stabilizing the first rib, continues to add additional compression and tension in the scalene muscles. Patients must be instructed in lateral flexion with slight rotation along with using a towel or a strap to hold the rib in a caudal position.

A total wellness concept of good eating habits and aerobic conditioning should also be followed. Many TOS patients are in poor aerobic condition causing decreased respiratory function and overuse of the scalene, trapezius and sternocleidomastoid muscles. Postural correction, including spinal extension, will allow better chest expansion with inspiration resulting in diaphragmatic excursion and will decrease the use of the accessory respiratory muscles (Mackinnon & Novak 2002).

Clinical experience has shown that by identifying the mechanical origin of symptoms, a successful treatment programme consisting of symptom alleviation is most helpful along with empowering the patient to be in charge of their own symptoms. Educating the patient in proper posture and breathing patterns at both work and leisure is the cornerstone for designing a treatment programme. Physical therapy that addresses postural abnormalities, neural mobility, joint mobility, and muscle imbalances is effective in relieving symptoms of TOS.

REFERENCES

Atasoy, E., 2004. Thoracic outlet syndrome: anatomy. Hand Clin. 20, 7–14.

Beyer, J.A., Wright, I.S., 1951. The hyperabduction syndrome: with special reference to its relationship to Raynaud's syndrome. Circulation 4, 161–172.

Brantigan, C.O., Roos, D.B., 2004. Diagnosing thoracic outlet syndrome. Hand Clin. 20, 17–36.

Brismée, J.M., Gilbert, K., Isom, K., et al., 2004. Rate of false positive using the Cyriax release test for thoracic outlet syndrome in an asymptomatic population. J. Man. Manip. Ther. 12, 73–81.

Brismée, J.M., Phelps, V., Sizer, P.S., 2005. Differential diagnosis and treatment of chronic neck and upper trapezius pain and upper extremity paresthesia: A case study involving the management of an elevated first rib and unco-vertebral joint dysfunction. J. Man. Manip. Ther. 13, 79–90.

Browder, D.A., Erhard, R.E., Piva, S.R., 2004. Intermittent cervical traction and thoracic manipulation for management of mild cervical compressive myelopathy attributed to cervical herniated disc: a case series. J. Orthop. Sports Phys. Ther. 34, 701–712.

Casey, R.G., Richards, S., O'Donahoe, M., 2003. Exercise induced clinical ischaemia of the upper limb secondary to a cervical rib. British Journal of Sports Medicine. 37, 455–456.

Colachis, S.C., Strohm, B.R., 1966. Effect of duration of intermittent cervical traction on vertebral separation. Arch. Phys. Med. Rehabil. 47, 353–359.

Cyriax, J., 1978. Textbook of orthopedic medicine: diagnosis of soft tissue lesions, seventh ed. Vol 1. Baillière Tindall, London.

Demondion, X., Herbinet, P., Van Sint Jan, S., 2006. Imaging assessment of thoracic outlet syndrome. Radiographics 26, 1735–1750.

Edgelow, P.L., 2004. Neurovascular consequences of cumulative trauma disorders affecting the thoracic outlet: a patient-centered treatment approach. Neurologic considerations. In: Donatelli, R.A. (Ed.), Physical Therapy of the Shoulder. fourth ed. Churchill Livingstone, Edinburgh, pp. 205–238.

Fugate, M.W., Rotellini-Coltvet, L., Freischlag, J.A., 2009. Current management of thoracic outlet syndrome. Curr. Treat. Options Cardiovasc. Med. 11, 176–183.

Gillard, J., Perez-Cousin, M., Hachulla, E., et al., 2001. Diagnosing thoracic outlet syndrome: Contribution of provocative tests, ultrasonography, electrophysiology, and helical computed tomography in 48 patients. Joint Bone Spine 68, 416–424.

Greenman, P.E., 1996. Principles of manual medicine. Lippincott Williams & Wilkins, Philadelphia, PA.

Gross, A.R., Hoving, J.L., Haines, T.A., et al., 2004. Manipulation and mobilization for mechanical neck disorders. Cochrane Database System Review CD004249.

Hall, T.M., Elvey, R.L., 1999. Nerve trunk pain: physical diagnosis and treatment. Man. Ther. 4, 63–73.

Hursh, L.F., Thanki, A., 1985. The TOS. Postgrad. Med. 77, 197–199.

Kaymak, B., Ozcakar, L., 2004. Complex regional pain syndrome in thoracic outlet syndrome. Br. J. Sports Med. 38, 364–368.

Leffert, R.D., 1991. Thoracic outlet syndrome. In: Tubiana, R. (Ed.), The Hand. fourth ed. WB Saunders Co., Philadelphia, pp. 343–351.

Lundborg, G., 1970. Iscli nerve injury. Scand. J. Plast. Reconstr. Surg. Hand Surg. 65, 1–113.

Mackinnon, S.E., Patterson, G.A., Novak, C.B., 1996. Thoracic outlet syndrome: a current overview. Seminars in Thoracic and Cardiovascular Surgery 8 (2), 176–182.

Mackinnon, S.E., Novak, C.B., 2002. Thoracic outlet syndrome. Curr. Probl. Surg. 39, 1070–1145.

MediFocus Guide, 2009. Thoracic outlet syndrome. #RT017 Available: http://www.medifocus.com (accessed 19.07.09.).

Nord, K.M., Kappor, P., Fisher, J., et al., 2008. False positive rate of thoracic outlet syndrome diagnostic maneuvers. Electromyogr. Clin. Neurophysiol. 48, 67–74.

Norlander, S., Gustavsson, B.A., Lindell, J., Nordgren, B., 1997. Reduced mobility in the cervico-thoracic motion segment – a risk factor for musculoskeletal neck-shoulder pain: a two-year prospective follow-up study. Scand. J. Rehabil. Med. 29, 167–174.

Plewa, M., Delinger, M., 1998. The false-positive rate of thoracic outlet syndrome shoulder maneuvers in healthy subjects. Academy of Emergency Medicine 5, 337–342.

Ryan, G.M., Jensen, C., 1995. Thoracic outlet syndrome: provocative examination maneuvers in a typical population. J. Shoulder Elbow. Surg. 4, 113–117.

Saal, J.S., Saal, J.A., Yurth, E.F., 1996. Nonoperative management of herniated cervical intervertebral disc with radiculopathy. Spine 21, 1877–1883.

Sahrmann, S.A., 2002. Diagnosis and treatment of movement impairment syndromes. Mosby, St. Louis, pp. 193–261.

Samarasam, I., Sadhu, D., Agarwal, S., et al., 2004. Surgical management of thoracic outlet syndrome: a 10-year experience. J. Surg. 74, 450–454.

Sanders, R.J., Hammond, S.L., Rao, N.M., 2008. Thoracic outlet syndrome: a review. Neurologist 14, 365–373.

Sanders, R.J., Haug, C.E., 1991. Thoracic outlet syndrome: A common sequela of neck injuries. In: Thoracic Outlet Syndrome. Lippincott, Philadelphia, pp. 26–73.

Sanders, R.J., 1990. Scalene muscle abnormalities in traumatic thoracic outlet syndrome. Am. J. Surg. 159, 231–236.

Schwartzman, R.J., 1987. Clinical Syndromes of RSD and TOS. Greater

Philadelphia Pain Society, Philadelphia.

Stralka, S.W., 2010. Thesis: effects of mobilization of fourth thoracic vertebra on pain and hand skin temperature in adult women with complex regional pain syndrome.

Talu, G.K., 2005. Thoracic outlet syndrome: A Review. Agri 17, 5–9.

Taskaynatan, M.A., Balaban, B., Yasar, E., Ozgul, A., Kalyon, T.A., 2007. Cervical traction in conservative management of thoracic outlet syndrome. Journal of Musculoskeketal Pain 15, 89–94.

Vanti, C., Natalini, L., Romeo, A., Tosarelli, D., et al., 2007. Conservative treatment of thoracic outlet syndrome. A review of the literature. Eura. Medicophys. 43, 55–70.

Watson, L.A., Pizzari, T., Balster, S., 2009. Thoracic outlet syndrome part 1: clinical manifestations, differentiation and treatment pathways. Man. Ther. 14, 586–595.

Yip-Menck, J., Mais, S., Kulig, K., 2000. Consideration of thoracic spine dysfunction in upper extremity Complex Regional Pain Syndrome Type I: A case report. J. Orthop. Sports Phys. Ther. 30, 401–409.

Chapter | 11 |

Thoracic spine manipulation

William Egan, Paul E Glynn, Joshua A Cleland

INTRODUCTION

For individuals with upper quarter musculoskeletal disorders, the thoracic spine is infrequently the primary source of symptoms. However, taking into account the concept of regional interdependence, the thoracic spine and rib cage can play a significant role in the perpetuation and management of upper quarter pain (Wainner et al 2007). For instance, a 45-year-old female presents to your clinic with mechanical neck pain. Her pain is of recent onset, occurring insidiously within the last 2 weeks, and she denies any symptoms radiating to the upper extremity below the shoulder. After a clinical examination which identified no signs of serious disease or contraindications, the clinician elects to perform thrust manipulation targeting her upper and middle thoracic spine. You also instruct her on mobility exercises for her cervical spine as well as deep neck flexor retraining. The patient returns 3 days later and reports a 3-point reduction on the numerical rating of pain scale (NPRS) and a 25% decrease on the Neck Disability Index (NDI).

© 2011 Elsevier Ltd.
DOI: 10.1016/B978-0-7020-3528-9.00011-X

You are also referred a 37-year-old male with right shoulder pain. Your examination is consistent with sub-acromial impingement syndrome and you also identify mobility impairments of his thoracic spine and rib cage. You perform a thrust manipulation of the patient's upper and middle thoracic spine in addition to non-thrust mobilization of the patient's rib cage. Immediately following the manipulation the patient reports a 50% decrease in resting pain and his pain-free active shoulder elevation is increased by 10°. You instruct the patient in thoracic extension mobility exercises as well as strengthening exercises for the lower trapezius and serratus anterior muscles. Upon return to the clinic 5 days later the patient's score on the Shoulder Pain and Disability Index (SPADI) is decreased by 25%. These two hypothetical clinical scenarios are based on the findings from recent clinical trials (Bergman et al 2004b, Gonzalez-Iglesias et al 2009b). Therefore, addressing impairments in the thoracic region can lead to improvements in pain and disability in patients with different upper quarter musculoskeletal disorders including the neck, shoulder, and elbow regions.

In the management of patients with upper quarter disorders the thoracic spine has been traditionally overlooked. However, there is evidence suggesting a strong biomechanical relationship between the thoracic spine, rib cage and the upper quarter (Sobel et al 1996, Kebaetse et al 1999, Theodoridis & Ruston 2002, Crosbie et al 2008). Further, studies have shown that manual therapy treatment directed towards the thoracic spine can have a positive impact on the outcomes of individuals with disorders of the upper extremity and cervical spine (Winters et al 1997, Bergman et al 2004b, Cleland et al 2007a, Gonzalez-Iglesias et al 2009b, Young et al 2009). This chapter covers anatomic and biomechanical related aspects of the thoracic spine, scientific and clinical evidence for the relevance of the thoracic spine for upper quarter pain syndromes, thoracic spine and rib cage exploration and manipulative interventions.

primary complaints of neck pain, headaches, or upper extremity pain syndromes (Sobel et al 1997, Piva et al 2006, Cleland et al 2007a, Berglund et al 2008). The posture of the thoracic spine has been shown to influence the posture of cervical spine and upper extremity (Kebaetse et al 1999). For instance, an increase in the thoracic kyphosis, which is common in the typical office worker, is associated with a forward head posture as well as an abducted and anteriorly tipped scapular position. To achieve full functional movement of the cervical spine and upper extremities, concomitant motion of the thoracic spine and rib cage and an erect, neutral thoracic posture is required. For example, full upper extremity elevation is accompanied by thoracic extension and ipsilateral side-bending (Theodoridis & Ruston 2002). Theoretically this would also require external rotation of the ipsilateral ribs which has been associated with thoracic spine extension (Cropper 1996). It has been shown that a slouched or flexed thoracic posture leads to decreased scapular posterior tipping during maximum glenohumeral abduction motion and decreased abduction force at 90° of abduction compared to an erect thoracic posture (Kebaetse et al 1999). Key postural muscles span from the thoracic spine to scapular regions. These muscles include the middle and lower portions of the trapezius and the serratus anterior. Postural or movement impairments in the thoracic region could play a role in dysfunction of these muscles and therefore have a direct influence on movement impairments and pain in the cervical and upper extremity regions. Two studies found that lower trapezius muscle strength increased after either thrust manipulation or non-thrust mobilization targeting the middle to lower thoracic spine (Liebler et al 2001, Cleland et al 2004a). Although both of these studies involved asymptomatic subjects and measured immediate changes in strength only, they suggest a clinically significant relationship between the thoracic spine and the lower trapezius muscle.

REGIONAL INTERDEPENDENCE OF THE THORACIC SPINE, RIB CAGE AND THE UPPER QUARTER

Biomechanical relationship between the thoracic spine and upper quarter

The structure and function of the thoracic spine and rib cage creates a symbiotic relationship with the cervical spine and upper extremity. The thoracic column serves as the base of support for the cervical spine and is intimately involved with the neck at the region of the cervico-thoracic junction. Stiffness and movement impairments of the cervico-thoracic junction are common findings in patients with

Pain referral patterns of the thoracic spine

It is uncommon for the thoracic spine to cause referred pain to the cervical or upper extremity regions. The cervical spine and upper extremities do not receive direct innervation from the thoracic roots with the exception of the first thoracic nerve root. However, the sympathetic nervous system via the sympathetic chain, running anterior to the costo-vertebral joints, can have a systemic affect and contribute to symptoms in the neck and upper extremities. A clinical syndrome referred to as the T4 syndrome has been described as a constellation of signs and symptoms associated with stiffness of the upper to middle thoracic region (Conroy & Schneiders 2005). Typical signs and symptoms include headaches, neck pain and arm pain, and bilateral 'stoking glove' paraesthesias. It is thought that these signs and symptoms could be resulting in part from the dysfunction of the thoracic spine and its influence on the sympathetic nervous system.

Furthermore, a published case report described a decrease in symptoms in a patient with upper extremity complex regional pain syndrome after a thrust manipulation directed to the upper thoracic spine (Menck et al 2000). In pain mapping studies of the thoracic spine facet joints and costo-transverse joints, local pain adjacent to the injected site is most commonly reported (Dreyfuss et al 1994, Fukui et al 1997, Young et al 2008). Subjects in these studies have not reported referred pain into the neck or upper extremity regions. Given the lack of a neuro-anatomical relationship with the cervical spine or upper extremities, this is not surprising. Patients with symptomatic thoracic disc herniation typically report thoracic spine and chest wall pain and do not report neck or arm pain (Wood et al 1999). With the exception of symptoms originating from the upper two thoracic segments and the thoracic sympathetic chain, the thoracic spine as a direct source of referred pain or symptoms to the cervical spine or upper extremity regions is unlikely.

Association between thoracic spine impairments and upper quarter pain syndromes

Postural impairments and movement dysfunctions of the thoracic spine have been found in patients with upper quarter musculoskeletal disorders. In a series of studies Norlander et al (1996, 1997) found that movement dysfunction of the upper thoracic spine was associated with upper quarter symptoms in a group of laundry workers. In their initial study and 2-year follow-up Norlander et al (1996, 1997) found that a decrease in forward flexion mobility of C7–T1 compared to T1–T2 predicted complaints of neck and shoulder pain. They referred to this finding as an inverse C7–T1 relationship, because in healthy subjects they found that C7–T1 had greater flexion mobility than T1–T2. In a third study, Norlander et al (1998) found that a reduction in forward flexion mobility of C7–T1 and T1–T2 was associated with a three-fold increase in complaints of neck pain, headaches, shoulder pain, and bilateral hand weakness in a group of electrical and laundry workers. These authors hypothesized that sensory input from joint receptors of the dysfunctional thoracic segments could potentially contribute to the neck and shoulder symptoms. Further research is required to make definitive conclusions.

Movement dysfunction of the thoracic spine, rib cage and shoulder girdle has been associated with patients reporting shoulder pain in primary care practices. In a 12–18-month follow up of patients with shoulder complaints, Winters et al (1999) found that patients who

reported that their shoulder pain was not 'cured' were more likely to have pain or limited mobility of the shoulder girdle. These authors defined the shoulder girdle as the cervical and upper thoracic spine, or upper ribs. This was in comparison to patients diagnosed with a synovial disorder originating from the gleno-humeral, acromio-clavicular or sub-acromial joints without dysfunction of the shoulder girdle. In another study, it was shown that patients presenting with shoulder girdle disorders respond well to manipulative therapy targeting impairments in this region whereas patients with synovial disorders respond best to steroid injection (Winters et al 1997).

Lateral elbow pain, a common upper extremity musculoskeletal disorder, has been associated with several impairments. Among these impairments are pain and mobility restrictions of the cervical and thoracic spine. A recent study found that subjects with lateral elbow pain had significantly higher frequency of positive responses with spring testing over the T1–T7 regions compared to subjects without elbow pain (Berglund et al 2008). Definitive conclusions could not be drawn about the association between pain with thoracic spring testing and lateral elbow pain in this study, and this finding may be attributed to the phenomenon of central sensitization of pain. However assessment and management of thoracic spine impairments in patients with elbow pain is the consideration in the clinic. In a small pilot study and a larger retrospective study Cleland et al (2004b, 2005a) found that patients who received manual therapy procedures targeting the cervical and thoracic region in addition to treatment of the elbow achieved more favourable outcomes than patients who received management of the elbow only.

EVIDENCE FOR MANUAL THERAPY MANAGEMENT OF THE THORACIC SPINE AND RIB CAGE IN UPPER QUARTER PAIN SYNDROMES

Due to the relatively small number of patients with primary complaints of thoracic spine and chest wall pain, there is only low quality evidence supporting the use of manual therapy procedures in the management of thoracic spine and chest wall pain. In a pilot study, Schiller (2001) found that patients with mechanical thoracic spine pain showed a significantly greater reduction in pain scores after six treatments of manipulative therapy targeting the thoracic spine compared to a placebo control group. Techniques utilized in the study were short lever thrusts with direct contact on the transverse processes. In a case report Kelley & Whitney (2006) described the immediate relief of right lower chest wall pain after a non-thrust manipulation of the middle thoracic spine in an adolescent athlete. Fruth (2006) reported a case of a patient with right upper thoracic pain that was resolved after seven physical therapy visits including non-thrust manipulation of the ribs, ischemic compression of trigger points and therapeutic exercise. In a retrospective review of 73 patients reporting to a rheumatology clinic with a primary complaint of thoracic spine pain, Bruckner et al (1987) reported that the majority of the patients were either pain-free (77%) or noted slight improvement (15%) after postural advice and manipulative treatment of the thoracic spine. The majority of patients (75%) in this retrospective review reported mid thoracic pain and about half also complained of anterior chest wall pain. Patients with chest wall pain should receive a differential diagnosis to rule out cardiac and visceral disorders. Musculoskeletal pain involving the thoracic spine can potentially cause pseudo-anginal or pseudo-visceral pain.

There have been two reports in the literature concerning patients with anterior chest or abdominal pain who have been worked up for cardiac and visceral disorders with negative findings (Hamberg & Lindahl 1981, Benhamou et al 1993). These patients were found to have mechanical thoracic pain that responded to either manipulation of the thoracic spine or injection of the costo-vertebral joints. Another study identified historical questions which assist the clinician in determining the source of a patient's abdominal pain as being musculoskeletal in origin (Sparkes et al 2003). For abdominal pain to be considered of musculoskeletal origin, the patient should answer yes to two questions and no to one question. This leads to a positive likelihood ratio of 4.2 that the patient's pain is of musculoskeletal origin.

The 'yes' questions are:

- Does coughing, sneezing, or taking a deep breath make your pain feel worse?
- Do activities such as bending, sitting, lifting, twisting, or turning over in bed make your pain feel worse?

The 'no' question is:

- Has there been any change in your bowel habits since the start of your symptoms?

There has been a recent emergence in the literature of studies investigating the effect of manual therapy procedures targeting the thoracic spine in patients with neck disorders. Given the small risk of serious adverse events associated with cervical thrust manipulation, some authors advocate thoracic thrust manipulation as a safe alternative to cervical manipulation especially in the presence of severe symptoms, radiculopathy, or post whiplash (Piva et al 2000, Pho & Godges 2004, Childs et al 2005). There are several studies showing that patients with mechanical neck pain benefit from thrust manipulation of the thoracic spine. This includes two case series, six randomized clinical trials and a preliminary clinical prediction rule study (Savolainen et al 2004, Cleland et al 2005b, 2007a,c, Fernandez-de-las-Peñas et al 2007, Krauss et al 2008, Gonzalez-Iglesias et al 2009a,b). These studies are of varying quality but in sum provide substantial evidence that patients with mechanical neck pain can experience clinically meaningful improvement in pain and disability following thrust manipulation of the thoracic spine. It is important to note that in several of the studies the thoracic spine manipulation was augmented by a therapeutic exercise programme. In these studies various techniques were utilized including seated, prone, and supine thrusts targeting both the middle and upper thoracic spine. Table 11.1 provides an overview of these studies involving patients with mechanical neck pain.

Neck pain after a whiplash injury is very common. There has been one randomized clinical trial and one case report concerning manipulation of the thoracic spine in patients with neck pain after a whiplash injury. In a two-part study, Fernandez-de-las-Peñas et al (2004) first compared the incidence of thoracic spine dysfunction in patients with mechanical neck pain compared to those with neck pain from a whiplash. Thoracic spine dysfunction was identified by palpation for asymmetry in thoracic flexion and pain or hypomobility associated with spring testing of the thoracic spine. Sixty-nine percent of patients with whiplash had thoracic joint dysfunction compared

Table 11.1 Overview of studies involving thoracic spine manipulation for patients with mechanical neck pain.

Author	Study design	Subjects	Interventions	Outcomes
Cleland et al 2005b	RCT	36 patients with mechanical neck pain	Supine thoracic thrust manipulation vs placebo	Immediate clinically significant reduction in neck pain following thrust compared to placebo.
Cleland et al 2007c	RCT	60 patients with mechanical neck pain	Six sessions of thoracic thrust manipulation and exercise vs non-thrust manipulation and exercise	At the completion of six sessions the thrust group achieved clinically significant more reduction in pain and disability as measured by the NDI compared to the non-thrust group

Table 11.1 Overview of studies involving thoracic spine manipulation for patients with mechanical neck pain.—cont'd

Author	Study design	Subjects	Interventions	Outcomes
Cleland et al 2007a	Prospective cohort study	78 patients with mechanical neck pain	All subjects received up to two sessions of thoracic thrust manipulation targeting both the middle and upper thoracic spine & ROM exercise for the cervical spine Patients achieving at least three of six variables have a positive likelihood ratio of 5.5 for a successful outcome with the intervention.	The following variables comprised the clinical prediction rule for patients who would achieve clinically meaningful improvement on the Global rating of Change Scale: 1. Symptoms < 30 days. 2. No symptoms below the shoulder. 3. Looking up does not aggravate symptoms 4. FABQPA Score < 12 5. Diminished Upper Thoracic Spine Kyphosis 6. Cervical extension ROM $< 30°$.
Fernandez-de-las-Peñas et al 2007	Case series	7 patients with mechanical neck pain	All patients received a single thrust manipulation in sitting targeting the upper thoracic spine	All patients achieved an immediate reduction in resting pain and improved cervical range of motion following the manipulation.
Flynn et al 2001	Case series	26 patients with neck pain	All patients received thrust manipulation targeting hypomobile segments including the upper and middle thoracic spine and rib cage.	Immediately post intervention, patients experienced a clinically meaningful improvement in cervical range of motion and a reduction in resting pain.
Gonzalez-Iglesias et al 2009a	RCT	45 patients with mechanical neck pain	Six sessions of TENS, exercise, and massage versus the same programme plus thoracic spine thrust manipulation in sitting 1/week for 3 weeks	Patients in the manipulation group achieved a clinically significant greater reduction in pain and disability scores and increased cervical range of motion compared to the non-manipulation group at the completion of the intervention.
Gonzalez-Iglesias et al 2009b	RCT	45 patients with mechanical neck pain	Five sessions on electro-thermal therapy versus the same treatment plus a seated thoracic thrust manipulation 1/week for 3 weeks	Patients in the manipulation group achieved a clinically significant greater reduction in pain and disability scores than the non-manipulation group at the end of the intervention, and at 2-week follow-up. The manipulation group continued show a clinically meaningful improvement in pain compared to the non-manipulation group at the 4 week follow up.
Krauss et al 2008	RCT	22 patients with mechanical neck pain	Thoracic thrust manipulation to the T1–T4 segments in supine versus a control group	The manipulation group experienced a clinically meaningful increase in right and left cervical rotation range of motion and a decrease in pain with right cervical rotation compared to the control group.
Savolainen et al 2004	RCT	75 subjects with mechanical neck pain	Four sessions of thoracic manipulation versus instruction in an exercise programme	Subjects in the manipulation group reported a significantly lower level of worst perceivable pain at 12-month follow-up.

to 13% with mechanical neck pain based on these criteria. In the second part of the study, 88 patients with whiplash were randomized to either receive 15 sessions of physiotherapy consisting of electro-thermal modalities, ultrasound, massage, and exercise or the same physiotherapy with the addition of two sessions of thoracic manipulation. The manipulation technique utilized was a supine thrust technique targeting the T4–5 segment. At the completion of the study, the group receiving the thoracic manipulation experienced significantly greater reduction in neck pain, measured on a VAS, compared to the physiotherapy group.

Pho & Godges (2004) presented a case report of a patient with neck pain after a whiplash injury. Initial management of the patient included thoracic spine thrust and non-thrust manipulation during the first two treatment sessions as the cervical spine was deemed too irritable for assessment and treatment in the initial stages. The patient experienced a full resolution of symptoms, disability, and range of motion deficits after four sessions of physical therapy. There is emerging evidence that thrust and non-thrust manipulation of the thoracic spine comprise an integral part of multimodal approaches in the management of patients with cervical radiculopathy. Cleland et al (2005c) and Waldrop (2006) published case series of patients diagnosed with cervical radiculopathy using a similar multi-modal interventional approach. Interventions included thrust manipulation of the thoracic spine, non-thrust manipulation of the cervical spine, intermittent traction, and therapeutic exercise. In both case series, the majority of patients experienced a clinically meaningful reduction in pain and disability at the end of the physical therapy intervention and at medium term follow-up. In a prospective cohort study involving patients with cervical radiculopathy, Cleland et al (2007b) identified variables that predicted short term success with physical therapy management. Success was defined as surpassing the minimally clinically important difference on the Neck Disability Index, the Patient Specific Functional Scale, the Numerical Rating of Pain Scale, and the Global Rating of Change Scale. The predictor variables were age < 54, looking down does not worsen symptoms, dominant arm is not affected, and the patient received multimodal therapy including cervical traction, manual therapy which typically included thoracic spine manipulation, and deep neck flexor strengthening during at least 50% of the visits. Patients meeting three of these four variables had a positive likelihood ratio of 5.2 for success. In a high quality randomized controlled trial, Young et al (2009) compared a multimodal approach including thoracic spine thrust manipulation, cervical non-thrust manipulation, and therapeutic exercises with and without mechanical cervical traction in patients with cervical radiculopathy. Patients received an average of two treatment sessions per week for 4 weeks. Therapists were required to include at least one manual therapy

intervention targeting both the middle and upper thoracic spine during each visit. Thrust techniques were conducted in sitting, supine, and prone. Both groups experienced a clinically meaningful decrease in pain and disability at 2 and 4 weeks with no differences between the groups.

In addition to cervical radiculopathy there is some evidence that thrust manipulation of the thoracic spine can assist with the management of patients with mild, grade I cervical compressive myelopathy. In a case series involving seven patients, Browder et al (2004) reported that a multimodal management programme of thoracic spine thrust manipulation and intermittent mechanical cervical traction resulted in a clinically meaningful reduction in pain and disability in all patients with an average of nine treatment sessions. Although it is difficult to parcel out the individual effects of thoracic spine manipulation from these studies, it was included in all of them and likely plays an integral part of the multi-modal management of patients with cervical radiculopathy. In the authors' experience most patients with cervical radiculopathy report significant relief of symptoms, especially in the scapular region, and improvement in cervical range of motion immediately following thoracic thrust manipulation.

Patients with cervicogenic headache form a clinically important sub-group for the clinician specializing in musculoskeletal disorders. Conservative management involving manual therapy and exercise has been shown to produce clinically meaningful benefits for patients in this sub-group (Jull et al 2002). Postural and mobility impairments involving the thoracic region can play a role in the perpetuation of these headaches. Furthermore, thrust and non-thrust manipulation of the thoracic spine could cause a reduction in headache pain by alternating the tension of multi-segmental muscle spanning from the thoracic to the upper cervical region. In the randomized trial conducted by Jull et al (2002) patients receiving manual therapy, exercise, or a combination of the two achieved a clinically meaningful reduction in headache frequency and intensity. Manual therapy procedures were selected by the clinician and included both thrust and non-thrust manipulation of the cervical and upper thoracic spine based on the patient's impairments, signs, and symptoms. The exercise programme included postural, motor control, and endurance exercises targeting the deep cervical flexors and scapular stabilizing muscles. In a case report of a patient with a headache, Viti & Paris (2000) reported a reduction in the patient's headache pain 4 days following a thrust manipulation of the upper thoracic spine. Previous management of the patient's impairments of the upper cervical region over five visits had failed to produce a change in symptoms. Preliminary evidence suggests that thrust and non-thrust manipulation of the thoracic spine can play a role in the multimodal management of patients with cervicogenic headache; however additional high quality research is required to further investigate this hypothesis.

As mentioned above the thoracic spine is intimately involved with the shoulder region due to the concomitant motion of the thoracic spine during movements of the shoulder. Additionally a neutral, erect posture is required for full range of motion of the shoulder. Three high quality studies have investigated the use of thrust and non-thrust manipulation of the thoracic region in patients with shoulder disorders (Winters et al 1997, Bang & Deyle 2000, Bergman et al 2004a). In two separate randomized clinical trials Winters et al (1997) and Bergman et al (2004a) both reported that manipulative therapy targeting the cervical spine, upper thoracic spine, and upper rib cage led to a clinically meaningful reduction in pain and disability, at short and medium term follow up, in patients with shoulder pain with signs and symptoms of shoulder girdle dysfunction. Comparison groups included non-manipulative physiotherapy, usual medical care, or steroid injection. Patients in both studies received up to six sessions of manipulative therapy provided by experienced manual physical therapists. Bang & Deyle (2000) compared exercise alone to exercise with manual therapy in patients with sub-acromial impingement syndrome. Patients in both groups received six sessions of treatment. At the completion of the study, patients in the manual therapy group experienced a clinically meaningful reduction in pain, disability and improvement in strength compared to the exercise group. Manual therapy included both thrust and non-thrust manipulation of the glenohumeral joint, clavicle, cervical spine, thoracic spine, and rib cage.

These three studies provide evidence that manual therapy management of the thoracic spine, as part of a multimodal treatment programme, can lead to positive outcomes for patients with shoulder pain. However it is unclear how much manual therapy of the thoracic spine, in isolation, contributes to the outcome. Boyles et al (2009) addressed this question in a prospective case series of 54 patients with shoulder impingement syndrome. They reported that pain, disability, and global rating of change was improved 48 hours after performing thrust manipulation of the upper and middle thoracic spine and rib cage. Seated thrust techniques were utilized to manipulate the thoracic spine and a supine technique was used to manipulation the ribs. Although it is unlikely that the thoracic and rib joints can directly refer pain to the shoulder region, Boyle (1999) reported that two patients' shoulder symptoms were completely resolved after non-thrust manipulation of the ipsilateral second rib.

As described above, mobility impairments and tenderness of the thoracic spine is common in patients reporting lateral elbow pain (Berglund et al 2008). Manual therapy management of the cervico-thoracic spine in addition to local treatment directed to the elbow has been shown to lead to improved outcomes in fewer visits compared to local treatment of the elbow alone (Cleland et al 2004b, 2005a).

EXAMINATION AND SCREENING OF THE THORACIC SPINE AND RIB CAGE IN PATIENTS WITH UPPER QUARTER MUSCULOSKELETAL PAIN

A full comprehensive musculoskeletal examination involving medical screening, patient history and a physical examination should be undertaken for all patients with upper quarter region complaints. What follows are the selected examination procedures that assist with identifying impairments that would be amenable to manipulation of the thoracic spine and rib cage. The reader is referred to other chapters of this book for other examination procedures. The examination is described by the patients' position.

Postural screen of the thoracic spine and rib cage

The examination of the thoracic spine begins with a postural screen aiming to identify regions of the thoracic spine that deviate from what is considered a normal, smooth thoracic kyphosis. Areas of increased or decreased kyphosis involving the upper, middle, and lower thoracic regions can be recorded. Observation for thoracic postural deviation in this fashion has fair to moderate reliability (Cleland et al 2006). For the clinical prediction rule developed by Cleland et al (2007a), a reduction in the upper thoracic kyphosis emerged as a predictor variable for success with thoracic manipulation in patients with mechanical neck pain. The examiner can palpate for alterations in the normal thoracic curvature by running his or her fingers along either side of the thoracic spine in the region of the paraspinal muscles. Areas of altered soft tissue tension and tenderness suggestive of underlying segmental dysfunction can be detected. Additionally the examiner can palpate the rib angles for tenderness by having the patient place his or her ipsilateral hand on the opposite shoulder to abduct the scapular out of the way. Tenderness of the rib angle is suggestive of underlying dysfunction of the rib (Flynn et al 2001).

Thoracic spine active range of motion

Active mobility testing of the thoracic spine in sitting commences with testing the patients' active range of motion in cardinal planes. Overpressure is applied if the motion is not pain provoking. Range of motion can be recorded using a bubble inclinometer over selected thoracic levels. The inclinometer is placed in the sagittal plane for flexion/extension and in the frontal plane for side-bending (Molina et al 2000). Seated active thoracic rotation followed by clinician overpressure can serve as a clinically efficient screen of thoracic spine. Pain and a visual gross judgment of range of motion can be recorded quickly with this test.

Mobility testing of the first rib

Screening for elevation of the first rib is completed in sitting with the examiner palpating the relative height of the first rib. The first rib is found and palpated by standing behind the patient and pulling back the upper trapezius muscle. The clinician can then rest his or her fingers on the posterior superior aspect of the first rib and make a visual judgment of the relative height of the first rib. The cervical rotation lateral flexion test (CRLF) advocated by Lindgren et al (1989) can also be performed to screen for elevation of the first rib. During this test the cervical spine is passively rotated to the contralateral side and then maximally side-bent in the sagittal plane. A reduction in side-bending mobility is suggestive of an elevated first rib on the side opposite from which the cervical spine was rotated.

Mobility testing of the first rib with the patient in supine is undertaken by the clinician applying a caudal glide to the posterior, superior aspect of the first rib using the palmar side of the second metacarpal phalangeal joint. Mobility or pain are recorded and are suggestive of dysfunction of the first rib. The clinician can also screen the first rib during inspiration and expiration by palpating the anterior aspect underneath the medial clavicle. A relative reduction in the excursion of motion during inspiration and expiration is suggestive of hypomobility of the first rib.

Segmental mobility testing of the thoracic spine and rib cage

The remaining ribs can be screened in a similar fashion and conventionally, they are examined in groups of three to four dividing the rib cage into the upper, middle, and lower regions. The clinician can also perform passive accessory mobility of the anterior ribs by springing in an anterior to posterior direction over the costo-sternal joints utilizing the thumbs (Maitland et al 2001). The clinician records the presence or absence of pain and notes whether the mobility is normal, hypomobile, or hypermobile for each rib (Heiderscheit & Boissonnault 2008).

Segmental mobility testing of the thoracic spine, utilizing posterior to anterior spring testing, is conducted with the patient prone. The clinician screens the thoracic spine for mobility and pain by applying his or her hypothenar eminence to the thoracic spinous process and producing a graded posterior to anterior force. The examiner records the presence or absence of pain and notes whether the mobility is normal, hypomobile, or hypermobile for each thoracic segment (Cleland et al 2006, Heiderscheit & Boissonnault 2008). The clinician can spring unilaterally over the thoracic transverse processes in a similar fashion. The ribs are also screened for mobility and pain. Using a crossed handed technique the clinician stabilizes the opposite side of the thoracic spine with his or her hypothenar eminence lateral to the spinous process and springs over each rib angle utilizing the hypothenar eminence of the opposite hand. Segmental mobility testing of the thoracic spine has poor-to-fair inter-rater reliability for both pain and mobility assessment in patients with neck pain (Cleland et al 2006). In two studies involving subjects without symptoms, reliability of segmental mobility testing of the thoracic spine and ribs improved when an expanded definition of agreement was utilized (Christensen et al 2002, Heiderscheit & Boissonnault 2008). Due to the potential inaccuracy of identifying a specific thoracic spinal level, these authors allowed for mobility agreement within and between raters to within ± 1 vertebral level.

Interpretation of the examination and reassessment

Using a compilation of the above examination procedures, the clinician can make a reasonable clinical judgment regarding the presence/absence of thoracic spine mobility impairments. Clinically, mobility impairments of the thoracic spine and rib cage are common in patients with upper quarter musculoskeletal pain and also in those without symptoms (Heiderscheit & Boissonnault 2008). Similar to other spinal regions, with increasing age, thoracic spine mobility becomes reduced (Edmondston & Singer 1997). Previous experts in manipulative therapy have described a detailed examination scheme in attempts to identify segment and direction of specific mobility impairments of the thoracic spine and rib cage. Following these biomechanical diagnoses, a manipulative procedure is then selected that matches the specified movement dysfunction. As stated above, reliability of segmental mobility testing of the thoracic spine and rib cage is fair. Additionally, research has shown that examination and manual therapy intervention procedures affect a region of the spine rather than a specific segment (Powers et al 2003, Ross et al 2004). We therefore propose a parsimonious examination process based on recent evidence. For example, to identify mobility impairments of a region of the thoracic spine, the examiner should find increased or decreased thoracic kyphosis in that region, limited active range of motion, soft tissue hyper-tonicity or tenderness, and hypomobility with spring testing. This examination scheme is also applied to the rib cage. Tenderness over the rib angle, reduced excursion during respiration, and hypomobility with spring testing over the anterior or posterior aspect of the rib suggest a mobility impairment of the rib. To identify a mobility impairment of the first rib, the examiner could use a combination of reduced mobility with spring testing, reduced excursion during respiration, tenderness over the rib angle, the presence of perceived superior elevation of the rib, and a positive CRLF test. To identify the thoracic spine as a pain generator or source of the patient's symptoms, the patient's familiar symptoms should be reproduced with examination procedures. For example, in the case report by Boyle (1999) the clinician reproduced the patient's familiar shoulder pain with posterior to anterior spring over the shaft of the ipsilateral second rib.

Often clinicians apply manual therapy procedures to an asymptomatic region of the thoracic spine in patients with neck or upper extremity disorders. Therefore, we recommend that the clinician bases the success or value of a particular technique on the effect it has on functional movement of the region of symptoms. For example, following manipulation of the thoracic spine, the clinician can then reassess the pain and range of motion associated with shoulder elevation in a patient with sub-acromial impingement syndrome. Likewise, pain-free grip strength could be retested after thoracic or rib thrust manipulation for a patient with lateral elbow pain. For patients with primary complaint of thoracic spine pain, functional reassessment procedures involving the thoracic spine, such as seated trunk rotation, are utilized.

MANUAL THERAPY INTERVENTIONS FOR THE THORACIC SPINE AND RIB CAGE

Complications from thrust or non-thrust manipulation of the thoracic spine are rare. As part of a comprehensive examination, a patient should be screened for conditions that require medical referral or contraindicate manipulation. Typical contraindications for manipulation in the thoracic region would include bone weakness or demineralization resulting from neoplasms, trauma, infection, or metabolic conditions (osteoporosis). The presence of signs of central cord compression, suggesting a possible massive thoracic disc herniation also contraindicate manipulation until diagnostic imaging is obtained. When deciding if an individual patient would benefit from thoracic manipulation, it is helpful to consider the inclusion and exclusion criteria of clinical trials involving thoracic manipulation. For example several trials had an age limit of 18–60 (Cleland et al 2005b, 2007a,c) while in others the limit was 18–45 (Gonzalez-Iglesias et al 2009a,b). With proper patient screening, thoracic spine manipulation is inherently safe provided that the clinician is properly trained in the techniques and avoids the unnecessary use of excessive force or amplitude. Minor side effects of temporary soreness are common after manipulation, so it is helpful to warn the patient so they are not alarmed (Cleland et al 2007c).

Biomechanical theories abound to explain the mechanisms by which spinal manipulation produces clinically important reduction in pain and disability. Specifically for the thoracic spine, it is thought that an improvement in mobility in the thoracic region following manipulation allows for enhanced pain-free mobility of the cervical or upper extremity region. It has also been proposed that improving mobility in the thoracic spine will take stress off adjacent, hyper-mobile cervical spine or shoulder joints. However, evidence is emerging that mechanisms behind the effects of manual therapy procedures have a predominantly neurophysiological component (Bialosky et al 2009). Analgesic effects after manipulation are thought to occur at the peripheral, spinal cord, and central nervous system levels. Effects include a reduction in reflexive muscular activity surrounding the spinal region manipulated, inhibition of pain production through gaiting mechanisms and activation of endogenous opioids, and alteration of pain processing in the brain. Non-specific effects involving a placebo response and patient's expectations of the treatment likely play a role in the effects of manual therapy (Bialosky et al 2008). With this in mind, clinicians can select particular manipulative techniques based on patient comfort, clinician experience and skill, and evidence from high quality research as opposed to selecting a procedure that matches a particular biomechanical lesion. What follows are descriptions of manual techniques for both the thoracic spine and ribs. Techniques for this chapter were selected based on what has been utilized in published clinical trials and the authors' clinical experience. For a comprehensive description of other thoracic spine manipulation techniques readers are referred to others texts (Flynn et al 2001, Maitland et al 2001, Gibbons & Tehan 2006). In keeping with the recent recommendations for manual therapy terminology all procedures will be referred to as manipulations (Mintken et al 2008). Thrust manipulation will refer to those techniques involving a quick or high velocity thrust. Non-thrust manipulations are techniques applied with lower velocity in a graded fashion.

Seated upper thoracic thrust manipulation

The patient sits on a treatment table with his or her hands clasped behind the neck as low down on the cervical spine as possible (Fig. 11.1). The clinician stands behind the patient and loops the hands through the patient's arms and places the hands clasped over the patient's hands. The clinician leans backwards to take up slack in a superior direction. A thrust is delivered by the clinician thrusting upwards towards the ceiling in an attempt to create a distraction force in the patient's upper thoracic region. The thrust should be generated by the clinician's legs. Care is taken with this procedure to not strain to

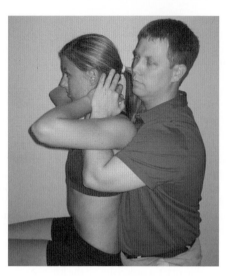

Fig 11.1 Seated upper thoracic thrust manipulation.

the patient's shoulder girdle. If the patient experiences shoulder discomfort or is unable to attain the position with his or her arms this technique is abandoned.

Seated mid thoracic thrust manipulation

The patient sits on the treatment table with his or her arms across the body with the hands grasping the opposite posterior shoulder region (Fig 11.2). Clinical experience suggests that the most comfortable position is with the elbows in parallel and this also allows for the clinician

to attempt the technique on a larger patient. The clinician applies the sternum to the patient's mid thoracic spine. Alternately a rolled towel can be placed horizontally on the caudal vertebra of the segment of interest between the patient and the clinician in attempt to be segment specific. The clinician reaches around the patient and grasps the patient's lower elbow. If possible the clinician interlocks the hands. The clinician takes up slack by adducting the arms, retracting the shoulder girdle, and pushing the chest towards the patient's thoracic spine. A high velocity thrust is performed by the clinician thrusting through the patient's arms in an anterior to posterior direction while at the same time keeping the chest pushed forward. Some clinicians attempt to produce a distractive force by lifting the patient during this procedure although this could potentially injure the clinician with a larger patient. If the clinician cannot reasonably reach the arms around the patient, another technique should be selected.

Prone upper thoracic thrust manipulation

With the patient lying prone, the clinician stands to one side of the patient. The clinician rotates the patient's head and neck to the opposite side (Fig 11.3). The clinician applies either the thumb or pisiform to the lateral aspect of the spinous process of the caudal vertebra of the segment of interest. Slack is taken up by the clinician applying the other hand to the patient's head and gently applying further rotation, contralateral side-bending, and extension until the spinous process of the segment begins to first move. The clinician delivers the thrust to the spinous process by translating it across the table in attempt to gap the joint on the opposite side. During the thrust the clinician maintains the patient's head and neck

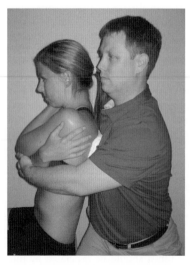

Fig 11.2 Seated mid thoracic thrust manipulation.

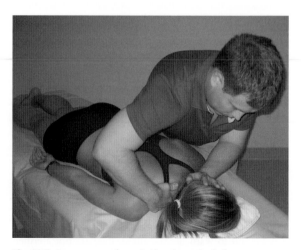

Fig 11.3 Prone upper thoracic thrust manipulation.

position with the opposite hand. Care is taken not to thrust through the patient's head and neck. If the patient experiences pain in the cervical region during the technique it can be attempted from the other side with the cervical spine rotated in the opposite direction or another technique should be selected.

Prone mid thoracic thrust and non-thrust manipulation

With the patient prone the examiner applies the hypothenar eminences just lateral to the spinous processes over the mid thoracic region (Fig 11.4). Slack is taken up by the examiner slightly twisting his or her hands in order to obtain a soft tissue or skin lock. From this position graded non-thrust manipulations or a thrust manipulation can be delivered in a posterior to anterior direction towards the table. The thrust can deliver after the patient exhales. Care is taken to not produce excessive force or amplitude with this procedure. The clinician should ensure that the contact is just lateral to the spinous process to avoid injury to the patient's ribs. The clinician should adjust the angle of the hand placement based on the contour of the patient's kyphosis in order to remain perpendicular to the spine.

Supine upper and middle thoracic thrust manipulation

With the patient supine the clinician instructs the patient to roll to his or her side. The clinician places one hand on the caudal vertebra of the segment of interest in the upper or middle thoracic region. The clinician's hand then serves as the fulcrum for the manipulation. A number of hand holds are possible including either a pistol grip or open hand technique. With the pistol grip the transverse processes of the thoracic segment are stabilized by the

clinician's hypothenar eminence and second metacarpophalangeal joint with the spinous process in between (Fig 11.5). With the open hand technique, the clinician applies his thenar eminence to one side of the thoracic spine just lateral to the spinous process (Fig 11.6). The clinician then rolls the patient back to the fully supine position while maintaining the hand position. The patient is instructed to either clasp his or her hands behind the neck (Fig 11.7) or cross the arms across the chest with the elbows parallel (Fig 11.8). Patient arm positioning is based on patient and clinician preference. Some patients prefer the hands clasped behind the neck to avoid pressure on the chest or breast tissue. Others report discomfort in the cervical region or are unable to obtain this position due to inflexibility of the upper extremities. From this position the clinician uses the other hand to flex or extend the patient down the region of interest so pressure is felt just over the clinician's bottom hand serving as the fulcrum. This is accomplished by the clinician either cradling the patient's head and neck (Fig 11.9) or by using the patients' arm (Fig 11.10).

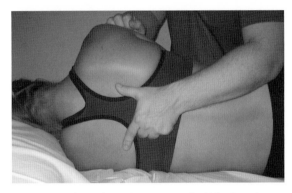

Fig 11.5 Pistol grip for supine upper and middle thoracic thrust manipulation.

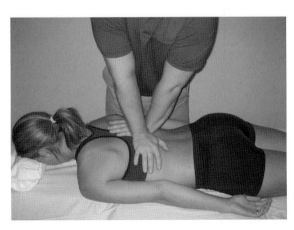

Fig 11.4 Prone mid thoracic thrust and non-thrust manipulation.

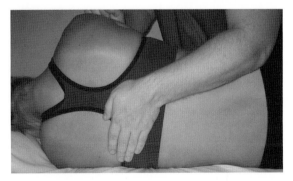

Fig 11.6 Open hand for supine upper and middle thoracic thrust manipulation.

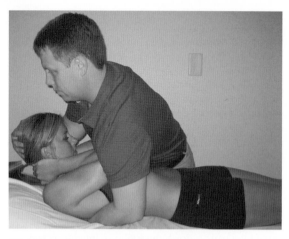

Fig 11.7 Supine upper and middle thoracic thrust manipulation with hands behind the neck.

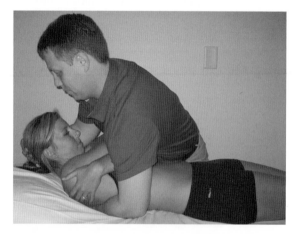

Fig 11.8 Supine upper and middle thoracic thrust manipulation with arms across the chest.

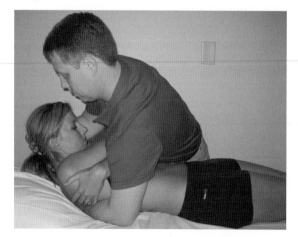

Fig 11.9 Supine upper and middle thoracic thrust manipulation with head flexion.

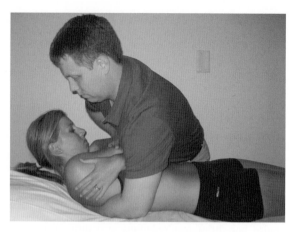

Fig 11.10 Supine upper and middle thoracic thrust manipulation with hand flexion.

Clinical experience suggests that extension is usually utilized in the upper thoracic region from T1–T3, whereas flexion is usually utilized in the middle thoracic region T4–T9. The clinician then takes up the slack by applying an anterior to posterior and slightly cranial force through the patient's arms and towards the fulcrum on the table. A thrust is delivered by the clinician through the patient's arms and towards the table. The thrust can be delivered after patient exhalation. Care is taken to not produce excessive force or amplitude with this technique. If the patient experiences pain in the shoulder the technique can be modified so that one of the patient's arms is crossed over the chest while the painful shoulder is left comfortably on the table (Fig 11.11).

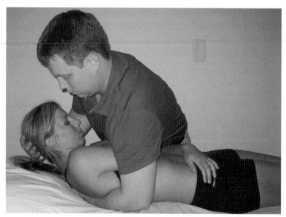

Fig 11.11 Supine upper and middle thoracic thrust manipulation adapted for patients with painful shoulder.

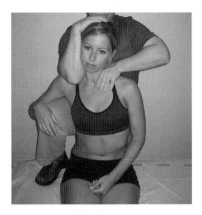

Fig 11.12 Seated first rib thrust and non-thrust manipulation.

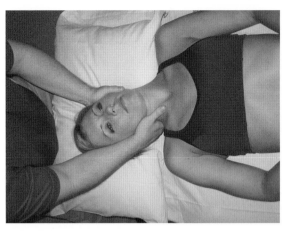

Fig 11.13 Supine first rib thrust and non-thrust manipulation.

Seated first rib thrust and non-thrust manipulation

The patient sits on the table and clinician stands behind the patient with the foot on the table with the knee in the patient's axilla on the side opposite from the side of the manipulation (Fig 11.12). The clinician applies the chest to the patient's thoracic region and places the forearm along the patient's head and cervical region on the side opposite of the manipulation. The clinician contacts the posterior, superior aspect of the patient's first rib with either the palmar aspect of the second metacarpophalangeal joint or the hypothenar eminence. The clinician, using the whole body, translates the patient toward the knee to produce side-bending of the cervical and thoracic region towards the side to be manipulated. This places the scalene muscles on slack and brings the first rib towards the clinician's thrusting hand. Further localization is achieved by slightly retracting the cervical spine and rotating it to the opposite side. The clinician can then deliver graded non-thrust manipulations or a thrust in a caudal and medial direction. Care is taken not to compress the patient's cervical spine with the non thrusting hand.

Supine first rib thrust and non-thrust manipulation

With the patient supine, the clinician contacts the posterior, superior aspect of the patient's first rib with the palmar aspect of the second metacarpophalangeal joint (Fig 11.13). With the opposite hand the clinician sidebends the patient's neck towards the side to be manipulated to put the scalene muscles on slack. The clinician performs graded non-thrust manipulation or a thrust in a caudal and medial direction. The thrust can be performed after patient exhalation.

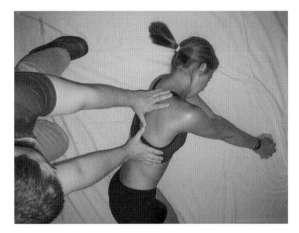

Fig 11.14 Side-lying ribs non-thrust manipulation.

Prone or side-lying ribs non-thrust manipulation

To perform non-thrust manipulation of the ribs the clinician can contact either the rib angle in prone or the costosternal joints in supine, and apply non-thrust mobilizations. These non-thrust manipulations can also be performed in side-lying with the patient's trunk rotated to either side in order to improve thoracic spine rotation (Fig 11.14).

Supine ribs thrust manipulation

This technique is almost identical to the supine thoracic thrust manipulation. To manipulate the rib the clinician stands on the opposite side of the rib to be manipulated. The clinician instructs the patient to roll to the side and contacts the rib just lateral to the transverse process with

165

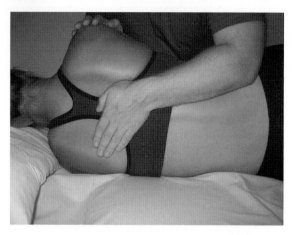

Fig 11.15 Contact for supine ribs thrust manipulation.

the thenar eminence (Fig 11.15). The patient is rolled back into the supine position. The patient is instructed to either clasp the hands behind the neck or place the arms across the chest. The clinician then flexes or extends the patient's trunk to localize the force towards the rib. The clinician delivers a thrust to the rib through the patient's arms and towards the table. The thrust can be delivered after patient exhalation. Care is taken to not use excessive amplitude or force. This technique tends to be less comfortable than the supine thoracic thrust so it is best to perform it quickly so pressure is not applied to the patient's rib for a long period of time.

Exercise interventions to augment the manual therapy techniques

Typically both thoracic thrust and non-thrust manipulations are augmented by patient self-mobilization exercises. In the authors' clinical experience, it is advantageous to immediately follow manual therapy procedures with active exercise. It has been suggested that manual therapy provides a window of opportunity after which exercise is facilitated (Raney et al 2007). The reader is directed to other chapters of this book for upper quarter strengthening and stretching exercises and for mobility exercises involving other upper quarter regions. What follows are descriptions of exercises to improve thoracic spine and rib cage mobility.

For the patient who lacks extension range of motion, an extension mobilization exercise can be utilized. The patient is instructed to clasp the hands behind the neck in order to stabilize the cervical spine. A fulcrum is placed in the region to be mobilized and the patient performs thoracic extension over the fulcrum. Several objects can be utilized as a fulcrum including the arm of a couch, the back of a chair, a foam roller, a rolled towel, or a mobilization wedge.

For the patient lacking thoracic spine flexion, a flexion mobilization exercise is utilized. This can be accomplished in either quadruped or with the patient's hands on the wall in a push-up position. The patient is instructed to flex the cervical and thoracic spine and protract the scapulae. This exercise has the added benefit of activating the serratus anterior muscles.

Patients with rib mobility restrictions can be instructed in the barrel hug exercise. With the patient seated, the clinician instructs the patient to pretend that he/she is holding onto a large barrel which produces thoracic flexion and shoulder girdle protraction. The patient is instructed to side-bend and rotates the trunk away from the side of the hypo-mobile rib. The patient can be instructed to perform this during full exhalation. The side-lying arm sweep exercise can be used for general thoracic spine and rib cage mobility. The patient lies on either side and, starting with the arm overhead, sweeps the arm downward towards the legs and the back up and around to the starting position. The patient can pause in areas where stiffness or a stretching sensation is felt and oscillate the shoulder girdle into protraction/retraction and trunk into rotation.

First rib hypomobility is addressed by the patient applying a downward pressure to the rib with a rolled towel or sheet. The sheet or towel is looped over the patient's shoulder and onto the first rib. The patient is instructed to drop the ipsilateral shoulder down and side-bend the cervical spine towards the rib to put the scalene muscles on slack. Using the towel the patient can apply a mobilization to the rib in a caudal direction.

CONCLUSION

In patients with upper quarter musculoskeletal disorders the thoracic spine and rib cage may play a significant role. The thoracic spine and rib cage are biomechanically linked to the cervical spine and upper extremity. Mobility impairments of the thoracic spine and rib cage are common in patients with upper quarter disorders. Evidence has shown that manual therapy interventions targeting the thoracic spine and rib cage can lead to positive outcomes in patients with a variety of upper quarter musculoskeletal disorders. Utilizing the concept of regional interdependence, the clinician should screen the thoracic spine and rib cage and address impairments found in patients presenting with neck, shoulder and elbow disorders. Thoracic spine manual therapy procedures are rarely used in isolation, but instead comprise part of a comprehensive, multimodal treatment programme utilizing manual therapy for other upper quarter regions, exercise, and patient education. Future research will assist the clinician in identifying patients who will benefit from thoracic manipulation and also in determining the optimal dosage of manipulation.

REFERENCES

Bang, M.D., Deyle, G.D., 2000. Comparison of supervised exercise with and without manual physical therapy for patients with shoulder impingement syndrome. J. Orthop. Sports Phys. Ther. 30 (3), 126–137.

Benhamou, C.L., Roux, C., Tourliere, D., et al., 1993. Pseudovisceral pain referred from costovertebral arthropathies. Twenty-eight cases. Spine 18 (6), 790–795.

Berglund, K.M., Persson, B.H., Denison, E., 2008. Prevalence of pain and dysfunction in the cervical and thoracic spine in persons with and without lateral elbow pain. Man. Ther. 13 (4), 295–299.

Bergman, G.J., Winters, J.C., Groenier, K.H., et al., 2004a. Manipulative therapy in addition to usual medical care for patients with shoulder dysfunction and pain: a randomized, controlled trial. Ann. Intern. Med. 141 (6), 432–439.

Bergman, G.J., Winters, J.C., Groenier, K.H., et al., 2004b. Manipulative therapy in addition to usual medical care for patients with shoulder dysfunction and pain: a randomized, controlled trial. Ann. Intern. Med. 141 (6), 432–439.

Bialosky, J.E., Bishop, M.D., Robinson, M.E., Barabas, J.A., George, S.Z., 2008. The influence of expectation on spinal manipulation induced hypoalgesia: an experimental study in normal subjects. BMC Musculoskelet. Disord. 9, 19.

Bialosky, J.E., Bishop, M.D., Price, D.D., Robinson, M.E., George, S.Z., 2009. The mechanisms of manual therapy in the treatment of musculoskeletal pain: A comprehensive model. Man. Ther. 14 (5), 531–538.

Boyle, J.J., 1999. Is the pain and dysfunction of shoulder impingement lesion really second rib syndrome in disguise? Two case reports. Man. Ther. 4 (1), 44–48.

Boyles, R.E., Ritland, B.M., Miracle, B.M., et al., 2009. The short-term effects of thoracic spine thrust manipulation on patients with shoulder impingement syndrome. Man. Ther. 14 (4), 375–380.

Browder, D.A., Erhard, R.E., Piva, S.R., 2004. Intermittent cervical traction and thoracic manipulation for management of mild cervical compressive myelopathy attributed to cervical herniated disc: a case series. J. Orthop. Sports Phys. Ther. 34 (11), 701–712.

Bruckner, F.E., Allard, S.A., Moussa, N.A., 1987. Benign thoracic pain. J. R. Soc. Med. 80 (5), 286–289.

Childs, J.D., Flynn, T., Fritz, J., et al., 2005. Screening for vertebrobasilar insufficiency in patients with neck pain: manual therapy decision-making in the presence of uncertainty. J. Orthop. Sports Phys. Ther. 35 (5), 300–306.

Christensen, H.W., Vach, W., Vach, K., et al., 2002. Palpation of the upper thoracic spine: an observer reliability study. J. Manipulative Physiol. Ther. 25 (5), 285–292.

Cleland, J.A., Selleck, B.S., Stowel, T.E.A., 2004a. Short-term effects of thoracic manipulation on lower trapezius muscle strength. J. Man. Manip. Ther. 12 (1), 82–90.

Cleland, J.A., Whitman, J.M., Fritz, J.M., 2004b. Effectiveness of manual physical therapy to the cervical spine in the management of lateral epicondylalgia: a retrospective analysis. J. Orthop. Sports Phys. Ther. 34 (11), 713–722; discussion 722–724.

Cleland, J.A., Flynn, T.W., Palmer, J., 2005a. Incorporation of manual therapy directed at the cervico-thoracic spine in patients with lateral epicondylalgia: A pilot clinical trial. J. Man. Manip. Ther. 13 (3), 143–151.

Cleland, J.A., Childs, J.D., McRae, M., Palmer, J.A., Stowell, T., 2005b. Immediate effects of thoracic manipulation in patients with neck pain: a randomized clinical trial. Man. Ther. 10 (2), 127–135.

Cleland, J.A., Whitman, J.M., Fritz, J.M., Palmer, J.A., 2005c. Manual physical therapy, cervical traction, and strengthening exercises in patients with cervical radiculopathy: a case series. J. Orthop. Sports Phys. Ther. 35 (12), 802–811.

Cleland, J.A., Childs, J.D., Fritz, J.M., Whitman, J.M., 2006. Inter-rater reliability of the history and physical examination in patients with mechanical neck pain. Arch. Phys. Med. Rehabil. 87 (10), 1388–1395.

Cleland, J.A., Childs, J.D., Fritz, J.M., Whitman, J., Eberhart, S.L., 2007a. Development of a clinical prediction rule for guiding treatment of a subgroup of patients with neck pain: use of thoracic spine manipulation, exercise, and patient education. Phys. Ther. 87 (1), 9–23.

Cleland, J.A., Fritz, J.M., Whitman, J.M., Heath, R., 2007b. Predictors of short-term outcome in people with a clinical diagnosis of cervical radiculopathy. Phys. Ther. 87 (12), 1619–1632.

Cleland, J.A., Glynn, P., Whitman, J.M., et al., 2007c. Short-term effects of thrust versus non-thrust mobilization/manipulation directed at the thoracic spine in patients with neck pain: a randomized clinical trial. Phys. Ther. 87 (4), 431–440.

Conroy, J.L., Schneiders, A.G., 2005. The T4 syndrome. Man. Ther. 10 (4), 292–296.

Cropper, J.R., 1996. Regional anatomy and biomechanics. In: Flynn, T.W. (Eds.), The Thoracic Spine and Ribcage. Butterworth-Heinemann, Boston, pp. 3–30.

Crosbie, J., Kilbreath, S.L., Hollmann, L., York, S., 2008. Scapulo-humeral rhythm and associated spinal motion. Clin. Biomech. 23 (2), 184–192.

Dreyfuss, P., Tibiletti, C., Dreyer, S.J., 1994. Thoracic zygapophyseal joint pain patterns. A study in normal volunteers. Spine 19 (7), 807–811.

Edmondston, S.J., Singer, K.P., 1997. Thoracic spine: anatomical and biomechanical considerations for manual therapy. Man. Ther. 2 (3), 132–143.

Fernandez-de-las-Peñas, C., Fernandez-Carnero, J., Fernandez, A.P., Lomas-Vega, R., Miangolarra-Page, J.C., 2004. Dorsal manipulation in whiplash injury treatment: a randomized controlled trial. Journal of Whiplash & Related Disorders 3 (2), 55–72.

Fernandez-de-las-Peñas, C., Palomeque-del-Cerro, L., Rodriguez-Blanco, C., Gomez-Conesa, A., Miangolarra-

Page, J.C., 2007. Changes in neck pain and active range of motion after a single thoracic spine manipulation in subjects presenting with mechanical neck pain: a case series. J. Manipulative Physiol. Ther. 30 (4), 312–320.

Flynn, T., Whitman, J., Magel, J., 2001. Orthopaedic manual physical therapy management of the cervical-thoracic spine & ribcage. Evidence in Motion, Louisville, KY.

Fruth, S.J., 2006. Differential diagnosis and treatment in a patient with posterior upper thoracic pain. Phys. Ther. 86 (2), 254–268.

Fukui, S., Ohseto, K., Shiotani, M., 1997. Patterns of pain induced by distending the thoracic zygapophyseal joints. Reg. Anesth. 22 (4), 332–336.

Gibbons, P., Tehan, P., 2006. Manipulation of the spine thorax and pelvis, second ed. Churchill Livingstone, Edinburgh.

Gonzalez-Iglesias, J., Fernandez-de-las-Peñas, C., Cleland, J.A., et al., 2009a. Inclusion of thoracic spine thrust manipulation into an electro-therapy/thermal program for the management of patients with acute mechanical neck pain: a randomized clinical trial. Man. Ther. 14 (3), 306–313.

Gonzalez-Iglesias, J., Fernandez-de-las-Peñas, C., Cleland, J.A., Gutierrez-Vega, M.R., 2009b. Thoracic spine manipulation for the management of patients with neck pain: a randomized clinical trial. J. Orthop. Sports Phys. Ther. 39 (1), 20–27.

Hamberg, J., Lindahl, O., 1981. Angina pectoris symptoms caused by thoracic spine disorders: Clinical examination and treatment. Acta Med. Scand. 644 (Suppl.), 84–86.

Heiderscheit, B., Boissonnault, W., 2008. Reliability of joint mobility and pain assessment of the thoracic spine and rib cage in asymptomatic individuals. J. Man. Manip. Ther. 16 (4), 210–216.

Jull, G., Trott, P., Potter, H., et al., 2002. A randomized controlled trial of exercise and manipulative therapy for cervicogenic headache. Spine 27 (17), 1835–1843.

Kebaetse, M., McClure, P., Pratt, N.A., 1999. Thoracic position effect on shoulder range of motion, strength,

and three-dimensional scapular kinematics. Arch. Phys. Med. Rehabil. 80 (8), 945–950.

Kelley, J.L., Whitney, S.L., 2006. The use of non-thrust manipulation in an adolescent for the treatment of thoracic pain and rib dysfunction: a case report. J. Orthop. Sports Phys. Ther. 36 (11), 887–892.

Krauss, J., Creighton, D., Ely, J.D., Podlewska-Ely, J., 2008. The immediate effects of upper thoracic translatoric spinal manipulation on cervical pain and range of motion: a randomized clinical trial. J. Man. Manip. Ther. 16 (2), 93–99.

Liebler, E.J., Tufano-Coors, L., Douris, P., Makofsky, H., 2001. The effect of thoracic spine mobilization on lower trapezius strength testing. J. Man. Manip. Ther. 9 (3), 207–212.

Lindgren, K.A., Leino, E., Manninen, H., 1989. Cineradiography of the hypomobile first rib. Arch. Phys. Med. Rehabil. 70 (5), 408–409.

Maitland, G.D., Banks, K., English, K., Hengveld, E., 2001. Maitland's Vertebral Manipulation, sixth ed. Butterworth, London.

Menck, J.Y., Requejo, S.M., Kulig, K., 2000. Thoracic spine dysfunction in upper extremity complex regional pain syndrome type I. J. Orthop. Sports Phys. Ther. 30 (7), 401–409.

Mintken, P.E., DeRosa, C., Littl, T., Smith, B., American Academy of Orthopaedic Manual Physical Therapists, 2008. AAOMPT clinical guidelines: A model for standardizing manipulation terminology in physical therapy practice. J. Orthop. Sports Phys. Ther. 38 (3), A1–A6.

Molina, C., Robbins, D., Roberts, H., et al., 2000. Reliability and validity of single inclinometer measurements for thoracic spine range of motion (abstract). J. Man. Manip. Ther. 8 (3), 143.

Norlander, S., Aste-Norlander, U., Nordgren, B., Sahlstedt, B., 1996. Mobility in the cervico-thoracic motion segment: an indicative factor of musculo-skeletal neck-shoulder pain. Scandinavian Journal of Rehabilitation Medicine. 28 (4), 183–192.

Norlander, S., Gustavsson, B.A., Lindell, J., Nordgren, B., 1997. Reduced mobility in the cervico-thoracic motion segment—a risk

factor for musculoskeletal neck-shoulder pain: a two-year prospective follow-up study. Scandinavian Journal of Rehabilitation Medicine. 29 (3), 167–174.

Norlander, S., Nordgren, B., 1998. Clinical symptoms related to musculoskeletal neck-shoulder pain and mobility in the cervico-thoracic spine. Scandinavian Journal of Rehabilitation Medicine. 30 (4), 243–251.

Pho, C., Godges, J., 2004. Management of whiplash-associated disorder addressing thoracic and cervical spine impairments: a case report. J. Orthop. Sports Phys. Ther. 34 (9), 511–519.

Piva, S.R., Erhard, R.E., Al-Hugail, M., 2000. Cervical radiculopathy: a case problem using a decision-making algorithm. J. Orthop. Sports Phys. Ther. 30 (12), 745–754.

Piva, S.R., Erhard, R.E., Childs, J.D., Browder, D.A., 2006. Inter-tester reliability of passive inter-vertebral and active movements of the cervical spine. Man. Ther. 11 (4), 321–330.

Powers, C.M., Kulig, K., Harrison, J., Bergman, G., 2003. Segmental mobility of the lumbar spine during a posterior to anterior mobilization: assessment using dynamic MRI. Clin. Biomech. 1 (1), 80–83.

Raney, N.H., Teyhen, D.S., Childs, J.D., 2007. Observed changes in lateral abdominal muscle thickness after spinal manipulation: a case series using rehabilitative ultrasound imaging. J. Orthop. Sports Phys. Ther. 37 (8), 472–479.

Ross, J.K., Bereznick, D.E., McGill, S.M., 2004. Determining cavitation location during lumbar and thoracic spinal manipulation: is spinal manipulation accurate and specific? Spine 29 (13), 1452–1457.

Savolainen, A., Ahlberg, J., Nummila, H., Nissinen, M., 2004. Active or passive treatment for neck-shoulder pain in occupational health care? A randomized controlled trial. Occup. Med. 54 (6), 422–424.

Schiller, L., 2001. Effectiveness of spinal manipulative therapy in the treatment of mechanical thoracic spine pain: a pilot randomized clinical trial. J. Manipulative Physiol. Ther. 24 (6), 394–401.

Sobel, J.S., Kremer, I., Winters, J.C., Arendzen, J.H., de Jong, B.M., 1996. The influence of the mobility in the cervicothoracic spine and the upper ribs (shoulder girdle) on the mobility of the scapulohumeral joint. J. Manipulative Physiol. Ther. 19 (7), 469–474.

Sobel, J.S., Winters, J.C., Groenier, K., et al., 1997. Physical examination of the cervical spine and shoulder girdle in patients with shoulder complaints. J. Manipulative Physiol. Ther. 20 (4), 257–262.

Sparkes, V., Prevost, A.T., Hunter, J.O., 2003. Derivation and identification of questions that act as predictors of abdominal pain of musculoskeletal origin. Eur. J. Gastroenterol. Hepatol. 15 (9), 1021–1027.

Theodoridis, D., Ruston, S., 2002. The effect of shoulder movements on thoracic spine 3D motion. Clin. Biomech. 17 (5), 418–421.

Viti, J.A., Paris, S.V., 2000. The use of upper thoracic manipulation in a patient with headache. J. Man. Manip. Ther. 8 (1), 25–28.

Wainner, R.S., Whitman, J., Cleland, J.A., Flynn, T.W., 2007. Regional interdependence: a musculoskeletal examination model whose time has come. J. Orthop. Sports Phys. Ther. 37 (11), 658–660.

Waldrop, M.A., 2006. Diagnosis and treatment of cervical radiculopathy using a clinical prediction rule and a multimodal intervention approach: a case series. J. Orthop. Sports Phys. Ther. 36 (3), 152–159.

Winters, J.C., Sobel, J.S., Groenier, K.H., et al., 1997. Comparison of physiotherapy, manipulation, and corticosteroid injection for treating shoulder complaints in general practice: randomised, single blind study. Br. Med. J. 314 (7090), 1320–1325.

Winters, J.C., Jorritsma, W., Groenier, K.H., Sobel, J.S., Meyboom-de Jong, B., Arendzen, H.J., 1999. Treatment of shoulder complaints in general practice: long term results of a randomised, single blind study comparing physiotherapy, manipulation, and corticosteroid injection. BMJ (Clinical Research Ed.) 318 (7195), 1395–1396.

Wood, K.B., Schellhas, K.P., Garvey, T.A., Aeppli, D., 1999. Thoracic discography in healthy individuals. A controlled prospective study of magnetic resonance imaging and discography in asymptomatic and symptomatic individuals. Spine 24 (15), 1548–1555.

Young, B.A., Gill, H.E., Wainner, R.S., Flynn, T.W., 2008. Thoracic costotransverse joint pain patterns: a study in normal volunteers. BMC Musculoskelet. Disord. 9, 140.

Young, I.A., Michener, L.A., Cleland, J.A., Aguilera, A.J., Snyder, A.R., 2009. Manual therapy, exercise, and traction for patients with cervical radiculopathy: A randomized clinical trial. Phys. Ther. 89 (7), 632–642.

Chapter | 12 |

Cervical spine mobilization and manipulation

John R Krauss, Douglas S Creighton

INTRODUCTION

It is estimated that 18–250 million manipulations are performed in the United States each year (Shekelle & Coulter 1997, Licht et al 2003) with over 2 million cervical manipulations performed on the cervical spine in Britain alone (Thiel & Bolton 2004). The use of manipulation and mobilization of the spine was documented as far back as 400BCE (Sigerist 1951) and continues to be used by modern medical professionals including physical therapists, chiropractors and osteopaths in the treatment of neck and head pain. Despite the historic and continued use of these manual therapy interventions there remains debate surrounding the safety, and efficacy of manipulative treatment for head and neck pain.

ADVERSE REACTIONS TO CERVICAL MANIPULATION AND MOBILIZATION

When considering the issue of safety, adverse reactions associated with manipulation and mobilization range from minor and self-limiting injuries such as headaches, stiffness, and limitations in motion (Senstad et al 1996, Lebouef-Yde et al 1997, Cagnie et al 2004, Hurwitz et al 2005) to serious injuries including permanent neurological deficits, dissection of a carotid or vertebral artery, and death (Di Fabio 1999, Ernst 2002, Haldeman et al 2002, Licht et al 2003, Oppenheim et al 2005). Evidence from the

DOI: 10.1016/B978-0-7020-3528-9.00012-1

literature suggests that adverse reactions are more likely following manipulation than mobilization and occur in the cervical spine more often than in other spinal regions (Senstad et al 1996, Lebouef-Yde et al 1997, Hurwitz et al 2005). An estimated 35–65% of patients report minor symptoms following their first manipulation (Senstad et al 1996, Lebouef-Yde et al 1997, Cagnie et al 2004, Hurwitz et al 2005). In general, it appears that minor adverse responses occur at a higher rate (one incident for every 476 to 1573 manipulations) (Di Fabio 1999) as compared to serious adverse response which occur at an estimated rate of one incident per 20,000 to 3,000,000 manipulations (Hurwitz et al 1996, Lebouef-Yde et al 1997, Shekelle & Coulter 1997, Di Fabio 1999, Gross et al 2002a, Haldeman et al 2002, Licht et al 2003, Oppenheim et al 2005). The actual number of adverse responses to cervical manipulation is difficult to estimate due to factors such as practitioner under-reporting, failure to follow-up with patients who do not return for treatment after receiving manipulation, and the potential delay in symptom onset following manipulation (Assendelft et al 1996, Di Fabio 1999, Norris et al 2000, Ernst 2002, Oppenheim et al 2005).

In order to assist the clinician in recognizing the implications of adverse responses on patient care it is necessary to include the associated loss of patient function and the need for follow-up treatment when reporting the degree of adverse response. With the exception of the most severe cases, the classification of adverse responses within the literature has lacked clear and consistent nomenclature especially regarding loss of function and follow-up treatment. To address this, Carnes et al (2010) suggests a three-layered pragmatic approach to the qualification of adverse events that includes the duration, severity, description, treatment and functional implications of the adverse response. Using these qualifiers, major, moderate and minor adverse events would be described as follows: (1) major adverse events are medium to long term in duration, moderate to severe in severity, described as unacceptable by the patient, and require further treatment for resolution, (2) moderate adverse events are the same as major adverse events in all aspects except that they are moderate in severity and (3) mild adverse events are of short duration, mild in severity, self limiting, and require no further treatment (Carnes et al 2010).

EVIDENCE FOR CERVICAL MANIPULATION AND MOBILIZATION

While there appears to be potential for post-manipulative adverse reactions, there is evidence suggesting that manipulation and mobilization are effective in immediately improving cervical range of motion and decreasing neck pain when applied to the cervical (Pikula 1999, Martinez-Segura et al 2006) and thoracic (Cleland et al 2005, Fernandez-de-las-Peñas et al 2007, Krauss et al 2008) spine. In addition, current evidence suggests that single applications of manipulation are more effective than single applications of mobilization in immediately reducing acute cervical pain and increasing range of motion (Martinez-Segura et al 2006). However, multiple applications of either treatment appear to yield similar results in terms of effects (Cassidy et al 1992, Hurwitz et al 2002). When managing chronic pain (pain lasting greater than 6 months) multimodal intervention combining manipulation or mobilization with exercise results in superior outcomes than using either in isolation (Evans et al 2002, Gross et al 2002b, 2004). Finally, the early use of mobilization and manipulation in the management of acute neck disorders appears to be associated with better outcomes than when these treatments are delayed (Boissonnault & Badke 2008).

HYPOTHESIZED MECHANISMS OF EFFECT

Historically, several potential mechanisms have been hypothesized to account for the outcomes associated with manipulation and mobilization. Biomechanical effects have been speculated to occur due to one or more of the following mechanisms: (1) release of entrapped synovial folds or plica, (2) relaxation of hypertonic muscle by sudden stretching, (3) disruption of articular or periarticular adhesions, (4) restoration of the proper mid position at rest, and (5) restoration of normal physiologic range of motion in joints that are 'stuck' in an end range position (Shekelle 1994, Evans 2002). Anatomical structures (Bogduk & Jull 1985, Giles & Taylor 1987, Mercer & Bogduk 1993) and biomechanical mechanisms (Palfrey & Newton 1970, Semlak & Ferguson 1970) have been identified that partially support mechanisms 1–3, however, supportive evidence for mechanisms 4 and 5 still remains lacking (Gal et al 1995, 1997, Evans 2002). One event that has been hypothesized to account for some of the biomechanical mechanisms associated with the positive results of spinal manipulation and mobilization is the formation and release of gas bubbles within the synovial fluid during manipulation. This event generates a 'cracking, popping or clicking' noise termed a cavitation and has been viewed as a sign that the manipulation was applied correctly (Evans & Breen 2006). However, recent studies suggest that improvements in pain and range of motion following manipulation is not dependent on the generation of joint cavitation (Herzog et al 1995, Flynn et al 2003, 2006, Ross et al 2004). Finally, other non-biomechanical mechanisms such as changes in dorsal horn activation in the spinal cord (Malisza et al 2003a), endogenous opioid responses (Vernon et al 1986), and improved psychological outcomes (Williams et al 2007) have also been associated with joint mobilization and manipulation.

Changes in dorsal horn activity, opioid responses and psychological outcomes are examples of neurophysiological effects from mobilization and manipulation and are theorized to originate from peripheral nervous system mechanisms, spinal cord mechanisms, and supraspinal mechanisms (Sterling et al 2001, Pickar 2002). Recent research suggests that manipulation and mobilization may account for peripheral nervous system mechanisms associated with reduction of blood and serum level cytokines, changes in β-endorphin, N-palmitoylethanolamide, anandamide, serotonin, endogenous cannabinoids and substance P levels (McPartland et al 2005, Teodorczyk-Injeyan et al 2006, Degenhardt et al 2007). In addition to peripheral nervous system mechanisms, manipulation and mobilization are proposed to generate a counter irritation effect through spinal cord mechanisms (Pickar & Wheeler 2001, Malisza et al 2003b, Boal & Gillette 2004). Last, manipulation and mobilization may reduce spinal cord responses through supraspinal descending inhibition through the anterior cingular cortex, amygdale, periaqueductal grey, and the rostral ventromedial medulla (Hsieh et al 1995, Vogt et al 1996, Derbyshire et al 1997, Iadarola et al 1998, Peyron et al 2000, Moulton et al 2005, Guo et al 2006, Bee & Dickenson 2007, Oshiro et al 2007, Staud et al 2007).

SPECIFICITY OF MANIPULATION AND MOBILIZATION

Based on the available scientific literature, it is likely that both biomechanical and neurophysiological mechanisms account for the principle outcomes (pain reduction and motion improvement) associated with mobilization and manipulation (Bialosky et al 2009). Accepting this notion, the question has been raised whether manipulation need be, and can be specific in terms of the movements and outcomes generated in the spine during treatment (Cleland & Childs 2005, Flynn 2006, Aquino et al 2009, Schomacher 2009). Regarding these questions, some studies have examined the effects of manipulative techniques using centrally applied posterior to anterior pressures (central PAs) on the spinous processes in the lumbar and cervical spines (Powers et al 2003, Kulig et al 2004, Lee et al 2005). These authors concluded that the greatest motion was generated at the point of contact. They also concluded that motion was generated at segments both cranial and caudal to the point of contact. Outcomes studies using the same mobilization technique concluded that there was no difference in levels of pain based on whether the most painful segment was treated or whether a randomly selected segment was treated (Beneck et al 2000, Lande et al 2008, Aquino et al 2009). When evaluating

the outcomes based studies which used the central PA technique only one of the studies indicated the amount of force used during mobilization (Maitland grade IV) (Beneck et al 2000, Hengeveld et al 2005, Lande et al 2008) the other left the decision of force to the discretion of the therapist which was not specified (Aquino et al 2009). Finally, the outcomes which were reported were immediate in nature and do not provide insight regarding the implications of repeated applications of these techniques in terms of adverse responses.

Caution should be used when generalizing the results of these studies to all mobilization and manipulation techniques. While these studies provide valuable insights into the inter-relationship of movement between vertebrae when a single central force is applied to the spine in a mid position they examine only one technique. In addition the technique makes no attempt to stabilize adjacent spinal levels leaving the degree of specificity in question. If the manual practitioner were to accept the assumption that it is not necessary or possible to be specific what would be the consequences? The most likely one would be unwanted and unanticipated adverse responses. The literature suggests that poorly localized and overly forceful manipulations may provoke adverse responses when applied through degenerative spinal segments (Assendelft et al 1996, Murphy 2006, Murphy et al 2006). For example, rotational manipulation of the cervical spine is associated with increased risk of carotid or vertebral artery dissection (Assendelft et al 1996, Smith et al 2003). It would therefore seem reasonable that in order to minimize the risk of adverse events occurring as a result of spinal manipulation it is necessary to either carefully select patients when using less specific manipulative techniques or use techniques which attempt to be more specific through the use of manual stabilization and/or spinal prepositioning.

SELECTING PATIENTS FOR CERVICAL MANIPULATION AND MOBILIZATION

Selecting patients who respond positively to manipulation and who will not experience adverse responses has traditionally been attempted through the use of a comprehensive history and physical exam and the use of pre-manipulative testing such as the vertebral artery test. Unfortunately tests and measures such as the vertebral artery test do not appear to accurately predict responses of these vascular structures to rotational manipulation (Arnold et al 2004, Thiel & Rix 2005). Recent attempts to improve patient selection include the development of clinical predication rules (CPRs) which in general attempt to match patient characteristics to patient interventions (Childs & Cleland 2006). In terms of manipulation, efforts in this area have resulted in CPRs that identify patient characteristics (e.g. number of days since onset of symptoms and joint hypomobility) and conditions (acute neck pain, cervicogenic headaches and radiculopathy) that respond favourably to manipulation in the lumbar, thoracic and cervical spines (Flynn et al 2002, Childs et al 2004, Cleland et al 2006, 2007a,b, Fleming et al 2007). While CPRs provide valuable insight into the connection between examination findings and treatment response, studies performed for neck related conditions have not been validated. In addition, the cervical CPRs are condition oriented (cervical radiculopathy and cervicogenic headache) and do not provide specifics regarding the mobilizations and manipulations associated with successful intervention (Cleland et al 2007b, Fleming et al 2007). Therefore, it has been recommended that further research is necessary before these CPRs can be generally applied with confidence (Hancock et al 2007, May & Resendale 2009).

An additional approach to minimizing adverse responses due to unwanted motion through adjacent spinal levels focuses more on technique design matched with patient selection. The principle behind these techniques is the notion that manual stabilization, segmental prepositioning, and the direction of force used during manipulation will impact the amount of force and direction of movement generated within the treatment segment and surrounding spinal levels (Krauss et al 2006). More specifically, techniques are applied which attempt to reduce pain and restore normal segmental motion using disc traction, facet separation or facet gliding as either sustained stretches (mobilizations) or impulses (manipulations). The selection of the specific type of technique (disc traction, facet separation, and facet gliding) and the degree to which manual stabilization and prepositioning of non-treatment segments are used depends on: (1) the amount and type of motion restriction, (2) the number of restricted spinal levels, (3) symptom duration and intensity, and (4) the degree of anatomical and pathomechanical changes at both the treatment segment and the adjacent spinal segments. Recent evidence supports the influence of prepositioning and manual stabilization in reducing movement in adjacent spinal levels for the upper cervical spine (Cattrysse et al 2007a,b). In addition, there is also limited evidence that techniques which use these principles can be applied without adverse response to patients with degenerative spinal conditions (Creighton et al 2005, Kondratek et al 2006).

TRANSLATORIC CERVICAL MANIPULATION AND MOBILIZATION

The techniques presented within this chapter were co-developed by Freddy Kaltenborn (PT, OMT) and Olaf Evjenth (PT, OMT) of Norway. The emphasis of these techniques is the avoidance of moderate to severe adverse responses as presented by Carnes et al (2010) and maximum outcomes in terms of pain reduction, motion restoration and disability reduction. Interestingly, the challenges Kaltenborn and Evjenth faced as they began developing these techniques in 1970 continues to be reflected today in terms of adverse responses, mechanisms of effect, specificity, and outcomes (Krauss et al 2006, Kaltenborn 2008). For the purposes of this chapter we use terminology consistent with an international perspective where: (1) manipulation is defined as a high velocity low amplitude movement delivered at the end of available restricted joint motion and within the normal anatomical range of joint motion, and (2) mobilization is defined as a low velocity varying amplitude (static holding, low amplitude, moderate amplitude) movement delivered at various points in the joints restricted range of motion or at the end of the available restricted joint motion and within the normal anatomical range of joint motion. More specifically, mobilization forces are applied within the available range of joint motion in a static or oscillatory manner when pain and/or orthopaedic conditions associated with tissue weakness are present. In contrast, mobilization, applied as a static hold, or manipulation (which is an impulse) is applied at the end of available joint motion when pain and/or orthopaedic conditions associated with tissue tightness are present.

Techniques presented in this chapter are grouped according to type and described using the American Academy of Orthopedic Manual Physical Therapy's recommended standardized terminology which includes: (1) the rate of application, (2) location in range of available movement, (3) direction of force, (4) target of force, (5) relative structural movement, and (6) patient position (Mintken et al 2008). Additional insights regarding the use of the techniques and errors to avoid are also provided.

Translatoric traction techniques

Translatoric traction techniques are used to unload/decompress the disc joint and inter-vertebral foramen contents (nerves, arteries, veins and lymphatics). Disc traction manipulations are performed at a right angle to the disc joint in what is essentially a cranially directed force. During disc traction bilaterally applied manipulative forces are used in an attempt to generate equal movement/traction of all parts of the inter-vertebral joint.

C2–C7 disc traction in supine (Fig 12.1)

The patient is supine in a position of greatest comfort where signs and symptoms are most minimal. The therapist stands facing the top of the patient's head. The therapist's left and right hands contact the posterior surface of

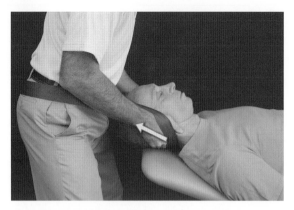

Fig 12.1 C2–C7 disc traction in supine.

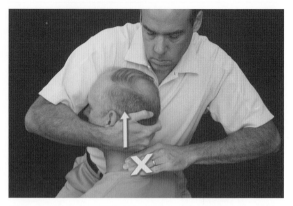

Fig 12.2 C2–C7 disc traction seated.

the transverse processes, lamina, inferior articular processes and spinous process of the cranial vertebra in the treatment segment. A belt may be placed around the therapist's waist and over the therapist's hands to assist in the generation of traction forces. The slack in the treatment segment is taken up in a cranial direction with both hands and the manipulation or mobilization is delivered using the same direction of motion. *Specificity*: Generally low, degree to which traction occurs in the spinal segments caudal to the point of contact is dependent on factors such as amount of force used and the amount of motion available at each spinal segment.

Note: In cases of cervical nerve irritation secondary to disc degeneration the authors recommend disc traction mobilization and manipulation. If radicular irritation is not stable, in other words the radicular discomfort is severe and variable; generally we recommend oscillatory disc traction mobilization. Above all, we feel that success in terms of immediate radicular symptom reduction with manual disc traction is often a matter of positioning as opposed to a matter of manipulative speed or force. We attempt to position the patient's involved segment using a combination of flexion, side bending and rotation such that the patient's symptoms lessen prior to the application of the disc traction mobilization procedure.

C2–C7 disc traction seated (Fig 12.2)

The patient is sitting in a position of greatest comfort where signs and symptoms are most minimal. The therapist stands in front of and to the right of the patient. The therapist's right hand holds around the left side of the inferior articular process and lamina of the cranial vertebra in the treatment segment. The right side of the therapist's chest is placed against the right side of the patient's head. The therapist's left hand contacts the bilateral laminae of the caudal vertebra. The slack in the treatment segment is taken up in a cranial direction with the right hand and chest. The therapist's left hand presses in a caudal direction as the slack is taken up. The manipulation or mobilization force

is directed cranially. *Specificity*: This technique is more specific than the supine version due to manual stabilization of the caudal vertebrae; however this would still be considered a lower specificity technique.

Note: We often use seated disc traction mobilization and manipulation in patients who present with single or multi-segment hypomobility. Patients who are less symptomatic, in other words more 'stiffness dominant' may benefit from the increased specificity and resultant increased manipulative force this technique allows. Note in Figure 12.2 how the non-manipulating hand manually stabilized the caudal vertebra in a ventral and caudal direction prior to applying either a cranially directed mobilization or manipulation.

Translatoric articular/facet separation techniques

Translatoric articular/facet separation techniques are used to unload/decompress the articular surfaces of occipito-atlanto (OA) and atlanto-axial (AA) joints and the facet joints in the lower cervical spine. Techniques grouped in this category generate separation of the articular surfaces (OA and AA articulations and C2–7 facets) that is unique from disc traction in that separation of all points of the articular surface is not equal. This is due in part to the use of unilaterally generated impulses in addition to the orientation of the facet surfaces. In the upper cervical spine, since the articular surfaces of the joints are positioned in the transverse plane the manipulation is directed cranially and slightly medially to maintain bony contact. In the lower cervical spine the facet joints are oriented approximately 45° from the horizontal. To generate the greatest amount of facet separation in the lower cervical spine the treatment segment is positioned in opposite side bending and rotation and the manipulation is directed in a ventral, medial and caudal direction. If applying this technique with a thrust the position of the segment and the facet joint should be such that the facet is in its most loose packed position for separation.

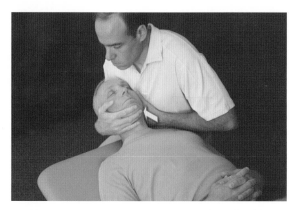

Fig 12.3 Occipito-atlanto (OA) separation in supine.

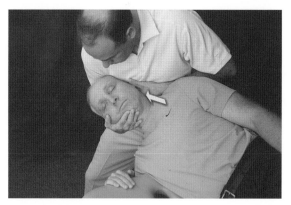

Fig 12.4 Atlanto-axial (AA) separation in side-lying.

Occipito-atlanto (OA) separation in supine (Fig 12.3)

The patient is positioned supine with slight left side bending, right rotation and dorsal flexion of the occiput on the atlas. The therapist is positioned to the left of the patient's head, neck and shoulder. The therapist's left hand and forearm are positioned behind the patient's head and against the right side of the patient's face. The therapist's left hand contacts the inferior edge of the patient's left mastoid process. The slack between occiput and atlas is taken up in a cranial direction by the therapist's right hand and chest. The manipulation/mobilization is delivered by the left hand in a cranial direction. *Specificity*: This is typically an articulation that responds with a cavitation when the technique is performed with the correct speed and prepositioning. No attempt is made to stabilize caudally so movement will occur below the point of contact.

Note: We feel that loosening the OA joint is often necessary in cases of upper cervical motion impairment. Only a few degrees of coupled side bending and rotation is available at the C0/C1 segment, but given the ligamentous connection (alar ligament) between the lateral masses of the occiput and the Dens Process of C2, improving mobility at C0/C1 can in some cases also improve coupled rotation at the C2 motion segment. Improving coupled rotation at either the C0/C1 segment or the C2/C3 segment will often improve upper cervical coupled rotation. Anecdotally, in patient cases where arthritic changes have limited the mobility at the OA joint and patients report an increase in occipital pain with active and passive upper cervical motion, the authors have found good reduction in occipital pain referral after application of OA traction manipulation.

Atlanto-axial (AA) separation in side-lying (Fig 12.4)

The patient is positioned side-lying with slight right side bending, left rotation and dorsal flexion of the atlas on the axis. The therapist is positioned behind the patient's head, neck and upper torso. The therapist's right hand and forearm are positioned under the right side of the patient's head with the index and middle fingers cupped around the patient's chin. The therapist's left hand contacts the inferior edge of the patient's transverse process and posterior arch of atlas. The slack between atlas and axis is taken up in a cranial direction by the therapist's right hand and chest. The manipulation/mobilization is delivered by the left hand in a cranial direction. *Specificity*: Generally low, degree to which traction occurs in the spinal segments caudal to the point of contact is dependent of factors such as amount of force used and the amount of motion available at each spinal segment

Note: We feel that rotational pre-positioning to the upper cervical segments using slow movement that is under the patient's control to stop is a safe and acceptable way to take up available capsule-ligamentous slack. Authors of this chapter discourage the use of high velocity rotational manipulation of the atlas on axis. Rather, after slow rotational pre-positioning of the upper cervical region, we recommend short amplitude translational movements in a cranial direction of atlas on axis as seen in Figure 12.4.

C2–C7 facet separation seated version 1 (Fig 12.5)

With the patient seated, the patient's cervical spine down through the treatment segment is positioned in right side bending and left rotation. The therapist stands to the left of the patient. The therapist's left hand supports the right posterior edge of the transverse process, articular process and lamina of the cranial vertebra in the treatment segment. The therapist's right thumb contacts the lamina and superior articular process of the caudal vertebra in the treatment segment. The slack in the treatment segment is taken up through prepositioning in right side bending and left rotation and by applying a slight cranial force

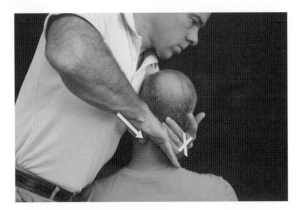

Fig 12.5 C2–C7 facet separation seated version 1.

on the cervical spine with the left hand and shoulder. The manipulation is delivered by the therapist's right thumb in a ventral, medial and caudal direction. *Specificity*: This technique is moderate to very specific in terms of the motion generated at the treatment segment and the direct manual contact point on the inferior facet. In addition the prepositioning and support of the cranial vertebra will reduce motion in segments cranial to the treatment segment. Movement of the caudal segments may occur towards a mid position.

Note: In complicated cervical presentations, e.g. mid-cervical symptomatic hypermobility with segmental hypomobility either above or below or radicular irritation with segmental hypomobility at segments either above or below, this version of facet joint distraction allows for simultaneous application of manual traction. This is applied with the therapist non-manipulating hand and the chest while the therapist thumb applies a specific facet joint distraction to the hypomobile level. Application of a

sustained manual traction takes up ligamentous slack and prevents excessive angular and translational movement at hypermobile segments during specific facet joint distraction mobilization/manipulation. This same manual traction which is generally applied throughout the entire neck can also prevent radicular irritation in patients presenting with this finding and segmental hypomobility.

C2–C7 facet separation seated version 2
(Fig 12.6)

With the patient seated, the patient's cervical spine down through the treatment segment is positioned in left side bending and right rotation. The therapist stands to the left of the patient. The therapist's left forearm is placed against the left side of the patient's face and neck supporting the head position. The radial border of the therapist's right second MCP contacts the lamina and superior articular process of the caudal vertebra in the treatment segment. The slack in the treatment segment is taken up through prepositioning in left side bending and right rotation. The manipulation/mobilization is delivered by the radial border of the therapist's right hand in a ventral, medial and caudal direction. *Specificity*: This technique is moderate to very specific in terms of the motion generated at the treatment segment and the direct manual contact point on the inferior facet. In addition the prepositioning and support of the cranial vertebra will reduce motion in segments cranial to the treatment segment. Movement of the caudal segments may occur towards a mid position.

Note: The authors often apply this version of facet distraction in the more 'stiffness dominant' patients, those whose cervical impairments are less symptomatic or perhaps only painful at or close to the end range of their active cervical motions. The mobilization version of this

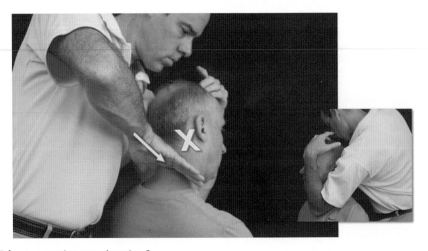

Fig 12.6 C2–C7 facet separation seated version 2.

technique can be applied with longer periods of sustained stretching for joints that are quite hypomobile.

C2–C7 facet separation in supine contralateral gap (Fig 12.7)

With the patient supine, the patient's cervical spine down through the treatment segment is positioned in right side bending and left rotation. The therapist stands to the left of the patient's head, neck and shoulder. The therapist's right forearm is placed against the right side of the patient's face supporting the head position. The radial border of the therapist's left second MCP contacts the left inferior and superior articular processes of the treatment segment. The slack in the treatment segment is taken up through prepositioning in left side bending and right rotation. The manipulation is delivered by the radial border of the therapist's left hand in a medial, slightly cranial and slightly dorsal direction. *Specificity*: This technique is moderately specific in terms of the motion generated at the treatment segment. Specificity is enhanced by taking up soft tissue slack in the treatment segment through pre-positioning in side bending and rotation. Impulses that are too long or movement of the support hand and therapist's body during the manipulation may generate unwanted movement in the spinal segments cranial and caudal to the treatment segment.

Note: We will often apply this mobilization/manipulation technique in patients who demonstrate facet joint hypomobility and overlying soft tissue tenderness on the same side. Figure 12.7 shows how the right facet joint is separated using a manual contact and manipulative force applied on the left side of the neck.

C7 facet separation in supine (Fig 12.8)

With the patient supine, the patient's C7 spinal segment is positioned in left side bending and right rotation. A large mobilization wedge (Norsk wedge pictured) is placed under the upper thoracic spine with the base facing cranial and positioned under T1. The therapist stands to the left of the patient's shoulder. The ulnar border of the therapist's left hand presses in the direction of the anterior surface of the patient's right transverse process of C7. The therapist's right hand is placed over the left to support the contact and wrist and hand position. The slack in the treatment segment is taken up through prepositioning. The manipulation or mobilization is delivered by the ulnar border of the therapist's left hand in a dorsal, lateral and cranial direction. *Specificity*: Due to the contact on C7 and the firm stabilization provided by the wedge this technique is considered moderately specific.

Note: In patients with hypo-mobile C7/T1 segments, this mobilization/manipulation technique provides a fairly strong stretch to the periarticular structures at the C7/T1 articulation. If a patient presents with symptomatic mid-cervical hypermobility or degenerative change we often choose to loosen the C7 segment with the patient's neck well supported and unloaded in a supine position.

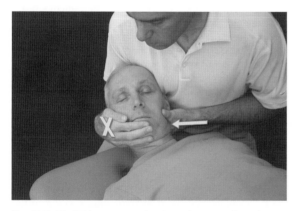

Fig 12.7 C2–C7 facet separation in supine contralateral gap.

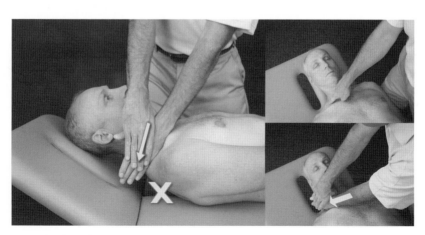

Fig 12.8 C7 facet separation in supine.

Translatoric facet gliding techniques

Translatoric facet gliding techniques are directed parallel to the articular surfaces in the upper and lower cervical spines. In the upper cervical spine the manipulative force is principally directed in a ventral and dorsal direction. In the lower cervical spine (C2–C7) the force is directed ventral, medial and cranial and dorsal, caudal. The decision regarding the direction of movement used for gliding techniques is determined by the direction of restricted motion. More specifically, dorsal gliding at the OA joint is used when ventral flexion of the joint is restricted and ventral gliding at the OA joint is used when dorsal flexion is restricted. In the lower cervical spine, ventral cranial gliding is used when ventral flexion is limited, or in the case of a right unilateral restriction when ventral flexion and left side bending and left rotation are restricted. Dorsal caudal gliding is used when dorsal flexion is restricted, or in the case of a right unilateral restriction when dorsal flexion and right side bending and rotation are restricted. During these techniques it is important that the compression forces are avoided during gliding. This is accomplished by applying a small amount (Kaltenborn Grade 1) traction to the joint prior to gliding.

Occipito-atlanto (OA) unilateral dorsal glide in supine (Fig 12.9)

The patient is positioned in supine with slight right side bending, left rotation and ventral flexion of the occiput on the atlas. The therapist stands facing the head of the patient. The therapist's left hand is placed posteriorly under the patient's occiput. The therapist's left shoulder is positioned anteriorly on the patient's forehead superior to the patient's left eye. The therapist's right hand contacts and stabilizes the right transverse process and posterior arch of atlas with the MCP and radial border of their index finger. The slack in the right OA joint is taken up by applying a dorsal and medial pressure with the therapist's left shoulder in the direction of the stabilizing hand. The mobilization force is applied in a dorsal and medial direction by the therapist's left shoulder. *Specificity*: This technique is considered moderate to very specific due to segmental prepositioning and the firm stabilization provided to the atlas by the therapist's hand positioned between the posterior arch of atlas and the treatment table.

Note: We have found that the occiput dorsal mobilization technique often reduces complaints of upper cervical pain and improves upper cervical flexion. This improved motion gives patients with the postural impairments an improved ability to bring their eyes into a more horizontal position.

C2–C6 facet ventral-cranial glide in supine (Fig 12.10)

The patient is positioned supine with the lower cervical spine in left side bending, right rotation and slight flexion. The treatment segment is positioned in right side bending, right rotation and slight ventral flexion. The therapist is positioned to the left of the patient's head, neck and left shoulder. The therapist's right hand and forearm are positioned under the right side of the patient's head with the ulnar side of the hand contacting the right inferior articular process, lamina and spinous process of the cranial vertebra in the treatment segment. The slack in the treatment segment is taken up during prepositioning. The manipulation is applied by the therapist's left hand in a ventral, medial and cranial direction. *Specificity*: Due to the use of spinal locking and manual reinforcement this technique is moderate to very specific. When applied correctly this technique typically generates a cavitation.

Note: Loosening coupled rotation and side bending at the C2 segment may assist in improving rotation of the dens within its osteo-ligamentous ring. This improves the ligamentous tensioning mechanism between the alar

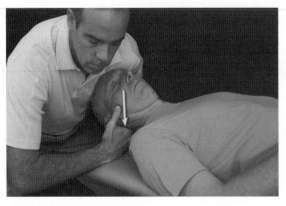

Fig 12.9 Occipito-atlanto (OA) unilateral dorsal glide in supine.

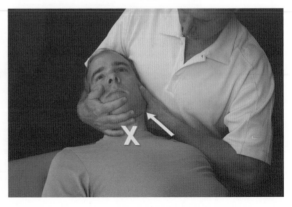

Fig 12.10 C2–C6 facet ventral-cranial glide in supine.

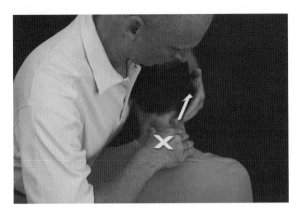

Fig 12.11 C2–C6 facet ventral-cranial glide seated.

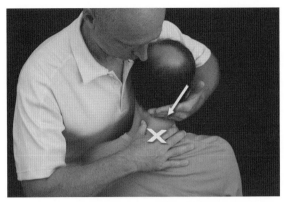

Fig 12.12 C2–C6 facet dorsal-caudal glide seated.

ligament and the occiput. As a result, improved coupled rotation at the C2 segment may enhance coupled motion at the OA segment.

C2–C6 facet ventral-cranial glide seated
(Fig 12.11)

The patient is seated with the lower cervical spine in right side bending, left rotation and slight flexion. The treatment segment is positioned in left side bending, left rotation and slight ventral flexion. The therapist is positioned to the left of the patient's head, neck and left shoulder. The radial border of the therapist's left hand contacts the right inferior articular process of the cranial vertebra in the treatment segment. The therapist's right thumb presses ventrally and medially against the left side of the caudal vertebra's lamina. The slack in the treatment segment is taken up during prepositioning. The manipulation is applied by the therapist's left hand in a ventral, medial and cranial direction. *Specificity*: Due to the use of spinal locking and manual reinforcement this technique is moderate to very specific.

Note: When manipulating the C2 segment, care must be taken that the manipulation hand is not placed on atlas. Anterior translation of atlas may cause unwanted stresses to the upper cervical ligamentous and vascular structures including the transverse ligament and vertebral artery.

C2–C6 facet dorsal-caudal glide seated
(Fig 12.12)

The patient is seated with the lower cervical spine in left side bending, right rotation and slight extension. The treatment segment is positioned in right side bending, right rotation and dorsal flexion. The therapist is positioned to the left of the patient's head, neck and left shoulder. The radial border of the therapist's left hand contacts the right inferior articular process of the cranial

vertebra in the treatment segment. The therapist's left thumb presses ventrally and medially against the left side of the caudal vertebra's lamina. The slack in the treatment segment is taken up during prepositioning. The manipulation is applied by the therapist's left hand in a dorsal, medial and caudal direction. *Specificity*: This technique is moderately specific due to spinal prepositioning and manual stabilization. Some movement may occur above and below the treatment segment.

Note: This mobilization appears to be effective in improving cervical rotation restriction but may increase symptoms from an infra-adjacent segmental irritation, if the segment/facet is compressed, and if manual stabilization is not correctly applied.

C7 facet ventral-cranial glide in supine
(Fig 12.13)

The patient is positioned supine with the C7 in left side bending, left rotation and slight flexion. The therapist is positioned to the left of the patient's head, neck and left shoulder. The radial border of the therapist's right hand

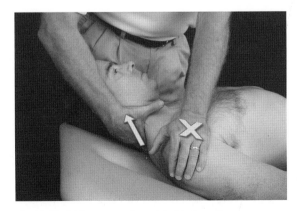

Fig 12.13 C7 facet ventral-cranial glide in supine.

contacts the right inferior articular process of C7. The therapist's left hand presses dorsally on the patient's right shoulder to stabilize T1. The slack in the treatment segment is taken up during prepositioning. The manipulation is applied by the therapist's right hand in a ventral, medial and cranial direction. *Specificity*: This technique is moderately specific. Some movement may occur in the spinal segments cranial to C7, however very little motion should occur in the spinal segments below.

Note: In patients with hypo-mobile C7/T1 segments, this technique provides a fairly strong stretch to the periarticular structures at the C7/T1 articulation. If a patient presents with symptomatic mid-cervical hypermobility or degenerative change we often choose to loosen the C7 segment with the patient's neck well supported and unloaded in a supine position.

C7 facet ventral-cranial glide seated
(Fig 12.14)

The patient is seated with the C7 in slight left side bending, left rotation and slight flexion. The therapist is positioned in front of the patient with his left knee positioned anteriorly contacting the patient's right shoulder and chest. The ulnar border of the therapist left hand contacts the posterior surface of the transverse process of C7 on the right. The radial border of the therapist's right hand contacts the left posterior laminae and facets of C7 and T1. The slack in the treatment segment is taken up during prepositioning. The manipulation is applied by the therapist's left hand in a ventral, medial and cranial direction. *Specificity*: This technique is moderate to very specific. Little movement should occur above or below the treatment segment.

Note: Patients whose cervical conditions are less painful and more stiffness dominates or perhaps only presenting with cervical discomfort closer to the end range of an active cervical movement often respond well to this

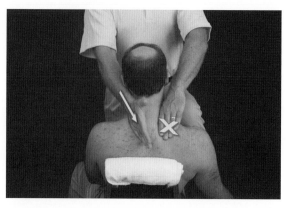

Fig 12.15 C7 facet dorsal-caudal glide seated.

technique. This technique provides a strong stretch to the periarticular structures at the C7/T1 articulation.

C7 facet dorsal-caudal glide seated (Fig 12.15)

The patient is seated with the C7 in slight left side bending, left rotation and dorsal flexion. The therapist is positioned in front of the patient with his left knee positioned anteriorly contacting the patient's right shoulder and chest. The ulnar border of the therapist right hand contacts the posterior surface of the transverse process of C7 on the left. The radial border of the therapist's left hand contacts the right posterior laminae and facets of C7 and T1. The slack in the treatment segment is taken up during prepositioning. The manipulation is applied by the therapist's right hand in a dorsal, medial and caudal direction. *Specificity*: This technique is moderate to very specific. Little movement should occur above or below the treatment segment.

Note: Patients whose cervical conditions are less painful and more stiffness dominates or perhaps only presenting with cervical discomfort closer to the end range of an active cervical movement often respond well to this technique. This technique provides a strong stretch to the periarticular structures at the C7/T1 articulation.

CONCLUSIONS

In summary, recent years have seen great advances in our understanding of the factors associated with successful management of neck and arm pain through the use of mobilization and manipulations of the neck. However, questions and challenges still remain unanswered and require continued open discussion by all practitioners of these interventions. Advancement in our understanding of the possibilities and pitfalls of the clinical practice of mobilization and manipulation requires continued careful examination of practitioner beliefs whether they are based on emerging literature or expert opinion.

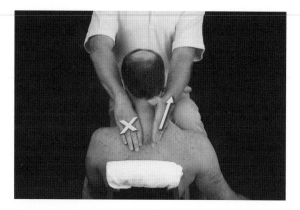

Fig 12.14 C7 facet ventral-cranial glide seated.

REFERENCES

Aquino, R.L., Caires, P.M., Furtado, F.C., Loureiro, A.V., Ferreira, P.H., Ferreira, M.L., 2009. Applying joint mobilization at different cervical vertebral levels does not influence immediate pain reduction in patients with chronic neck pain: A randomized clinical trial. J. Man. Manip. Ther. 17, 95–100.

Arnold, C., Bourassa, R., Langer, T., Stoneham, G., 2004. Doppler studies evaluating the effect of a physical therapy screening protocol on vertebral artery blood flow. Man. Ther. 9, 13–21.

Assendelft, W.J., Bouter, L.M., Knipschild, P.G., 1996. Complications of spinal manipulation: a comprehensive review of the literature. J. Fam. Pract. 42, 475–480.

Bee, L.A., Dickenson, A.H., 2007. Rostral ventromedial medulla control of spinal sensory processing in normal and pathophysiological states. Neuroscience 147, 786–793.

Beneck, G., Kulig, K., Landel, R., Powers, C., 2000. The relationship between lumbar segmental motion and pain response produced by a posterior-to-anterior force in persons with nonspecific low back pain. J. Orthop. Sports Phys. Ther. 35, 203–209.

Bialosky, J.E., Bishop, M.D., Price, D., Robinson, M., George, S., 2009. The mechanisms of Manual Therapy in the treatment of musculoskeletal pain: a comprehensive model. Man. Ther. 14, 531–538.

Boal, R.W., Gillette, R.G., 2004. Central Neuronal Plasticity, Low Back Pain and Spinal Manipulative Therapy. J. Manipulative Physiol. Ther. 27, 314–326.

Bogduk, N., Jull, G., 1985. The theoretical pathology of acute locked back: a basis for manipulative therapy. Manual Medicine 1, 78–82.

Boissonnault, W.G., Badke, M.B., 2008. Influence of acuity on physical therapy outcomes for patients with cervical disorders. Arch. Phys. Med. Rehabil. 89, 81–86.

Cagnie, B., Vinck, E., Beernaert, A., Cambier, D., 2004. How common are side effects of spinal manipulation and can these side effects be predicted? Man. Ther. 9, 151–156.

Carnes, D., Mullinger, B., Underwood, M., 2010. Defining adverse events in manual therapies: A modified Delphi consensus study. Man. Ther. 15, 2–6.

Cassidy, J.D., Lopes, A.A., Yong-Hing, K., 1992. The immediate effect of manipulation versus mobilization on pain and range of motion in the cervical spine: a randomized controlled trial. J. Manipulative Physiol. Ther. 15, 570–575.

Cattrysse, E., Baeyens, J.P., Clarys, J.P., Van Roy, P., 2007a. Manual fixation versus locking during upper cervical segmental mobilization. Part 1: an in vitro three-dimensional arthrokinematic analysis of manual flexion-extension mobilization of the atlanto-occipital joint. Man. Ther. 12, 342–352.

Cattrysse, E., Baeyens, J.P., Clarys, J.P., Van Roy, P., 2007b. Manual fixation versus locking during upper cervical segmental mobilization. Part 2: an in vitro three-dimensional arthrokinematic analysis of manual axial rotation and lateral bending mobilization of the atlanto-axial joint. Man. Ther. 12, 353–362.

Childs, J.D., Cleland, J.A., 2006. Development and application of clinical prediction rules to improve decision making in physical therapist practice. Phys. Ther. 86, 122–131.

Childs, J.D., Fritz, J.M., Flynn, T.W., et al., 2004. A clinical prediction rule to identify patients with low back pain most likely to benefit from spinal manipulation: a validation study. Ann. Intern. Med. 141, 920–928.

Cleland, J.A., Childs, J.D., 2005a. Does Manual Therapy technique matter? Orthopedics Division Reviews 27–28.

Cleland, J.A., Childs, J.D., McRae, M., Palmer, J.A., Stowell, T., 2005b. Immediate effects of thoracic manipulation in patients with neck pain: a randomized clinical trial. Man. Ther. 10, 127–135.

Cleland, J.A., Fritz, J.M., Whitman, J.M., Childs, J.D., Palmer, J.A., 2006. The use of a lumbar spine manipulation technique by physical therapists in patients who satisfy a clinical prediction rule: a case series. J. Orthop. Sports Phys. Ther. 36, 209–214.

Cleland, J.A., Childs, J.D., Fritz, J.M., Whitman, J.M., Eberhart, S.L., 2007a. Development of a clinical prediction rule for guiding treatment of a subgroup of patients with neck pain: use of thoracic spine manipulation, exercise, and patient education. Phys. Ther. 87, 9–23.

Cleland, J.A., Fritz, J.M., Whitman, J.M., Heath, R., 2007b. Predictors of short-term outcome in people with a clinical diagnosis of cervical radiculopathy. Phys. Ther. 87, 1619–1632.

Creighton, D., Viti, J., Krauss, J., 2005. Use of translatoric mobilization in a patient with cervical spondylotic degeneration: A case report. J. Man. Manip. Ther. 13, 12–26.

Degenhardt, B.F., Darmani, N.A., Johnson, J.C., et al., 2007. Role of Osteopathic Manipulative Treatment in Altering Pain Biomarkers: A Pilot Study. J. Am. Osteopath. Assoc. 107, 387–400.

Derbyshire, S.W., Jones, A.K., Gyulai, F., Clark, S., Townsend, D., Firestone, L.L., 1997. Pain processing during three levels of noxious stimulation produces differential patterns of central activity. Pain 73, 431–445.

Di Fabio, R.P., 1999. Manipulation of the cervical spine: risks and benefits. Phys. Ther. 79, 50–65.

Ernst, E., 2002. Manipulation of the cervical spine: a systematic review of case reports of serious adverse events. Med. J. Aust. 176, 376–380.

Evans, D.W., 2002. Mechanisms and effects of spinal high-velocity, low-amplitude thrust manipulation: previous theories. J. Manipulative Physiol. Ther. 25, 251–262.

Evans, D.W., Breen, A.C., 2006. A biomechanical model for mechanically efficient cavitation production during spinal manipulation: prethrust position and the neutral zone. J. Manipulative Physiol. Ther. 29, 72–82.

Evans, R., Bronfort, G., Nelson, B., Goldsmith, C.H., 2002. Two-year follow-up of a randomized clinical trial of spinal manipulation and two types of exercise for patients with chronic neck pain. Spine 27, 2383–2389.

Fernandez-de-las-Penas, C., Palomeque-del-Cerro, L., Rodriguez-Blanco, C., Gomez-Conesa, A., Miangolarra-Page, J.C., 2007. Changes in neck pain and active range of motion after a single thoracic spine manipulation in subjects presenting with mechanical neck pain: a case series. J. Manipulative Physiol. Ther. 30, 312–320.

Fleming, R., Forsythe, S., Cook, C., 2007. Influential variables associated with outcomes in patients with cervicogenic headache. J. Man. Manip. Ther. 15, 155–164.

Flynn, T., Fritz, J., Whitman, J., et al., 2002. A clinical prediction rule for classifying patients with low back pain who demonstrate short-term improvement with spinal manipulation. Spine 27, 2835–2843.

Flynn, T.W., 2006a. There's more than one way to manipulate a spine. J. Orthop. Sports Phys. Ther. 36, 198–199.

Flynn, T.W., Fritz, J.M., Wainner, R.S., Whitman, J.M., 2003. The audible pop is not necessary for successful spinal high-velocity thrust manipulation in individuals with low back pain. Arch. Phys. Med. Rehabil. 84, 1057–1060.

Flynn, T.W., Childs, J.D., Fritz, J.M., 2006b. The audible pop from high-velocity thrust manipulation and outcome in individuals with low back pain. J. Manipulative Physiol. Ther. 29, 40–45.

Gal, J., Herzog, W., Kawchuk, G., Conway, P.J., Zhang, Y.T., 1997. Movements of vertebrae during manipulative thrusts to unembalmed human cadavers. J. Manipulative Physiol. Ther. 20, 30–40.

Gal, J.M., Herzog, W., Kawchuk, G.N., Conway, P.J., Zhang, Y.T., 1995. Forces and relative vertebral movements during SMT to unembalmed post-rigor human cadavers: peculiarities associated with joint cavitation. J. Manipulative Physiol. Ther. 18, 4–9.

Giles, L.G., Taylor, J.R., 1987. Human zygapophyseal joint capsule and synovial fold innervation. Br. J. Rheumatol. 26, 93–98.

Gross, A., Kay, T., Kennedy, C., et al., 2002a. Clinical practice guidelines on the use of manipulation or mobilization in the treatment of adults with mechanical neck disorders. Man. Ther. 7, 193–2005.

Gross, A.R., Kay, T., Hondras, M., et al., 2002b. Manual therapy for mechanical neck disorders: a systematic review. Man. Ther. 7, 131–149.

Gross, A.R., Hoving, J.L., Haines, T.A., et al., 2004. A Cochrane review of manipulation and mobilization for mechanical neck disorders. Spine 29, 1541–1548.

Guo, W., Robbins, M.T., Wei, F., Zou, S., Dubner, R., Ren, K., 2006. Supraspinal brain-derived neurotrophic factor signaling: a novel mechanism for descending pain facilitation. J. Neurosci. 26, 126–137.

Haldeman, S., Kohlbeck, F.J., McGregor, M., 2002. Unpredictability of cerebrovascular ischemia associated with cervical spine manipulation. Spine 27, 49–55.

Hancock, M.J., Maher, C.G., Latimer, J., et al., 2007. Assessment of diclofenac or spinal manipulative therapy, or both, in addition to recommended first-line treatment for acute low back pain: a randomised controlled trial. Lancet 370, 1638–1643.

Hengeveld, E., Banks, K., Maitland, G.D., 2005. Maitland's vertebral manipulation. Elsevier Butterworth-Heinemann, Oxford.

Herzog, W., Conway, P.J., Zhang, Y.T., Gal, J., Guimaraes, A.C., 1995. Reflex responses associated with manipulative treatments on the thoracic spine: a pilot study. J. Manipulative Physiol. Ther. 18, 233–236.

Hsieh, J.C., Belfrage, M., Stone-Elander, S., Hansson, P., Ingvar, M., 1995. Central representation of chronic ongoing neuropathic pain studied by positron emission tomography. Pain 63, 225–236.

Hurwitz, E.L., Aker, P.D., Adams, A.H., Meeker, W.C., Shekelle, P.G., 1996. Manipulation and mobilization of the cervical spine. Spine 21, 1746–1759.

Hurwitz, E.L., Morgenstern, H., Harber, P., Kominski, G.F., Yu, F., Adams, A.H., 2002. A randomized trial of chiropractic manipulation and mobilization for patients with neck pain: clinical outcomes from the UCLA neck-pain study. Am. J. Public Health 92, 1634–1641.

Hurwitz, E.L., Morgenstern, H., Vassilaki, M., Chiang, L.M., 2005. Frequency and clinical predictors of adverse reactions to chiropractic care in the UCLA neck pain study. Spine 30, 1477–1484.

Iadarola, M., Berman, K., Zeffiro, T., et al., 1998. Neural activation during acute capsaicin-evoked pain and allodynia assessed with PET. Brain 121, 931–947.

Kaltenborn, F., 2008. Traction-Manipulation of the Extremities and Spine. vol. III. Norli, Oslo.

Kondratek, M., Creighton, D., Krauss, J., 2006. Use of translatoric mobilization in a patient with cervicogenic dizziness and motion restriction: a case report. J. Man. Manip. Ther. 14, 140–151.

Krauss, J., Evjenth, O., Creighton, D.S., 2006. Translatoric Spinal Manipulation for Physical Therapists. Lakeview Media L.L.C. Publications.

Krauss, J., Creighton, D., Podlewska-Ely, J., 2008. The immediate effects of upper thoracic translatoric spinal manipulation on cervical pain and range of motion: a randomized clinical trial. J. Man. Manip. Ther. 16, 93–99.

Kulig, K., Landel, R., Powers, C.M., 2004. Assessment of lumbar spine kinematics using dynamic MRI: a proposed mechanism of sagittal plane motion induced by manual posterior-to-anterior mobilization. J. Orthop. Sports Phys. Ther. 34, 57–64.

Lande, R., Kulig, K., Fredericson, M., Li, B., Powers, C.M., 2008. Intertester reliability and validity of motion assessments during lumbar spine accessory motion testing. Phys. Ther. 88, 43–49.

Lebouef-Y de, C., Hennius, B., Rudberg, E., Leufvenmark, P., Thunman, M., 1997. Side effects of chiropractic treatment: a prospective study. J. Manipulative Physiol. Ther. 20, 223–228.

Lee, R.Y., McGregor, A.H., Bull, A.M., Wragg, P., 2005. Dynamic response of the cervical spine to posteroanterior mobilisation. Clin. Biomech. 20, 228–231.

Licht, P.B., Christensen, H.W., Hoilund-Carlsen, P.F., 2003. Is cervical spinal manipulation dangerous? J. Manipulative Physiol. Ther. 26, 48–52.

Malisza, K.L., Gregorash, L., Turner, A., et al., 2003a. Functional MRI involving painful stimulation of the ankle and the effect of physiotherapy joint mobilization. J. Magn. Reson. Imaging 21, 489–496.

Malisza, K.L., Stroman, P.W., Turner, A., Gregorash, L., Foniok, T., Wright, A., 2003b. Functional MRI of the rat lumbar spinal cord involving painful stimulation and the effect of peripheral joint mobilization. J. Magn. Reson. Imaging 18, 152–159.

Martinez-Segura, R., Fernandez-de-las-Penas, C., Ruiz-Saez, M., Lopez-Jimenez, C., Rodriguez-Blanco, C., 2006. Immediate effects on neck pain and active range of motion after a single cervical high-velocity low-amplitude manipulation in subjects presenting with mechanical neck pain: a randomized controlled trial. J. Manipulative Physiol. Ther. 29, 511–517.

May, S., Resendale, R., 2009. Prescriptive clinical predication rules in back pain research: A systematic review. J. Man. Manip. Ther. 17, 36–45.

McPartland, J.M., Giuffrida, A., King, J., Skinner, E., Scotter, J., Musty, R.E., 2005. Cannabimimetic effects of osteopathic manipulative treatment. J. Am. Osteopath. Assoc. 105, 283–291.

Mercer, S., Bogduk, N., 1993. Intra-articular inclusions of the cervical synovial joints. Br. J. Rheumatol. 32, 705–710.

Mintken, P.E., DeRosa, C., Little, T., Smith, B., 2008. AAOMPT clinical guidelines: A model for standardizing manipulation terminology in physical therapy practice. J. Orthop. Sports Phys. Ther. 38, A1–A6.

Moulton, E.A., Keaser, M.L., Gullapalli, R.P., Greenspan, J.D., 2005. Regional intensive and temporal patterns of functional MRI activation distinguishing noxious and innocuous contact heat. J. Neurophysiol. 93, 2183–2193.

Murphy, D.R., 2006. Herniated disc with radiculopathy following cervical manipulation: nonsurgical management. Spine J. 6, 459–463.

Murphy, D.R., Hurwitz, E.L., Gregory, A.A., 2006. Manipulation in the presence of cervical spinal cord compression: a case series. J. Manipulative Physiol. Ther. 29, 236–244.

Norris, J.W., Beletsky, V., Nadareishvili, Z.G., 2000. Sudden neck movement and cervical artery dissection. The Canadian Stroke Consortium. Can. Med. Assoc. J. 163, 38–40.

Oppenheim, J.S., Spitzer, D.E., Segal, D.H., 2005. Nonvascular complications following spinal manipulation. Spine J. 5, 660–667.

Oshiro, Y., Quevedo, A.S., McHaffie, J., Kraft, R., Coghill, R.C., 2007. Brain mechanisms supporting spatial discrimination of pain. J. Neurosci. 27, 3388–3394.

Palfrey, A.J., Newton, M., 1970. The viscosity of synovial fluid at high shear rates. J. Anat. 106, 404.

Peyron, R., Laurent, B., García-Larrea, L., 2000. Functional imaging of brain responses to pain. A review and meta-analysis. Clin. Neurophysiol. 30, 263–288.

Pickar, J.G., 2002. Neurophysiological effects of spinal manipulation. Spine J. 2, 357–371.

Pickar, J.G., Wheeler, J.D., 2001. Response of muscle proprioceptors to spinal manipulative-like loads in the anesthetized cat. J. Manipulative Physiol. Ther. 24, 2–11.

Pikula, J., 1999. The effect of spinal manipulation therapy (SMT) on pain reduction and range of motion in patients with acute unilateral neck pain: a pilot study. J. Can. Chiropr. Assoc. 43, 111–119.

Powers, C.M., Kulig, K., Harrison, J., Bergman, G., 2003. Segmental mobility of the lumbar spine during a posterior to anterior mobilization: assessment using dynamic MRI. Clin. Biomech. 18, 80–83.

Ross, J.K., Bereznick, D.E., McGill, S.M., 2004. Determining cavitation location during lumbar and thoracic spinal manipulation: is spinal manipulation accurate and specific? Spine 29, 1452–1457.

Schomacher, J., 2009. The effect of analgesic mobilization technique when applied at symptomatic or asymptomatic levels of the cervical spine in subjects with neck pain: A randomized controlled trial. J. Man. Manip. Ther. 17, 101–108.

Semlak, K., Ferguson Jr., A.B., 1970. Joint stability maintained by atmospheric pressure. An experimental study. Clin. Orthop. Relat. Res. 68, 294–300.

Senstad, O., Lebouef-Y, C., Borchgrevink, C., 1996. Predictors of side effects to spinal manipulative therapy. J. Manipulative Physiol. Ther. 19, 441–445.

Shekelle, P.G., 1994. Spinal manipulation. Spine 19, 858–861.

Shekelle, P.G., Coulter, I., 1997. Cervical spine manipulation: summary report of a systematic review of the literature and a multidisciplinary expert panel. J. Spinal Disord. Tech. 10, 223–228.

Sigerist, H.E., 1951. A History of Medicine, Vol. I: Primitive and Archaic Medicine. vol. I. Oxford University Press, New York.

Smith, W.S., Johnston, S.C., Skalabrin, E.J., et al., 2003. Spinal manipulative therapy is an independent risk factor for vertebral artery dissection. Neurology 60, 1–24–1428.

Staud, R., Craggs, J.G., Robinson, M.E., Perlstein, W.M., Price, D.D., 2007. Brain activity related to temporal summation of C-fiber evoked pain. Pain 129, 130–142.

Sterling, M., Jull, G., Wright, A., 2001. Cervical mobilisation: concurrent effects on pain, sympathetic nervous system activity and motor activity. Man. Ther. 6, 72–81.

Teodorczyk-Injeyan, J.A., Injeyan, H.S., Ruegg, R., 2006. Spinal manipulative therapy reduces inflammatory cytokines but not substance P production in normal subjects. J. Manipulative Physiol. Ther. 29, 14–21.

Thiel, H., Bolton, J., 2004. Estimate of the number of treatment visits involving cervical spine manipulation carried out by members of the British and Scottish Chiropractor Associations over a one-year period. Clinical Chiropractic 7, 163–167.

Thiel, H., Rix, G., 2005. Is it time to stop functional pre-manipulation testing of the cervical spine? Man. Ther. 10, 154–158.

Vernon, H., Dhami, M., Howley, T., Annett, R., 1986. Spinal manipulation and betaendorphin: a controlled study of the effect of a spinal manipulation on plasma beta-endorphin levels in normal males. J. Manipulative Physiol. Ther. 9, 115–123.

Vogt, B.A., Derbyshire, S., Jones, A.K., 1996. Pain processing in four regions of human cingulate cortex localized with co-registered PET and MR imaging. J. Neurosci. 8, 1461–1473.

Williams, N.H., Hendry, M., Lewis, R., Russell, I., Westmoreland, A., Wilkinson, C., 2007. Psychological response in spinal manipulation (PRISM): A systematic review of psychological outcomes in randomised controlled trial. Complement. Ther. Med. 15, 271–283.

Chapter | 13 |

Therapeutic exercise for mechanical neck pain

Carol Kennedy

INTRODUCTION

The use of specific therapeutic exercise as an adjunct to manual therapy treatment has been a major emphasis of physiotherapy in recent years as part of the multimodal approach to management of acute and chronic mechanical neck pain (MNP). It can be challenging to develop a comprehensive exercise programme, attempting to address the many factors involved, yet not overload or irritate the neck.

In a systematic review of the conservative management of MNP, Gross et al (2007) found strong evidence of benefit for long term pain reduction, improved function, and positive global perceived benefit for a combination of manual therapy and exercise for sub-acute and chronic mechanical neck disorders. There was also moderate evidence for long term improved function for neck strengthening and stretching exercises in chronic subjects. For the use of vertigo exercises, there was moderate evidence for high global perceived effect. Sarig-Bahat (2003) in a review of the use of exercise alone concluded that there was strong evidence supporting the effectiveness of dynamic resisted strengthening and proprioceptive exercises. There was also moderate evidence to support the use of early mobility exercises for acute whiplash associated disorder (WAD). Several studies (Jull et al 2002, Ylinen et al 2006, Walker et al 2008) have shown improvements to be maintained over the long term of 1 to 3 years, even though continuation of home exercises following the initial training was inconsistent (Ylinen et al 2007a).

Supervised exercise programmes have been found to be more effective than home exercise or exercise advice in

© 2011 Elsevier Ltd.
DOI: 10.1016/B978-0-7020-3528-9.00013-3

improving self efficacy, fear of movement/re-injury, and pain disability (Taimela et al 2000, Bunketorp et al 2006).

Conley et al (1997) demonstrated that exercises focusing on the upper extremity did not result in hypertrophy of the cervical musculature; strengthening had to be directed specifically to the neck.

Although it is clear that cervical exercise programmes are an effective component in the management of neck pain, which type of exercise that is most effective has not yet been determined. Various programmes of low load cranio-cervical flexion (CCF) exercises, higher load head lift exercises and resisted static and dynamic exercises have all been found to be effective in terms of reducing pain and improving function, but not necessarily superior to each other (Jordan et al 1998, Randlov et al 1998, Bronfort et al 2001, Jull 2000, Falla et al 2006, Vassiliou et al 2006). Higher loaded exercises do seem to be more effective in increasing overall strength and decreasing fatigability (Falla et al 2006, Ylinen et al 2006). The lower load exercise has been shown to be superior for postural control (Falla et al 2007a) and normalizing patterning during cranio-cervical flexion. The higher load programmes have not been tested in groups with higher pain levels and may not be appropriate for that patient population.

This chapter describes various therapeutic exercise interventions for the common impairments seen with MNP patients.

EXERCISES FOR MOTOR FUNCTION

Abnormal recruitment patterning of the anterior cervical muscles occurs in subjects with neck pain with a tendency toward over-dominance of the superficial muscle groups, and inhibition of the deep spinal stabilizers (Jull 2000, Sterling et al 2003, 2004, Falla et al 2004a, Jull et al 2004, 2007a). In low load situations, this imbalance is more apparent, although there is also true weakness and lack of endurance of both deep and superficial muscle groups (Falla et al 2003, O'Leary et al 2007). A timing delay of the neck stabilizers occurs during arm motion, most noticeably the deep neck flexors (DNF), compromising spinal control during upper extremity function (Falla et al 2004b). Studies have shown a tendency toward over-activity in the upper trapezius muscle (UFT) and anterior superficial neck muscles during repetitive arm activities and head lift, with prolonged relaxation times post activity (Nederhand et al 2000, 2002, Falla et al 2004c, Szeto et al 2005). On imaging, subjects with neck pain or headache exhibit atrophy and histological changes of the deep neck extensor muscles at the effected segment (Hallgren et al 1994, Uhlig et al 1995, Kristjansson 2004, Elliot et al 2006, 2008, Fernandez-de-las-Peñas et al 2007, 2008).

Clinically then, it seems important to begin motor retraining in MNP patients by focusing on the ability to recruit and isolate the deep neck flexors and extensors in low load situations. Prolonged holds emphasize the endurance function. During any upper extremity exercises, a pre-set DNF recruitment would help retrain the timing impairment. It is important to encourage complete relaxation of all muscle groups, particularly superficial, following exercise and activity. Progression onto higher load exercises will then regain strength of the full synergy, but must ensure that there is contribution from the deeper muscle groups. Depending on the patient's occupation and activities, this may require additional load beyond the weight of the head.

Recruitment

Deep neck flexors

The basic exercise used to retrain the DNF is the head nod of cranio-cervical flexion (CCF). Although longus capitus and colli muscles are often considered together as the DNF, Cagnie et al (2008) showed that longus capitus is the primary muscle during this motion. The patient is instructed in the proper technique of CCF. Through palpation of the anterior neck both SCM and anterior/middle scalene are monitored, nodding as far into range as possible without activating these muscles. If the cervical extensors are particularly tight, the superficial flexors will contract early to overcome the resistance, making it more effective to lengthen those first to allow a freer nod motion. Unwanted hyoid muscle activity is minimized by having the tongue rest in the roof of the mouth, the jaw relaxed. The head must remain in contact with the surface, but retraction avoided. Cues like 'slide the back of your head up the surface' or 'look down with your eyes as you initiate the nod' may help the patient recruit the deep muscles in isolation. The nod should be held for a 10 count and repeated 10 times, twice daily (Jull et al 2002).

DNF recruitment and isolation can be performed in either supine or up against the wall. Theoretically the wall position is easier because of gravity-assist, but some patients will relax the superficial muscles more effectively in lying and patients with poor posture are often better supported in that position. In standing, the head must remain in contact with the wall throughout the exercise to ensure the use of the flexors, rather than eccentric extensor activity (Fig 13.1). In supine, the use of a towel roll helps to support the normal lordosis of the cervical spine. However, some patients find the roll uncomfortable or will tend to press back against it using retraction instead of the correct CCF motion. Pillow support tends to be easier than without. Clinical reasoning should be utilized to determine which option is optimal for any given patient.

In patients with longstanding bracing patterns of their neck, the scalene muscles often become so facilitated that they are used as primary muscles of respiration. Down-training may start with diaphragmatic breathing

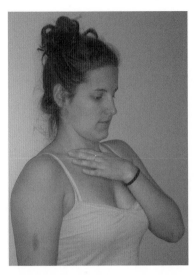

Fig 13.1 Wall slide deep neck flexor recruitment exercise. Keeping the head in contact with the wall, the head is nodded as far as possible without any activity in the superficial muscles, palpated at the anterior neck.

exercises, encouraging lateral costal motion while monitoring the scalene to reduce their excessive activity.

Deep neck extensors

Isolated recruitment of a segmental muscle is difficult, but a 'muscle energy' type technique or electrical muscle stimulation may help teach the patient to feel the desired localized contraction of multifidus or a posterior suboccipital muscle (Fig 13.2). The patient can then practise an auto-resisted contraction at the affected level. Resistance must be light to encourage deep rather than superficial muscle contraction. In supine, a towel roll under the neck may

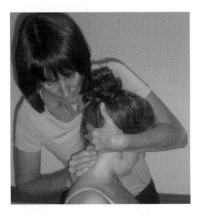

Fig 13.2 Muscle energy recruitment technique. Recruitment of the right C2/3 multifidus muscle is achieved by utilizing a muscle energy type technique.

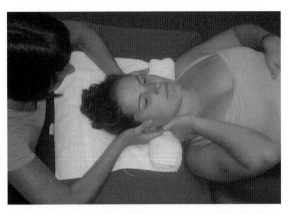

Fig 13.3 Auto-resisted deep neck extensors. In supine with a towel roll, the patient is taught to resist extension/side-flexion at the effected level to recruit the multifidus muscle segmentally.

help the patient perform a unilateral extension quadrant motion to facilitate multifidus contraction (Fig 13.3).

Another method to recruit the DNE is to use a segmental extension motion from a slump position starting in the thorax and moving cranially (Fig 13.4). If the chin is kept tucked initially, the superficial muscles will be less active during this motion (Mayoux-Benhamou et al 1997). As motion is performed segmentally focus is on the deeper muscle layers. The motion must also be kept fluid and relaxed, as bracing will only encourage the rigidity which is so often seen in patients with chronic neck pain.

Strength and endurance

As stated previously, although both low load (CCF nod) and higher load (head lift) exercises appear equally as effective in reducing pain and disability, higher load exercise using added resistance may be more effective in regaining full strength and endurance. Therefore, to optimize return of normal neck muscle function, higher load exercise progressions should be included at some point in the rehabilitation programme. However, in cases of more severe neck pain, higher load exercises, if done too early, tend to exacerbate the pain, which would further inhibit normal muscle function. In those patients with longstanding protective bracing and rigidity, it would seem counterintuitive to add higher loads which encourage even more superficial muscle activation. On the other hand, patients with low intensity neck pain and generalized muscle weakness would tolerate and benefit from fairly rapid progression to higher load exercises as long as they demonstrate appropriate muscle balance. As the deep musculature should contract to stabilize the spine prior to any loading, initiating and maintaining a DNF nod throughout the higher loaded exercises would encourage optimal patterning.

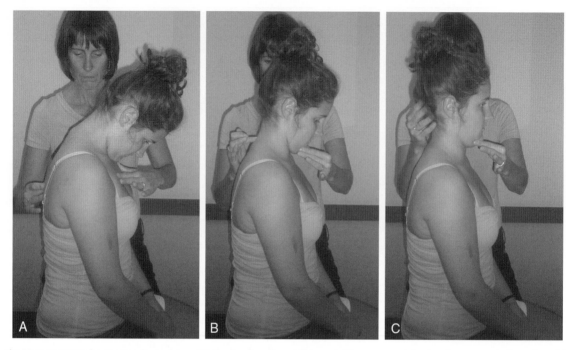

Fig 13.4 Segmental extension from slump. (A) Starting in a flexed slump position, segmental extension proceeds from the mid thoracic spine cranially. (B) Once the thorax is in neutral, segmental extension continues from the lower cervical spine to the cranio-vertebral region. (C) In the erect position, the nod is released to the neutral neck position.

Higher load flexor progressions

Auto-resisted exercises can be graded and are lower load than head lift exercises. Hands or a ball under the chin to resist an isometric or concentric contraction encourages the CCF pattern. An isometric holding contraction can be progressed by having the patient nod to cervical neutral and maintain this as they lean back at the hips to add gravity resistance. This can be further progressed by performing the sit back on an exercise ball, moving farther back into range (Fig 13.5).

A nod lift-off motion can be performed on an incline (Fig 13.6). The patient uses a nod motion to lift the head just off the surface to a neutral position. Endurance can be emphasized by progressively increasing the hold time and the exercise made more difficult by gradually reducing the angle of the incline.

Theraband can be used to add resistance. As an isometric exercise in sitting, the patient adopts a cervical neutral nod with the band around the forehead, and while maintaining neutral, leans forward at the hips to add resistance (Fig 13.7). Alternately, the band can be used to resist a through range isotonic exercise, ensuring that forward translation is controlled.

In supine, a head lift exercise can be performed in two different ways. As an isometric contraction, the patient

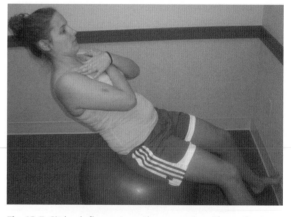

Fig 13.5 Sit back flexor strength progression. The patient can increase loading for the cervical flexors doing sit back exercises on the ball, maintaining a neutral deep neck flexor nod.

maintains a neutral nod and lifts the head off the surface, holding for progressively longer periods of time. Another option is an isotonic segmental flexion curl up exercise, continuing the nod through to inner range (Fig 13.8). In an MRI study, Cagnie et al (2008) showed that longus capitus and colli along with SCM were all more active

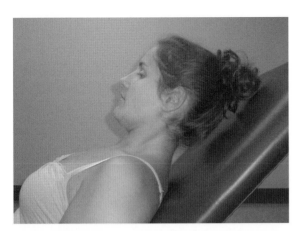

Fig 13.6 Nod lift-off on an incline. The patient lifts the head off the incline using a deep neck flexor nod action, holding a cervical neutral posture.

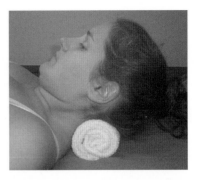

Fig 13.8 Curl up head lift. The patient initiates the exercise with a cranio-cervical flexion motion and continues to flex through to inner range. The towel roll can facilitate the segmental nature of the motion.

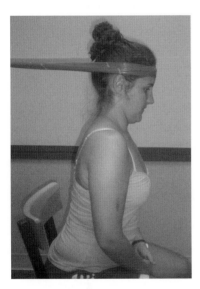

Fig 13.7 Elastic band resisted flexors. Maintaining a cervical nod, the body is leaned forward at the hips to increase the tension in the band to strengthen the cervical flexor synergy.

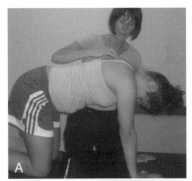

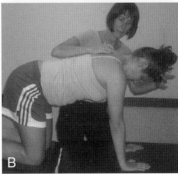

Fig 13.9 Segmental extension in 4-point kneeling. (A) Lumbo-sacral neutral is found and then thoracic neutral achieved by pressing up through the arms. (B) Subsequently the cervical spine is extended segmentally starting at the cervico-thoracic junction until the head and neck reaches neutral.

with this second exercise. It may be beneficial to use a towel roll under the neck to encourage the curl up action.

Higher load extensor progressions

DNE strengthening can be progressed by increasing the load effect of gravity in 4-point kneeling (4PK). The start position is with the head dropped into full flexion and the back sagged (Fig 13.9A). The patient is first instructed to find neutral lumbo-pelvic posture. Then they are taught to obtain a neutral thorax by pressing up through the arms to a slight kyphosis, not over-flexing. Keeping the chin tucked initially, and starting at the lower cervical spine, the head is brought in line with the trunk through segmental extension. The chin tuck is relaxed slightly at the end of the motion to ensure a neutral cervical lordosis is obtained rather than over retraction, with the plane of the face parallel to the floor (Fig 13.9B). This position is held for the count of 10 seconds. By reversing the motion,

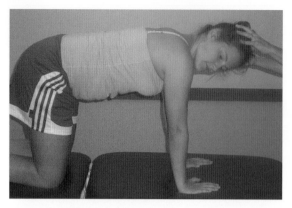

Fig 13.10 Pure rotation in neutral 4-point kneeling. Pure rotation is added, ensuring no compensatory side-flexion/extension, to challenge the posterior suboccipital muscles, practise motor control, and address asymmetrical muscle weakness.

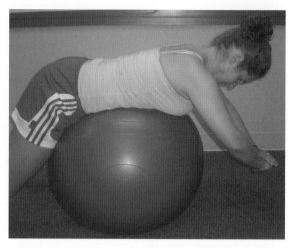

Fig 13.11 Integrated extension. Prone on a ball, the head and neck are brought up into cervical neutral, the arms lifted off the ball to activate scapular stabilized, and then the sternum lifted off the ball to recruit thoracic extensors.

starting with segmental flexion at the upper cervical spine until the head is hanging in full flexion, eccentric loading of the cervical extensors occurs. For less loading, the position is modified to a forward lean at either the wall or a counter. If the patient is unable to tolerate the load through the wrists, the prone on elbows position may be used or the patient can lie just over the end of the bed to perform the cervical component of the motion. Once a patient can accomplish this motion, the exercise is progressed into hyperextension, controlling any collapse into anterior translation. Adding pure rotation in the neutral 4PK position will focus on retraining the posterior suboccipitals as the upper cervical spine is responsible for the majority of cervical spine rotation (Fig 13.10).

An alternate exercise can be done prone over an exercise ball (Fig 13.11). The head is brought up into cervical neutral, the arms lifted using the scapular stabilizers, and then the trunk is lifted off the ball into thoracic extension. This incorporates the essential interaction between the head, neck, shoulder girdle and thoracic spine.

Elastic band resistance can be used to obtain a graded increase in load in the 4PK position. In sitting, the patient adopts a cervical neutral nod with the band around the back of the head, and while maintaining neutral, leans backward at the hips to add resistance. The patient could also hold the band in front and resist a retraction motion to neutral (Fig 13.12). Clinical reasoning should be used to determine which of these exercises would optimally address a patient's specific dysfunction.

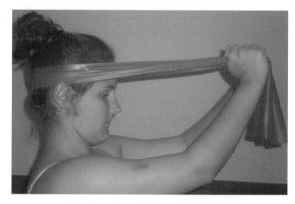

Fig 13.12 Band retraction. The band is held looped around the back of the head to apply resistance to a nod/retract motion to strengthen the cervical extensors.

Side flexion/rotation exercises for asymmetric weakness

In many patients with side dominant symptoms, atrophy and weakness will be more profound on that side. Although the previously described exercises often regain strength bilaterally, there may be certain situations where loading asymmetrically through rotation and side flexion may be more appropriate. Many of these exercises would also be considered motion control exercises.

Using a foam wedge pillow, the slope can act as resistance when the head is placed in an offset position. The patient is instructed to maintain a pre-set DNF nod throughout the exercise (Fig 13.13A). In the right offset position, the head is slowly lowered down the slope into right rotation, utilizing eccentric control of the muscles on the left side of the neck (Fig 13.13B). The motion is then reversed, using the left muscles concentrically to bring the head back to the start position and continue up the slope into full left rotation. The head is then returned to neutral and the nod relaxed before repeating.

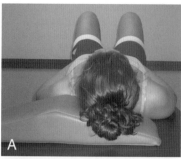

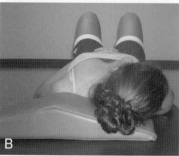

Fig 13.13 Wedge pillow offset. (A) The head is placed in the right offset position on the wedge pillow. (B) Maintaining a deep neck flexor nod throughout, the head is slowly rotated down the slope, working the left sided muscles eccentrically. The exercise is completed by returning the head back up the slope continuing to full left rotation and then back to neutral.

Pure rotation performed in either the nod lift-off on the incline, or the 4PK position will add asymmetric load to the flexors or extensors respectively (Figs 13.10 & 13.14). The patient is instructed to avoid the common compensations of either side flexion or cranio-vertebral extension, particularly toward the end of range. Diagonal motion

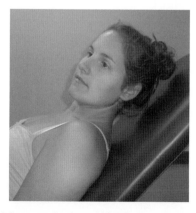

Fig 13.14 Pure rotation in nod lift-off. Pure rotation is added to the nod lift-off exercise on an incline to increase the loading, target asymmetric weakness, and practise higher load spinal motor control.

into a flexion quadrant during a supine curl up exercise, or an extension quadrant in 4PK will also bias the load unilaterally.

Isometrics can be performed into the weak rotation or side flexion. Wall support and a preset nod will help prevent unwanted translation. An elastic band can be used as resistance for isometric or isotonic contractions.

The weight of the head can be used as load in a side lying position, with or without a pillow or towel roll under the neck to act as a fulcrum. Once again the preset nod is performed prior to tilting the head up into side flexion, emphasizing the angular motion rather than translation.

Motor control

For upper quadrant function, it is necessary to have the ability to maintain cervical neutral during upper limb motion and loading. Deep and superficial muscle balance, timing, as well as relaxation post activity need to be addressed. Falla et al (2008) found that neither low nor higher load flexor exercise programmes resulted in improvement of the muscle recruitment abnormalities during arm lift, so perhaps this needs to be practised as a specific functional exercise. It is also important to have segmental control during head and neck movements, as many daily activities require a mobile neck.

Cervical neutral during limb load

Clinical reasoning must be applied to each patient presentation to determine which arm movements, in which positions, with which load, are best suited for that patient at that stage of their rehabilitation. The patient must be cued on how to achieve optimal posture, and to use a pre-set DNF nod to activate the stabilizers prior to any limb load motion. They may be asked to release and reset this nod prior to each repetition to focus on the timing pattern, or if endurance is the goal the patient would hold the nodded, cervical neutral position throughout all repetitions for each set of the exercise.

(a) *Positions*: In a patient with an irritable neck and poor motor control, arm movements may be performed with the patient in supine on a mat before progressing to a full or half foam roll. In the lying position, gravity along with head contact on the surface helps to prevent the tendency to protrude the head during overhead limb motion. When progressing into sitting and then standing, support against the wall can give feedback of head position. Sitting can be progressed to unsupported sitting on a ball, and standing progressed onto a wobble board. The 4PK position particularly challenges control of the anterior head drift so commonly seen with forward head posture (FHP), and is similar to the loads experienced by those who lean forward for their occupation or activities.

(b) *Arm motions*: Arm movements are chosen starting with those that are the least provocative, progressing to those which challenge spinal control. Bilateral flexion stresses anterior translation in the neck, whereas unilateral flexion or abduction stresses lateral translation. Starting with movements below shoulder level is less of a challenge. Reciprocal movements of the arms create a perturbation at the neck which increases as the speed of movement increases. Often there is an associated muscle imbalance at the shoulder girdle that needs to be addressed and then these arm motions are used to improve the scapular resting position, muscle balance and control, and simultaneously challenge maintenance of cervical neutral. If before each arm movement the patient is reminded to perform a pre-set DNF nod, both the timing and motor control is emphasized. Care must be taken to ensure that these shoulder girdle exercises are not at too high a level for the patient to maintain cervical neutral. Often the focus is on down-training those muscles that are over-active, as much as true strengthening of the weak muscles.

(c) *Resistance*: Weight may be added to the limb motions through free weights, elastic tubing and pulleys. Initially keeping weights low and emphasizing proper movement patterns will do more for motor control than the strengthening effect of higher loads. It is most efficient if the resisted exercises are focused on strengthening those scapular stabilizers required to improve shoulder girdle function (Fig 13.15).

Segmental control during neck motion

The neutral zone is that portion of the range of motion in which there is minimal resistance to movement by the inert stabilizing structures of the spine (Panjabi 1992).

The joints of the cervical spine, particularly the craniovertebral joints, have a large neutral zone as compared to other regions of the spine. Motion within this portion of the range relies heavily on the dynamic control of the stabilizing musculature.

Some segmental motor control exercises are low load and can be integrated into the exercise programme at the early stages of rehabilitation. Using the foam wedge pillow with the head starting on the peak allows controlled non-weight-bearing motion. The patient begins the exercise by performing the DNF pre-set nod and then controls the neck motion as the head moves down the slope in one direction, back to the peak, and then to the opposite side. As described previously for strengthening, the offset position would add a further load to challenge the motor control (Fig 13.13).

Pure eye-level rotation and pure side flexion can be practised through the maximal range that can be performed without losing controlled uniplanar motion. They can be done at the wall, with the head in contact to give feedback for the maintenance of cervical neutral. For side flexion, mirror feedback can also be added. Higher load pure rotation exercises can be done in both the incline nod lift-off and 4PK positions (Figs 13.10 & 13.14). This ensures that these positions are being maintained without rigidity, as the neck is still free to move.

Controlled flexion/extension has been previously described as a segmental motion from a slump position up to neutral and returning to flexion. This can be performed initially in sitting and then progressed to 4PK (Figs 13.4 & 13.9). Controlled hyperextension can be practised in sitting or 4PK, ensuring that there is no collapse into anterior translation during the motion (Fig 13.16). Controlled hyperextension in the seated lean back position is a further challenge to the flexor group and is a useful exercise for patients that need to work looking overhead.

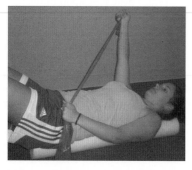

Fig 13.15 Motor control with limb load. Positioned on a foam roll, a deep neck flexor nod is maintained while strengthening lower trapezius muscle to improve both spinal and scapular control.

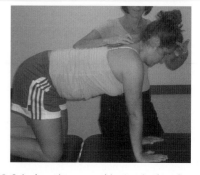

Fig 13.16 Spinal motion control in 4-point kneeling. Hyperextension is practised in 4PK controlling for collapse into anterior translation.

MOBILITY EXERCISES

Reduced cervical spine mobility is a feature of subjects with neck pain (Dall'Alba et al 2001, Dumas et al 2001, Kasch et al 2001, Oginco et al 2007). Potential sources of this mobility impairment include the joint structures, myofascial extensibility or abnormal tension within the neuro-meningeal system. Pain and fear avoidance may play a role in limiting the patient's willingness to move actively. Cervical mobility may also be affected by the starting position of the shoulder girdle. If retesting the cervical active range of motion with the scapula position corrected immediately results in increased range, then motor control around the shoulder needs to be addressed. As a multimodal approach including both manual therapy and exercise is the most effective in managing neck pain (Gross et al 2007), motion regained by manual therapy should be maintained with specific exercise

Generalized active range of motion

Even in the earliest stages of acute WAD, patients can be instructed in active pain-free mobility exercises. Initially these movements may be performed non-weight bearing in supine with pillow support. A foam wedge pillow can be used to assist the motion down the slope of the wedge. This exercise does tend to combine ipsilateral side bending and rotation with slight extension. If there is a concern regarding foramenal compression, the exercise should be modified, perhaps only utilizing the movement to the side opposite from the symptoms to encourage 'opening' of the intervertebral foramen.

In a series of studies, Rosenfeld et al (2000, 2003, 2006) found that WAD subjects who performed repeated cervical rotation 10 times per hour, had less pain, less sick time and better range of motion at 3 years than controls, more so if the movements were started early (within 96 hours) rather than later (> 2 weeks).

Movement may start uniplanar, but combined movements into the flexion ovoid of motion will bias lengthening of structures unilaterally. When attempting to regain a loss of extension, consideration must be given to the effects on vascular and neurological tissues, particularly in the extension quadrant. Often the problem with extension range is compression pain rather than decreased length, and perhaps a motor control approach would be more appropriate. Segmental joint restrictions of extension can be addressed with localized self-mobilization exercises described below.

Although the focus here is on mobility, practising correct movement patterns should be emphasized from the start. Integrating mobility exercises with motor control will achieve greater success in obtaining pain-free functional movement.

Articular/self-mobilization

Segmental mobility restrictions are best treated with manual therapy with specific self mobilization exercises to maintain the range gained. The patient can be taught to localize the motion to the involved segment with his fingers or the edge of a towel. An atlanto-axial (AA) towel rotation mobilization exercise has been found to be effective in the treatment of cervicogenic headaches (Hall et al 2007). The following are instructions for segmental self mobilization exercises (Fig 13.17):

Cranio-vertebral region

OA flexion (bilateral/unilateral):

* Sitting tall in a chair
* Stabilize the neck by placing clasped hands just under the skull, being careful not to pull the neck forward
* Nod the head on the neck, tucking the chin back, lifting the skull at the back (Fig 13.17a)
* To bias to one side, tilt the head away from the stiff side and rotate the chin toward the armpit on that stiff side (Fig 13.17b)

OA extension (unilateral):

* Sitting tall in a chair
* Stabilize the neck by placing clasped hands around the neck holding back, just under the angle of the jaw on the stiff side
* Tip the head toward the stiff side, rotating away, poking the chin forward towards the opposite elbow (Fig 13.17c)

AA joint rotation (right rotation restriction):

* Sitting tall in a chair
* Stabilize the neck by placing clasped hands behind the neck with little fingers at the large bump at the top of the neck below the skull, being careful not to pull the neck forward
* Turn the head into pure right rotation, keeping the eyes level, not allowing any tilt or chin poke
* To bias to right joint:
  ■ tuck chin into a bit of flexion before rotating
  ■ hold forward with right hand behind neck on the right side (Fig 13.17e)
* To bias to left joint:
  ■ tip chin up slightly before rotating
  ■ hold backward with left hand slightly in front of neck on the left side (Fig 13.17f)
* A towel can also be used to stabilize and over-press the rotation motion (Fig 13.17d)

Mid-cervical spine

* Use one hand to find the stiff joint (thick, tender spot at back/side of neck)
* Stabilize the bottom bone of that joint by pushing in gently with the fingers

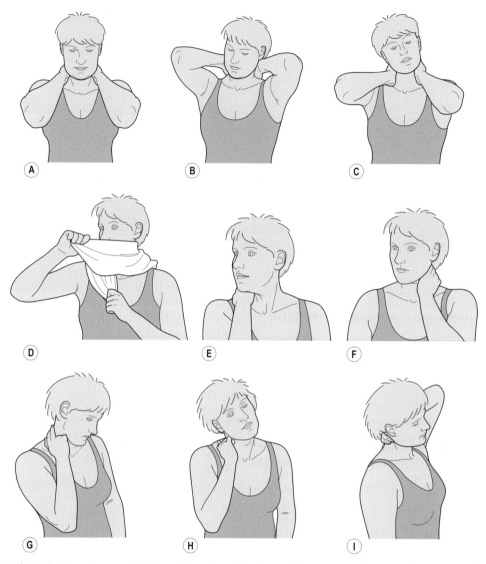

Fig 13.17 Self mobilization exercises. (A) Bilateral OA flexion. (B) Unilateral OA flexion. (C) Unilateral OA extension. (D) AA right rotation. (E) Bias right lateral AA joint. (F) Bias left lateral AA joint. (G) Mid C unilateral flexion. (H) Unilateral extension. (I) Left lateral glide.

- A towel can be used to fixate the joint and apply overpressure
- For flexion:
  - nod head into flexion, tilt and rotate away from the stiff joint
  - a tug should be felt at the stiff joint (Fig 13.17g)
- For extension:
  - tip the head back, side bend and rotate toward the stiff joint
  - use pressure up and in with fingers to focus the motion to the stiff joint

- the whole of the head and neck should not have to go into extension (Fig 13.17h)
- For left lateral glide right side flexion:
  - the left hand reaches around from the opposite side to pull the top bone across into left lateral glide as the head is tipped toward the stiff right side (Fig 13.17i)
  - *or*
  - as the head is tilted toward the right, the top bone is pushed laterally to the left to encourage the lateral glide required for side bending

Myofascial extensibility

Individuals with neck pain, particularly cervicogenic headache, have a higher incidence of muscle tightness as compared to controls (Zito et al 2006, Jull et al 2007a). Stretching exercises have been found to be effective in reducing neck pain in some populations (Gross et al 2007, Ylinen et al 2007b). For WAD individuals, excessive activity and prolonged relaxation times have been found for several muscle groups. In these cases, focus on motor patterning and relaxation following activity may be more valuable than stretching. The resting position of the scapula may place a muscle in a lengthened position, making it feel tight to the patient, even though it is not short. Likely as a protective mechanism, UFT has been found to be tighter in subjects with adverse tension in the neuromeningeal system (Edgar et al 1994) and so this should be addressed prior to any lengthening exercises for the UFT.

Muscles that tend to tighten are posterior suboccipitals, long cervical extensors, anterior and middle scalene, SCM, levator scapula, and upper trapezius (Janda 1994). Length tests are well described elsewhere (Kendall & McCreary 1983), and should be used to confirm true muscle shortening before instituting a stretching programme. The effects of a specific muscle lengthening exercise on either stiff or hyper-mobile joints should also be considered, and exercises modified as indicated. To elongate tissue, the exercise should be performed as a prolonged hold for 20–30 seconds, repeated 3–5 times.

In patients with tight cervical extensors, there is often a region of relative flexibility in the upper or mid thoracic spine. Performing the lengthening exercise at the wall with the thoracic spine in contact with the wall or towel roll will focus the stretch to the upper and mid cervical regions. For the sub-occipital group, the nod motion is the focus, and a fist placed under the chin may improve the localization as a passive stretch is added (Fig 13.18). As the long extensors attach at the base of the skull, this nod must be maintained as the head is dropped further forward to lengthen the rest of the long cervical extensors (Fig 13.19). Tilting the head to the right or left is indicated for asymmetric tightness.

As the scalene muscles tend to be over-dominant in patients with neck pain, active lengthening with a focus on 'letting go' may be the most appropriate approach. When performed at the wall in a neutral pre-set DNF nod, the tendency to collapse into extension during lengthening is minimized (Fig 13.20). For middle scalene, pure side flexion is performed. For anterior scalene, adding rotation toward the stiff side localizes stretch to that portion of the muscle. Either manually stabilizing the first rib, or breathing out, will prevent the rib from elevating as the muscle is lengthened. If the muscle is truly short, the patient may use the opposite hand to passively increase the stretch.

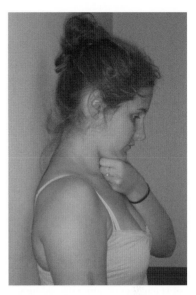

Fig 13.18 Suboccipital lengthening exercise. Standing at the wall, using a nod motion and a fist under the chin helps to focus the stretch to the suboccipital muscles.

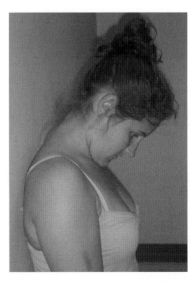

Fig 13.19 Cervical extensor lengthening exercise. Maintaining the thorax against the wall and keeping a chin tuck position helps focus the stretch to the long cervical extensors.

SCM also has a tendency toward over-activity but often regains its normal length by focusing on DNF recruitment. The muscle can be lengthened by side flexion away, rotation toward, and extension of the head on trunk with the chin held tucked.

To stretch levator scapula, the neck must be flexed, side flexed and rotated away. There are two bands described in

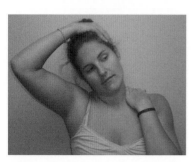

Fig 13.20 Scalene medius lengthening exercise. Standing at the wall and maintaining a chin nod helps prevent collapse into extension while lengthening the scalene as a group into pure side flexion. The first rib is fixated on the stiff side. To bias to the anterior scalene, the head can be rotated slightly to the stiff side.

the literature (Behrsin & Maguire 1986, Diener 1998). The vertical band is lengthened more by adding upward rotation and depression of the scapula with the arm overhead. The horizontal fibres may be more effectively lengthened by depression and downward rotation with the arm behind the back.

The UFT are lengthened by dropping the head into flexion, side flexing away, and rotating toward the stiff side. The scapula is depressed and downwardly rotated by reaching the hand down behind the back.

Neurodynamics

Adverse tension in the neuromeningeal system can affect cervical spine mobility. The assessment and interventions focused on this component is dealt with in Chapter 38.

POSTURAL CORRECTION EXERCISES

Optimal posture is that of cervical neutral, where the head is located directly above the shoulders and trunk. The cranio-vertebral region is in relative flexion and the mid cervical spine maintains a slightly lordotic position, with the plane of the face being vertical. A slightly kyphotic curve is considered neutral for the thoracic spine. The most common postural impairment of the cervical spine is the forward head posture (FHP).

Historically FHP has been associated with an increased likelihood of neck pain, although the research is inconsistent (Watson & Trott 1993, Treleaven et al 1994, Michaelson et al 2003, Yip et al 2008). Harman et al (2005) found that a postural correction exercise programme resulted in significant improvement in static measures of FHP. Falla et al (2007a) investigated the ability to maintain erect posture over time while completing a computer type task. There was an increase in thoracic flexion and

forward drift of the head over time in subjects with neck pain as compared to controls which showed a similar but lesser tendency. Low load CCF training or higher load strength exercise both resulted in improved control of the thoracic posture, but only the CCF training group showed improvement in cervical posture. Both groups showed a similar decrease in pain and disability. Activation of the DNF is higher in subjects instructed in lumbo-pelvic postural correction with verbal and handling cues than in those subjects merely told to 'sit straight', suggesting that specific postural instruction is important (Falla et al 2007b).

Patients must be individually assessed to determine the cause of their FHP and therefore the focus of their specific postural correction. The following areas need to be addressed with exercise intervention, much of which has already been discussed in previous sections of this chapter.

Muscle imbalance

The following muscles tend to weaken and require recruitment, strength or endurance exercises: deep neck flexors and extensors, scapular stabilizers and upper thoracic extensors. With FHP, the following muscles tend to tighten and require lengthening exercises: cervical extensors (suboccipital and long superficial extensors), scalene, upper trapezius, levator scapula, and pectoralis major and minor.

Articular system

The following regions tend to become hypo-mobile and require mobility exercises to regain range: upper cervical flexion, cervico-thoracic extension, upper & mid thoracic extension, and patients with lordotic upper thoracic spines must regain flexion to a neutral kyphosis.

Neuromeningeal system

Adverse tension in the neuromeningeal system may also contribute to postural abnormalities in the upper quadrant and must be assessed and addressed depending on the specific dysfunctions found (see Chapter 38).

Postural correction exercises

Depending on exactly which mechanisms caused the impaired posture, specific cues can be used to teach the patient how to attain a more optimal resting position. This can be reinforced throughout their exercise programme. Often after cuing a neutral lumbo-pelvic lordosis and a sternal lift, the head automatically comes back in line with the trunk. Depending on how the head has drifted forward, varying degrees of retraction, occipital lift or nod can be added. Pearson & Walmsley (1995) showed that repeated retractions in asymptomatic subjects improved cervical resting posture. Care must be taken to avoid over-retraction. It is also important to educate the

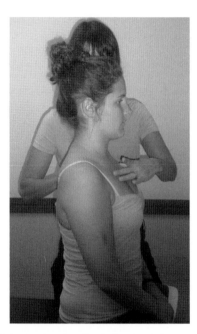

Fig 13.21 Postural cueing. Physical and verbal cues are used to assist the patient to find both lumbo-sacral and thoracic neutral. Any further correction required for the head and neck is achieved through a combination of nod, occipital lift and retraction as needed.

patient on neutral scapular positioning. The patient can practise these corrections in multiple positions, many times a day (Fig 13.21).

The DNF nod exercise can be utilized to address many of the dysfunctions seen with postural impairment and when done at the wall can also improve proprioceptive awareness. It will mobilize CV flexion, lengthen the tight posterior structures and begin to recruit the DNF shown to improve the ability to prevent forward drift of the head. The segmental extension from a slump position in sitting and 4PK is also an effective exercise to control FHP. Often thoracic extension mobility must be regained, and then the muscles that help maintain optimal thoracic and shoulder girdle posture must be re-educated and strengthened. Alternatively, those patients with a flattened or lordotic upper thoracic spine and excessive bracing of the long, superficial thoracic extensors must learn to relax by dropping the sternum down slightly to regain a neutral kyphotic spine.

The patient then practises the maintenance of optimal posture while incorporating arm movements, initially unloaded, but then adding free weights, tubing or pulleys. Progressing to an unstable base will increase the challenge and also assist in balance control. Using movements and positions required for work or sport will help carry over the postural control to functional activity. These types of exercises and their progressions have been described in the Motor Control section of this chapter (see Fig 13.15).

SOMATO-SENSORY DYSFUNCTION

Subjects with neck pain, particularly those with WAD and symptoms of dizziness, exhibit impairments of balance, kinaesthetic awareness and eye movement control (Revel et al 1991, Heikkila & Astrom 1996, Loudon et al 1997, Treleaven et al 2003, 2005a, 2005b, 2006, Kristjansson & Falla 2009). This has been described in detail earlier in the text and the reader is directed to Chapter 8 for further information.

Specific exercise focusing on sensory-motor control can be used to improve these impairments, and have also been found to improve pain, mobility and disability as a secondary gain (Revel et al 1994, Hansson et al 2006, Jull et al 2007b). Manual therapy also improves sensorimotor function and so should be included with exercise for optimal management of this patient subgroup (Karlberg et al 1996, Palmgren et al 2006, Reid et al 2008).

Balance retraining can be progressed through various levels of challenge starting with narrowed or tandem stance on a firm surface with eyes open, progressing at the other end of the continuum to single leg stance on an unstable surface with eyes closed. Physiotherapists are familiar with the multitude of options that can be employed to retrain balance, and should use clinical reasoning to develop a progressive exercise programme suited to the needs of the specific patient.

Kinasthetic awareness can be trained in several ways. Recruitment exercises for the posterior sub-occipital muscles such as pure rotation in 4PK may be useful as these muscles have substantial proprioceptive input. Using the pressure biofeedback cuff, the patient can practise nodding to specific points in range with eyes closed, checking and correcting the position on the guage once they open their eyes. Head repositioning to neutral or specific points in

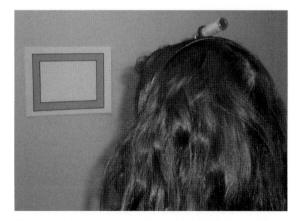

Fig 13.22 Kinaesthetic awareness and eye movement control. Tracing a figure with a laser pointer attached to the head facilitates both position sense and eye/head control.

range can be practised with a laser pointer and target. Tracing a figure with the pointer would combine eye/head control with position sense (Fig 13.22).

Eye movement control exercises include, for example, following a moving target, gaze fixation while moving the head, as well as eye/head co-ordination movements.

Several components of sensorimotor function can be combined in a single exercise to increase the challenge and assist in carry-over to more functional activities. For example the patient can practise gaze fixation or eye movement control while tandem walking and changing directions.

REFERENCES

Behrsin, J., Maguire, K., 1986. Levator Scapula action during shoulder movement: A possible mechanism for shoulder pain of cervical origin. Aust. J. Physiother. 32, 101–106.

Brontfort, G., Evans, R., Nelson, B., et al., 2001. A randomized clinical trial of exercise and spinal manipulation for patients with chronic neck pain. Spine 26, 788–797.

Bunketorp, L., Carlsson, L., Stener-Victorin, E., 2006. The effectiveness of a supervised physical training model tailored to the individual needs of patients with whiplash-associated disorder: a randomized controlled trial. Clin. Rehabil. 20, 201–217.

Cagnie, B., Dickx, N., Peeters, I., et al., 2008. The use of functional MRI to evaluate cervical flexor activity during different cervical flexion exercises. J. Appl. Physiol. 104, 230–235.

Conley, M.S., Stone, M.H., Nimmons, M., et al., 1997. Specificity of resistance training responses in neck muscle size and strength. Eur. J. Appl. Physiol. Occup. Physiol. 75, 443–448.

Dall'Alba, P.T., Sterling, M., Treleaven, J., et al., 2001. Cervical range of motion discriminates between asymptomatic persons and those with whiplash. Spine 26, 2090–2094.

Diener, I., 1998. The effect of levator scapula tightness on the cervical spine: proposal of another length test. J. Man. Manip. Ther. 6, 78–86.

Dumas, J.P., Arsenault, A.B., Boudreau, G., et al., 2001. Physical impairments in cervicogenic headache: traumatic vs. nontraumatic onset. Cephalgia 21, 884–893.

Edgar, D., Jull, G., Sutton, S., 1994. The relationship between upper trapezius muscle length and upper quadrant neural tissue extensibility. Aust. J. Physiother. 40, 99–103.

Elliott, J., Jull, G., Noteboom, J., et al., 2006. Fatty infiltration in the cervical extensor muscles in persistent whiplash-associated disorders: a magnetic resonance imaging analysis. Spine 31, 847–855.

Elliot, J., Jull, G., Noteboom, J., et al., 2008. MRI study of the cross sectional area for the cervical extensor musculature in patients with persistent whiplash associated disorders (WAD). Man. Ther. 13, 258–265.

Falla, D., Rainoldi, A., Merletti, R., et al., 2003. Myoelectric manifestations of sternocleidomastoid and anterior scalene muscle fatigue in chronic neck pain patients. Clin. Neurophysiol. 114, 488–495.

Falla, D., Jull, G., Hodges, P., et al., 2004a. Patients with neck pain demonstrate reduced electromyographic activity of the deep cervical flexor muscles during performance of the craniocervical flexion test. Spine 29, 2108–2114.

Falla, D., Jull, G., Hodges, P., 2004b. Feedforward activity of the cervical flexor muscles during voluntary arm movements is delayed in chronic neck pain. Exp. Brain Res. 157, 43–48.

Falla, D., Bilenkij, G., Jull, G., 2004c. Patients with chronic neck pain demonstrate altered patterns of muscle activity during performance of an upper limb task. Spine 29, 1436–1440.

Falla, D., Jull, G., Hodges, P., et al., 2006. An endurance-strength training regime is effective in reducing myoelectric manifestations of cervical flexor muscle fatigue in females with chronic neck pain. Clin. Neurophysiol. 117, 828–837.

Falla, D., Jull, G., Russell, T., et al., 2007a. Effect of neck exercise on sitting posture in patients with chronic neck pain. Phys. Ther. 87, 408–417.

Falla, D., O'Leary, S., Fagan, A., et al., 2007b. Recruitment of the deep cervical flexors during a postural–correction exercise performed in sitting. Man. Ther. 12, 139–143.

Falla, D., Jull, G., Hodges, P., et al., 2008. Training the cervical muscles with prescribed motor tasks does not change muscle activation during a functional activity. Man. Ther. 13, 507–512.

Fernandez-de-las-Penas, C., Bueno, A., Ferrando, J., et al., 2007. Magnetic resonance imaging study of the morphology of the cervical extensor muscles in chronic tension-type headache. Cephalgia 27, 355–362.

Fernandez-de-las-Penas, C., Alber-Sanchis, C., Buil, M., et al., 2008. Cross-sectional area of the cervical multifidus muscle in females with chronic bilateral neck pain compared to controls. J. Orthop. Sports Phys. Ther. 38, 175–180.

Gross, A.R., Goldsmith, C., Hoving, J., et al., 2007. Conservative management of mechanical neck disorders: a systematic review. J. Rheumatol. 34, 1083–1102.

Hall, T., Chan, H., Christensen, L., et al., 2007. Efficacy of a C1-2 self sustained natural apophyseal glide (Snag) in the management of cervicogenic headache. J. Orthop. Sports Phys. Ther. 37, 100–107.

Hallgren, R.C., Greenman, P.E., Rechtien, J.J., 1994. Atrophy of suboccipital muscles in patients with chronic pain: a pilot study. J. Am. Osteopath. Assoc. 94, 1032–1038.

Hansson, E.E., Nils-Ove Månsson, A., Karin, A.M., Ringsberg, A., Anders Håkansson, A., 2006. Dizziness among patients with whiplash-associated disorder: a randomized controlled trial. J. Rehabil. Med. 38, 387–390.

Harman, K., Hubley-Kozey, C.L., Butler, H., 2005. Effectiveness of an exercise program to improve head forward posture in normal adults: a randomized controlled 10 week trial. J. Man. Manip. Ther. 13, 163–176.

Heikkila, H., Astrom, P.G., 1996. Cervicocephalic kinesthetic sensibility in patients with whiplash injury. Scand. J. Rehabil. Med. 28, 133–138.

Janda, V., 1994. Muscles and motor control in cervicogenic disorders: assessment and management. In: Grant, R. (Ed.), Physical Therapy for the Cervical and Thoracic Spine. Churchill Livingstone, Melbourne.

Jordan, A., Bendix, T., Nielsen, H., et al., 1998. Intensive training, physiotherapy, or manipulation for patients with chronic neck pain. A prospective, single-blinded, randomized clinical trial. Spine 23, 311–318.

Jull, G., 2000. Deep neck flexor dysfunction in whiplash. Journal of Musculoskeletal Pain 8, 143–154.

Jull, G., Trott, P., Potter, H., et al., 2002. A randomized controlled trial of exercise and manipulative therapy for cervicogenic headache. Spine 27, 1835–1843.

Jull, G., Kristjansson, E., Dall'Alba, P., 2004. Impairment in the cervical flexors: a comparison of whiplash and insidious onset neck pain patients. Man. Ther. 9, 89–94.

Jull, G., Amiri, M., Bullock-Saxton, J., et al., 2007a. Cervical musculoskeletal impairment in frequent intermittent headache. Part 1: subjects with single headaches. Cephalgia 27, 793–802.

Jull, G., Falla, D., Treleaven, J., et al., 2007b. Retraining cervical joint position sense: the effect of two exercise regimes. J. Orthop. Res. 25, 404–412.

Karlberg, M., Magnusson, M., Malmstrom, E., et al., 1996. Postural and symptomatic improvement after physiotherapy in patients with dizziness of suspected cervical origin. Arch. Phys. Med. Rehabil. 77, 874–882.

Kasch, H., Stengaard-Pedersen, K., Arendt-Nielsen, L., et al., 2001. Headache, neck pain and neck mobility after acute whiplash injury. Spine 26, 1246–1251.

Kendall, F.P., McCreary, E.K., 1983. Muscles, Testing and Function,

third ed. Williams & Wilkins, Baltimore.

Kristjansson, E., 2004. Reliability of ultrasonography for the cervical multifidus muscle in asymptomatic and symptomatic subjects. Man. Ther. 9, 83–88.

Kristjansson, E., Falla, D., 2009. Sensorimotor function and dizziness in neck pain: implications for assessment and management. J. Orthop. Sports Phys. Ther. 39, 364–377.

Loudon, J.K., Ruhl, M., Field, E., 1997. Ability to reproduce head position after whiplash injury. Spine 22, 865–868.

Mayoux-Benhamou, M.A., Revel, M., Vallee, 1997. Selective electromyography of dorsal neck muscles in humans. Exp. Brain Res. 113, 353–360.

Michaelson, P., Michaelson, M., Jaric, S., et al., 2003. Vertical posture and head stability in patients with chronic neck. Journal of Rehabilitative Medicine 35, 229–235.

Nederhand, M.J., IJerman, M.J., Hermens, H.J., et al., 2000. Cervical muscle dysfunction in the chronic whiplash associated disorder grade II (WAD-II). Spine 25, 1938–1943.

Nederhand, M.J., Hermens, H.J., IJerman, M.J., et al., 2002. Cervical muscle dysfunction in chronic whiplash-associated disorder grade 2. Spine 27, 1056–1061.

Ogince, M., Hall, T., Robinson, K., et al., 2007. The diagnostic validity of the cervical flexion-rotation test in C1/2-related cervicogenic headache. Man. Ther. 12, 256–262.

O'Leary, S., Jull, G., Kim, M., et al., 2007. Cranio-cervical flexor muscle impairment at maximal, moderate and low loads is a feature of neck pain. Man. Ther. 12, 34–39.

Palmgren, P.J., Sandstrom, P.J., Lundqvist, F.J., et al., 2006. Improvement after chiropractic care in cervicogenic kinesthetic sensibility and subjective pain intensity in patients with nontraumatic neck pain. Journal of Manipulative Physiological Therapy 29, 100–106.

Panjabi, M., 1992. The stabilizing system of the spine. Part 1: Function, adaptation, and enhancement. Part 2: Neutral zone and instability

hypothesis. J. Spinal Disord. 5, 383–397.

Pearson, N., Walmsley, R., 1995. Trial into the effects of repeated neck retractions in normal subjects. Spine 20, 1245–1250.

Randlov, A., Ostergaaed, M., Manniche, C., et al., 1998. Intensive dynamic training for females with chronic neck/shoulder pain. A randomized controlled trial. Clin. Rehabil. 12, 200–210.

Reid, S., Rivett, D., Katekar, M., et al., 2008. Sustained natural apophyseal glides (SNAGs) are an effective treatment for cervicogenic dizziness. Man. Ther. 13, 357–366.

Revel, M., Andre-Deshays, C., Minguet, M., 1991. Cervicocephalic kinesthetic sensibility in patients with cervical pain. Arch. Phys. Med. 72, 288–291.

Revel, M., Minguet, M., Gergoy, P., et al., 1994. Changes in cervicocephalic kinesthesia after a proprioceptive rehabilitation program in patients with neck pain. Arch. Phys. Med. Rehabil. 75, 895–899.

Rosenfeld, M., Gunnarsson, R., Borenstein, P., 2000. Early intervention in whiplash-associated disorders. Spine 25, 1782–1787.

Rosenfeld, M., Seferiadis, A., Carlsson, J., et al., 2003. Active intervention in patients with whiplash-associated disorders improves long term prognosis. Spine 28, 2491–2498.

Rosenfeld, M., Seferiadis, A., Gunnarsson, R., 2006. Active involvement and intervention in patients exposed to whiplash trauma in automobile crashes reduces costs. Spine 31, 1799–1804.

Sarig-Bahat, H., 2003. Evidence for exercise therapy in mechanical neck disorders. Man. Ther. 8, 10–20.

Sterling, M., Jull, G., Vicenzino, B., et al., 2003. Development of motor dysfunction following whiplash injury. Pain 103, 65–73.

Sterling, M., Jull, G., Vicenzino, B., et al., 2004. Characterization of acute whiplash associated disorders. Spine 29, 182–188.

Szeto, G., Straker, L., O'sullivan, P., 2005. comparison of symptomatic and asymptomatic office workers performing monotonous keyboard work. Man. Ther. 10, 270–291.

Taimela, S., Takala, E.P., Asklof, T., et al., 2000. Active treatment of chronic neck pain: a prospective randomized intervention. Spine 25, 1021–1027.

Treleaven, et al., 1994. Cervical Musculoskeletal Dysfunction in Post-concussional Headache. Cephalgia 14, 273–279.

Treleaven, J., Jull, G., LowChoy, N., 2003. Dizziness and unsteadiness following whiplash injury: characteristic features and relationship with cervical joint position error. Journal of Rehabilitative Medicine 35, 36–43.

Treleaven, J., Jull, G., LowChoy, N., 2005a. Standing balance in persistent whiplash: A comparison between subjects with dizziness and without dizziness. Journal of Rehabilitative Medicine 37, 224–229.

Treleaven, J., Jull, G., LowChoy, N., 2005b. Smooth pursuit neck torsion test in whiplash associated disorders: relationship to self-reports of neck pain and disability, dizziness and anxiety. J. Rehabil. Med. 37, 219–223.

Treleaven, J., Jull, G., LowChoy, N., 2006. The relationship of cervical joint position error to balance and eye movement disorders in persistent whiplash. Man. Ther. 11, 99–106.

Uhlig, Y., Weber, B., Grob, D., et al., 1995. Fibre composition and fibre transformation in neck muscles of patients with dysfunction of the cervical spine. Journal of Orthopedic Research 13, 240–249.

Vassiliou, T., Kaluza, G., Putzke, C., et al., 2006. Physical Therapy and active exercises – An adequate treatment for prevention of late whiplash syndrome? Pain 124, 69–76.

Walker, M., Boyles, R., Young, B., et al., 2008. The effectiveness of manual physical therapy and exercise for mechanical neck pain. Spine 33, 2371–2378.

Watson, D., Trott, P., 1993. Cervical headache: an investigation of natural head posture and upper cervical flexor muscle performance. Cephalgia 13, 272–282.

Yip, C., Chiu, T., Poon, A., 2008. The relationship between head posture and severity and disability of patients with neck pain. Man. Ther. 13, 148–154.

Ylinen, J., Häkkinen, A., Takala, E., et al., 2006. Effects of neck muscle strengthening in women with chronic neck pain: one year follow-up study. J. Strength. Cond. Res. 20, 6–13.

Ylinen, J., Häkkinen, A., Takala, E., et al., 2007a. Neck muscle training in the treatment of chronic neck pain: a three-year follow-up. Eura Medicophysi 43, 161–169.

Ylinen, J., Häkkinen, A., Takala, E., et al., 2007b. Stretching exercises vs manual therapy in treatment of chronic neck pain: a randomized controlled cross-over trial. Journal of Rehabilitative Medicine 39, 126–132.

Zito, G., Jull, G., Story, I., 2006. Clinical tests of musculoskeletal dysfunction in the diagnosis of Cervicogenic headache. Man. Ther. 11, 118–129.

Chapter | 14 |

Acromio-clavicular joint

Janette W Powell, Ian Shrier, Peter A Huijbregts

INTRODUCTION

Shoulder pain is the third most common cause for musculoskeletal consultation in primary care (Docimo et al 2008). Acromio-clavicular joint (ACJ) pathology and dysfunction is a common component of shoulder pain (Hutchinson & Ahuja 1996, Magee & Reid 1996, Auge & Fischer 1998, Shaffer 1999, Debski et al 2001, Garretson & Williams 2003, Renfree & Wright 2003, Kiner 2004, Walton et al 2004, Powell & Huijbregts 2006, Codsi 2007, Docimo et al 2008, Simovitch et al 2009). The ACJ accounts for approximately 9–12% of shoulder injuries presenting for general medical care (Rudzki et al 2003, Docimo et al 2008, Fraser-Moodie et al 2008, Macdonald & Lapointe 2008, White et al 2008) and is one of the most frequently injured joints in certain sports, e.g. football, ice hockey, skiing, snowboarding, skating, and rugby (Magee & Reid 1996, Renfree & Wright 2003, Powell & Huijbregts 2006, Petron & Hanson 2007, Fraser-Moodie et al 2008, White et al 2008). Overall, ACJ sprains/separations have been described as

accounting for 40–50% of all athletic shoulder injuries (Debski et al 2001, Petron & Hanson 2007, Simovitch et al 2009) and are noted to be twice as common as complete ACJ disruptions (Fraser-Moodie et al 2008, Petron & Hanson 2007), which account for 12% of all dislocations affecting the shoulder girdle (Magee & Reid 1996). In addition to the ACJ, the clavicle is frequently injured with an incidence of 23 per 1000 athletic exposures for ice hockey and 17 per 1000 athletic exposures for lacrosse (Hutchinson & Ahuja 1996). The prevalence of atraumatic osteolysis of the distal clavicle has been reported to be as high as 27% in weightlifters (Auge & Fischer 1998). These numbers likely underestimate the true prevalence, as individuals with minor injuries or dysfunction might not seek medical care (Mehrberg et al 2004, Fraser-Moodie et al 2008). ACJ injuries are more common in males (Beim 2000, Mehrberg et al 2004, Petron & Hanson 2007, White et al 2008, Fraser-Moodie et al 2008) and over half occur in the under-30 population (Kiner 2004, Mehrberg et al 2004).

ANATOMY OF ACROMIO-CLAVICULAR JOINT

Fraser-Moodie et al (2008) described the ACJ as the 'keystone' link between the scapula and the clavicle. It suspends the upper extremity from the axial skeleton (Buss & Watts 2003, Nuber & Bowen 2003, Renfree & Wright 2003, Shaffer 1999). A thin capsule surrounds the diarthrodial ACJ, which typically contains a fibrocartilaginous disk (Lemos 1998, Shaffer 1999, Beim 2000, Buss & Watts 2003, Garretson & Williams 2003, Renfree & Wright 2003, Docimo et al 2008, Fraser-Moodie et al 2008, Macdonald

DOI: 10.1016/B978-0-7020-3528-9.00014-5

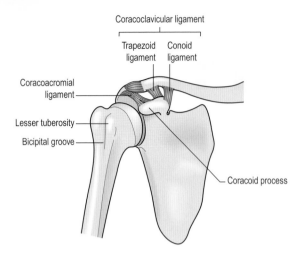

Fig 14.1 Normal anatomy of the acromio-clavicular joint.

& Lapointe 2008, Rios & Mazzocca 2008, White et al 2008, Simovitch et al 2009). This intra-articular disk is variable in size and shape and may sometimes undergo rapid degeneration beginning as early as the second decade of life (Beim 2000, Renfree & Wright 2003, Mehrberg et al 2004, Docimo et al 2008, White et al 2008 Simovitch et al 2009). The ACJ is reinforced by the acromio-clavicular (AC) ligaments (superior, inferior, anterior and posterior), the robust coraco-clavicular (CC) ligaments (conoid and trapezoid), the coraco-acromial ligament, and the delto-trapezius aponeurosis (Fig. 14.1) (Lemos 1998, Shaffer 1999, Beim 2000, Buss & Watts 2003, Garretson & Williams 2003, Renfree & Wright 2003, Petron & Hanson 2007, Docimo et al 2008, Fraser-Moodie et al 2008, Macdonald & Lapointe 2008, White et al 2008, Rios & Mazzocca 2008, Simovitch et al 2009, White et al 2008). Dynamic stabilization is provided by the deltoid and trapezius muscles (Lizaur et al 1994, Beim 2000, Buss & Watts 2003, Renfree & Wright 2003, Garretson & Williams 2003, Petron & Hanson 2007, Macdonald & Lapointe 2008, Rios & Mazzocca 2008, Docimo et al 2008, White et al 2008, Simovitch et al 2009).

BIOMECHANICS OF ACROMIO-CLAVICULAR JOINT

Few studies have been published on ACJ kinematics (Teece et al 2008) but more recent 3D imaging studies that quantify its motion suggest that movement has historically been underestimated (Sahara et al 2006, 2007, Fraser-Moodie et al 2008, Teece et al 2008). Sahara et al (2007) have noted that during abduction of the shoulder there is significant rotation of the clavicle and within the ACJ, with the clavicle acting as a screw axis (Sahara 2006). For example, in the antero-posterior direction, the clavicle translated most posteriorly (1.9 ± 1.3 mm) at 90° of abduction and most anteriorly (1.6 ± 2.7 mm) at maximum abduction. When defining motion of the scapula with respect to the clavicle, the scapula generally rotated about a specific screw axis passing through the insertions of both the acromio-clavicular and the coraco-clavicular ligaments on the coracoid process (Sahara et al 2006). Teece et al (2008) found that significant motion (internal rotation, upward rotation, and posterior tilting) occurs at the ACJ during active humeral elevation, and discussed how abnormal motions at the ACJ will affect the position of the scapula on the thorax, and contribute to shoulder pathology and dysfunction. Teece et al (2008) observed during active scapular plane abduction from rest to 90°, average ACJ angular values demonstrated increased internal rotation (approximately 4.3°), increased upward rotation (approximately 14.6°), and increased posterior tilting (approximately 6.7°). Teece et al (2008) did not analyse motion beyond 90° abduction, due to technical limitations with clavicular tracking. These ACJ motions are of sufficient magnitude to warrant clinical attention with manual mobilization when these motions are abnormal or dysfunctional.

PATHOLOGY OF ACROMIO-CLAVICULAR JOINT

Box 14.1 contains pathologies that may affect the ACJ (Hutchinson & Ahuja 1996, Magee & Reid 1996, Auge & Fischer 1998, Lemos 1998, Shaffer 1999, Lehtinen et al 1999, Santis et al 2001, Debski et al 2001, Garretson & Williams 2003, Renfree & Wright 2003, Kiner 2004 Walton et al 2004, Simovitch et al 2009). The ACJ can be acutely injured by direct blows to the shoulder or falls on an upper extremity (ligament sprain/separations/dislocations). The ACJ is also vulnerable to repetitive overuse (osteolysis and degenerative joint disease) (Lemos 1998, Debski et al 2001, Kiner 2004, Nuber & Bowen 2003, Petron & Hanson 2007, Rios & Mazzocca 2008, Macdonald & Lapointe 2008, Simovitch et al 2009).

Acute injuries to the ACJ typically involve a direct fall onto the outer aspect of the shoulder, usually with the arm adducted (Beim 2000, Buss & Watts 2003, Garretson & Williams 2003, Rudzki et al 2003, Petron & Hanson 2007, Fraser-Moodie et al 2008, Simovitch 2009). This force drives the acromion inferiorly under the clavicle. The greater stability of the sternoclavicular joint (discussed in the following chapter) results in the majority of the impact dissipated in the ACJ structures which leads to a systematic failure of stabilizing structures with progressive force (Beim 2000, Bradley & Elkousy 2003, Rudzki et al 2003, Petron & Hanson 2007, Fraser-Moodie et al 2008,

Macdonald & Lapointe 2008, Rios & Mazzocca 2008, Simovitch et al 2009). The downward force with this injury initially stretches the AC ligaments; then, as the force continues, the AC ligaments tear and the CC ligaments are stressed (Tom et al 2009). As the downward force continues the CC ligaments tear, followed by the muscle attachments of the deltoid and trapezius muscles, resulting in a complete disruption to the ACJ (Tom et al 2009).

These sequential acute injuries have been defined and described by Tossy et al (1963). Rockwood et al (1996) modified and expanded these injury types to the system commonly used today (Fig 14.2):

- Type I: AC ligament sprain, CC ligament intact, deltoid and trapezius muscles intact
- Type II: AC ligaments & ACJ disrupted, CC ligament sprain, deltoid and trapezius muscles intact
- Type III: AC ligaments & ACJ disrupted and displaced, CC ligaments disrupted with CC interspace 25–100% larger than normal shoulder, deltoid and trapezius muscles usually detached;
- Type IV: AC ligaments disrupted & ACJ displaced, clavicle displaced posteriorly, CC ligaments disrupted with wider CC interspace, deltoid and trapezius muscles detached
- Type V: AC & CC ligaments disrupted, ACJ grossly displaced (100–300% more than normal shoulder), deltoid and trapezius muscles detached
- Type VI: AC & CC ligaments disrupted & ACJ displaced, clavicle displaced inferiorly, deltoid and trapezius muscles detached (Tossy et al 1963, Simovitch et al 2009, Tom et al 2009)

A less common mechanism of acute injury to the ACJ would involve a fall onto an outstretched hand, or a direct blow to the elbow. These mechanisms drive the humeral head superiorly into the acromion (Beim 2000, Garretson & Williams 2003, Petron & Hanson 2007, White et al 2008). These indirect forces may result in the same injury patterns described above (Simovitch et al 2009), or may spare the CC ligaments when the scapula is driven superiorly and medially injuring the AC ligaments in isolation (Mehrberg et al 2004, White et al 2008). Additionally the ACJ may be injured by a traction force applied to the upper extremity (Beim 2000, Garretson & Williams 2003).

Rios & Mazzocca (2008) describe an acute 'internal derangement' whereby the intra-articular disk is torn. Magee & Reid (1996) propose that intra-articular disk injuries are implicated in the 'clicking' that is sometimes heard and in some of the post-traumatic pain syndromes following ACJ injuries.

Although many ACJ injuries are due to a sudden force, repetitive loads may also cause injury to the region. Non-contact sports such as cycling, baseball, and weightlifting have been associated with degenerative ACJ injuries (Bowen & Nuber 2003). For example, the compressive forces across the ACJ that are created during repeated forceful contraction by the deltoid, trapezius, and pectoralis major muscles may contribute to osteolysis of the distal clavicle (Nuber & Bowen 2003, Renfree & Wright 2003). This repetitive stress to the subchondral bone can cause fatigue fractures and a hypervascular response leading to absorption of bone and an eventual clinically relevant osteolysis. The sequelae include demineralization, osteopenia, subchondral cyst formation, and distal clavicle erosion (Nuber & Bowen 2003). It is often noted that the ACJ is required to transmit large loads across a very small surface area and this may contribute to failure with repetitive activity and overuse (Shaffer 1999, Beim 2000, Nuber & Bowen 2003, Renfree & Wright 2003, Docimo et al 2008).

In addition, degeneration of the ACJ intra-articular disk commences in the second decade of life and may be significant by the fourth decade (Garretson & Williams 2003). An incomplete fibrocartilaginous disk may play a significant role in the development of arthrosis (Beim 2000, Powell & Huijbregts 2006, Docimo et al 2008). Primary osteoarthritis and post-traumatic arthritis are noted to be prevalent in 50–60% of asymptomatic elderly individuals (Shaffer 1999, Docimo et al 2008, Rios & Mazzocca 2008). ACJ arthrosis, joint degradation, may be idiopathic, or result from injury and/or instability of this joint (Rios & Mazzocca 2008). The ACJ is also prone to inflammatory, septic, and crystalline arthropathy (Garretson & Williams 2003, Renfree & Wright 2003).

DIAGNOSIS OF ACROMIO-CLAVICULAR JOINT

The clinical presentation of an individual with acute ACJ injury typically involves a history of one of the mechanisms of injury described above: direct trauma to the

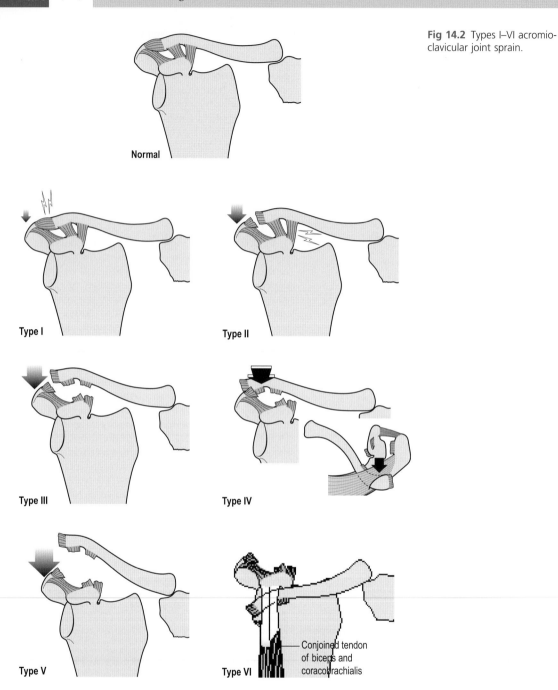

Fig 14.2 Types I–VI acromio-clavicular joint sprain.

Normal

Type I

Type II

Type III

Type IV

Type V

Type VI — Conjoined tendon of biceps and coracobrachialis

shoulder with the arm adducted, fall onto an outstretched hand or elbow, or a traction injury to the upper extremity (Hutchinson & Ahuja 1996, Lemos 1998, Beim 2000, Buss & Watts 2003, Garretson & Williams 2003, Petron & Hanson 2007, Macdonald & Lapointe 2008, Rios & Mazzocca 2008, White et al 2008, Simovitch et al 2009). Individuals with isolated ACJ lesions typically note pain over the anterior and/or superior aspect of the shoulder.

Although the pain is often localized to the region directly over the ACJ, it may radiate to the anterolateral neck, the trapezius-supraspinatus region, and to the anterolateral deltoid (Gerber et al 1998, Shaffer 1999, Petron & Hanson 2007, Macdonald & Lapointe 2008, Rios & Mazzocca 2008, Fraser-Moodie et al 2008).

Swelling, ecchymosis/erythema, and deformity, if present, are easily observed as the ACJ is just under the skin

(Hutchinson & Ahuja 1996, Shaffer 1999, Beim 2000, Mehrberg et al 2004, Petron & Hanson 2007, Fraser-Moodie et al 2008, Macdonald & Lapointe 2008, White et al 2008, Simovitch et al 2009, Tom et al 2009). Tenderness on palpation of the ACJ is reported as a common clinical finding associated with ACJ dysfunction (Hutchinson & Ahuja 1996, Magee & Reid 1996, Shaffer 1999, Beim 2000, Tallia & Cardone 2003, Buss & Watts 2003, Nuber & Bowen 2003, Mehrberg et al 2004, Walton et al 2004, Brukner & Khan 2006, Petron & Hanson 2007, White et al 2008, Docimo et al 2008, Fraser-Moodie et al 2008, Macdonald & Lapointe 2008, Rios & Mazzocca 2008, Park et al 2009, Simovitch et al 2009, Tom et al 2009). A number of physical examination tests have been proposed to stress the structures of the ACJ and assist in the clinical diagnosis of ACJ pathology. These include the active compression test (also known as O'Brien's sign) (Fig 14.3) (O'Brien et al 1998, Maritz & Oosthuizen, 2002, Chronopoulos et al 2004, Walton et al 2004), cross-body adduction test (also known as Scarf sign) (Fig 14.4) (Maritz & Oosthuizen 2002, Chronopoulos et al 2004), acromio-clavicular resisted extension test (Fig 14.5) (Chronopoulos et al 2004), ACJ tenderness test (Maritz & Oosthuizen 2002, Walton et al 2004), and Paxinos sign (Fig 14.6) (Walton et al 2004, Brukner & Khan 2006). Table 14.1 provides psychometric data on these clinical tests.

Powell & Huijbregts (2006) noted that research evidence supports the inclusion of the following tests, with the following interpretation, for the diagnosis of painful ACJ dysfunction:

- A negative finding on *ANY* of the following tests would *rule out* ACJ dysfunction: cross-body adduction test; tenderness on palpation of the ACJ; Paxinos sign

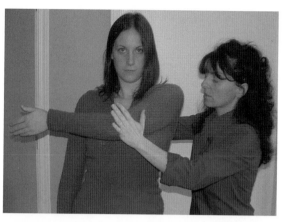

Fig 14.4 Cross-body adduction test: the client's arm is forward flexed to 90° and then horizontally adducted across the body. Literature is unclear on whether this test is active or passive. This test is considered positive if it causes pain localized to the ACJ (from Powell & Huijbregts, 2006, with permission).

- A positive finding on *ANY* of the following tests would *rule in* ACJ dysfunction: active compression test; the cross-body adduction test; acromio-clavicular resisted extension test
- A positive finding on *ALL* three tests used to rule in ACJ dysfunction (the cross-body adduction stress, active compression, and resisted acromio-clavicular extension tests) may be relevant when considering a medical-surgical referral and associated higher-risk interventions

A number of authors note the value of ACJ local anaesthetic injections to assist and/or confirm the involvement of ACJ dysfunction in the clinical presentation when other

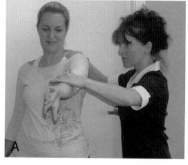 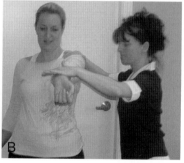

Fig 14.3 Active compression test: (A) maximal internal rotation: the client stands with the involved arm straight and forward flexed to 90°. The arm is then horizontally adducted 10–15° and maximally internally rotated. The client then resists a downward force applied by the examiner to the distal arm. (B) Maximal external rotation: the test is then repeated in the same position with the arm maximally externally rotated: O'Brien et al (1998) did not quantify the amount of force used. This test is considered positive for ACJ dysfunction if the pain is localized to the ACJ on the first position and relieved or eliminated on the second position. Pain 'deep inside the shoulder', with or without a click, in the first position and eliminated or reduced in the second position is considered indicative of a glenoid labrum tear (from Powell & Huijbregts 2006, with permission).

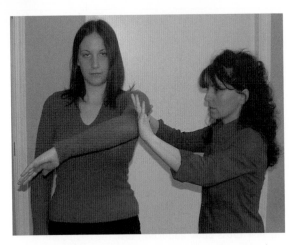

Fig 14.5 **Acromio-clavicular resisted extension test**: the client's shoulder is flexed to 90°, then combined with maximal internal rotation and 90° of elbow flexion. The client is then asked to horizontally abduct the arm against resistance. This test is considered positive if it causes pain at the ACJ (from Powell & Huijbregts, 2006, with permission).

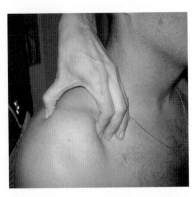

Fig 14.6 **Paxinos sign:** the patient sits with the arm relaxed by his/her side. The examiner's thumb is placed under the postero-lateral aspect of the acromion; the index and long fingers (same or contralateral hand) are then placed superior to the mid-portion of the ipsilateral clavicle. The thumb applies an antero-superior force concurrently while the fingers apply an inferior force. This test is considered positive if it causes or increases pain localized to the ACJ (from Powell & Huijbregts, 2006, with permission).

Table 14.1 Psychometric data for ACJ physical examination tests (Powell & Huijbregts 2006)

	Active compression	Cross-body adduction	AC resisted extension	ACJ tenderness	Paxinos sign
Accuracy	0.53[1]; 0.92[2]; 0.97[3]	0.79[2]	0.84[2]	0.53[1]	0.65[1]
Sensitivity	0.16[1]; 0.41[2]; 0.68[4]; 1.0[3]	0.77[2];1.0[4]	0.72[2]	0.95[4]; 0.96[1]	0.7[1]
Specificity	0.90[1]; 0.93[3]; 0.95[2]	0.79[2]	0.85[2]	0.1[1]	0.5[1]
Positive predictive value	0.29[2]; 0.62[1]; 0.92[3]	0.2[2]	0.2[2]	0.52[1]	0.61[1]
Negative predictive value	0.52[1]; 0.97[2];1.0[3]	0.98[2]	0.98[2]	0.71[1]	0.7[1]
Positive likelihood ratio	1.6[1]; 8.2[2]; 13.3[3]	3.7[2]	4.8[2]	1.1[1]	1.6[1]
Negative likelihood ratio	0.0[3]; 0.6[2]; 0.9[1]	0.3[2]	0.3[2]	0.4[1]	0.4[1]

[1]Walton & Sadi (2008);
[2]Chronopoulos et al (2004)
[3]O'Brien et al (1998);
[4]Maritz & Oosthuizen (2002)

associated shoulder injuries may be present (Parlington & Broome 1998, Shaffer 1999, Maritz & Oosthuizen 2002, Nuber & Bowen 2003, Tallia & Cardone 2003, Walton et al 2004, Chronopoulos et al 2004, Codsi 2007, Docimo et al 2008, Rios & Mazzocca 2008, Park et al 2009) and some consider it the criterion reference (gold standard) for the diagnosis of ACJ injury/pathology (Parlington & Broome 1998, Maritz & Oosthuizen 2002, Walton et al 2004, Chronopoulos et al 2004). If pain ceases with injection, only the ACJ is involved if pain decreases with injection, then other pathologies likely co-exist; if pain is unaffected, the ACJ is likely not involved (Parlington & Broome 1998, Shaffer 1999, Maritz & Oosthuizen 2002, Tallia & Cardone 2003, Walton et al 2004, Chronopoulos et al 2004, Codsi 2007, Docimo et al 2008, Rios & Mazzocca 2008, Park et al 2009). However, injection into the ACJ is noted to have its challenges. It may be unsuccessful, particularly with injection targeting, due to its variable anatomy, variability in the obliquity of the joint, the small intra-articular region, and substantial joint space narrowing when diminished by osteophyte formation (Shaffer 1999, Parlington & Broome 1998, Bisbinas et al 2006, Codsi 2007, Rios & Mazzocca 2008). Parlington & Broome (1998) noted that non-image guided intra-articular infiltrations were placed successfully in the ACJ in only 16/24 (67%) of cadaveric shoulders. Bisbinas et al (2006) found that only 40% of ACJ injections will be placed in the joint if performed without imaging guidance.

As a general principle, imaging is only necessary when it will change management. For acute injuries, history and clinical examination will usually rule out a fracture or an ACJ injury severe enough to require surgical intervention and therefore imaging is often not recommended. If a fracture cannot be ruled out, or if the injury may benefit from surgery, standardized radiographs are essential to both the diagnosis and classification (Shaffer 1999, Fraser-Moodie et al 2008, Nuber & Bowen 2003, Docimo et al 2008, White et al 2008, Simovitch et al 2009). These routine images include: true AP views, axillary views, and the Zanca view (10–15° cephalic tilt) (Shaffer 1999, Beim 2000, Garretson & Williams 2003, Nuber & Bowen 2003, Mehrberg et al 2004, Rios & Mazzocca 2008, Docimo et al 2008, Fraser-Moodie et al 2008, Macdonald & Lapointe 2008, White et al 2008, Simovitch et al 2009). Ideally views would be taken of the uninvolved shoulder to provide normative comparison images (Shaffer 1999, Beim 2000, Garretson & Williams 2003, Simovitch et al 2009). Although stress views of the ACJ have been described to differentiate between Type II and Type III injuries, they are costly, uncomfortable, rarely add diagnostic information, do not affect management, and are thus no longer recommended for routine use (Shaffer 1999, Beim 2000, Buss & Watts 2003, Garretson & Williams 2003, Petron & Hanson 2007, Rios & Mazzocca 2008, White et al 2008, Simovitch et al 2009). Rios & Mazzocca (2008) proposed the use of an AP radiograph of the involved shoulder with the arm adducted across the chest as a prognostic tool. Normal positioning, where the acromion does not overlap the clavicle, indicates a stable joint and directs the clinician to non-surgical management. Superimposition of the acromion and distal clavicle suggests instability and may indicate the need for surgical intervention (Rios & Mazzocca 2008).

Contrary to acute injuries, standardized radiographs are often essential to both the diagnosis and classification of non-acute injuries (Shaffer 1999, Nuber & Bowen 2003, Docimo et al 2008, Fraser-Moodie et al 2008, White et al 2008, Simovitch et al 2009). Computed tomography can be utilized when investigating arthritic osseous changes (joint narrowing, erosions, subchondral cysts) (Docimo et al 2008, Macdonald & Lapointe 2008). Some authors recommend magnetic resonance imaging and ultrasound when investigating capsular hypertrophy, effusions, subchondral edema, subchondral fractures, and ligamentous/aponeurosis injury (Shaffer 1999, Nuber &

Bowen 2003, Petron & Hanson 2007, Docimo et al 2008, Fraser-Moodie et al 2008, Macdonald & Lapointe 2008). A recent study utilized ultrasound to identify abnormal movements in an injured ACJ that were not identified on standard imaging or stress radiographs (Peetrons & Bédard 2007, Rios & Mazzocca 2008). Isotope bone scanning may be useful in discriminating the source of symptoms (Shaffer 1999, Nuber & Bowen 2003, Fraser-Moodie et al 2008). Walton et al (2004) found bone scans had relatively high sensitivity (82%) and specificity (70%) in the diagnosis of ACJ-related pain.

MANAGEMENT OF ACROMIO-CLAVICULAR JOINT

The goals of treatment for ACJ injuries are achieving painless range of motion of the shoulder, obtaining full strength, and exhibiting no limitation in activity (Fraser-Moodie et al 2008, Macdonald & Lapointe 2008, White et al 2008). Conservative management is considered the standard of care for non-acute ACJ dysfunction and for types I and II ACJ injuries (Magee & Reid 1996, Bradley & Elkousy 2003, Buss & Watts 2003, Hootman 2004, Mehrberg et al 2004, Petron & Hanson 2007, Spencer 2007, Ceccarelli et al 2008, Docimo et al 2008, Fraser-Moodie et al 2008, Macdonald & Lapointe 2008, Rios & Mazzocca 2008, White et al 2008, Tom et al 2009). Although there is some controversy over the treatments of type III injuries, most authors now favour non-surgical intervention (Magee & Reid 1996, Bradley & Elkousy 2003, Buss & Watts 2003, Rudzki et al 2003, Hootman 2004, Mehrberg et al 2004, Brukner & Khan 2006, Petron & Hanson 2007, Spencer 2007, Ceccarelli et al 2008, Fraser-Moodie et al 2008, Macdonald & Lapointe 2008, Rios & Mazzocca 2008, White et al 2008, Simovitch et al 2009, Tom et al 2009, Murena et al 2009). Treatment of type III ACJ injuries is dependent on the injury severity and activity level of the patient. Surgical intervention is recommended for types IV, V, and VI and for protracted pain/disability with ACJ dysfunction (Urist 1963, Bradley & Elkousy 2003, Hootman 2004, Mehrberg et al 2004, Macdonald & Lapointe 2008, Petron & Hanson 2007, Rabalais & McCarty 2007, Rios & Mazzocca 2008, White et al 2008, Simovitch et al 2009).

Conservative management can involve rest, splinting/bracing, physical therapy (including, but not limited to manual therapy, active rehabilitation, taping, modalities including cold, heat, ultrasound, laser, electrical stimulation, and iontophoresis), ACJ corticosteroid injections, and anti-inflammatory and/or analgesic medication (Magee & Reid 1996, Shaffer 1999, Bradley & Elkousy 2003, Buss & Watts 2003, Rudzki et al 2003, Lemos & Tolo 2003, Buttaci et al 2004, Mehrberg et al 2004, Brukner & Khan 2006, Codsi 2007, Petron & Hanson

2007, Spencer 2007, Docimo et al 2008, Fraser-Moodie et al 2008, Macdonald & Lapointe 2008, White et al 2008, Rios & Mazzocca 2008, Simovitch et al 2009, Tom et al 2009). A structured active rehabilitation programme that involves the strengthening of the shoulder girdle muscles, including the deltoid, trapezius, sternocleido-mastoid, and subclavius, as well as the rotator cuff and periscapular stabilizers, is recommended to prevent on-going disability in individuals with AJC dysfunction/injury (Shaffer 1999, Bradley & Elkousy 2003, Buss & Watts 2003, Fraser-Moodie et al 2008, Simovitch et al 2009).

The literature suggests 80–90% of conservatively managed individuals have good/satisfactory outcomes with regards to strength, motion, and return to pre-injury levels of function (Rudzki et al 2003, Hootman 2004, Macdonald & Lapointe 2008, Rios & Mazzocca 2008, White et al 2008, Simovitch et al 2009). These studies used a variety of 'conservative treatments'. Simovitch et al (2009) proposed that non-surgical management often translates into benign neglect and suggested that inadequate rehabilitation explains some of the failures seen in non-surgical management. First, a good/satisfactory outcome in 80–90% of individuals does not necessarily mean these subjects are free of pain or dysfunction (Bjerneld et al 1983, Rawes & Dias 1996, Schlegel et al 2001): up to one-third of those with type I and type II ACJ injuries had pain on activity at longer term follow-up (Galpiri et al 1985, Rawes & Dias 1996). Bergfeld et al. (1978) found that 30% of individuals with type I ACJ injury and 42% of individuals with type II ACJ injury reported clicking and pain with push-ups and dips. An additional 9% and 23% of individuals with type I and II injuries, respectively, reported severe pain and limitation of activities. Mouhsine et al (2003) reported similar results noting 27% of individuals with type I & II ACJ injuries treated non-surgically developed chronic ACJ symptoms at a mean of 26 months post injury and required subsequent surgery. Unsatisfactory results have been reported in 10% to 50% of individuals undergoing conservative management, at times leading to a change of job and/or modification of recreational activities, even potentially requiring subsequent surgery (Fraser-Moodie et al 2008). These results underscore the need for investigators and clinicians to provide detailed information about 'conservative management' when reporting their results, just as a proper evaluation of studies on pharmaceuticals require details on type, dose, and frequency.

The importance of adequate rehabilitation was shown in a study of the non-surgical management of type III ACJ injuries (Simovitch et al 2009). Glick et al (1977) investigated 35 unreduced ACJ dislocations that were managed conservatively in a professional and competitive recreational athletic population and noted all individuals who had a supervised rehabilitation programme were pain-free. They concluded that the predominant reason for persistent pain and disability after a type III ACJ injury

managed conservatively was inadequate rehabilitation. This proposition is supported by Gurd (1941) who noted that the shoulder can function normally despite an absent clavicle, as long as the shoulder girdle muscles are strengthened and maintained.

Despite the success of conservative treatment for the vast majority of injuries, there are indications for surgery. These include: ACJ tenderness with (1) evident abnormal signs on ACJ imaging results such as those seen on types IV, V & VI ACJ injuries, (2) a lack of response to conservative management, and (3) an unwillingness or inability to modify or refrain from demanding physical activity (overhead sports, weight training, manual labour) (Shaffer 1999, Schwarzkopf et al 2008, White et al 2008). When indicated, surgical outcomes are also successful but tend to have higher rates of complications, longer convalescence, and longer time away from work and sports (Petron & Hanson 2007, Spencer 2007). There are many surgical options for managing ACJ dysfunction and injury, including but not limited to open or arthroscopic procedures, distal clavicle resection, primary fixation of the ACJ, secondary stabilization of the ACJ via a linkage between the clavicle and coracoid process, dynamic stabilization of the ACJ via a musculo-tendinous (inferiorly directed force) transfer from distal clavicle to the coracoid process, ligament transfers and soft tissue reconstructions, and anatomic reconstruction (Magee & Reid 1996, Shaffer 1999, Bradley & Elkousy 2003, Buss & Watts 2003, Nuber & Bowen 2003, Kwon & Iannotti 2003, Mehrberg et al 2004, Buttaci et al 2004, Docimo et al 2008, Petron & Hanson 2007, Rabalais & McCarty 2007, Macdonald & Lapointe 2008, White et al 2008, Simovitch et al 2009, Murena et al 2009, Tom et al 2009).

A wide variety of surgical techniques have been described, but none have been shown to be significantly superior (Fraser-Moodie et al 2008). The later minimally-invasive techniques are reported to show promise, but well-designed prospective studies need to be performed (Fraser-Moodie et al 2008, White et al 2008). Timing of surgery is controversial with some authors advocating early reconstruction and others advocating surgery be reserved for chronic symptomatic patients (Weinstein et al 1995, Bradley & Elkousy 2003, Buss & Watts 2003). Weinstein et al (1995) noted a trend to better outcomes when ligament reconstruction was done within the first 3 weeks after injury. Dumontier et al (1995) found no difference between early (< 3 weeks) and late ligamentous reconstruction.

The evaluation of success or failure for a surgical intervention must include complications. Surgical complications include, but are not limited to: hardware failure and migration, neurovascular injury, infection, fracture, and osteolysis (Shaffer 1999, Bradley & Elkousy 2003, Kwon & Iannotti 2003, Lemos & Tolo 2003, Nuber & Bowen 2003, Rudzki 2003, Petron & Hanson 2007, Fraser-Moodie et al 2008, Rios & Mazzocca 2008, White et al 2008, Simovitch et al 2009). Many surgical options exist for the ACJ region and their goal is to minimize symptoms and maximize long-term function (Bradley & Elkousy 2003, Kwon & Iannotti 2003). Bradley & Elkousy (2003) note there is no correlation in the literature between anatomic reduction and improvements in pain, strength or motion. Fraser-Moodie et al (2008) note that even though the many varied surgical techniques record a low rate of failure the multiplicity of procedures, the lack of a generally-accepted surgical method, and the number of reports outlining the specific surgical complications infer that all ACJ surgical techniques carry a substantial risk of failure of the implant, leading to re-subluxation of the joint. Partial re-subluxation is not necessarily associated with poor outcomes and is often managed conservatively (Fraser-Moodie et al 2008). Complete re-subluxation is associated with residual symptoms, and there are reports of successful revision operations (Fraser-Moodie et al 2008).

CONCLUSION

The vast majority of ACJ injuries are minor (Grades I–II, with CC ligaments intact) and recover fully with adequate conservative management. Studies comparing adequate rehabilitation to surgery for Grade III injuries (CC ligaments disrupted) also support the role of adequate rehabilitation as the primary treatment. The more severe injuries (e.g. posterior or inferior displacement of the clavicle) are rarer and there is some research suggesting these injuries should be treated surgically. Areas that are most likely to benefit from more research include:

- Long-term prognosis: Studying the sequelae of ACJ injury with validated relevant outcome measures (Hootman 2004).
- Diagnostic testing: Study of the validity of the newer diagnostic manoeuvres such as Paxinos sign and the cross-arm adduction AP radiographs (Rios & Mazzocca 2008) and understanding how best to combine the results of different tests for making management decisions.
- Conservative treatment: The comparison of different types of supervised rehabilitation in the management of types I, II and III ACJ injury and in chronic ACJ dysfunction (Hootman 2004, Spencer 2007, Macdonald & Lapointe 2008, Ceccarelli et al 2008, Simovitch et al 2009).
- Surgical treatment: The timing of surgical interventions, including whether there are sometimes indications for early surgical intervention with type III ACJ injury (Rios & Mazzocca 2008).

REFERENCES

Auge, W.K., Fischer, R.A., 1998. Arthroscopic distal clavicle resection for isolated atraumatic osteolysis in weight lifters. Am. J. Sports Med. 26, 189–192.

Beim, G.M., 2000. Acromio-clavicular joint injuries. J. Athl. Train. 35, 261–267.

Bergfeld, J.A., Andrish, J.T., Clancy, W. G., 1978. Evaluation of the acromio-clavicular joint following first- and second-degree sprains. Am. J. Sports Med. 6, 153–159.

Bisbinas, I., Belthur, M., Said, H.G., et al., 2006. Accuracy of needle placement in ACJ injections. Knee Surg. Sports Traumatol. Arthrosc. 14, 762–765.

Bjerneld, H., Hovelius, L., ThoHing, J., 1983. Acromioclavicular separations treated conservatively: a 5-year follow-up study. Acta Orthop. Scand. 54, 743–745.

Bowen, M.K., Nuber, G.W., 2003. Acromioclavicular and sternoclavicular injuries. Clin. Sports Med. 22, xiii.

Bradley, J.P., Elkousy, H., 2003. Decision making: operative versus nonoperative treatment of acromio-clavicular joint injuries. Clin. Sports Med. 22, 277–290.

Brukner, P., Khan, K., 2006. Clinical Sports Medicine. McGraw-Hill Australia, Sydney.

Buss, D.D., Watts, J.D., 2003. Acromioclavicular injuries in the throwing athlete. Clin. Sports Med. 22, 327–341.

Buttaci, C.J., Stitik, T.P., Yonclas, P.P., et al., 2004. Osteoarthritis of the acromio-clavicular joint: a review of anatomy, biomechanics, diagnosis, and treatment. Am. J. Phys. Med. Rehabil. 83, 791–797.

Ceccarelli, E., Bondì, R., Alviti, F., et al., 2008. Treatment of acute grade III acromioclavicular dislocation: a lack of evidence. Journal of Orthopedics and Traumatology 9, 105–108.

Chronopoulos, E., Kim, T.K., Park, H.B., et al., 2004. Diagnostic value of physical tests for isolated chronic acromioclavicular lesions. Am. J. Sports Med. 32, 655–661.

Codsi, M.J., 2007. The painful shoulder: when to inject and when to refer. Cleve. Clin. J. Med. 74, 473–488.

Debski, R.E., Parsons, I.M., Woo, S.L.Y., et al., 2001. Effect of Capsular Injury on acromio-clavicular joint mechanics. J. Bone Joint Surg. 83B, 1344–1351.

Docimo, S., Kornitsky, D., Futterman, B., et al., 2008. Surgical treatment for acromio-clavicular joint osteoarthritis: patient selection, surgical options, complications, and outcome. Curr. Rev. Musculoskelet. Med. 1, 154–160.

Dumontier, C., Sautet, A., Man, M., et al., 1995. Acromioclavicular dislocations: treatment by coracoacromial ligamentoplasty. J. Shoulder Elbow Surg. 4, 130–134.

Fraser-Moodie, J., Shortt, N.L., Robinson, C.M., 2008. Injuries to the acromio-clavicular joint. J. Bone Joint Surg. 90B, 697–707.

Galpiri, R.D., Hawkins, R.J., Grainger, R. W., 1985. A comparative analysis of operative versus nonoperative treatment of grade III acromioclavicular separations. Clin. Orthop. Relat. Res. 193, 150–155.

Garretson 3rd, R.B., Williams Jr., G.R., 2003. Clinical evaluation of injuries to the acromioclavicular and sternoclavicular joints. Clin. Sports Med. 22, 239–254.

Gerber, C., Galantay, R.V., Hersche, O., 1998. The pattern of pain produced by irritation of the acromio-clavicular joint and the subacromial space. J. Shoulder Elbow Surg. 7, 352–355.

Glick, J.M., Milburn, L.J., Haggerty, J.F., et al., 1977. Dislocated acromio-clavicular joint: follow-up study of 35 unreduced acromioclavicular dislocations. Am. J. Sports Med. 5, 264–270.

Gurd, F.B., 1941. The treatment of complete dislocation of the outer end of the clavicle: An hitherto undescribed operation. Ann. Surg. 113, 1094–1098.

Hootman, J.M., 2004. Acromioclavicular dislocation: Conservative or surgical therapy. J. Athl. Train. 39, 10–11.

Hutchinson, M.R., Ahuja, G.S., 1996. Diagnosing and treating clavicle injuries. Phys. Sportsmed. 24, 26–36.

Kiner, A., 2004. Diagnosis and management of grade II acromio-clavicular joint separation. Clinical Chiropractic 7, 24–30.

Kwon, Y.W., Iannotti, J.P., 2003. Operative treatment of acromio-clavicular joint injuries and results. Clin. Sports Med. 22, 291–300.

Lehtinen, J.T., Lehto, M.U.K., Kaarela, K., et al., 1999. Radiographic joint space in rheumatoid acromio-clavicular joints: A 15 year prospective follow-up study in 74 patients. Rheumatology 38, 1104–1107.

Lemos, M.J., 1998. The evaluation and treatment of the injured acromio-clavicular joint in athletes. Am. J. Sports Med. 26, 137–144.

Lemos, M.J., Tolo, E.T., 2003. Complications of the treatment of the acromio-clavicular and sternoclavicular joint injuries, including instability. Clin. Sports Med. 22, 371–385.

Lizaur, A., Marco, L., Cebrian, R., 1994. Acute dislocation of the acromio-clavicular joint. Traumatic anatomy and the importance of deltoid and trapezius. J. Bone Joint Surg. 76B, 602–606.

Macdonald, P.B., Lapointe, P., 2008. Acromioclavicular and sternoclavicular joint injuries. Orthop. Clin. North Am. 39, 535–545.

Magee, D.J., Reid, D.C., 1996. Shoulder injuries. In: Zachazewski, J.E., Quillen, W.S. (Eds.), Athletic injuries and rehabilitation. W.B. Saunders, Philadelphia.

Maritz, N.G.J., Oosthuizen, P.J., 2002. Diagnostic criteria for acromio-clavicular joint pathology. J. Bone Joint Surg. 84A, 78.

Mehrberg, R.D., Lobel, S.M., Gibson, W.K., 2004. Disorders of the acromio-clavicular joint. Phys. Med. Rehabil. Clin. N. Am. 15, 537–555.

Mouhsine, E., Garofalo, R., Crevoisier, X., et al., 2003. Grade I and II acromio-clavicular dislocations: results of conservative treatment. J. Shoulder Elbow Surg. 12, 599–602.

Murena, L., Vulcano, E., Ratti, C., et al., 2009. Arthroscopic treatment of acute acromio-clavicular joint dislocation with double flip button. Knee Surg. Sports Traumatol. Arthrosc. 17 (12), 1511–1515.

Nuber, G.W., Bowen, M.K., 2003. Arthroscopic treatment of acromio-clavicular joint injuries and results. Clin. Sports Med. 22, 301–317.

O'Brien, S.J., Pagnani, M.J., Fealy, S., et al., 1998. The active compression test: a new and effective test for diagnosing labral tears and acromio-clavicular joint abnormality. Am. J. Sports Med. 26, 610–613.

Park, G.Y., Park, J.H., Bae, J.H., 2009. Structural changes in the acromio-clavicular joint measured by ultrasonography during provocative tests. Clin. Anat. 22, 580–585.

Parlington, P.F., Broome, G.H., 1998. Diagnostic injection around the shoulder: Hit and miss. A cadaveric study of injection accuracy. J. Shoulder Elbow Surg. 7, 147–150.

Peetrons, P., Bédard, J.P., 2007. Acromio-clavicular joint injury: enhanced technique of examination with dynamic maneuver. J. Clin. Ultrasound 35, 262–267.

Petron, D.J., Hanson Jr., R.W., 2007. Acromio-clavicular joint disorders. Curr. Sports Med. Rep. 6, 300–306.

Powell, J.W., Huijbregts, P.A., 2006. Concurrent criterion-related validity of acromio-clavicular joint physical examination tests: A systematic review. J. Man. Manip. Ther. 14, E19–E29.

Rabalais, R.D., McCarty, E., 2007. Surgical treatment of symptomatic acromio-clavicular joint problems: a systematic review. Clin. Orthop. Relat. Res. 455, 30–37.

Rawes, M.L., Dias, J., 1996. Long-term results of conservative treatment for acromio-clavicular dislocation. J. Bone Joint Surg. 78B, 410–412.

Renfree, K.J., Wright, T.W., 2003. Anatomy and biomechanics of the acromio-clavicular and sternoclavicular joints. Clin. Sports Med. 22, 219–237.

Rios, C.G., Mazzocca, A.D., 2008. Acromio-clavicular joint problems in athletes and new methods of management. Clin. Sports Med. 27, 763–788.

Rockwood Jr., C.A., Williams, G.R., Young, D.C., 1996. Injuries to the acromio-clavicular joint. In: Rockwood Jr., C.A., Bucholz, R.W., Green, D.P. (Eds.), Fractures in adults. Lippincott-Raven, Philadelphia, pp. 1341–1413.

Rudzki, J.R., Matava, M.J., Paletta Jr., G. A., 2003. Complications of treatment of acromio-clavicular and sternoclavicular joint injuries. Clin. Sports Med. 22, 387–405.

Sahara, W., Sugamoto, K., Murai, M., et al., 2006. 3D kinematic analysis of the acromio-clavicular joint during arm abduction using vertically open MRI. J. Orthop. Res. 24, 1823–1831.

Sahara, W., Sugamoto, K., Murai, M., et al., 2007. Three-dimensional clavicular and acromioclavicular rotations during arm abduction using vertically open MRI. J. Orthop. Res. 25, 1243–1249.

Santis, D.D., Palazzi, C., D'Amico, E., et al., 2001. Acromioclavicular cyst and 'porcupine shoulder' in gout. Rheumatology 40, 1320–1321.

Schlegel, T.F., Burks, R.T., Marcus, R.I., et al., 2001. A prospective evaluation of untreated acute grade iii acromioclavicular separations. Am. J. Sports Med. 29, 699–703.

Schwarzkopf, R., Ishak, C., Elman, M., et al., 2008. Distal clavicular osteolysis: A review of the literature. Bull. NYU Hosp. Jt. Dis. 66, 94–101.

Shaffer, B.S., 1999. Painful conditions of the acromio-clavicular joint. J. Am. Acad. Orthop. Surg. 7, 176–188.

Simovitch, R., Sanders, B., Ozbaydar, M., et al., 2009. Acromio-clavicular joint injuries: diagnosis and management. J. Am. Acad. Orthop. Surg. 17, 207–219.

Spencer Jr., E.E., 2007. Treatment of grade III acromio-clavicular joint injuries: A systematic review. Clin. Orthop. Relat. Res. 455, 38–44.

Tallia, A.F., Cardone, D.A., 2003. Diagnostic and therapeutic injection of the shoulder region. Am. Fam. Physician 67, 1271–1278.

Teece, R.M., Lunden, J.B., Lloyd, A.S., et al., 2008. Three-dimensional acromio-clavicular joint motions during elevation of the arm. J. Orthop. Sports Phys. Ther. 38, 181–190.

Tom, A., Mazzocca, A.D., Pavlatos, C.J., 2009. Acromio-clavicular joint Injuries. In: Wilk, K.E., Reinold, M.M., Andrews, J. (Eds.), The athlete's shoulder. Churchill Livingstone-Elsevier, Philadelphia, pp. 303–313.

Tossy, J.D., Mead, N.C., Sigmond, H.M., 1963. Acromioclavicular separations: Useful and practical classification for treatment. Clin. Orthop. Relat. Res. 28, 111–119.

Urist, M.R., 1963. Complete dislocation of the acromio-clavicular joint. J. Bone Joint Surg. 45A, 1750–1753.

Walton, D.M., Sadi, J., 2008. Identifying SLAP lesions: A meta-analysis of clinical tests and exercise in clinical reasoning. Phys. Ther. Sport 9, 167–176.

Walton, J., Mahajan, S., Paxinos, A., et al., 2004. Diagnostic values of tests for acromio-clavicular joint pain. J. Bone Joint Surg. 86A, 807–812.

Weinstein, D.M., McCann, P.D., McIlveen, S.J., et al., 1995. Surgical treatment of complete acromioclavicular dislocations. Am. J. Sports Med. 23, 324–331.

White, B., Epstein, D., Sanders, S., et al., 2008. Acute acromioclavicular injuries in adults. Orthopedics 31, 1219–1226.

Chapter | 15 |

Sterno-clavicular joint

Erland Pettman

INTRODUCTION

A literature search on the sterno-clavicular joint rapidly makes the reader aware that there are a very limited number of publications on this joint and these predominantly cover medical and surgical concerns. Anatomical and biomechanical references are designed, most often, to support medical or surgical interventions. From a physical therapy perspective this joint would appear to be the 'poor cousin' of the shoulder girdle in both interest and research. However, whilst bemoaning this fact the reason almost certainly lies in the joint's inherent strength and stability. These factors will be covered in the sections on anatomy and biomechanics.

What is most interesting to the writer, however, is this joint's proposed ability to work in concert with the thoracic spine to facilitate the function of elevation through flexion/abduction without compromise to the neurovascular structures that supply the upper limb. In view of our upper limbs we must accept the fact that they enable us to be primate 'brachiates', i.e. we are able to locomote with our upper limbs. Whilst, as we get older and heavier this seems an unlikely premise we need merely to view children at a playground or study gymnasts to realize this is at least one of the functions of the human upper limb and something we have in common with all other primates.

In all anatomy texts the author of the chapter has read that the shoulder girdle 'ends' at the manubrium. Emphasis is, therefore, placed on how the clavicle moves at the sternomanubrial articulation. The writer's paper entitled 'The functional shoulder girdle' (Pettman 1984) inferred that during functional movements of the shoulder girdle there is indeed another biomechanical component to this joint that needs to be considered, and that is *manubrio-sternal* motion, i.e. that dictated by the thoracic spine. Given the dearth of biomechanical research regarding this joint the writer must at least present a proposed biomechanical model, based on observation and palpation, which might lead to further research. Within this proposal will be a clinically reasoned explanation as to how thoracic and/or sterno-clavicular dysfunction may directly affect gleno-humeral joint function.

© 2011 Elsevier Ltd.
DOI: 10.1016/B978-0-7020-3528-9.00015-7

ANATOMY OF THE STERNO-CLAVICULAR JOINT

Descriptive anatomy of this joint is well covered in texts such as Gray's Anatomy (Standring 2004). Therefore, the emphasis here should be on functional and comparative anatomy. In embryological development the clavicle is present in almost all mammals. However, in quadrupeds the clavicle becomes a vestigial or rudimentary structure helping to provide muscle attachments that produce a muscular 'sling' to support the weight of the thorax, neck and head. A fully developed, osseous clavicle that connects the scapula to the manubrium only exists in primates. This bony strut enables primates to enjoy a very large range of upper limb motion, especially away from the midline of the body. Such motion gives primates the functional advantages of grasping, thrusting (throwing or punching), and brachiation (swinging).

Specialization of function within different primate groups appears to depend upon the position of the scapula bone (lateral or posterior to the thorax) (Chan 2007) and the curvature(s) of the clavicle (Voisin 2006). The distinctive 'S' shape of the human clavicle has been likened to a 'crank'. This enables our muscles to support a relatively heavier body weight during brachiation but also to increase the power and velocity of upper limb movements such as throwing. However, that same 'S' shaped clavicle does poorly with compressive loading, its weak spot being the junction between the medial convexity and its lateral concavity. This fact is underscored by this mid-shaft region being the most prevalent site for clavicular fractures during compressive loading such as a fall directly on the shoulder or on the outstretched hand (Denard et al 2005). Most fractures of this region are uncomplicated but on rare occasion may lead to brachial plexus involvement, pulmonary dysfunction or even death (Kendall et al 2000).

The medial end of the clavicle bone presents a large, bulbous head. Its surface is concave horizontally and convex vertically giving it a saddle-shaped appearance. Histological analysis of the clavicular head (Ellis & Carlson 1986), at least developmentally, shows plates of cartilage within the bone. This is a direct comparison with the head of the mandible (Wolford et al 1994), both designed presumably to absorb extreme stresses and strains. The corresponding surface of the sternum reciprocally has an obvious concave surface vertically and a slight convexity horizontally. Since the articulating surface of the clavicular head is over twice that of the manubrial surface this apparent incongruence, whilst enabling large amplitude of motion makes the joint potentially very unstable. It is the role of the joint's ligamentous structures to maintain stability (Iannotti & Williams 1999). Ligaments of the sterno-clavicular joint include the intra-articular ligament or disc, the inter-clavicular ligament, the capsular (superior) ligament, and the costo-clavicular ligament.

There is some disagreement as to whether this intra-articular ligament serves primarily as a ligament or as an intra-articular disc and this will be discussed later. This dense fibrous structure has a strong peripheral capsular attachment that completely divides the joint into separate cavities (DePalma 1959), which in itself hints at a discrete function for each of the joint's cavities. Occasionally, there may be some central connection between the two joint cavities but this is believed to be secondary to wear and tear. Inferiorly, the disc arises from the synchondrosis of the first rib cartilage and the manubrium. Superiorly, it attaches to the superior and medial aspects of the medial clavicle at the lateral joint margin but blends with the fibres of the capsular (superior) ligament.

The interclavicular ligament, as its name suggests, blends with the same ligament of the opposite side. Also, it is attached to the superior part of the manubrium and blends with the ipsilateral capsular (superior) ligament.

The capsular (superior) ligament, perhaps the strongest of the sterno-clavicular joint ligaments, really represents antero-superior and posterior reinforcement (or thickening) of the articular capsule, the antero-superior being the thickest.

Working in concert these above three ligaments afford both strength and static stability to the sterno-clavicular joint with the shoulder girdles in a resting, weight dependent position. This has been referred to as 'shoulder poise' where the distal end of the clavicle is passively supported slightly higher than its medial end. As a passive support mechanism they represent a significant saving in muscular energy expenditure to help carry objects on the shoulder girdles (for example, a yoke, satchel, and even a child) or carry objects by hand (hunted game, water containers, and suitcases). Also, passive shoulder poise is essential for efficiency of manual activities that require minimal shoulder girdle excursion (for example, moulding clay, cooking and using the computer mouse). With regard to stability, the most important of the three ligaments appears to be the capsular (superior) ligament. Cadaveric experiments (Bearn 1967) have clearly demonstrated that static 'clavicular poise' is independent of myofascial support, or even support from the interclavicular and intra-articular disc ligaments. Once the capsular ligament is torn minimal force is needed to tear the intra-articular ligament, leading to superior dislocation and disruption of the sterno-clavicular joint. If the posterior part of the capsular ligament also fails then posterior dislocation is possible which may lead to more serious health or even life-threatening complications due to compression of mediastinal structures.

The costo-clavicular ligament is also called the rhomboid ligament because of the orientation of its fibres. For this ligament there appears to be some disagreement as to its actual morphology (Tubbs et al 2009). Traditionally this ligament has been described as a 'flattened' cone.

The best way to visualize this is to take a polystyrene paper cup and draw oblique parallel lines around its perimeter. Now squash it flat. The drawn lines would resemble a rhomboid if viewed from anterior and posterior. However the lateral and medial margins of the cup would appear to continue the spiralling lines originally drawn. As such, the fibres of the ligament would indeed be capable of resisting clavicular motion in all directions and planes, except for one and that is depression of the clavicle in neutral. The argument within the literature as to its morphology is whether there is an interposing bursa (or space) between the anterior and posterior sets of fibres or if they form one solid mass. Regardless the orientation this ligament's fibres are clearly designed to resist any motion of the clavicle away from its neutral 'poise'. The anterior fibres appear particularly vulnerable to excessive elevation and protraction of the shoulder girdle, which this author feels, from cadaveric observation, is the close-packed position of the sterno-clavicular joint.

During full elevation of the humerus (through flexion/abduction) the shoulder girdle (scapula and clavicle) moves into depression and retraction. The disagreement as to whether the clavicle elevates or depresses (Ludewig et al 2004) is probably the result of different instructions to the observed models. If the model is asked to elevate their hand as high as they can, then elevation of the clavicle will result. However, this author believes that functional elevation requires a stable, depressed clavicle.

During full elevation recruitment of lower trapezius coincides with activation of subclavius muscle (Konstant et al 1982). This would make sense since the motion probably coincides with the greatest stress placed on the sterno-clavicular joint for either throwing or brachiation. The 'shunt' action of subclavius would be most appropriate now for stability of the sterno-clavicular joint. In this author's experience most costo-clavicular ligament injuries (treatable by physical therapy) occur when there is forceful elevation thrust of the arm with a corresponding elevation and protraction of the shoulder girdle. This forced lateral displacement of the clavicle would not be resisted by the appropriate reflex shunt action of subclavius rendering the anterior fibres susceptible to damage. Individuals who might perform such an action are limited to certain athletes (for example, shot putters, javelin throwers, racquet players) but also those performing household tasks (for example, cleaning a bathtub, painters).

BIOMECHANICS OF THE STERNO-CLAVICULAR JOINT

At the sterno-clavicular joint, the clavicle is clearly capable of moving through at least two cardinal planes, i.e. the horizontal (35° of combined protraction and retraction) and vertical plane (30–35° degrees of elevation) (Iannotti & Williams 1999). The joint is therefore considered to possess two degrees of freedom that are both pure swings. The largest displacement, however, is 45–50° of rotation (Iannotti & Williams 1999, Ludewig et al 2004) around the long axis of the clavicle (that is, motion through a sagittal plane) but this author wonders if this can truly be considered a degree of freedom?

The joint is clearly divided into two separate anatomical compartments suggesting two separate functions (similar to the temporomandibular joint). If the posterior edge of the lateral end of the clavicle is palpated during inspiration and expiration rotation of the bone is clearly felt. This is because the clavicle is 'crank' shaped, and as the manubrium rises with inspiration elevation of the medial end of the clavicle produces a posterior rotation around its longitudinal axis. Since there is no other displacement of the clavicle (shoulder girdle) obvious it is assumed that the rotational motion at the sterno-clavicular joint occurs within the medial component (disc/manubrium) of the joint. So it could well be argued that the sterno-clavicular joint complex has indeed got three degrees of freedom of motion.

The large, superficial head of the clavicle is easily palpated during motion of the shoulder girdle on a relatively stationary manubrium. From full retraction towards protraction the most obvious motion initially appears as a posterior male (convex on concave) glide but this glide only occurs through the first two-thirds of the range (from full retraction to neutral poise). After that, as protraction continues an anterior rotation is apparent, representing a female (concave on convex) glide.

A similar change in glides is apparent when the joint is palpated from full depression to full elevation of the shoulder girdle where there is initial inferior male glide followed by a superior anterior female glide. Understanding that the male motion occurs at the disc/clavicle component and the female from the disc/manubrium component allows for a very simple palpatory assessment technique to discern which component is in dysfunction, or indeed whether the whole complex might be deranged.

Considering the dearth of biomechanical research relevant to physical therapy, at this point the author sees fit to propose an interaction between clavicular motion and manubrial motion during elevation of the arm through flexion and abduction based on clinical experience and extrapolation of anatomical knowledge. As the arm is elevated through flexion/abduction the initial motion appears to occur at the gleno-humeral and acromio-clavicular joints on a relatively fixed clavicle. The inferior angle of the scapula displaces laterally and anteriorly to produce an upward rotation of the scapula and its glenoid surface, the motion occurring at the acromio-clavicular joint. At about 150° of elevation the inferior angle stops moving. Presumably fixated by an isometric contraction of lower serratus anterior muscle, the axis of shoulder girdle motion now shifts from the acromio-clavicular joint to the sterno-clavicular joint and the shoulder girdle is seen to depress and retract in the last 30–50° of arm elevation. It might be reasonably assumed that the clavicle should significantly rotate posteriorly. However, if the clavicle is palpated during this terminal range minimal, if any, rotation is sensed. To solve this apparent conundrum one must now study what is occurring at the manubrium.

As the arm is elevated beyond 150° upper thoracic motion can be both seen and palpated. The upper thoracic spine extends, ipsilaterally rotates, and side-bends towards the moving arm. The first thoracic vertebra, first rib, and manubrium now all move in concert, dictated by thoracic spine motion. This is easily felt at the manubrium by palpating bilaterally just below the first rib cartilage. The manubrium also side-bends and rotates towards the elevating arm. So the manubrium is now moving under the clavicle producing a relative anterior rotation of the sterno-clavicular joint. This simultaneous motion of both the clavicle and the manubrium ensures that there is no resultant posterior rotation of the clavicle. The main question now is: why would this be necessary?

The deep cervical fascia blends with the posterior and superior periosteum of the clavicle. If the clavicle were to rotate posteriorly up to 45°, as has been suggested, the deep cervical fascia would undergo an extreme increase in tension potentially compromising the neuro-vascular tissue passing through it, a distinct disadvantage for a brachiator.

Although not strictly a sterno-clavicular joint disruption or injury, an inability for the thoracic spine to move appropriately during the final stages of arm elevation would prevent the disk/manubrium component of the sterno-clavicular joint from de-rotating the clavicle. Clinically, those who perform habitual or sustained arm elevation in their recreational or work environment would potentially complain of signs or symptoms of abnormal neural tension within the arm and/or damage to distal shoulder girdle structures from mechanical compensation. For this reason assessment of thoracic and manubrial motion should be a routine part of shoulder girdle assessment.

PATHOLOGY OF THE STERNO-CLAVICULAR JOINT

For the physical therapist pathologies of the sterno-clavicular joint are best divided into two main sections, i.e. those requiring a medical/surgical consult and those with an indication for physical therapy intervention.

Patients requiring a medical/surgical consult

The sterno-clavicular joint is susceptible to any of the pathologies that affect synovial joints (Iannotti &

Williams 1999, Higginbotham & Khun 2005). Whilst not attempting an exact medical diagnosis, the therapist needs to be able to identify patients suffering from serious traumatic injuries and non-traumatic or degenerative arthritic conditions. Dislocations, although uncommon, represent the greatest threat to articular function. They can occur in anterior, superior, and posterior directions. Dislocations can be the result of direct trauma to the clavicle or manubrium as may occur in motor vehicle accidents or sports. They also result from indirect trauma, especially to the postero-lateral shoulder (superior and posterior dislocations) and antero-lateral shoulder (anterior dislocations) (Iannotti & Williams 1999).

The posterior dislocation is of greatest concern because of the threat to retro-sternal structures such as the trachea and major blood vessels (Rodrigues 1843, Worman & Laegus 1967, Cooper et al 1992). If these structures are involved the patient may well be observed as having breathing problems and changes in skin colour due to vascular or airway compromise.

Dislocations tend not to be subtle. The therapist may suspect them from a history of extreme trauma, a gross loss of motion of the upper limb, and an obvious observable and palpable change in the natural contours of the sterno-clavicular joint. During palpation of motion (described later) the therapist may detect gross disruption of the anticipated (male to female) motion sequence.

Although the clavicle is the first long bone to begin ossification, it is the last to complete it. The epiphysis of the medial end of the clavicle ossifies in the 18th–20th year and fuses with the shaft between the 23rd–25th years. Direct and indirect trauma to the medial end of the clavicle may result in epiphyseal disruption, even fracture. Closely resembling the presentation of a dislocation, only medical examination can provide an accurate diagnosis (Iannotti & Williams 1999).

Hyperostosis at the sterno-clavicular joint (Dihlmann et al 1993, Noble 2003), felt initially by the therapist as an apparent bony hypertrophy of either the clavicular head or the manubrium could signify serious pathology, and a medical consult is certainly warranted (Fritz et al 1992). However, the author has seen two cases of physeal trauma where fracture or disruption were ruled out but the trauma resulted in benign hyperostosis of the head of the clavicle. Apart from the distressing cosmetic appearance, joint function and stability in these two cases appeared normal.

The sterno-clavicular joint has been shown to suffer from almost all potential causes of non-traumatic arthritis, the more common including septic arthritis, rheumatoid arthritis, tuberculosis, and ankylosing spondylitis. The author has rarely seen gouty arthritis as is mentioned in the literature (Kearn et al 1999) but clearly it cannot be ruled out. The presentation of a painful, hot, and swollen joint with no history of injury should immediately raise enough concern for the therapist to request a medical consult.

Patients with indication for physical therapy intervention

These patients will include those with sprains and strains of the sterno-clavicular joint. Acute traumatic arthritis may present with enough pain, swelling and dysfunction that a medical consult should be sought. They are most effectively treated with a resting sling and subsequent referral to physical therapy.

The location of pain from sterno-clavicular joint injury is most commonly in the joint itself, but distal referral for example to the neck, shoulder, and arm is also possible (Hassett & Barnsley 2001). With sub-acute and chronic (traumatic) arthritis the therapist's main concern is whether joint motion has been lost, and if so assess which component of the joint is responsible.

Another concern would be the possibility of any ligamentous sprain. The author is unaware of any confirmed discrete tests for the intra-articular disc ligament, capsular ligament, or inter-clavicular ligament. However if articular motion is normal but localized pain is reproduced by overpressure of shoulder girdle movements, a ligamentous injury must be suspected. Accurate palpation followed by deep transverse friction massage (DTFM) and ultrasound would appear to be the treatment of choice.

Unlike the other ligaments the costo-clavicular ligament can be stressed discretely. With the patient in contralateral side-lying, the therapist moves the (affected side) glenohumeral joint into extension and adduction. Applying pressure through the elbow the therapist then pushes the shoulder girdle into full elevation and protraction. Continued pressure through the patient's elbow now provides a lateral distractive force to the sterno-clavicular joint, maximally stressing the costo-clavicular ligament. In this author's opinion and experience, the anterior fibres are the most likely to be injured. They are accessible to DTFM if the shoulder girdle is positioned into depression and retraction (posterior rotation of the clavicle).

Osteoarthrosis is suspected when crepitation or even 'clunking' are detected during motion palpation. One paper on cadaveric dissection of the sterno-clavicular joints suggested that 80% of people over 50 may have osteoarthrosis of this joint (Hagemann & Ruttner 1979). Since cadaveric dissection can rarely be correlated with symptoms it is unclear how much symptomatology this condition is responsible for. In the author's experience minor, asymptomatic joint crepitation is common in the presence of normal joint function and should probably be ignored. However, if the crepitation or clunking is significant, or corresponds to the reproduction of the patient's symptoms then a medical consult should be sought. The degenerative state of the joint may help in an eventual prognosis, but also in determining the appropriate magnitude of force used in physical therapy procedures (Frosi et al 2004). It is worth remembering that all resisted forces on the upper limb must ultimately be transferred to the sterno-clavicular joint.

DIAGNOSIS OF THE STERNO-CLAVICULAR JOINT

As was inferred earlier the size of the clavicular head, coupled with the fact it is located so superficial, enables the therapist to easily palpate sterno-clavicular joint motion. Following the taking of a history and observation the therapist palpates the anterior surface of the head of the clavicle.

From a position of full retraction the patient is instructed to pull their shoulder girdles into protraction. In normal motion the therapist should be able to feel the head of the clavicle move initially posteriorly (male clavicular/disc motion). At the position of neutral 'poise' the motion should be felt to change to a female (disc/manubrial motion) anterior glide (roll). From a position of full depression the patient is instructed to lift their shoulder girdles into elevation. In normal motion the therapist should be able to feel the head of the clavicle move initially inferiorly (male clavicular/disc motion). At mid-range this motion is felt to change to a female superior/anterior roll. This simple test enables the therapist to decide which articular component is lacking.

MANAGEMENT OF THE STERNO-CLAVICULAR JOINT

Options for physical therapy management have been provided above in the section on pathology. The emphasis in this section will be on manual therapy intervention and adjunct exercises for patients with mechanical sterno-clavicular joint dysfunction. Techniques address either disc/manubrial restrictions (anterior and posterior rotation) or clavicular/disc estrictions (inferior glide and posterior glide).

Anterior disc/manubrial rotation mobilization (left shoulder)

The patient is placed on the right side lying facing the therapist. The therapist is standing, facing the patient. The therapist's left middle and ring finger tips are tucked posterior and inferior to the lateral edge of the patient's left clavicle. The therapist's right hand grasps the inferior angle of the scapula. Passively draws the patient's left shoulder girdle into elevation and protraction until anterior rotation is sensed to cease (Fig 15.1).

The therapist instructs the patient to take a short breath in followed by a long breath out. As the patient breathes

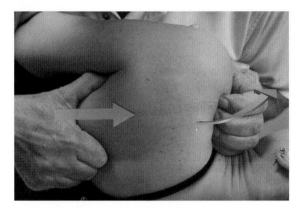

Fig 15.1 Mobilization for anterior rotation of the female component (elevation and protraction).

out increased anterior rotation of the clavicle is taken up by passively increasing elevation and protraction and also by the therapist's left hand pulling the posterior edge of the clavicle upward and forward. The procedure is repeated until no further motion can be elicited.

Posterior disc/manubrial rotation mobilization (left shoulder)

The patient's starting position is the same as described above. In this technique and in contrast to the above technique for anterior rotation, the therapist's middle and ring fingers are over the superior aspect of the posterior edge of the lateral clavicle. The therapist moves the shoulder girdle into depression and retraction until posterior rotation of the clavicle ceases (Fig 15.2).

The patient is instructed to take a short breath out followed by a long breath in. As increased posterior rotation of the clavicle is detected the therapist pushes the patient's shoulder girdle into further depression and retraction

with an accompanying push on the posterior edge of the clavicle inferiorly by the therapist's left fingers. This procedure is repeated until no further motion can be elicited.

Inferior clavicular/disc glide (right shoulder)

The patient is supine. The therapist is standing adjacent to the patient's opposite shoulder girdle. The therapist's left thumb pad or thenar eminence is placed over the superior aspect of the head of the patient's right clavicle. The therapist's right hand draws the patient's right shoulder girdle into elevation until the inferior glide of the clavicular head ceases (Fig 15.3).

The therapist instructs the patient to resist an attempt to push the right shoulder girdle into depression. An inferior glide of the right clavicular head will be detected and this motion slack is taken up by pressure from the therapist's left thumb. Any slack in right girdle elevation is now taken up by the therapist's right hand. This procedure is repeated until no further motion is perceived.

Posterior clavicular/disc glide (right shoulder)

The patient is supine. The therapist is standing on the opposite side to the joint being treated. The therapist grasps the patient's right shoulder with their left hand and instructs the patient to place their right hand on therapist's left arm. The therapist's right thumb or thenar eminence is placed over the anterior surface of the head of the patient's right clavicle (Fig 15.4).

The patient is instructed to resist the therapist's attempt to push the patient's right shoulder girdle into retraction. A posterior motion of the clavicular head will be noted and therapist's right thumb takes up the slack. Any increased protraction is taken up by therapist's left hand. This procedure is repeated until no further motion is perceived.

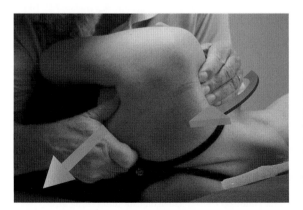

Fig 15.2 Mobilization of posterior rotation of the female component (depression and retraction).

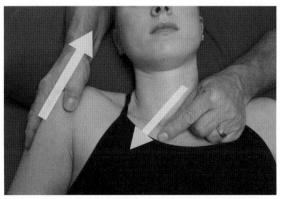

Fig 15.3 Mobilization of the inferior male glide (elevation).

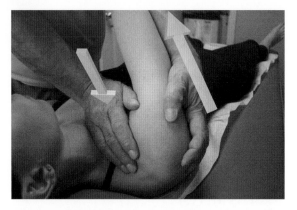

Fig 15.4 Mobilization of the posterior male glide (protraction).

Adjunct exercises

Active exercises to maintain range of motion of the sterno-clavicular joint gained by passive mobilizations should simply be instructed in functional sets, that is, they should have an emphasis on either a combination of elevation and protraction or on a combination of depression and retraction. With regard to normal sterno-clavicular joint function, however, the author cannot overemphasize the need for normal thoracic joint motion. Manual mobilization and manipulation techniques to restore mobility in

this region have been described in Chapter 11 and should be reviewed and included for optimal management of patients with sterno-clavicular joint dysfunction as indicated by the examination findings. Addressing this component of sterno-clavicular joint dysfunction may also necessitate additional thoracic spine exercises to facilitate shoulder girdle depression and retraction (extension and ipsilateral side bending/rotation of the thoracic spine) or girdle elevation and protraction (flexion and contralateral side bending/rotation of the thoracic spine).

CONCLUSION

The sterno-clavicular joint seems poorly understood and more poorly researched, but it is accepted that this is, in part, due to the rarity of significant injury to the joint. However, as physical therapists continue to gain the privilege of direct access to patients it is essential they become aware of how to differentiate between pathological conditions of this joint that may be either health or life threatening demanding a medical consult or that require a physical therapy intervention. Also, much more work is required by all interested parties to investigate the biomechanical role of the thorax in sterno-clavicular joint function and its potential patho-biomechanical interaction with upper limb function.

REFERENCES

Bearn, J.G., 1967. Direct observations on the function of the capsule of the sterno-clavicular joint in the clavicular support. Anatomy 101, 159–170.

Chan, L.K., 2007. Scapular position in primates. Folia Primatol. 7, 19–35.

Cooper, G.J., Stubbs, D., Walker, D.A., et al., 1992. Posterior sterno-clavicular joint dislocation: a novel method of external fixation. Injury 23, 565–567.

Denard, P.J., Koval, K.J., Cantu, R.V., et al., 2005. Management of midshaft clavicle fractures in adults. Am. J. Orthop. 34 (11), 527–536.

DePalma, A.F., 1959. The role of the disks of the sterno-clavicular and the acromioclavicular joints. Clin. Orthop. Relat. Res. 13, 222–233.

Dihlmann, W., Schnabel, A., Gross, W.L., 1993. The acquired hyperostosis syndrome: a little known skeletal disorder with distinctive radiological

and clinical features. J. Clin. Invest. 72, 4–11.

Ellis, E., Carlson, D.S., 1986. Histological comparison of the costochondral, sterno-clavicular and temporomandibular joints during growth in *Macaca mulatta*. J. Oral Maxillofac. Surg. 44, 312–321.

Fritz, P., Baldauf, G., Whilke, H.J., et al., 1992. Hyperostosis: its progression and radiological features. Ann. Rheum. Dis. 51, 658–664.

Frosi, G., Sulli, A., Testa, M., et al., 2004. The sterno-clavicular joint: anatomy, biomechanics, clinical features and aspects of manual therapy. Rheumatismo 56, 82–88.

Hagemann, R., Ruttner, J.R., 1979. Arthrosis of the sterno-clavicular joint. Z. Rheumatol. 38, 27–28.

Hassett, G., Barnsley, L., 2001. Pain referral from the sterno-clavicular joint: A study in normal volunteers. Rheumatology 40, 859–862.

Higginbotham, T.O., Khun, J.E., 2005. Atraumatic disorders of the sternoclavicular joint. J Am Acad Orthop Surg 13, 138–145.

Iannotti, J.P., Williams, G.R., 1999. Disorders of the shoulder. Lippincott Williams and Wilkins, Philadelphia.

Kearn, A., Schunk, A., Thelan, M., 1999. Gout in the area of the cervical area and sterno-clavicular joint. Rofo 170, 515–517.

Kendall, K.M., Burton, J.H., Cushing, B., 2000. Fatal subclavian artery transection from isolated clavicle fracture. Trauma 42, 316–318.

Konstant, W., Stern, J., Fleagle, J., et al., 1982. Function of the subclavius muscle in a non-human primate, the spider monkey. Folia Primatol. 38, 170–182.

Ludewig, P., Bahrens, S., Spoden, S., et al., 2004. Three-dimensional clavicular motion during arm elevation: reliability and descriptive data. J. Orthop. Sports Phys. Ther. 34, 140–149.

Noble, J.S., 2003. Degenerative sterno-clavicular arthritis and hyperostosis. Clin. Sports Med. 22, 407–422.

Pettman, E., 1984. The functional shoulder girdle. International Federation of Orthopaedic Manipulative Therapists (IFOMT), Vancouver.

Rodrigues, H., 1843. Case of dislocation, inwards, of the internal extremity of the clavicle. Lancet 1, 309–310.

Standring, S. (Ed.), 2004. Gray's anatomy: The anatomical basis of clinical practice. thirtyninth ed Churchill Livingstone, Edinburgh.

Tubbs, S.R., Shah, N.A., Sullivan, B.P., et al., 2009. The costoclavicular ligament revisited: A functional and anatomical study. Journal of Morphology and Embryology 50, 475–479.

Voisin, J.L., 2006. Clavicle, a neglected bone: Morphology and relation to arm movements and shoulder

architecture in primates. Anat. Rec. A 288A, 944–953.

Wolford, L.M., Cottrell, D.A., Henry, C., 1994. Sterno-clavicular grafts for temporomandibular reconstruction. J. Oral Maxillofac. Surg. 52, 119–128.

Worman, L.W., Laegus, C., 1967. Intrathoracic injury following retrosternal dislocation of the clavicle. J. Trauma 7, 416–423.

Chapter | 16 |

Rotator cuff lesions: shoulder impingement

Peter A Huijbregts, Carel Bron

INTRODUCTION

Shoulder complaints are common. A Dutch study indicated a point-prevalence in the general population of 20.9% (Picavet et al 2000). Another Dutch study indicated a yearly incidence of 11.2 per 1000 patients in general medical practice with 41% of the patients seeking care for shoulder complaints diagnosed with impingement (van der Windt et al 1995). A UK study found that at 16%, shoulder problems were the third most common cause of musculoskeletal disease in primary care (Urwin et al 1998). Shoulder complaints are also a common reason for patients to seek therapy. In a survey of US outpatient physical therapy services 11% of 1258 patients indicated the shoulder as their chief area of complaints (Boissonnault 1999).

Although descriptions of rotator cuff tears can be found in the medical literature as early as the 18th century (Limb & Collier 2000) and Codman (1906, 1934) and Goldthwait (1909) in the early 20th century had made significant contributions to our understanding of anatomy and pathology of the subacromial region, the description and classification by Neer (1972) into stage I (oedema and haemorrhage), II (tendonitis with fibrosis), and III (partial to full thickness rotator cuff tears) impingement truly brought subacromial impingement to the diagnostic forefront. However, the development in our understanding of impingement has not stopped there and today in addition to primary or subacromial impingement we recognize secondary, internal, and coracoid impingement as distinct and relevant clinical presentations. Similarly, an understanding of relevant intrinsic pathological mechanisms has complemented the sole emphasis by Neer on extrinsic aetiology. Together with this increased knowledge has come an increasing role for conservative management of patients with these conditions.

ANATOMY

Anatomical structures relevant to the various types of impingement are the rotator cuff tendons, the tendon of the long head of the biceps, the subacromial/subdeltoid bursa, the coraco-acromial arch, the glenohumeral capsulo-ligamentous structures (Chapter 17), and the glenoid labrum (Chapter 18). With movement of the shoulder dependent on the other components of the shoulder girdle but also the cervical and thoracic spine, the reader is also referred to the other relevant chapters in this text for more details on anatomy.

The rotator cuff consists of the supraspinatus, infraspinatus, teres minor, and subscapularis muscles. Even macroscopically the tendons of these muscles can be seen to fuse into a single structure. The supraspinatus and infraspinatus join some 1.5 cm proximal to their insertion, whereas the infraspinatus in turn merges with the teres

© 2011 Elsevier Ltd.
DOI: 10.1016/B978-0-7020-3528-9.00016-9

minor proximal to their musculotendinous junction (Clark & Harryman 1992). Even though the anterior portion of the supraspinatus and the superior portion of the subscapularis are separated by the rotator interval, through which the coracoid process projects medially, the fibres from the supraspinatus and subscapularis also merge and interweave to form a sheath around the biceps tendon (Carr & Harvie 2005, Clark & Harryman 1992). These interconnected fibres from the subscapularis and supraspinatus tendons together with the superior glenohumeral and coracohumeral ligament form a tenoligamentous sling called the biceps pulley that keeps the long head of the biceps tendon stabilized, as it courses across the glenohumeral joint to the bicipital sulcus (Choi et al 2004, Habermeyer et al 2004).

Microscopically, an even greater anatomical interdependence becomes apparent. At the level of the supraspinatus, infraspinatus and subjacent capsulo-ligamentous structures, there are five distinct layers to the cuff-capsule complex (Clark & Harryman 1992):

1. The most superficial layer is 1 mm thick and consists of fibres of the coracohumeral ligament, coursing through the rotator interval and oriented obliquely to the axis of each muscle
2. The second layer is 3–5 mm thick and consists of closely packed parallel tendons fibres grouped in large bundles that also form the roof of the biceps tendon sheath
3. The third layer is 3 mm thick and consists of smaller tendon fascicles with a less uniform orientation where fibre bundles intersect at a 45° angle and extensive interdigitations occur between the supraspinatus and infraspinatus tendons
4. The fourth layer consists of loose connective tissue with some thick collagen fibre bands located mostly on the extra-articular side of this layer
5. The deepest layer is only 1.5–2 mm thick and is made up of interwoven collagen fibrils that make up the 'true' glenohumeral capsule

The subscapularis tendon consists of 4–6 thick collagen fibre bundles. The most proximal of these bundles passes under the biceps tendon to form the floor of its sheath interwoven with some fibres from the supraspinatus. In this groove these interwoven tendons become fibro-cartilaginous. The superior and middle glenohumeral ligaments run under the subscapularis tendon and separate the tendon from the capsule with a structure similar to that described for the fourth layer of the supraspinatus region above (Clark & Harryman 1992).

Although extensively interwoven with the other local structures as described above, the tendinous segments of the rotator cuff are thickened along the axes of the four muscles (Clark & Harryman 1992). Clinically most relevant is that the strong central tendon of the bipennate supraspinatus muscle along its course migrates anteriorly

leaving a stress riser at the junction of its thick leading edge and the weaker posterior two-thirds, which is where 96% of all rotator cuff tears initiate (Bunker 2002).

Vascular anatomy of the rotator cuff has been a contentious issue. Rathbun & Macnab (1970) reported an avascular area near the supraspinatus insertion, especially with adduction, that corresponds with the area where tears first occur. Biberthaler et al (2003) also noted a significant reduction in capillary density at the edge of degenerative rotator cuff lesions. Other sources have reported no such hypovascularity (Moseley & Goldie 1963, Bunker 2002, Carr & Harvie 2005) or have even shown hypervascularity in patients with symptomatic impingement (Chansky & Iannotti 1991). Impaired but also increased blood supply may be a secondary event rather than a factor in the aetiology of rotator cuff lesions (Carr & Harvie 2005).

The coraco-acromial arch defines the subacromial space and consists of the acromion and coracoid processes with spanned between them the coraco-acromial ligament. Between the head of the humerus and the coraco-acromial arch in a space measuring 1–1.5 cm on radiographs taken in the anatomical position are located the subacromial bursa, the rotator cuff tendons, and the tendon of the long head of the biceps (Limb & Collier 2000). Apart from its mechanical role, variations in the anatomy of the long head of the biceps have been associated with the aetiology of rotator cuff lesions. Dierickx et al (2009) noted the role of the double-origin biceps variant in causing impingement and tears in young patients. Variations in the shape of the acromion have been suggested as playing a role in impingement. Bigliani et al (1986) described a flat (type I), a curved (type II), and a hooked (type III) acromion and related these types with increasing occurrence of impingement.

BIOMECHANICS

Although a simplification, within the context of impingement we can divide the muscles of the glenohumeral joint into prime movers and stabilizers. Normal glenohumeral motion consists of a roll-gliding combination that keeps the humeral head centred on the glenoid. Due to their orientation, the large prime mover muscles impart not only rolling but also significant translational forces on the head of the humerus. The latissimus dorsi and the teres major, for example, can impart an inferior glide (Halder et al 2001), whereas the deltoid will cause a superior glide (Limb & Collier 2000). While a superior translation of the humeral head can be easily seen to cause narrowing of the subacromial space and subsequent impingement, de-centring of the humeral head on the glenoid in any direction will cause excessive tensile, compressive, and shear forces in active and passive structures predisposing the patient to eventual pathology.

Described in more detail in Chapter 17, the glenohumeral capsulo-ligamentous structures serve as stabilizers mainly near or at end-range of motions. Negative intra-articular pressure, lost in case of a full-thickness rotator cuff tear, further contributes to glenohumeral stability (Hurschler et al 2000). However, the main stabilizers of the glenohumeral joint are the rotator cuff muscles. In the context of this muscular stabilization, two force couples are relevant (Parsons et al 2002). In the coronal plane both the deltoid and supraspinatus muscles contribute to abduction. Whereas the supraspinatus throughout abduction has a predominant vector compressing the humeral head into the glenoid, this component increases for the deltoid as abduction progresses (Fig 16.1). However, during early abduction the predominant vector for the deltoid muscle is directed cranially thus compressing the humeral head against the subacromial structures and the coraco-acromial arch. Most relevant to keeping the humeral head centred throughout motion – and likely explaining the noted prevalence of asymptomatic rotator cuff tears involving solely the supraspinatus (Sher et al 1995) – is the transverse plane force couple formed by the subscapularis, infraspinatus, and teres minor muscles (Fig 16.2). Together the frontal and coronal plane force couples counteract the cranially directed force imposed by the deltoid muscle (Lo & Burkhart 2002).

Traditionally, the rotator cuff muscles were thought of as humeral head depressors maintaining a physiologic subacromial space against mainly the deltoid imparting superior translation. However, the rotator cuff muscles are poorly positioned to produce effective depression of the humeral head (Halder et al 2001). More likely, their true or main role is in producing the compressive forces required for concavity compression. Concavity compression is a mechanism in which compression of the convex humeral head into the concave glenoid fossa stabilizes it against translating forces. Glenohumeral stability is thereby related to the depth of the concavity as well as

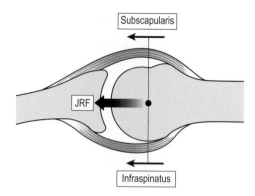

Fig 16.2 Transverse plane force couple.

the magnitude of the compressive force. This clarifies the important role in stability of the rotator cuff but also of glenoid morphology and an intact glenoid rim, labrum, and closely associated capsulo-ligamentous structures responsible for the glenoid concavity (Lippitt et al 1993).

Often functionally considered part of the rotator cuff, research evidence with regard to the biomechanical role of the tendon of the long head of the biceps is equivocal ranging from it having no role at the shoulder to considering it a major depressor of the humeral head (Krupp et al 2009). The most likely role of the biceps tendon (as well as the coraco-acromial arch) is that of a static restraint to superior translation of the humeral head. In normal shoulders the active role in stability for the biceps tendon seems limited to a position of abduction and maximal external rotation as occurs in the late cocking phase of an overhead throwing motion where contraction of the biceps add to torsional stiffness of the glenohumeral joint and reduces anterior translation (Itoi et al 1993, Rodosky et al 1994). However, confirming both authors' clinical observations the biceps tendon may have a greater role in shoulders with rotator cuff deficiency: Kido et al

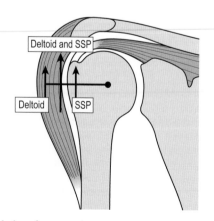

Fig 16.1 Frontal plane force couple.

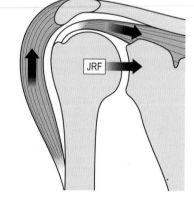

(2000) showed that it acted as a humeral head depressor limiting upward translation not just at 90° but also at 0° and 45° of abduction in patients with a rotator cuff tear.

Clinically, function and biomechanics of the glenohumeral joint cannot be discussed in isolation. The glenohumeral joint assumes the required positions in space by the grace of scapular movement. Scapulo-thoracic movement in turn is made possible by adequate mobility and neuromuscular function in the acromio-clavicular, sterno-clavicular, and upper thoracic joints discussed in greater detail in Chapters 14 and 15. Adequate neuromuscular function of the scapulo-thoracic joint, thoracic posture, and the degree of thoracic kyphosis also determine scapular movement (Ludewig & Reynolds 2009).

In the context of scapulo-thoracic contribution to shoulder motion clinicians often refer to the scapulo-thoracic rhythm. At its least complex, a normal scapulo-thoracic rhythm has been defined as a scapula that remains stable during the initial 30° of shoulder abduction or 60° of flexion and then smoothly and continuously rotates upwards during elevation followed by a smooth and continuous downward rotation when the arm moves back to neutral without evidence of scapular winging (Kelley 1995, McClure et al 2009). Normal relative contribution of glenohumeral and scapulo-thoracic motion to elevation motions of the shoulder are suggested to be 2:1 meaning that 120° occurs in the glenohumeral joint versus 60° in the scapulo-thoracic joint (Kelley 1995). However, research has shown that the exact contribution throughout motion has high inter-individual variability, is affected by adding resistance to motion, and differs between active and passive motions (Kelley 1995, Ludewig & Reynolds 2009). This makes reliable and valid clinical diagnosis of relevant scapulo-thoracic dyskinesis

problematic. Using a more 3-dimensional orthogonal biomechanical rather than clinical perspective to describe motion, normal shoulder function depends on the ability of the scapula to produce sufficient frontal plane upward rotation and sagittal plane posterior tilt during elevation motions (Fig 16.3); in a transverse plane initially the scapula may internally rotate some but in end-range it is externally rotated (Ludewig & Reynolds 2009).

PATHOLOGY OF THE ROTATOR CUFF

When Neer (1972) classified impingement into stages I–III he described what is now known as primary impingement. In primary impingement the combination of repetitive overhead activity and external narrowing of the subacromial space is thought responsible for tendon injury. Mechanical compression occurs between the tendons and the coraco-acromial arch. Causes of subacromial narrowing include acromial variants such as an unfused anterior acromial epiphysis or os acromiale, mal-union or nonunion after acromial fracture, and acromio-clavicular separation or degeneration with inferior osteophytic spurring (Pyne 2004). Although acromial morphology, especially a type II or III acromion, has been suggested as a cause of primary impingement, prevalence of these variants increases with age and it has been suggested that they are traction spurs due to tension in the coraco-acromial ligament resulting from rather than causing impingement (Bunker 2002, Shah et al 2001).

Secondary impingement is associated with glenohumeral instability. This primary instability has to be thought of as a continuum that ranges from minor or functional

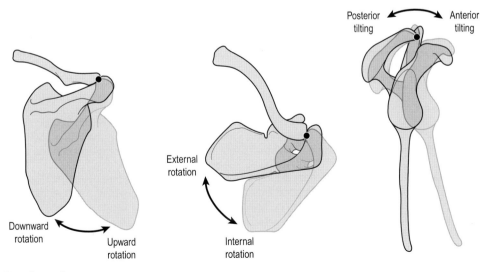

Fig 16.3 Scapular motions.

instability often indicated only by history findings to more pronounced instability that presents with physical examination and at times even imaging findings (Belling-Sørensen & Jørgensen 2000). Congenital laxity, labral and rotator cuff tears, and posterior glenohumeral capsular tightness have all been implicated in secondary impingement (Pyne 2004). Neuromuscular insufficiency (initially without musculotendinous lesions) can lead to decreased efficiency of the concavity compression mechanism. Likely indicative of insufficient active stabilization, glenohumeral proprioceptive acuity is decreased in patients with impingement (Machner et al 2003) but also with muscle fatigue in asymptomatic subjects, especially in the injury-prone late cocking position (Carpenter et al 1998, Tripp et al 2004). Neuromuscular insufficiency may go beyond decreased proprioception, coordination, and endurance. Ganssen & Irlenbusch (2002) showed selective fast-twitch muscle fibre atrophy in the supraspinatus more so than the deltoid muscle with progressively worse rotator cuff lesions. Especially relevant for the active older population is that with age there seems to be an increase in muscle activity in the rotator cuff (infraspinatus and supraspinatus) and deltoid muscles required for shoulder motions (Gaur et al 2007). Higher demand may lead to earlier fatigue and impaired active stabilization in the elderly as compared to younger subjects.

Reflecting the role of the glenohumeral joint as part of the multi-joint shoulder girdle, scapular dyskinesis has been suggested as a cause for secondary but also internal impingement (Ludewig & Reynolds 2009). We discussed the role of the acromio-clavicular, sterno-clavicular, and upper thoracic joints and the influence of increased thoracic kyphosis and thoracic flexion postures above. Soft tissue tightness as often found in, for example, the pectoralis minor muscle and the levator scapulae muscle might result in inadequate posterior scapular tilt. We also need to consider the role of scapulo-thoracic neuromuscular fatigue and dyscoordination. Ludewig & Reynolds (2009) described decreased serratus anterior and increased upper trapezius muscle activity. External rotator fatigue significantly reduced scapular upward rotation, posterior tilt, and external rotation during shoulder elevation thereby decreasing the amount of subacromial space (Tsai et al 2003). Cools et al (2003) showed significant delays in muscle activation of the middle and lower trapezius muscle in subjects with impingement as compared to asymptomatic controls. Indicating the possible role of pain-related inhibition in scapular dyskinesis, Falla et al (2007) demonstrated that an acute bout of upper trapezius pain was sufficient to result in altered motor control of this muscle, not only locally at the site of pain but also in non-painful regions within the muscle and on the contralateral side. A modification of motor strategy that results in compensatory muscle activity is likely to lead to muscle overload and perpetuate pain and dyskinesis.

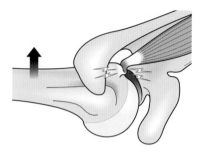

Fig 16.4 Postero-superior glenoid impingement.

The most common type of internal impingement is postero-superior internal impingement whereby the articular side of the supraspinatus tendon is impinged between the postero-superior labrum and glenoid and the greater tuberosity (Fig 16.4) (Belling-Sørensen & Jørgensen 2000). This contact between the supraspinatus and the postero-superior structures is actually a normal and physiologic occurrence during abduction-external rotation but likely in higher-level throwing athletes – perhaps secondary to concurrent minor instability or scapular dyskinesis – may lead to fraying of the tendon and labrum and symptoms especially located in the posterior shoulder during the late cocking phase of throwing (Pyne 2004). Of differential diagnostic relevance is that shoulder pain in the late cocking phase may also be due to the overstretching of the subscapularis muscle. Myofascial trigger points in the subscapularis may produce referred pain in the posterior shoulder. Trigger points in the posterior deltoid and the teres minor muscle may also produce posterior shoulder pain due to their concentric contraction in a shortened position during late cocking (Simons et al 1999).

Although very infrequently encountered in both authors' clinical practice, with antero-superior internal impingement, contact occurs between the biceps pulley and the antero-superior labrum when the shoulder is flexed and internally rotated. This causes damage to the antero-superior labrum, the tendon of the long head of the biceps, the biceps pulley, the superior part of the insertion of the subscapularis, and sometimes the anterior fibres of the insertion of supraspinatus that are normally unaffected in degenerative or tensile rotator cuff lesions. Antero-superior internal impingement may be responsible for the infrequent (4%) anterosuperior rotator cuff tear (Bunker 2002, Habermeyer et al 2004).

With coracoid impingement, the tendon of the subscapularis and occasionally the long head of the biceps tendon are impinged between the lesser tuberosity and the coracoid process. This impingement occurs especially during flexion, internal rotation, and cross-body adduction of the shoulder. Coracoid impingement may occur after arthroscopy, glenoplasty, tenodesis of the long head of the biceps, acromioplasty, coracoid or glenoid fracture with mal-union but can also be related to congenital or acquired deformities of the humeral head or coracoid apophysis, anterior glenohumeral instability, and chronic overuse in a flexion-adduction-internal rotation position (Ferrick 2000, Radas & Pieper 2004).

Impingement can produce or contribute to lesions that vary across a spectrum that includes inflammatory tendonitis, bursitis, degenerative tendinosis, and partial or full-thickness rotator cuff tears. We discussed the stress riser at the junction of the thick leading edge and the weaker posterior two-thirds of the supraspinatus tendon where most tears due to primary impingement initiate. Located some 7 mm behind the biceps pulley an articular side rim-rent tear starts at this weak point and gradually peels back further off its insertion into the superior facet of the greater tuberosity until it emerges on the bursal side and has thus evolved from a partial to a full-thickness tear. Decreased concavity compression allows for superior subluxation of the humeral head and secondary impingement. The cuff tear can extend either slowly over time or give way more suddenly with trauma progressing from a small (< 1 cm) to a moderate tear (1–3 cm). The superior capsule loosened from its humeral insertion contracts and pulls the cuff to which it is merged back toward the glenoid. As the coracohumeral ligament, which reinforces the superior capsule, retracts towards the coracoid it pulls the strong leading edge of the supraspinatus tendon with it. As the tear thus evolves into a large (3–5 cm) tear, the humeral head 'pops' up through the hole and causes an inferior subluxation of the leading edge of the supraspinatus tendon anteriorly and the infraspinatus tendon posteriorly.

Although the infraspinatus tendon rarely tears, even surgically it is hard to retrieve from behind the acromion and therefore by many surgeons often assumed torn. Either way, in its new mechanically disadvantageous position and due to atrophy it becomes non-functional making the question whether or not it really tears a moot point. The tendon of the long head of the biceps starts to hypertrophy and fray. As the lesion extends into a massive tear (> 5 cm) in some 16% of patients with cuff tearing the biceps pulley and the superior margin of the subscapularis also give way, which can lead to the biceps tendon subluxing or even tearing, thus taking away one more stabilizing force in the rotator cuff-deficient shoulder. As the humeral head subluxes anteriorly and superiorly through the now massive tear, arthritic changes between the humeral head and acromion may ensue. This leads to the end stage of cuff tear arthropathy or Milwaukee shoulder, identified on radiograph by massive rotator cuff calcifications (Bunker 2002, Hughes & Bolton-Maggs 2002). Isolated subscapularis tendon tears are very rare and may be solely associated with antero-superior internal impingement (Bunker 2002), although one might, with its impingement of the subscapularis, implicate coracoid impingement as well.

Although all above types of impingement would seem to strongly favor an extrinsic mechanical aetiology for rotator cuff lesions, intrinsic mechanisms are likely to also play a role, especially in the more chronic degenerative tendinopathies. As we discussed, evidence for the role of hypovascularity as an intrinsic factor is equivocal. However, immobilization, age-related changes, genetic disorders, endocrine and metabolic influences, rheumatic diseases, nutritional deficiencies, and tensile overload need all be considered as relevant intrinsic factors in the aetiology of rotator cuff injuries but with their impact also on prognosis these will be discussed in more detail in that section.

DIAGNOSIS OF SHOULDER IMPINGEMENT

Shoulder impingement often presents with a poorly localized pain in the anterior to lateral shoulder. The pain may be present at rest or at night, but is most pronounced with motion, especially overhead. Associated symptoms may include weakness, crepitus, and stiffness. A history of repetitive overhead use in sports or work (throwing, painting, carpentry) may be elicited (Pyne 2004, Boyles et al 2009). Secondary and postero-superior internal impingement occurs mostly in athletes under 35 years of age with overhead activity as in throwing or racket sports, gymnastics, and swimming (Belling-Sørensen & Jørgensen 2000). Antero-superior internal impingement is more prevalent in middle-aged men, who are still active in sports with pain especially on flexion and internal rotation movements (Bunker 2002). Chronic overuse in a flexion-adduction-internal rotation position, pain more consistently in mid range than end range of shoulder flexion, and tenderness indicated over the coracoid may suggest coracoid impingement (Ferrick 2000).

Northover et al (2007) studied risk factors for primary impingement. Activities that increased the risk of primary impingement included occupations with heavy manual labour (OR 3.81; 95% CI 1.93–7.51) and/or overhead work (OR 3.83; 95% CI 2.15–6.84), weight training (OR 2.39; 95% CI 1.07–5.05), and swimming (OR 1.98; 95% CI 1.11–3.53). Work involving hammering (OR 2.47; 95% CI 1.12–5.44) and using vibrating tools (OR 1.95; 95% CI 0.973–3.93) also increased odds of impingement but these risk factors may have not been independent risk factors but rather associated with heavy labor. A medical history that included diabetes (OR 3.34; 95% CI 1.26–8.85) and generalized osteoarthritis (OR 2.39; 95% CI 1.41–4.07) also served as a risk factor.

Generally pain levels in patients with impingement are at best moderate and severe pain may indicate pathology requiring referral for medical diagnosis and (co) management, if for no other reason than adequate pain control.

The build-up of calcium hydroxyapatite crystals within the tendon is characteristic for calcifying tendinopathy. In the shoulder, the supraspinatus tendon is most commonly affected with deposits located 1–1.5 cm proximal to its humeral insertion. Although calcific deposits in the rotator cuff tendons are often asymptomatic, in case of sudden-onset severe pain where the patient is reluctant to move the shoulder actively or passively and where increased temperature is noted on palpation the clinician needs to consider calcifying tendinopathy during its resorption phase. Symptoms are due to exudation of cells, rupture of the calcific deposit into the bursa, and vascular proliferation. This acute episode can last up to 2 weeks, whereas the subsequent subacute episode with pain and restricted movement lasts 3–8 weeks (Hughes & Bolton-Maggs 2002).

With data on diagnostic accuracy of history items not available and the above-mentioned history items obviously not very specific, the clinician needs to depend to a greater extent on physical examination. Patients with pathology ranging from impingement to massive tears have noted decreases in shoulder flexion and external rotation (at 0° and 90°) range of motion compared to the contralateral shoulder (McCabe et al 2005). Clinically both authors also find noted painfully decreased mobility for the hand-behind-the back test for the full spectrum of impingement.

A painful arc sign is defined as pain on active frontal or scapular plane elevation that is most pronounced during midrange (60–120°). Sensitivity of the painful arc sign in the diagnosis of rotator cuff tears was 0.45–0.98 and for impingement sensitivity was 0.33–0.71. Specificity for rotator cuff tears was 0.10–0.79 and for impingement was 0.47–0.81 (Çalis et al 2000, Litaker et al 2000, Park et al 2005). Considering the wide range of diagnostic accuracy statistics this sign can hardly be considered (as it often is) pathognomonic for rotator cuff lesions.

Rotator cuff lesions can affect findings on strength tests due to pain and/or tearing. Patients with the full spectrum of impingement have significant decreases in shoulder strength in abduction (at 10° and 90°), external rotation (at 90°), and on the empty can test (resisted scapular plane elevation with internal rotation) when compared to the contralateral shoulder. Note that weakness of greater than 50% compared to the other arm for abduction at 10° is indicative of a large or massive rotator cuff tear (McCabe et al 2005). Weakness on the empty can test, weakness on external rotation, and a positive impingement sign provides a 98% (95% CI 89–100%) probability that a (partial or full-thickness) rotator cuff tear is present. Any two of three positive tests in a patient over 60 also provide the exact same post-test probability of a rotator cuff tear (Murrell & Walton 2001).

Although originally described by Neer with a retest after subacromial anaesthetic infiltration (Northover et al 2007), in physical therapy literature the Neer impingement test is generally described as the clinician preventing scapular rotation with one hand while passively elevating the patient's arm in the scapular of sagittal plane. Pain at end-range is considered a positive finding. The Hawkins–Kennedy impingement test involves the clinician facing the patient and raising the arm to 90° flexion followed by internal rotation with pain again considered a positive finding. Hegedus et al (2008) did a meta-analysis and provided a pooled sensitivity of 0.79 (95% CI 0.75–0.82) and a pooled specificity of 0.53 (95% CI 0.48–0.58) for the Neer test; for the Hawkins–Kennedy test pooled sensitivity and specificity were 0.79 (95% CI 0.75–0.82) and 0.59 (95% CI 0.53–0.64). As Dinnes et al (2003) also have indicated this means that these special tests can be helpful when negative in ruling out but not diagnosing impingement when positive.

After eliminating diagnostic accuracy studies of insufficient methodological quality, Hegedus et al (2008) noted the external rotation lag sign as a specific test for infraspinatus tears (98%) (although as noted above the infraspinatus likely does not truly tear but rather subluxes and atrophies) or any rotator cuff tear (98%). For the external rotation lag sign the patient is seated. The clinician stands behind the patient. The elbow is passively flexed to 90° with the shoulder at 90° of scapular plane elevation. The shoulder is placed in maximal external rotation less 5° (to avoid elastic recoil in the shoulder). The patient is asked to actively maintain this position as the clinician releases the wrist while maintaining support of the arm at the elbow. The test is positive when lag or angular drop occurs.

The Hornblower or Patte sign was noted as specific (92%) for absence or severe degeneration of the teres minor (Hegedus et al 2008). For this test the clinician supports the patient's arm at 90° of scapular plane elevation with the elbow also flexed to 90°. The patient is asked to rotate the forearm externally against the resistance of the clinician's hand. If unable, the test is considered positive.

Hegedus et al (2008) noted the bear hug (92%) and belly press test (98%) as specific for subscapularis tears. The bear hug test places the palm of the involved side on the opposite shoulder with the fingers extended so that the patient cannot resist by grabbing the shoulder. The patient is asked to hold the hand on the opposite shoulder as the clinician attempts to pull the patient's hand off the shoulder with an external rotation force applied perpendicular to the forearm. The test is positive if the patient cannot hold the hand against the shoulder; a 20% deficit with a 5-second static strength test compared to the opposite side measured with a tensiometer has also been described as a positive finding (Barth et al 2006). The belly press test has the patient press a flat hand on the abdomen while maintaining maximal internal rotation at the shoulder. If the patient is unable to maintain active internal rotation and the elbow drops back behind the frontal plane, the test is considered positive.

With bicipital injury defined as a tear, instability, or intra-substance tendinopathy, Kibler et al (2009) reported the bear hug (79%) and upper cut test (73%) as the most sensitive. The belly press test was noted as most specific (85%). The upper cut test also produced the highest positive likelihood ratio (3.38). The upper cut test is performed with the involved shoulder in a neutral position, the elbow flexed 90°, the forearm supinated, and the patient making a fist. The patient is then asked to rapidly bring the hand up and toward the chin mimicking an upper cut punch as the clinician resists this motion with his or her hand on the patient's fist. Pain or a painful pop over the anterior portion of the shoulder indicates a positive test.

In young athletes with shoulder pain, Meister et al (2004) validated the posterior impingement sign whereby the shoulder is brought into 90–110° of abduction, 10–15° of extension, and maximal external rotation. Pain reproduced in the posterior shoulder constituted a positive finding. Sensitivity and specificity for the diagnosis of a posterior labral and/or articular side rotator cuff tear were 75.5% and 85%, respectively. When only athletes with a gradual onset of pain were considered, sensitivity increased to 95% and specificity to 100% making this the only test described in the literature with established diagnostic accuracy relevant to internal impingement. Although admittedly not validated and solely based on biomechanical extrapolation and clinical experience, the first author attaches further diagnostic relevance to relief of posterior shoulder symptoms on adding a posterior glide (relocation) to the test position.

Medical diagnostic options include diagnostic anaesthetic infiltration and imaging (Pyne 2004). Imaging relevant for patients with impingement includes plain radiography, ultrasonography, magnetic resonance imaging (MRI), and magnetic resonance arthrography (MRA). Plain radiography shows calcific deposits in the rotator cuff tendons in 2.7–20% of asymptomatic adults. Calcific deposits at the edge of some full-thickness rotator cuff tears indicate poor prognosis. Massive calcifications as in Milwaukee shoulder or cuff arthropathy indicate end-stage rotator cuff disease and severe glenohumeral osteoarthritis (Bunker 2002, Hughes & Bolton-Maggs 2002). Sclerosis of the underside of the acromion and upper greater tuberosity together with superior migration of the humeral head may indicate the presence of a large to massive rotator cuff tear. Lesions associated with frank instability such as a Hill-Sachs lesion, acromio-clavicular abnormalities narrowing the subacromial space, acromial or coracoid abnormalities, and acromial shape can all be identified with plain radiography (Limb & Collier 2000, Pyne 2004).

Ultrasonography is portable and offers high-resolution, the option of dynamic imaging, and the ability to directly correlate imaging with physical findings, all at a relatively low cost (Pyne 2004). Dinnes et al (2003) did a systematic review of the literature on diagnostic accuracy of tests for soft tissue disorders of the shoulder including the rotator cuff. If partial and full-thickness cuff tears were combined, sensitivity for ultrasound was 0.33–1.00 and specificity was 0.43–1.00. For full-thickness tears, both sensitivity and specificity were higher than for diagnosis of all tears combined but ranges were still wide with sensitivity at 0.58–1.00 and specificity at 0.78–1.00. For detection of partial-thickness tears pooled sensitivity of ultrasonography was low (0.67, 95% CI: 0.61–0.73) but specificity remained high (0.94, 95% CI: 0.92–0.96). Ultrasound, therefore, can be used with greater confidence for diagnosing than for ruling out partial and full-thickness rotator cuff tears.

For any tear, pooled sensitivity of MRI was 0.83 (95% CI: 0.79–0.86) and specificity was 0.86 (95% CI: 0.83–0.88). For diagnosis of partial-thickness tears pooled sensitivity was low (0.44, 95% CI: 0.36–0.51) but specificity remained high (0.90, 95% CI: 0.87–0.92) (Dinnes et al 2003). MRI can be used with confidence for diagnosing partial and full-thickness tears and for ruling out full but not partial-thickness tears. It should be noted that MRI produces many false-positives. For example, Sher et al (1995) found in asymptomatic subjects that under the age of 40 nobody had a tear, whereas between the ages of 40 and 60, 4% had a tear and over the age of 60, 24% of subjects had a tear. Milgrom et al (1995) showed a similar correlation between age and incidence of asymptomatic rotator cuff tears. Further questioning the diagnostic relevance of MRI, Krief & Huguet (2006) reported no correlation between pain or function and size or location of rotator cuff tears on MRI.

In the diagnosis of full-thickness tears MRA had a pooled sensitivity of 0.95 (95% CI: 0.82–0.98) and a specificity of 0.93 (95% CI: 0.84–0.97) making it a useful tool to both diagnose and rule out full-thickness tears. Despite limited research evidence, Dinnes et al (2003) noted that for partial tears diagnostic accuracy of MRA exceeded that of ultrasonography or MRI.

PROGNOSIS

Research on prognostic indicators for patients with impingement syndrome is very limited. Brox & Brevik (1996) reported on indicators for success or failure with treatment in patients with stage II impingement. The best independent prognostic indicators for success were active treatment in the sense of arthroscopic surgery or supervised exercise (4.8; 95% CI 1.7–13.6), not being on sick leave (4.4; 95% CI 1.6–12.1), and not being on regular medication (OR 4.2; 95% CI 1.5–11.1). Reported shoulder-related work demands did not impact sick leave. Taking regular medication was a prognostic factor for treatment failure that was particularly high in those

Box 16.1 Prognostic factors: diseases and conditions associated with tendon degeneration

- Genetic disorders
- Ehlers–Danlos syndrome
- Marfan syndrome
- Osteogenesis imperfecta
- Homocystinuria
- Hypercholesterolaemia
- Hypertriglyceridaemia
- Aspartylglycosaminuria
- Haemochromatosis
- Menke syndrome
- Larsen syndrome
- Congenital muscle dystrophies
- Endocrine and metabolic diseases/conditions
- Diabetes mellitus
- Stress
- Overtraining
- Premature menopause
- Diminished oestrogen levels
- Premenopausal hysterectomy

- Oral contraceptive use (increased oestradiol)
- Hyperthyroidism
- Hyperparathyroidism
- Renal disease
- Dialysis
- Rheumatic diseases
- Rheumatoid arthritis
- Seronegative spondylarthropathies
- Nutritional deficiencies
- Decreased levels of vitamin A
- Decreased levels of vitamin C
- Decreased levels of copper
- Medications
- Corticosteroids
- Indomethacin
- Naproxen
- Parecoxib used during early tendon healing
- Immobilization
- Aging

patients, who had no disease apart from the painful shoulder (OR 17.0) indicating the need for careful pharmacological management.

Under pathology we briefly discussed intrinsic causes for rotator cuff tendon pathology. In addition to a role in aetiology these causes predisposing the rotator cuff to degenerative tendon lesions will likely also affect prognosis and management choices, although specific quantitative study into their prognostic relevance has not been done. Box 16.1 lists diseases and conditions associated with tendon degeneration relevant not only to the rotator cuff tendons but to all tendons (Leadbetter 1992, Archambault et al 1995, Buckwalter 1995, Jósza & Kannus 1997, Curwin 1998, Almekinders & Deol 1999, Dahners & Mullis 2004, Virchenko et al 2004, Broughton et al 2006, Hansen et al 2008).

MANAGEMENT

Physical therapy management options for patients with impingement syndrome include education, modalities, exercise, manual therapy, and also taping interventions. Common medical management includes non-steroidal anti-inflammatory medication (NSAID), subacromial steroid infiltration, and arthroscopic or open subacromial decompression surgery.

Considering the role of thoracic flexion on scapulothoracic motion, education with regard to appropriate posture seems an obvious component of patient education. Bullock et al (2005) noted a significant increase in patients with impingement for shoulder flexion range although not pain intensity with erect as compared to slouched sitting posture. Visual, manual, and verbal feedback combined with education on faulty movement patterns provided significantly decreased electromyographic activity in the upper and middle trapezius, infraspinatus, serratus anterior, and anterior and middle deltoid muscles of patients with impingement immediately and 24 hours after movement training, whereas trunk, shoulder, and clavicular kinematics improved during and immediately after training, especially in the subset of patients with elevated clavicular position supporting the role of educating patients on correct movement patterns (Roy et al 2009).

Taping patients may support retraining of correct movement patterns. However, using asymptomatic subjects Cools et al (2002) showed that tape application intended to inhibit the upper and facilitate the lower trapezius had no effect on electromyographic activity in the serratus anterior or all three portions of the trapezius with resisted or un-resisted flexion and abduction of the shoulder. The authors suggested altered timing as a possible explanation for the clinically observed effects of taping. In contrast, in patients with subacromial impingement Selkowitz et al (2007) did show that similar taping decreased upper trapezius and increased lower trapezius activity during a functional overhead-reaching task and that it decreased upper trapezius activity during shoulder abduction in the scapular plane. Mechanisms suggested to be involved

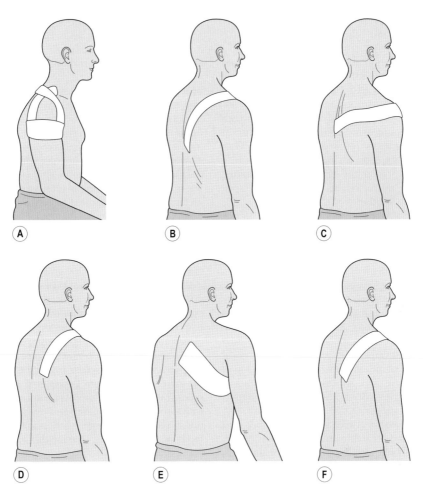

Fig 16.5 Taping techniques for the shoulder. (A) Elevation of the shoulder girdle. (B) Retraction/upward rotation. (C) Retraction of the shoulder. (D) Upper trapezius inhibition. (E) Serratus anterior facilitation and inferior angle abduction. (F) AC joint relocation.

in taping include facilitation or augmentation of proprioceptive cutaneous input, tension when movement occurs outside of the movement pattern allowed by the taping application, and inhibition or facilitation by taping shortened overactive muscles in a lengthened position, whereas the tape might be used hold lengthened under-active muscles in a shortened position. Various taping techniques appropriate for patients with impingement have been described in the literature (Morrissey 2000, Kneeshaw 2002) (Fig 16.5). Morrissey (2000) suggested that when the positive effect on the movement pattern or on symptoms was maintained, taping could be discontinued.

Laser therapy was not demonstrated to be superior to placebo for patients with rotator cuff tendinopathy (Green et al 2003). Ultrasound (RR 1.81, 95% CI 1.26–2.60) and pulsed electromagnetic field therapy (RR 19, 95% CI 1.16–12.43) resulted in improvement compared to placebo with regard to pain in patients with calcific tendinopathy. There is no evidence of an effect for ultrasound in patients with other tendinopathy. Ultrasound also provides no additional benefit when used in combination with exercise interventions over exercise alone (Green et al 2003). There is strong evidence that extracorporeal shock-wave therapy is no more effective than placebo in patients with impingement with regard to functional limitations (Faber et al 2006).

Exercise therapy interventions for patients with impingement are intended to restore the frontal and transverse plane glenohumeral force couples and normalize scapular motion. Generally they consist of progressive resistive exercises for the rotator cuff and scapular muscles and stretching of tight structures but they should also address the motor control deficits identified in patients with impingement. More detail on shoulder exercises is provided in Chapters 21 and 22. Exercise interventions have been supported in a number of recent randomized trials (Werner et al 2002, Walther et al 2004, Lombardi et al 2008) and systematic literature reviews for producing improvements in both pain and function (Green et al 2003, Trampas & Kitsios 2006, Faber et al 2006). In a Cochrane review (Green et al 2003), exercise was noted as effective in terms of short-term recovery in rotator cuff disease (RR 7.74; 95% CI 1.97–30.32) and for longer-term benefit with regard to function (RR 2.45; 95% CI 1.24–4.86). It should be noted that in patients with Neer stage I–II impingement there are no significant between-group differences (at 6 and 12 weeks) with regard to pain and function for patients treated with a supervised exercise programme or a home programme in which they are instructed by a physical therapist (Werner et al 2002, Walther et al 2004).

The presence and size of a full-thickness rotator cuff tear may limit potential for management with exercise and underscores the importance of correct diagnosis. However, at least in a subset of patients with impingement non-operative management is equally effective as open or arthroscopic decompression (Coghlan et al 2008). Haahr et al (2005) noted no between-group differences at 12 months for pain and function in patients treated with subacromial arthroscopic decompression or 19 sessions of rotator cuff and scapular strengthening augmented by thermotherapy and massage. Faber et al (2006) reported no significant difference between supervised exercise therapy and arthroscopic acromioplasty with regard to return to work status at 6 months and at 2.5 years.

Some systematic reviews (Green et al 2003, Faber et al 2006) have supported a combination of manual therapy and exercise for patients with impingement for improvements in pain and function. Manual therapy interventions may be appropriate for restrictions in the glenohumeral joint, shoulder girdle, cervical and thoracic spine, and ribs and are discussed in more detail in Chapters 11, 12, 15 and 20.

Senbursa et al (2007) compared a home programme of rotator cuff and scapular strengthening exercises, active range of motion, and stretching with 12 sessions of glenohumeral soft tissue and joint mobilization, ice application, stretching and strengthening exercises in patients with impingement. At 4 weeks there were significant between group differences with regard to pain and function favouring the manual therapy group. Kachingwe et al (2008) showed significant changes with regard to pain, pain-free range of motion, and function for patients with impingement treated with 6 sessions of supervised exercise only, supervised exercise with glenohumeral grade I–IV glide and traction mobilizations from midrange, supervised exercise with a Mulligan mobilization with movement (MWM) shoulder flexion technique, or a control group receiving only physician advice; there were no between-group differences. Although power in this pilot study was extremely limited, the three intervention groups had a greater improvement in function and both manual therapy groups improved more with regard to pain measures. Active range of motion increased most for the MWM and least for the mobilization group.

Bergman et al (2004) compared medical care (consisting of oral analgesics or NSAID, education, advice, corticosteroid infiltrations and physical therapy referral for exercise, modalities, massage after 6 weeks) to medical care with up to 6 treatments of thrust and non-thrust manipulative interventions to the ribs and cervical-thoracic spine over 12 weeks in patients with shoulder symptoms and dysfunction of cervico-thoracic spine and adjacent ribs. At 12 weeks, 43% of the manipulation group and 21% of the medical care group reported full recovery. A 17-percentage point difference favouring manipulation still existed at 52 weeks. During intervention and follow-up a consistent between-group difference in severity of the main complaint, shoulder pain and disability, and general health favoured the manual therapy group.

Bang & Deyle (2000) showed significant between-group differences on function, pain, and isometric strength of the shoulder in patients with impingement for the group that received thrust and non-thrust techniques to the glenohumeral joint, shoulder girdle, cervical and thoracic spine, and ribs and also manual muscle stretching, massage, and supervised exercise over the group receiving only the exercise intervention. Boyles et al (2009) showed significant within-group improvements at 48 hours for pain with provocative shoulder and resisted tests and functional scores in patients with impingement after only receiving mid-thoracic, cervico-thoracic, and rib thrust manipulation.

With regard to medical management, Green et al (2003) reported that for rotator cuff disease, corticosteroid injections might at times be superior to physical therapy. Buchbinder et al (2003) noted that for rotator cuff disease, subacromial steroid injection demonstrated a small benefit over placebo in some trials. Pooled results of three trials showed no benefit of subacromial steroid injection over NSAIDs. In the context of surgery it should be noted that no significant differences have been reported in outcome between arthroscopic and open subacromial decompression, although four trials did report earlier recovery with arthroscopic decompression (Coghlan et al 2008).

CONCLUSION

Hegedus et al (2008) called impingement the final common pathway for all shoulder disorders and we agree. It is not the diagnosis of impingement per se that is difficult but what is challenging is finding out what the underlying aetiology is. This requires a combination of clinical reasoning based on patho-physiological and patho-biomechanical extrapolation and a good command of relevant research knowledge thereby epitomizing the evidence-informed paradigm. Future research is required with regard to clinical diagnosis of the various types of impingement discussed in this chapter but also into implications of these various types with regard to optimal patient management and on prognostic factors that can guide management decisions for patients along the impingement spectrum.

REFERENCES

Almekinders, L.C., Deol, G., 1999. The effects of aging, anti-inflammatory drugs, and ultrasound on the in vitro response of tendon tissue. Am. J. Sports Med. 27, 417–421.

Archambault, D.M., Wiley, J.P., Bray, R.C., 1995. Exercise loading of tendons and the development of overuse injuries, a review of current literature. Sports Med. 20, 77–89.

Bang, M.D., Deyle, G.D., 2000. Comparison of supervised exercise with and without manual physical therapy for patients with shoulder impingement syndrome. J. Orthop. Sports Phys. Ther. 30, 126–137.

Barth, J.R., Burkhart, S.S., De Beer, J.F., 2006. The bear-hug test: A new and sensitive test for diagnosing a sub-scapularis tear. Arthroscopy 22, 1076–1084.

Belling Sørensen, A.K., Jørgensen, U., 2000. Secondary impingement in the shoulder: An improved terminology in impingement. Scand. J. Med. Sci. Sports 10, 266–278.

Bergman, G.J.D., Winters, J.C., Groenier, K.H., et al., 2004. Manipulative therapy in addition to usual medical care for patients with shoulder dysfunction and pain. Ann. Intern. Med. 141, 432–439.

Biberthaler, P., Wiedemann, E., Nerlich, A., et al., 2003. Microcirculation associated with degenerative rotator cuff lesions. J. Bone Joint Surg. 85A, 475–480.

Bigliani, L.U., Morrison, D.S., April, E.W., 1986. The morphology of the acromion and its relationship to rotator cuff tears. Orthopaedic Transactions 10, 228.

Boissonnault, W.G., 1999. Prevalence of comorbid conditions, surgeries, and medications in a physical therapy outpatient population: A multicentered study. J. Orthop. Sports Phys. Ther. 29, 506–525.

Boyles, R.E., Ritland, B.M., Miracle, B.M., et al., 2009. The short-term effects of thoracic spine thrust manipulation on patients with shoulder impingement syndrome. Man. Ther. 14, 375–380.

Broughton, G., Janis, J.E., Attinger, C.E., 2006. Wound healing: An overview. Plast. Reconstr. Surg. 117, 1eS–32eS.

Brox, J.I., Brevik, J.I., 1996. Prognostic factors in patients with rotator tendinosis (stage II impingement syndrome) of the shoulder. Scand. J. Prim. Health Care 14, 100–105.

Buchbinder, R., Green, S., Youd, J.M., 2003. Corticosteroid injections for shoulder pain. Cochrane Database Syst. Rev. (1), Art No CD004016. DOI: 10.1002/14651858.CD004016.

Buckwalter, J.A., 1995. Pharmacological treatment of soft-tissue injuries. J. Bone Joint Surg. 77A, 1902–1914.

Bullock, M.P., Foster, N.E., Wright, C.C., 2005. Shoulder impingement: The effect of sitting posture on shoulder pain and range of motion. Man. Ther. 10, 28–37.

Bunker, T., 2002. Rotator cuff disease. Current Orthopaedics 16, 223–233.

Çalis, M., Akgün, K., Birtane, M., Karacan, I., Çalis, H., Tüzün, F., 2000. Diagnostic values of clinical diagnostic tests in sub-acromial impingement syndrome. Ann. Rheum. Dis. 59, 44–47.

Carpenter, J.E., Blasier, R.B., Pellizzon, G.G., 1998. The effect of muscle fatigue on shoulder joint position sense. Am. J. Sports Med. 26, 262–265.

Carr, A., Harvie, P., 2005. Rotator cuff tendinopathy. In: Maffulli, N., Renström, P., Leadbetter, W.B. (Eds.), Tendon injuries: Basic science and clinical medicine. Springer, London, pp. 101–118.

Chansky, H.A., Iannotti, J.P., 1991. The vascularity of the rotator cuff. Clin. Sports Med. 10, 807–822.

Choi, C.H., Kim, S.K., Jang, W.C., Kim, S.J., 2004. Biceps pulley impingement. Arthroscopy 20, 80–83.

Clark, J.M., Harryman, D.T., 1992. Tendons, ligaments, and capsule of the rotator cuff: Gross and microscopic anatomy. J. Bone Joint Surg. 74A, 713–725.

Codman, E.A., 1906. On stiff and painful shoulders: The anatomy of the sub-deltoid and sub-acromial bursa and its clinical importance. Sub-deltoid bursitis. Boston Med. Surg. J. 154, 613–616.

Codman, E.A., 1934. The shoulder: Rupture of the supraspinatus tendon and other lesions in or about the sub-acromial bursa. Thomas Todd, Boston.

Coghlan, J.A., Buchbinder, R., Green, S., Johnston, R.V., Bell, S.N., 2008. Surgery for rotator cuff disease. Cochrane Database Syst. Rev. (1), Art No CD005619. DOI: 10.1002/14651858.CD005619.

Cools, A.M., Witvrouw, E.E., Danneels, L.A., Cambier, D.C., 2002. Does taping influence electromyographic muscle activity in the scapular rotators in healthy shoulder? Man. Ther. 7, 154–162.

Cools, A.M., Witvrouw, E.E., Declerq, G.A., Danneels, L.A., Cambier, D.C., 2003. Scapular muscle recruitment patterns: Trapezius muscle latency with and without impingement symptoms. Am. J. Sports Med. 31, 542–549.

Curwin, S.L., 1998. The aetiology and treatment of tendinitis. In: Harries, M., Williams, C., Stanish, W.D., Micheli, L.J. (Eds.), Oxford Textbook of Sports Medicine. Oxford University Press, Oxford, pp. 610–630.

Dahners, L.E., Mullis, B.H., 2004. Effects of non-steroidal anti-inflammatory drugs on bone formation and soft-tissue healing. J. Am. Acad. Orthop. Surg. 12, 139–143.

Dierickx, C., Ceccarelli, E., Conti, M., Vanlommel, J., Castagna, A., 2009. Variations of the intra-articular portion of the long head of the biceps tendon: A classification of embryologically explained variations. J. Shoulder Elbow Surg. 18, 556–565.

Dinnes, J., Loveman, E., McIntyre, L., Waugh, N., 2003. The effectiveness of diagnostic tests for the assessment of shoulder pain due to soft tissue disorders: A systematic review. Health Technol. Assess. 7 (29).

Faber, E., Kuiper, J.I., Burdorf, A., Miedema, H.S., Verhaar, J.A.N., 2006. Treatment of impingement syndrome: A systematic review of the effects on functional limitations and return to work. J. Occup. Rehabil. 16, 7–25.

Falla, D., Farina, D., Graven-Nielsen, T., 2007. Experimental muscle pain results in reorganization of coordination among trapezius muscle subdivisions during repetitive shoulder flexion. Exp. Brain Res. 178, 385–393.

Ferrick, M.R., 2000. Coracoid impingement: A case report with review of the literature. Am. J. Sports Med. 28, 117–119.

Ganssen, H.K., Irlenbusch, U., 2002. Die neuromuskuläre Insuffizienz der Rotatorenmanschette ala Ursache des funktionellen Impingement: Muskelbioptische Untersuchungen am Schultergelenk. Zeitschrift für Orthopädie 140, 65–71.

Gaur, D.G., Shenoy, S., Sandhu, J.S., 2007. Effect of aging on shoulder muscles during dynamic activities: An electromyographic analysis. Int. J. Shoulder Surg. 1, 51–57.

Goldthwait, J.E., 1909. An anatomic and mechanical study of the shoulder joint, explaining many of the cases of painful shoulder, many of the recurrent dislocations and many of the cases of brachial neuralgia or neuritis. Am. J. Orthop. Surg. 6, 579–606.

Green, S., Buchbinder, R., Hetrick, S.E., 2003. Physiotherapy interventions for shoulder pain. Cochrane Database Syst. Rev. (2), Art No CD004258. DOI: 10.1002/14651858.CD004258.

Haahr, J.P., Østergaard, S., Dalsgaard, J., et al., 2005. Exercises versus arthroscopic decompression in patients with sub-acromial impingement: A randomized, controlled study in 90 cases with a one year follow up. Ann. Rheum. Dis. 64, 760–764.

Habermeyer, P., Magosch, P., Pritsch, M., Scheibel, M.T., Lichtenberg, S., 2004. Antero-posterior impingement of the shoulder as a result of pulley lesions: A prospective arthroscopic study. J. Shoulder Elbow Surg. 13, 5–12.

Halder, A.M., Zhao, K.D., O'Driscoll, S.W., Morrey, B.F., An, K.N., 2001. Dynamic contributions to superior shoulder stability. J. Orthop. Res. 19, 206–212.

Hansen, M., Koskinen, S.O., Petersen, S.G., et al., 2008. Ethinyl oestradiol administration in women suppresses synthesis of collagen in tendon in response to exercise. J. Physiol. 586, 3005–3016.

Hegedus, E.J., Goode, A., Campbell, S., et al., 2008. Physical examination tests of the shoulder: A systematic review with meta-analysis of individual tests. Br. J. Sports Med. 42, 80–92.

Hughes, P.J., Bolton-Maggs, P., 2002. Calcifying tendonitis. Current Orthopaedics 16, 389–394.

Hurschler, C., Wülker, N., Mendila, M., 2000. The effect of negative intra-articular pressure and rotator cuff force on gleno-humeral translation during simulated active elevation. Clin. Biomech. 15, 306–314.

Itoi, E., Kuechle, D.K., Newman, S.R., Morrey, B.F., An, K.N., 1993. Stabilising function of the biceps in stable and unstable shoulders. J. Bone Joint Surg. 75B, 546–550.

Jósza, L., Kannus, P., 1997. Human tendons: Anatomy, physiology, and pathology. Human Kinetics, Champaign.

Kachingwe, A.F., Phillips, B., Sletten, E., Plunkett, S.W., 2008. Comparison of manual therapy techniques with therapeutic exercise in the treatment of shoulder impingement: A randomized controlled pilot clinical trial. J. Man. Manip. Ther. 16, 238–247.

Kelley, M.J., 1995. Biomechanics of the shoulder. In: Kelley, M.J., Clark, W.A. (Eds.), Orthopaedic therapy of the shoulder. J B Lippincott Company, Philadelphia.

Kibler, W.B., Sciascia, A.D., Hester, P., Dome, D., Jacobs, C., 2009. Clinical utility of traditional and new tests in the diagnosis of biceps tendon injuries and superior labrum anterior and posterior lesions in the shoulder. Am. J. Sports Med. 37, 1840–1847.

Kido, T., Etoi, E., Konno, N., Sano, A., Urayama, M., Sato, K., 2000. The depressor function of the biceps on the head of the humerus in shoulders with tears of the rotator cuff. J. Bone Joint Surg. 82B, 416–419.

Kneeshaw, D., 2002. Shoulder taping in the clinical setting. J. Bodyw. Mov. Ther. 6, 2–8.

Krief, O.P., Huguet, D., 2006. Shoulder pain and disability: Comparison with MRI findings. American Journal of Radiology 186, 1234–1239.

Krupp, R.J., Kevern, M.A., Gaines, M.D., Kotara, S., Singleton, S.B., 2009. Long head of the biceps tendon pain: Differential diagnosis and treatment. J. Orthop. Sports Phys. Ther. 39, 55–70.

Leadbetter, W.B., 1992. Cell-matrix response in tendon injury. Clin. Sports Med. 11, 533–578.

Limb, D., Collier, A., 2000. Impingement syndrome. Current Orthopaedics 14, 161–166.

Lippitt, S., Vanderhooft, J., Harris, S., Sidles, J., Harryman, D., Matsen, F., 1993. Gleno-humeral stability from concavity-compression: A quantitative analysis. J. Shoulder Elbow Surg. 2, 27–35.

Litaker, D., Pioro, M., Bilbeisi, H.E., Brems, J., 2000. Returning to bedside: Using the history and physical examination to identify rotator cuff tears. Journal of the American Geriatric Society 48, 1633–1637.

Lo, I.K., Burkhart, S.S., 2002. Sub-scapularis tears: Arthroscopic repair of the forgotten rotator cuff tendon. Techniques in Shoulder and Elbow Surgery 3, 282–291.

Lombardi, I., Magri, A.G., Fleury, A.M., Da Silva, A.C., Natour, J., 2008. Progressive resistance training in patients with shoulder impingement syndrome: A randomized controlled trial. Arthritis Rheum. 59, 615–622.

Ludewig, P.M., Reynolds, J.F., 2009. The association of scapular kinematics and gleno-humeral joint pathologies. J. Orthop. Sports Phys. Ther. 39, 90–104.

Machner, A., Merk, H., Becker, R., Rohkohl, K., Wissel, H., Pap, G., 2003. Kinesthetic sense of the shoulder in patients with impingement syndrome. Acta Orthop. Scand. 74, 85–88.

McCabe, R.A., Nicholas, S.J., Montgomery, K.D., Finneran, J.J., McHigh, M.P., 2005. The effect of rotator cuff size on shoulder strength and range of motion. J. Orthop. Sports Phys. Ther. 35, 130–135.

McClure, P., Tate, A.R., Kareha, S., Irwin, D., Zlupko, E., 2009. A clinical method for identifying scapular dyskinesis, part 1: Reliability. J. Athl. Train. 44, 160–164.

Meister, K., Buckley, B., Batts, J., 2004. The posterior impingement sign: Diagnosis of rotator cuff and posterior labral tears secondary to internal impingement in overhand athletes. Am. J. Orthop. 33, 412–415.

Milgrom, C., Schaffler, M., Gilbert, S., et al., 1995. Rotator cuff changes in asymptomatic adults: The effect of age, hand dominance and gender. J. Bone Joint Surg. 77B, 296–298.

Morrissey, D., 2000. Proprioceptive shoulder taping. J. Bodyw. Mov. Ther. 4, 189–194.

Moseley, H.F., Goldie, I., 1963. The arterial pattern of the rotator cuff of the shoulder. J. Bone Joint Surg. 45B, 780–789.

Murrell, G.A.C., Walton, J.R., 2001. Diagnosis of rotator cuff tears. Lancet 357, 769–770.

Neer, C.S., 1972. Anterior acromioplasty for the chronic impingement syndrome in the shoulder: A preliminary report. J. Bone Joint Surg. 54A, 41–50.

Northover, J.R., Lunn, P., Clark, D.I., Phillipson, M., 2007. Risk factors for development of rotator cuff disease. Int. J. Shoulder Surg. 1, 82–86.

Parsons, I.M., Apreleva, M., Fu, F.H., Woo, S.L., 2002. The effect of rotator cuff tears on reaction forces at the gleno-humeral joint. J. Orthop. Res. 20, 439–446.

Park, H.B., Yokota, A., Gill, H.S., El Rassi, G., McFarland, E.G., 2005. Diagnostic accuracy of clinical tests for the different degrees of sub-acromial impingement syndrome. J. Bone Joint Surg. 87A, 1446–1455.

Picavet, H.S.J., Van Gils, H.W.V., Schouten, J.S.A.G., 2000. Klachten van het bewegingsapparaat in de Nederlandse bevolking: Prevalenties, consequenties en risicogroepen. Centraal Bureau voor Statistiek, Bilthoven.

Pyne, S.W., 2004. Diagnosis and current treatment options of shoulder impingement. Curr. Sports Med. Rep. 3, 251–255.

Radas, C.B., Pieper, H.G., 2004. The coracoid impingement of the sub-scapularis tendon: A cadaver study. J. Elbow Shoulder Surg. 13, 154–159.

Rathbun, J.B., Macnab, I., 1970. The microvascular patter of the rotator cuff. J. Bone Joint Surg. 52B, 540–553.

Rodosky, M.W., Harner, C.D., Fu, F.H., 1994. The role of the long head of the biceps muscle and superior glenoid labrum in anterior stability of the shoulder. Am. J. Sports Med. 22, 121–130.

Roy, J.S., Moffett, H., MacFadyen, B.J., Lirette, R., 2009. Impact of movement training on upper limb motor strategies in persons with shoulder impingement syndrome. Sports Med. Arthrosc. Rehabil. Ther. Technol. 1, 8.

Senbursa, G., Baltasi, G., Atay, A., 2007. Comparison of conservative treatment with and without manual physical therapy for patients with shoulder impingement syndrome: a prospective, randomized clinical trial. Knee Surg. Sports Traumatol. Arthrosc. 15, 915–921.

Selkowitz, D.M., Chaney, C., Stuckey, S.J., Vlad, G., 2007. The effects of scapular taping on the surface electromyographic signal amplitude of shoulder girdle muscles during upper extremity elevation in individuals with suspected shoulder impingement syndrome. J. Orthop. Sports Phys. Ther. 37, 694–702.

Shah, N.N., Bayliss, N.C., Malcolm, A., 2001. Shape of the acromion: Congenital or acquired. A macroscopic, radiographic, and microscopic study of acromion. J. Shoulder Elbow Surg. 10, 309–316.

Sher, J.S., Uribe, J.W., Posada, A., et al, 1995. Abnormal findings on MRI of asymptomatic shoulders. J. Bone Joint Surg. 77B, 10–15.

Simons, D.G., Travell, J.G., Simons, L.S., 1999. Travell and Simons' myofascial pain and dysfunction: The trigger point manual. Vol. 1: Upper half of body, second ed. Williams & Wilkins, Baltimore.

Trampas, A., Kitsios, A., 2006. Exercise and manual therapy for the treatment of impingement syndrome of the shoulder: A systematic review. Physical Therapy Reviews 11, 125–142.

Tripp, B.L., Boswell, L., Gansneder, B.M., Schultz, S.J., 2004. Functional fatigue decreases 3-dimensional multi-joint position reproduction acuity in the overhead-throwing athlete. 39, 316–320.

Tsai, N.T., McClure, P.W., Karduna, A.R., 2003. Effects of muscle fatigue on 3-dimensional scapular kinematics. Arch. Phys. Med. Rehabil. 84, 1000–1005.

Urwin, M., Symmons, D., Allison, T., 1998. Estimating the burden of musculoskeletal disease in the community. Ann. Rheum. Dis. 57, 649–655.

Van der Windt, D.A., Koes, B.W., De Jong, B.A., Bouter, L.M., 1995. Shoulder disorders in general practice: Incidence, patient characteristics and management. Ann. Rheum. Dis. 54, 959–964.

Virchenko, O., Skoglund, B., Aspenberg, P., 2004. Parecoxib impairs early tendon repair but improves later remodeling. Am. J. Sports Med. 32, 1743–1747.

Walther, M., Werner, A., Stahlschmidt, T., Woelfel, R., Gohlke, F., 2004. The sub-acromial impingement syndrome of the shoulder treated by conventional physiotherapy, self-training, and a shoulder brace: Results of a prospective, randomized study. J. Shoulder Elbow Surg. 13, 417–423.

Werner, A., Walther, M., Ilg, A., Stahlschmidt, T., Gohlke, F., 2002. Zentrierende Kräftigungstherapie beim einfachen subakromialen Schmerzsyndrom: Eigentrainung versus Krankengymnastik. Zeitschrift fur Orthopädie 140, 375–380.

Chapter | 17 |

Glenohumeral instability

Steven C Allen, Russell S VanderWilde, Peter A Huijbregts

INTRODUCTION

In Chapter 16, glenohumeral instability was discussed in the context of secondary impingement. In the authors' combined experience, patients presenting with shoulder pain often have underlying instability of the glenohumeral joint. However, glenohumeral instability presents a wide spectrum. On the one end of the instability spectrum is the minor instability (more appropriately classified as atraumatic, involuntary, recurrent, mostly anterior-inferior subluxation) with often only history findings indicative of its presence that responds well to conservative management. On the other end of the spectrum is the traumatic dislocation at times with associated fractures and neurovascular or soft-tissue damage that often poses a surgical indication.

With regard to dislocation, Krøner et al (1989) reported an incidence of 0.17 per 1000 person-years in a general urban population. Owens et al (2009) reported an incidence for the general population of 0.08 versus 1.69 per 1000 person-years for military personnel. In about 98% of patients the shoulder dislocates anteriorly, whereas less than 2% of dislocations are posterior and only 0.5% inferior (Walton et al 2002, Cicak 2004, Camarda et al 2009).

The glenohumeral joint can be unstable in anterior, posterior, or multiple directions. Multi-directional instability (MDI) is symptomatic laxity in two or more directions, one of which is always inferior (Caplan et al 2007). It is important to distinguish instability from laxity, as the great majority of lax shoulders are not unstable

© 2011 Elsevier Ltd.
DOI: 10.1016/B978-0-7020-3528-9.00017-0

(McFarland et al 2010). Objectively, laxity describes the extent to which the humeral head can be translated on the glenoid (Schenk & Brems 1998). In contrast, instability is an abnormal increase in glenohumeral translation that causes symptoms related to subluxation or dislocation. Shoulder instability becomes a clinically relevant pathology in the presence of: (1) abnormal and usually asymmetric laxity, (2) correlating symptoms, and (3) correlating pathologic anatomy. When these three elements are present, an imbalance of the static and dynamic glenohumeral joint stabilizers occurs and the result is instability. Likely due to problems with definitive diagnosis, epidemiological data on shoulder instability are not available.

Many young athletic patients present to physical therapy with shoulder pain due to atraumatic, involuntary, recurrent, mostly anterior-inferior subluxation. However, therapists in a direct access role may also be confronted with patients with complaints on the other side of the spectrum and therefore need to also be familiar with the presentation of frank dislocations, so that they may recognize a patient in need of medical-surgical evaluation.

ANATOMY

The anterior shoulder joint capsule has distinct bands described as superior (SGHL), middle (MGHL) and inferior (IGHL) glenohumeral ligaments. The humeral attachment of the SGLH lies just superior to the lesser tuberosity near the bicipital groove. The ligament courses anterior to the biceps tendon to attach to the antero-superior labrum (Levine & Flatow 2000). The MGHL, the most variable (and at times absent) of the glenohumeral ligaments, arises off the humerus at the lesser tuberosity in association with the subscapularis tendon; its labral attachment lies just inferior to that of the SGHL. The humeral attachment of the inferior capsule or axillary pouch, which contains the anterior (AB-IGHL) and posterior (PB-IGHL) band of the IGHL, runs from the 4 to 8 o'clock position of the humeral head to attach to the inferior labrum (Suglaski et al 2005). The posterior capsule extends from the PB-IGHL to the posterior band of the tendon of the long head of the biceps. It has been subdivided into the superior (SC), middle, and posterior capsule. Although often assumed of minor biomechanical importance it should be noted that the SC has a tissue thickness similar to that of the AB-IGHL (Bey et al 2005).

The coraco-humeral ligament (CHL) arises off the lateral aspect of the coracoid process traversing horizontally beneath the coraco-acromial ligament (CAL). It attaches into the greater and lesser tuberosities on either side of the bicipital groove. In the rotator interval between the inferior margin of the supraspinatus and the superior margin of the subscapularis, the CHL blends with the

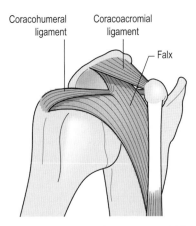

Fig 17.1 Falx attaching fibres of coraco-acromial ligament directly to conjoint tendon of the rotator cuff.

adjacent tendons and the underlying joint capsule. At the anterior joint capsule the anterior band of this ligament is superficial to and overlies the SGHL.

The coraco-acromial ligament (CAL) spans the superior aspect of the shoulder running from the coracoid process to the anterior and inferior acromion. Lee et al (2001) described a falx or band of tissue that directly connects the fibres of the CAL to the conjoint tendon of the rotator cuff without attaching to the coracoid process (Fig 17.1). In the rotator interval, the CHL is also connected via this falx to the CAL, and laxity or damage (also iatrogenic as occurs during acromioplasty) to the CAL may compromise the tension in the CHL.

The intact labrum (discussed in detail in Chapter 18) is fibrous throughout with a fibrocartilaginous transition zone at its attachment with the glenoid articular cartilage (Abboud & Soslowsky 2002). Firmly attached inferiorly and found to be looser superiorly and anteriorly, the labrum increases the depth of the glenohumeral socket by 50% (Cooper et al 1992). As noted above, it serves as the attachment sites for the glenohumeral ligaments and biceps tendon.

BIOMECHANICS

All three bands of the glenohumeral joint capsule serve as the primary passive restraints to external rotation (Turkel et al 1981, O'Connell et al 1990). The SGHL contributes a primary restraint to external rotation in 0° of abduction. The CHL, intimate anatomically to the SGHL, also contributes a primary source of passive restraint to external rotation in this position (Neer et al 1992, Kuhn et al 2005). The MGHL is believed to be a more important contributor to anterior shoulder stability in 45° of abduction, possibly implicating it in midrange shoulder instability (O'Connell et al 1990, Kuhn et al 2005). Together the SGHL and CHL also limit inferior translation and posterior translation in the flexed, adducted, and internally rotated shoulder (Levine & Flatow 2000).

The inferior portion of joint capsule acts as a 'hammock' that checks undue translation of the humeral head on the glenoid. In abduction, this entire complex moves beneath the humeral head and becomes taut. The AB-IGHL comes under the greatest tension in 90° of abduction, 10° of extension and end-range external rotation. The inferior complex moves anteriorly beneath the humeral head with external rotation limiting anterior translation (Levine & Flatow 2000). In cadaver tests of the AB-IGHL complex, the anterior drawer test at 60° abduction produced high strain at the insertion sites on both the humerus and glenoid. These two sites correspond to the most prevalent failure sites during tensile testing of the AB-IGHL; specifically the insertion site on the glenoid is a common site for an anterior labral tear (Bankart lesion). Kuhn et al (2005) reported that the entire IGHL, including the axillary pouch, was the most important restraint for external rotation in both positions of 15° and 60° abduction.

The PB-IGHL of the inferior recess comes under tension with abduction and internal rotation, as the complex moves posteriorly beneath the humeral head (Levine & Flatow 2000). The PB-IGHL has been implicated in the clinically observed stiff posterior shoulder. After the PB-IGHL, in the flexed and internally rotated shoulder the greatest tension is found in the posterior shoulder capsule indicating its role as another posterior stabilizer (Urayama 2001).

The CAL is a significant static stabilizer of the glenohumeral joint at lower elevations (Lee et al 2001). Previously thought to have no functional importance and surgically released during acromioplasty, compromise of the CAL allows for increased anterior and inferior translation of the internally and externally rotated shoulder in 0 and 30° of abduction indicating the potential for iatrogenic instability after acromioplasty.

The intact labrum contributes to the centring of the humeral head on the glenoid, and damage to the antero-inferior labrum allows migration of the humeral head toward the site of lesion. Fehringer et al (2003) concluded that precise centric position of the glenohumeral joint is well served by an intact labrum, especially in mid ranges where the majority of ligaments are lax. The glenohumeral labrum elevates the glenoid edge contributing to shoulder stability by effectively doubling the depth of the glenoid socket and serving as a 'chock block' to translation (Walton et al 2002) adding as much as 20% to the resistance to translation forces (Abboud & Soslowsky 2002). In the preceding chapter the role of the labrum in the concavity compression mechanism contributing to glenohumeral stability was discussed.

Stability, of course, is not solely provided by passive restraints. The transverse (subscapularis, infraspinatus,

and teres minor) and frontal plane (supraspinatus and deltoid) force couples of the concavity compression mechanism function as local stabilizers (Parsons et al 2002). Both the rotator cuff muscles and the prime movers of the shoulder provide muscle force vectors to the glenohumeral joint that have compressive and shear components (Lee et al 2000). The directions of these force vectors change substantially from 0° to 90° abduction, although the compressive component provided by the rotator cuff is consistently much larger than its shear component. The shear component can potentially stabilize or destabilize the joint, depending on its direction. The infraspinatus and teres minor generate a posterior shear in the late cocking phase of throwing, thereby contributing to anterior shoulder stabilization, whereas the supraspinatus generates a large anterior shear force in end-range thus destabilizing the joint in the anterior direction (Lee et al 2000). The pectoralis major similarly provides an anterior destabilizing force in the late cocking position (Labriola et al 2005). The latissimus dorsi and teres major produce more effective inferior shear forces than do infraspinatus and subscapularis; the role of the supraspinatus in this regard is only minimal (Halder et al 2001a). In Chapter 16 the equivocal evidence on the role of the long head of the biceps tendon in stabilization was discussed. The deltoid is a significant contributor to anterior stability in the position of apprehension, with all three heads contributing equally to stabilization (Kido et al 2003). The lateral deltoid is a key muscle restraint to inferior glenohumeral instability (Halder et al 2001b).

PATHOLOGY

Avulsion of the glenoid labrum in the antero-inferior quadrant called a Bankart or Perthes lesion is the most common pathology seen in anterior shoulder dislocation. It is disruption of the IGHL, and not solely the Bankart lesion that is thought to allow for dislocation (Robinson & Dobson 2004). Bigliani et al (1992) showed that an intra-substance ligament injury occurs before labral avulsion. An isolated IGHL injury renders the glenohumeral joint very unstable, even with intact dynamic stabilizers. The typical mechanism for anterior dislocation in the younger patient is indirect trauma to the abducted, extended, and externally rotated arm most commonly in overhead sports activities (Bohnsack & Wulker 2002). Primary anterior dislocation of the shoulder occurs commonly after low-energy falls in the elderly (Robinson & Dobson 2004). An impression fracture of the postero-lateral humeral head called a Hill-Sachs lesion is also present in most patients with anterior instability (Cicak 2004, Robinson & Dobson 2004).

At less than 2% of all dislocations, dislocation in a posterior direction is uncommon. Posterior dislocation can be caused by a fall onto the outstretched arm, a weight 'getting away' from a weight lifter at terminal extension of a bench press, a football lineman unable to hold off an opponent with forces axially transmitted through the forward flexed arms, or a hockey player attempting to slow down velocity of a hit into the boards. It may also result from epileptic seizure or electric shock. Posterior dislocation may be associated with fractures of the surgical neck of the humerus or fractures of the tuberosities. Posterior shoulder dislocations with posterior labral detachment (reverse Bankart lesion) and a humeral antero-medial impression fracture (reverse Hill-Sachs lesion) need to be considered for surgery. Indications for surgical repair include recurrent subluxations or dislocations or mechanical symptoms despite adequate rehabilitation (Seebauer & Keyl 1998, Cicak 2004, Kim et al 2005).

At 0.5% of all dislocations inferior dislocations are even less common. Mechanisms of injury include direct axial loading through the humerus as might occur when the patient tries to catch himself overhead when falling from a height. The other mechanism is violent forced abduction of an already abducted shoulder. Impingement of the neck or proximal shaft of the humerus against the acromion levers the humeral head inferiorly out of the glenoid. The term 'luxatio erecta' refers to the presentation of patient with the arm abducted, elbow flexed, forearms pronated, and hand above the head unable to lower the arm to the side. Associated injuries may include fractures of the acromion, clavicle, coracoid process, greater tuberosity, and humeral head. Associated vascular injuries to the axillary vessels are often serious and require surgery but are less common than axillary, radial, or ulnar nerve or brachial plexus injuries that mostly recover well indicating their neuropraxic nature (Baba et al 2007, Camarda et al 2009). Mallon et al (1990) reviewed 80 cases and reported greater tuberosity fracture or rotator cuff injuries in 80%, neurological involvement in 60%, and vascular compromise in 3.3% of cases.

Posterior subluxation is attributed to posterior compressive or tensile loading and forced hyperadduction (Kim et al 2005, Robinson & Dobson 2004) with pain attributed to excessive translation into the posterior recess. Recurrent posterior shoulder subluxation as a clinical entity has become increasingly recognized as a less common (2–5%) but important contributor to shoulder instability (Eckenrode et al 2009). A single traumatic event or repetitive cumulative trauma as may occur in contact sports with high-energy forces directed to the posterior capsule may lead to posterior glenohumeral instability. Glenoid retroversion and weakness of the external rotators have also been identified as potential contributors (Eckenrode et al 2009).

Excessive anterior translation of the humeral head during abduction-external rotation leads to plastic deformation of the AB-IGHL and anterior glenohumeral joint subluxation. This would also indicate that the degree of excessive laxity commonly found in the shoulder of throwing athletes might be on a progressive track of excessive motion and translation leading to symptoms that eventually manifest in labral injury and/or partial-thickness rotator cuff tears (Kuhn et al 2003). However, laxity and hypermobility is not instability and in fact is a prerequisite to achieve higher degrees of speed and torque in the throwing shoulder (Huijbregts 1998). Considering its frequent association with anterior shoulder instability and subluxation, we believe it is important to review the various phases of overhead throwing and apply clinical reasoning to the kinetic chain to allow for the diagnosis of possible relevant patho-biomechanical faults.

The overhead throw has five phases: wind-up, early cocking, late cocking phase, acceleration and follow-through (Fig 17.2). The wind-up phase in the overhead baseball pitch is a preparatory phase, centred on flexion. A right-handed thrower has a flexion pattern of the left lower extremity with considerable hip and knee flexion. There also will be a flexion movement of the spine. Both

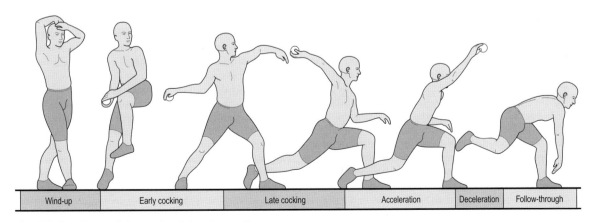

| Wind-up | Early cocking | Late cocking | Acceleration | Deceleration | Follow-through |

Fig 17.2 Five phases of the overhead throwing motion.

hands are in contact with the ball and the shoulders are in an internal rotation-adduction position with bilateral elbow flexion. The pitcher is facing the batter with the left side of the body. Early cocking starts when the left hand loses contact with the ball. The right shoulder moves from adduction and internal rotation to abduction and external rotation. The pitcher steps with the previously flexed left leg in the direction of the batter, and the trunk moves into extension, right rotation, and left side bending. The late-cocking phase starts when the left foot of the pitcher hits the ground. This is the start of a de-rotation movement of the trunk and legs that will contribute to accelerating the ball. The right arm and ball still move in the same direction of horizontal abduction and external rotation.

Acceleration starts with the switch over from shoulder external rotation to shoulder internal rotation. This rotation is the most important movement of the acceleration phase. In this phase, the shoulder also moves from horizontal abduction to horizontal adduction and back in the direction of horizontal abduction just prior to ball release. Ball release by the right hand marks the end of acceleration. The arm, which has been immensely accelerated for the throwing motion, now has to be decelerated. The left lower extremity moves into flexion and trunk into flexion and left rotation. The right arm is moving into adduction and internal rotation. The first phase of follow-through (deceleration) is marked by high activity in the muscle complex of the right shoulder with the second phase of follow-through requiring adequate trunk and lower extremity movement to decrease the force requirements about the shoulder and reduce the potential for injury (Huijbregts 1998). The overhead throw is an extremely fast activity. Fleisig et al (1995) measured an average time of 0.139 ± 0.017 (s) from foot contact to ball release, a period that corresponds to the late cocking and acceleration phases combined.

Two critical instants are identified in the overhead throw that place unusually high demands on the shoulder complex. The first phase identified in late cocking, reveals high torsional and compressive loads to the shoulder that may well exceed the plastic limit of the antero-inferior capsuloligamentous complex resulting in pain and instability in this quadrant. The second critical instant occurs just after ball release in the early deceleration phase. Although torsional loading is significantly reduced and shear forces to the anterior restraints are low in this phase of throwing, the compressive loading to the shoulder joint is highest at 1100 (N), constituting a more than 100% increase from compression during the first critical instant. Any unwanted translation of the humeral head in the presence of these compressive forces has the potential to produce damage to the capsule, the closely associated rotator cuff tendons, and the labrum. Enormous demands are placed on both the active and passive restraints of the shoulder with – in addition to these high torques and forces – an external rotation range of motion

of 140° at the end of late cocking, an internal rotation angular velocity of 7000°/s during acceleration and an angular deceleration of 500,000°/s^2 during deceleration (Huijbregts 1998).

In a throwing athlete with glenohumeral instability the clinician should not limit the search for causative or contributory dysfunctions to shoulder joint or even the shoulder girdle. As an example of relevant lower quadrant dysfunctions, a right sacral torsion present at left foot contact in the acceleration phase may lead to excessive compensation in the shoulder to attain the required arm velocity for competitive throwing. Also maximal lumbar extension and right side bending are required in this phase of throwing, implying that an unresolved, chronic right postero-lateral disc lesion may also place excessive demand on the shoulder girdle, as trunk motion in this quadrant may be limited. This same disc lesion in a more irritable back problem would compromise the de-rotation and deceleration of the throwing arm where flexion and left rotation of the trunk are required.

The overhead athlete may also be vulnerable in case of lumbar instability or an increase in the neutral zone of a spinal motion segment (Panjabi 1992). If this instability is in a rotational plane to the right in the overhead thrower, the critical zone of acceleration may result in compensation higher up in the kinetic chain and subsequent injury to the glenohumeral joint. Unilateral weakness of the multifidus muscles of the lumbar spine may lead to subsequent atrophy in patients with unilateral back pain (Hides et al 1996). Asymmetrical contraction of this group of segmental muscles would result in torsional loading with excessive translation of the spinal motion segment and loss of form closure in the lumbosacral region (Lee 1989) again exposing the glenohumeral joint higher up the kinetic chain to excessive shear or compression. A higher incidence of osteoarthrosis in the opposite hip from the throwing side in retired javelin throwers (Schmitt et al 2004) suggests the need to tolerate high torsional forces on the left hip in the right-handed overhead athlete. Weakness in the deep left hip rotators or gluteus medius in the deceleration phase of throwing or limited hip rotation mobility would likely compromise the safety margin for attenuating force requirements on the throwing shoulder that the contribution of the hip muscles in this phase would otherwise offer.

With regard to upper quadrant dysfunctions, scapular dynamics require adequate upward rotation, abduction and posterior tilting for optimal shoulder function in the throwing athlete (Magarey & Jones 1992). Muscle imbalances between the upper trapezius and serratus anterior may manifest in scapular winging due to serratus anterior inhibition (Sahrmann 2002) thus compromising the well-coordinated movement of the scapula and humerus and the maintenance of centric position of the humeral head on the labrum. A hypertonic or stiff levator scapulae muscle due to C4 facilitation from a cervical spine joint dysfunction would tilt the scapula into downward rotation and inhibit the 'chock-block' mechanism offered by the labrum (Fowler & Pettman 1992, Walton et al 2002). This would increase strain in the structures limiting inferior and anterior translation of the humeral head. The upper thoracic spine requires adequate rotation and side bending to the right in a right-handed thrower. Hypomobility in this region of the thoracic spine is common and will directly impact the degree of stress placed on the anterior restraints to the glenohumeral joint.

DIAGNOSIS OF GLENOHUMERAL INSTABILITY

Although it would be hard to imagine that a clinician would not recognize a luxatio erecta, the much more common patient with minor instability is much harder to diagnose and even most posterior dislocations are missed on initial examination (Cicak 2004).

History

Patients with shoulder instability most often present with pain as their primary complaint. Somatic pain described as deep, aching, and intermittent and located in the anterior or posterior shoulder joint is common. Trauma may suggest dislocation that may have spontaneously reduced, especially when in an anterior direction. Under pathology we discussed mechanisms of injury that should make the clinician consider anterior, posterior, and inferior dislocations. As noted above posterior dislocations are often missed on initial examination with the patient only complaining of subjective instability and pain with flexion, adduction, and internal rotation (Cicak 2004).

In the introduction we discussed how in physical therapy the commonly used diagnosis of minor instability would be more appropriately classified as atraumatic, involuntary, recurrent, mostly anterior-inferior subluxation. This type of instability is much more common but hard to definitively diagnose. It is most often seen in young, overhead throwing athletes or gymnasts. Trauma may play a role but is often more of a cumulative type with previous minor episodes of injury. Magarey & Jones (1992) have suggested the following (non-validated) history findings as indicative of minor shoulder instability: (1) apprehension with certain movements, (2) sensation of the joint slipping in and out, (3) pain worse with overhead activity, (4) painful catches through range, (5) painful intra-articular clicking or 'dead arm syndrome' during late cocking, (6) weakness in the late cocking position. Note, however, that at least some of these symptoms can hardly be considered specific. Schenk & Brems (1998) also noted that patients with MDI might present with pain in midrange positions.

Examination

As indicated above, examination of a patient with shoulder instability should not be limited to the shoulder girdle but include a search for causative or contributory dysfunctions throughout the kinetic chain in upper and lower quadrants. Specific to the shoulder, though, a scanning examination must include assessment of 3D posture. Winging of the scapula at rest and in 90° abduction can be appreciated with a posterior view and indicates the need for specific muscle strength and flexibility tests. A side view may suggest muscle length restriction in the pectoralis minor evidenced by the shoulder held in protraction and elevation with scapular inferior border winging. A patient with an unreduced anterior or inferior dislocation may present with the humeral head visible and palpable on the chest wall out of the glenoid socket. Patients with unreduced posterior dislocation may present with the arm held and fixed in adduction and internal rotation.

Active range of motion in cardinal planes with overpressure and discreet resistance to muscles while on stretch (Cyriax 1978) as well as combined motions begins to examine for provocation and assess integrity. Making them easy to spot, patients with luxatio erecta are not able to lower the arms from the elevated position (Camarda et al 2009). Patients with posterior dislocation may have the humeral head caught on the posterior glenoid rim locking the shoulder between 10–60° of internal rotation with no external rotation possible from this position (Cicak 2004). Should this initial screen not provoke the patient's symptoms, the clinician may suspect a remote source including referred mechanical pain from the cervical spine or a non-mechanical etiology. Note that unless there has been recent trauma there may well be a full or nearly full range of motion (ROM) in the shoulder girdle. A neurovascular examination for compromise especially in the patient with a possible dislocation will complete the seated examination. Close inspection of the scapula from a posterior viewpoint during arm elevation will be helpful for abnormal rhythm, lack of upward rotation, and abduction, or medial border winging as discussed in the chapter on impingement (Chapter 16).

Magarey & Jones (1992) have suggested the following (non-validated) physical examination findings as indicative of minor instability: (1) excessive mobility or loss of normal end-feel on instability tests with or without apprehension or intra-articular click, (2) full or excessive ROM with end-range pain, (3) loose end-feel with less of a ligamentous character, (4) external rotation at 90° abduction that is either limited by spasm or shows excessive range, (5) pain free and strong rotator cuff contractions with the exception of an often weak but pain free infraspinatus. Again note that many of these findings may not be very specific.

Stability tests

Special tests for clinical instability of the glenohumeral joint fall into two categories (Levy et al 1999, Ellenbecker et al 2002, Tibone et al 2002). Stability tests use provocation, apprehension, and end feel to determine joint integrity toward end-range, whereas laxity tests examine the mobility of a joint in functional and midranges of motion. Bahk et al (2007) concluded that special tests can add significantly to our assessment of the unstable shoulder but findings on clinical laxity examination and relevance to instability must be placed in perspective. If findings 'fit' they confirm and solidify the diagnosis. If findings on these tests do not fit with other history and examination findings, laxity alone means nothing except a 'loose shoulder', which is not a diagnosis, but rather a physical exam finding. In the clinic of the second author, throwing-related MDI is often superimposed upon an already genetically loose shoulder capsule that subsequently becomes too loose and 'decompensate'. An important paradox is that the genetic laxity is partly what initially allows these athletes to succeed at a high level in overhead athletics like throwing. Once they decompensate, the original advantage, however, becomes a detriment.

Apprehension test

The patient is supine on table, glenohumeral joint at the edge of the table but with the scapula supported by the table. The patient's shoulder is at 90° of abduction, the elbow is flexed to 90° and the examiner's knee supports the elbow to prevent extension of the shoulder. The examiner then applies external rotation progressively until the patient cannot tolerate any further rotation and the degree of rotation is recorded. In patients with anterior instability, a patient report of apprehension and a feeling that the shoulder will come out of joint is considered a positive test. Some authors note that pain in this maneuver may be indicative of more subtle anterior instability. Sensitivity for this test for the diagnosis of traumatic anterior instability has been established at 52.78% and specificity at 98.91% (Lo et al 2004).

Relocation test

First described by Jobe et al (1989), the relocation test applies a posterior force to the humeral head in the position of apprehension of the above test and is positive if it relieves the symptoms of apprehension. Although Lo et al (2004) proposed this test to differentiate a subtle instability in the overhead athlete from rotator cuff impingement, if pain was experienced in the apprehension exam and improved with the relocation test, the sensitivity and specificity with production and reduction of pain only were both low at 40% and 42.65%, respectively. However, when considering solely diminished apprehension a

positive test finding, specificity was 100% for anterior shoulder instability, although sensitivity stayed low at 31.94%. Reduction of symptoms is usually associated with an increase in external rotation range.

Surprise (release) test

While holding the final position of the relocation test, the examiner's hand is quickly removed from the proximal humerus and the patient's response elicited. A positive test is indicated by a sudden return of symptoms noted with the apprehension test. The surprise test had a sensitivity of 63.89% and specificity of 98.91% for the diagnosis of anterior instability (Lo et al 2004). Note that the surprise test finds the shoulder in a more vulnerable position of greater external rotation than in the apprehension test. For this reason to perform the surprise test safely and accurately, we recommend that the apprehension and relocation tests be performed first. This will give the examiner an initial impression of where the patient feels vulnerable and thus allows careful placement to apply and release the posterior directed force within the patient's comfort level. Performing a surprise test immediately may not only startle the patient but can also acutely dislocate the shoulder.

Posterior shoulder instability has typically been examined with a load-and-shift test producing posterior translation or by posterior joint line tenderness (Eckenrode et al 2009). Patients may also have a positive jerk test. This test is performed with the patient supine, arm to be tested in 90° abduction and internal rotation. An axial load is then applied as the arm is brought into horizontal adduction. The test is positive if the manoeuvre produces a palpable or audible clunk, as well as pain. Sensitivity and specificity were reported to be 73% and 98%, respectively, in the diagnosis of a postero-inferior labral lesion (Kim et al 2005).

Laxity tests

Motion in any simple plane of the glenohumeral joint results in coupled motion in two additional planes. A strain gauge analysis of the glenohumeral ligaments showed that for each ligament tested, a tension-sharing relationship existed with transfer of tension among all ligaments (Terry 1991). Still, Fowler & Pettman (1992) in their teaching at the North American Institute of Orthopaedic Manual Therapy (NAIOMT) have proposed that the capsuloligamentous complex of the glenohumeral joint can be tested in serial fashion to discriminate the predominant site of injury or loss of integrity. Using an electronic digital ruler, Sharp and Kisser (unpublished research 2009) in a physical therapy doctoral capstone research project at Andrews University in Berrien Springs, Michigan provided preliminary validation for the selective tensioning suggested as the rationale for NAIOMT tests for the SGHL, MGHL, and AB-IGHL.

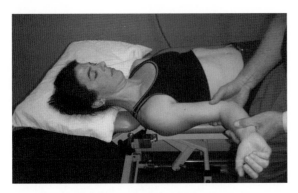

Fig 17.3 NAIOMT SGHL/posterior CHL test.

NAIOMT SGHL/CHL test

With the patient supine, the shoulder to be tested at the edge of the examination table with the scapula supported on the table, the shoulder is placed in 0° abduction and end-range external rotation followed by an anterior glide of the proximal humerus (Fig 17.3) to test the SGHL and the posterior or lateral band of the CHL. If the arm is now allowed to move into 10° extension, the anterior or medial band of the CHL comes more under tension (Fig 17.4).

NAIOMT MGHL test

From the test position of 0° abduction, 10° extension, and end-range external rotation, the examiner now moves the arm to 45° abduction and then applies an anterior medial glide in the plane of the glenohumeral joint surface (Fig 17.5) to test the MGHL.

NAIOMT IGHL test

From the MGHL test position, the examiner now moves the arm to 90° abduction and applies an anterior medial

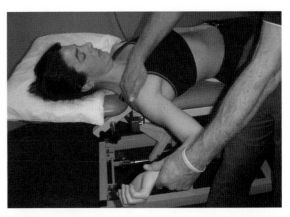

Fig 17.5 NAIOMT MGHL test.

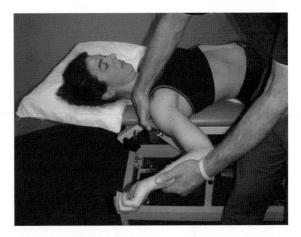

Fig 17.6 NAIOMT AB-IGHL test.

glide to the proximal humerus to test the AB-IGHL (Fig 17.6). The PB-IGHL is tested with the arm maintained in this position of 90° abduction and 10° extension but now with full internal rotation and a posterior lateral glide applied to the glenohumeral joint (Fig 17.7) (Fowler & Pettman 1992, Levine & Flatow 2000).

NAIOMT posterior capsule test

Bringing the arm to 90° flexion, followed by full internal rotation, then end-range horizontal adduction, and finally an axial stress applied to the proximal humerus in a posterior lateral direction tests the posterior capsule (Fig 17.8) (Fowler & Pettman 1992, Urayama 2001).

NAIOMT sulcus stability test for IGHL-AB/PB and inferior labrum

A sulcus sign or dimple created beneath the acromion when the subject's arm is axially tractioned inferiorly,

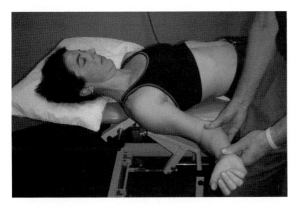

Fig 17.4 NAIOMT SGHL/anterior CHL test.

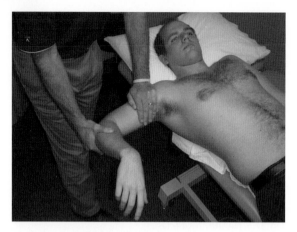

Fig 17.7 NAIOMT PB-IGHL test.

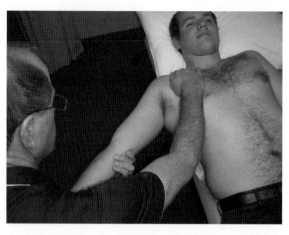

Fig 17.9 NAIOMT sulcus sign in external rotation.

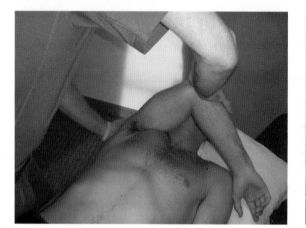

Fig 17.8 NAIOMT posterior capsule test.

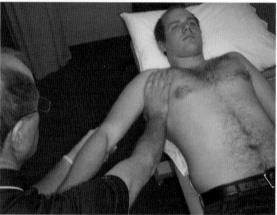

Fig 17.10 NAIOMT sulcus sign in internal rotation.

usually in a seated position, was first described as the hall-mark test for MDI if it also produced the patient's characteristic symptoms (Neer & Foster 1980). However, Bahk et al (2007) reported the test as provocative for patient's symptoms in only a small number of symptomatic patients. The degree of laxity considered relevant has also been arbitrary and McFarland et al (2003) suggested that the sulcus sign might lead to an over-diagnosis of MDI. Pettman (personal communication 2009) has suggested a modification of the sulcus sign. In this test the examiner stabilizes the scapula by stabilizing with one hand in the axilla. The other hand rotates the arm into external rotation and while holding this position applies an inferior force to assess for a sulcus sign suggested as consistent with a possible labral lesion in the AB-IGHL complex (Fig 17.9). If this sulcus sign is present in the same test with the arm in full internal rotation, a possible labral lesion in the PB-IGHL complex is suggested (Fig 17.10).

Imaging

From a medical-surgical perspective the diagnosis of instability in the vast majority of patients is based on the history and physical examination in combination with plane radiographs. Plain radiographs are also important in ruling out fractures often associated with dislocations. Whereas a standard AP view of the uncomplicated unstable shoulder may produce equivocal findings or may be hard to interpret, an axillary lateral view is helpful to visualize the presence and extent of a (reverse) Hill-Sachs lesion but may be near impossible to obtain in a patient whose abduction is severely limited due to pain. The lateral scapular plane view is particularly helpful in determining the relationship of the humeral head to the glenoid. In anterior dislocations of the shoulder, the humeral head lies anterior to the glenoid; in posterior dislocations it is posterior (Cicak 2004, Workman et al 1992).

With sensitivity of 97% and specificity of 91% magnetic resonance imaging (MRI) has been show to have greater accuracy in the diagnosis of Hill-Sachs lesions than plain radiography and arthroscopy (Workman et al 1992). MRI is most useful to visualize the rotator cuff in elderly patients, who have sustained a dislocation and are at risk for a rotator cuff tear as a result of the dislocation. The second author considers magnetic resonance arthrography (MRA), with gadolinium contrast injected into the joint, the imaging study of choice for patients with mechanical symptoms and a clinical concern for labral or intra-articular pathology. MRA can be particularly valuable in the young athlete suspected of a dislocation, but who clinically may have suffered only a subluxation. In the opinion of the second author, in the young overhand athlete, a clear labral detachment (either an anterior or posterior Bankart tear), and a clear Hill-Sachs lesion on MRA (Fig 17.11) would serve to confirm a dislocation and steer the treating physician toward a surgical repair due to the high risk of recurrent instability with non-operative management. Computed tomography (CT) can be a very useful tool to image bony defects like a Hill-Sachs lesion or an anterior glenoid bone deficiency (Cicak 2004). This can be useful in surgical planning and to help determine the need for alternative procedures to address bony defects.

PROGNOSIS

The challenge to the orthopaedic physical therapist is to determine which patients presenting with instability can be best managed on a conservative basis with a well-outlined and carefully managed programme, and which patients are best referred for further diagnostic testing and orthopaedic surgery consult. Patients that may require surgical stabilization must not be delayed or missed as the long-term outlook for recurrence and morbidity associated with further insult to the articular cartilage is a primary concern. Although the authors did not study the possible mitigating effect of conservative or surgical intervention, based on a case-control study Marx et al (2002) reported that the risk of developing severe arthrosis of the shoulder is between 10 and 20 times greater for patients who have had a previous dislocation.

In the clinical opinion of the second author, the young patient (less than age 20) with a first-time traumatic anterior dislocation with a Bankart tear and Hill-Sachs lesion is the most obvious high-risk patient and probably the only clear early surgery candidate after a single instability episode (Arciero et al 1994). In addition, the elderly patient with a rotator cuff tear and weakness should consider surgery due to risk of pain and weakness rather than due to risk of recurrent dislocation. All others should consider surgery when they fail non-operative management

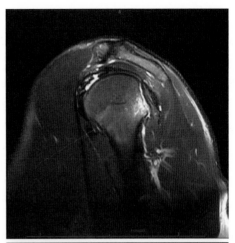

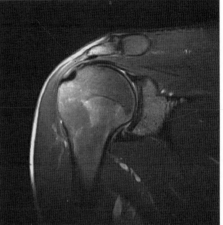

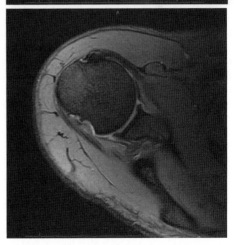

Fig 17.11 Hill-Sachs lesion on MRI.

with persisting symptoms or recurrent dislocations or sub-luxation symptoms. Although the exact risk of recurrent instability is impossible to determine for any individual, risk factors have been identified that help us classify those individuals who are at increased risk of recurrent instability. Risks of recurrence can be broken down into clinical and anatomic risk factors.

Clinical risk factors

Age of first dislocation is a very powerful prognosticator. In young patients under age 20, recurrence rates have ranged from 55% to 94%. Te Slaa et al (2004) reported 26% recurrence within 4 years. In their study, age was the most significant prognostic factor with recurrence in 64% of patients less than 20 years of age and in only 6% of those older than 40 years. Kralinger et al (2002) also reported age between 21 and 30 as the only factor associated with recurrence. Note that advancing age is however associated with an increased falling risk leading to recurrent dislocation and an increasing incidence of rotator cuff tears.

Chronicity refers to the number of times a patient has suffered a dislocation. Although rare a truly chronically dislocated shoulder is one that has dislocated and remains dislocated. An acute dislocation is a shoulder that has just dislocated and is in need of reduction. More common clinically is the recurrent dislocation. The recurrent dislocator is the patient, who reports both prior dislocations and subsequent reductions. The more frequently a patient has suffered with an instability episode, the more likely a subsequent recurrence will take place. There is, however, no consensus on the number of instability episodes after which the risk becomes a certainty.

A traumatic aetiology is associated with a higher recurrence risk than either micro-traumatic/overuse or atraumatic instability. Atraumatic instability, especially when associated with generalized ligamentous laxity, is in fact a risk factor for surgical failure. Volition is the patient's ability to reproduce the symptom or dislocation at will. Some describe their 'trick shoulder' and can voluntarily demonstrate the ability to dislocate or subluxate their joint. These voluntary dislocators need careful screening for emotional and mental health issues. Although not an absolute surgical contraindication, surgery in this subset of patients needs to be very carefully considered only after failure of non-operative management and careful counselling of the patient and family.

Although perhaps by some considered an indication of likely failure with conservative management, patients with MDI may benefit from conservative management. In addition, in a subset of patients with MDI natural history even without conservative intervention seems benign. Kuroda et al (2001) reported spontaneous recovery in 43 of 476 shoulders of patients followed for 3 years or longer. Although shoulder kinematics may not be restored with physical therapy in all patients with MDI but rather may

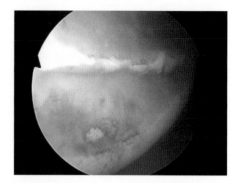

Fig 17.12 Hill-Sachs lesion.

require surgical intervention and postoperative physical therapy (Kiss et al 2009), conservative management has also been shown to be effective in an as of yet not clearly identified subset of these patients and ultimately may be the key to a successful outcome. Glenohumeral instability can occur as a complete separation of the humerus from the glenoid socket or as a partial separation or subluxation. Dislocations carry a higher risk of associated injury and recurrence.

Anatomic risk factors

Anatomic risk factors for recurrence include soft tissue and bony defects. Soft tissue defects include rotator cuff, labral, and capsular tears. Bony defects include glenoid rim fractures and (reverse) Hill-Sachs lesions. A Hill-Sachs lesion is basically a dent in the humeral head due to an impaction fracture that occurs as the head dislocates and impacts the anterior or posterior glenoid rim. An engaging Hill-Sachs lesion is a dent that hooks over the edge of the glenoid in a functional range of motion and by levering causes a high risk for recurrent anterior or posterior glenohumeral dislocation (Fig 17.12). A large or engaging Hill-Sachs lesion constitutes a higher risk for recurrent dislocation.

MANAGEMENT OF GLENOHUMERAL INSTABILITY

Inferior and anterior dislocations are generally addressed with closed reduction with the patient sedated (Baba et al 2007, Camarda et al 2009). Cicak (2004) suggested that closed reduction under general anaesthesia of a posterior dislocation is most likely to be successful in patients with a humeral head defect of less than 25% of the articular surface where the dislocation is present less than 3 weeks. If closed reduction is unsuccessful the surgeon may have to progress to an open reduction. Although in some jurisdictions such as most provinces in Canada it is within the physical therapy scope of practice to reduce acute dislocations of extremity joints, the risk of associated fractures and neurovascular and other soft tissue damage, the lack of access to imaging, and the inability to provide sedation however clearly indicate the need for medical-surgical referral and management where possible. Surgical management may also include addressing possibly present anatomic risk factors for recurrence addressed above.

In the past, patients post-dislocation were often temporarily immobilized with a sling and the arm in adduction and internal rotation. Bracing in 15–20° of external rotation has been suggested as anatomically more beneficial and leading to decreased recurrence (Itoi et al 2001, 2003, Funk & Smith 2005) but more recent research has pointed out that the evidence is insufficient to support use of one immobilization method over the other or even to support immobilization at all (Kralinger et al 2002, Handoll et al 2006, Smith 2006, Finestone et al 2009). It should be noted that patient compliance with the required 3 weeks of full-time bracing is often limited irrespective of the method used.

Although not providing sufficient operational definitions of specific interventions, Kralinger et al (2002) reported that whether the patient had participated in physical therapy did not reduce risk of recurrence. In general, insufficient evidence is available to guide physical therapy management after closed reduction of traumatic anterior dislocation perhaps reflective of insufficient methodological quality of studies in this area (Handoll et al 2006). A recent Cochrane review reported no differences with regard to renewed injury or function between open or arthroscopic stabilizing surgery for anterior shoulder instability in adults (Pulavarti et al 2009). Scheibel (2007) discussed the possibility of subscapularis dysfunction after open repairs and considering the important role of this muscle in the transverse plane stabilizing force couple this may present another reason to choose arthroscopic over open techniques. Limited evidence supports surgery in young predominantly male adults with a first acute traumatic dislocation, who are engaged in highly demanding physical activities for reducing recurrent dislocation or subluxation but no evidence is available to determine the best treatment for other patient groups (Handoll & Al-Maiyah 2004).

In the absence of research to guide conservative management of patients post-dislocation but also those patients with (minor) instability, therapists have to depend on clinical reasoning and extrapolation from basic science research. Te Slaa et al (2004) did not report sports participation as a risk factor for dislocation, yet Kuroda et al (2001) reported an 8.7-fold increase in incidence of spontaneous recovery for those patients with atraumatic shoulder instability who discontinued playing overhead sports. Education with regard to adaptation with regard to high-risk movements in sports seems a logical intervention. In

athletes, this includes modification of the often-ancillary weight-training activities. Fees et al (1998) suggested a grip width during the bench press of less than 1.5 times the bi-acromial distance in patients with anterior shoulder instability. Other suggested modifications included required assists when lifting the bar from and onto the rack, decreasing the shoulder abduction angle during the bench press, alternating flat and decline bench press to reduce the chance of micro-traumatic injury, and eliminating the incline bench press and the behind-the-neck press and pull-down exercises but also the back squat position where the hands stabilize the bar on the shoulders. In patients with posterior shoulder instability, Fees et al (1998) suggested a grip width during the bench press of > 2 times bi-acromial width, using a shoulder abduction angle > 80°, horizontal abduction > 15° at the start and horizontal adduction < 20° at the finish of the bench press motion. They also proposed mandatory assists with (un) racking the bar and using only the flat bench press or preferably no bench press at all.

As discussed in Chapter 16, proprioceptive deficits have also been identified in patients with anterior glenohumeral joint instability as well as altered muscle activation (Myers et al 2004). Decreased rotator cuff co-activation and slower biceps brachii and pectoralis major activation were identified and restoration of their normal function thus should be part of any targeted rehabilitation programme for anterior instability. A defect in proprioception also may be a factor in the pathophysiology of MDI (Schenk & Brems 1998). Dynamic exercises incorporating proprioceptive neuromuscular facilitation (PNF) have been found to be effective in the early phases of shoulder rehabilitation (Padua et al 2004). Utilizing well-established principles of PNF to the upper quadrant such as rhythmic stabilization, eccentric-to-concentric loading, and continuous movements associated with rotation (Knott & Voss 1968), therapists can easily implement and progress a programme even in early stages. Closed kinetic chain exercises initially on stable and later on unstable surfaces can increase accuracy of joint position sense and enhance stimulation of mechanoreceptors (Naughton et al 2005, Eckenrode et al 2009). Open-chain oscillatory exercises with the Body Blade can be used to provide more advanced open-chain dynamic stabilization (Buteau et al 2007). Exercises for muscular endurance and strength need to address both the local stabilizers in an attempt to restore at least the active (if not the passive) contribution to the concavity compression mechanism but also the prime movers required for functional movement and known to have an effect on glenohumeral stability. A careful progression needs to be adapted to the patient's functional demands and rehabilitation goals but also based on a careful and educated impression of the therapist with regard to rehabilitation potential. Chapters 21 and 22 provide examples of exercises for motor control and other exercises relevant to the shoulder.

CONCLUSION

Shoulder instability can present a challenge to the orthopedic physical therapist in differential diagnosis and management. Identification of patients at high risk for recurrence of shoulder dislocation indicates the need for referral to a shoulder specialist for likely surgical intervention. Further research on diagnostic and prognostic validity of our clinical tests such as those outlined above is necessary and would help drive outcome studies of conservative versus surgical management for possible subgroups of patients identified based on our clinical tests. A clear indication of glenohumeral instability should not limit the therapists to management solely of the shoulder area. Patients with a history of shoulder instability should be examined for underlying biomechanical faults in both the upper and lower quadrants that may contribute to the instability in more dynamic activities.

REFERENCES

Abboud, A.A., Soslowsky, J., 2002. Interplay of the static and dynamic restraints in glenohumeral instability. Clin. Orthop. Relat. Res. 400, 48–57.

Arciero, R.A., Wheeler, J.H., Ryan, J.B., McBride, J.T., 1994. Arthroscopic Bankart repair versus nonoperative treatment for acute, initial anterior shoulder dislocations. Am. J. Sports Med. 22, 589–594.

Baba, A.N., Bhat, J.A., Paljor, S.D., Mir, N.A., Majid, S., 2007. Luxatio erecta: Inferior glenohumeral dislocation–a case report. Int. J. Shoulder Surg. 1, 100–102.

Bahk, M., Keyurapan, E., Tasaki, A., 2007. Laxity testing of the shoulder: A review. Am. J. Sports Med. 35, 131–144.

Bey, M., Hunter, S., Kilambi, N., et al., 2005. The structural and mechanical properties of the glenohumeral joint capsule. J. Shoulder Elbow Surg. 14, 201–206.

Bigliani, L.U., Pollock, R.G., Soslowsky, L.J., Flatow, E.L., Pawluk, R.J., Mow, V.C., 1992. Tensile properties of the inferior glenohumeral ligament. J. Orthop. Res. 10, 187–197.

Bohnsack, M., Wulker, N., 2002. Arthroscopic anterior shoulder stabilization: Combined multiple suture repair and laser-assisted capsular shrinkage. Injury 33, 795–799.

Buteau, J.L., Eriksrud, O., Hasson, S.M., 2007. Rehabilitation of a glenohumeral instability utilizing the Body Blade. Physiotherapy Practice 23, 333–349.

Camarda, R., Martorana, U., D'Arienzo, M., 2009. A case of bilateral luxatio erecta. Journal of Orthopaedic Traumatology 10, 97–99.

Caplan, J., Julien, T.P., Michelson, J., Neviaser, R.J., 2007. Multidirectional instability of the shoulder in elite female gymnasts. Am. J. Orthop. 36, 660–665.

Cicak, N., 2004. Posterior dislocation of the shoulder. J. Bone Joint Surg. 86B, 324–332.

Cooper, D.E., Arnoczky, S.P., O'Brien, S.J., Warren, R.F., DiCarlo, E., Allen, A.A., 1992. Anatomy, histology and vascularity of the glenoid labrum: An anatomic study. J. Bone Joint Surg. 74A, 46–52.

Cyriax, J., 1978. Textbook of orthopaedic medicine, Vol. 1. Cassell, London.

Eckenrode, B.J., Logerstedt, D.S., Sennett, B.J., 2009. Rehabilitation and functional outcomes in collegiate wrestlers following a posterior shoulder stabilization procedure. J. Orthop. Sports Phys. Ther. 39, 550–559.

Ellenbecker, T., Bailie, D., Mattalino, A., et al., 2002. Intrarater and interrater reliability of a manual technique to assess anterior humeral head translation of the glenohumeral joint. J. Shoulder Elbow Surg. 11, 470–475.

Fees, M., Decker, T., Snyder-Mackler, L., Axe, M.J., 1998. Upper extremity weight-training modifications for the injured athlete. Am. J. Sports Med. 26, 732–742.

Fehringer, E.V., Schmidt, G.R., Boorman, R.S., et al., 2003. The anteroinferior labrum helps center the humeral head on the glenoid. J. Shoulder Elbow Surg. 12, 53–58.

Finestone, A., Milgrom, C., Radeva-Petrova, D.R., et al., 2009. Bracing in external rotation for traumatic anterior dislocation of the shoulder. J. Bone Joint Surg. 91, 918–921.

Fleisig, G., Andrews, J., Dillman, C., Escamilla, R., 1995. Kinetics of baseball pitching with implications about injury mechanisms. Am. J. Sports Med. 23, 233–239.

Fowler, C., Pettman, E., 1992. North American Institute Orthopaedic Manual Therapy (NAIOMT) Upper Quadrant Course 600A, Portland.

Funk, L., Smith, M., 2005. Best evidence report. How to immobilize after shoulder dislocation? Emerg. Med. J. 22, 814–815.

Halder, A.M., Zhao, K.D., O'Driscoll, S.W., Morrey, B.F., An, K.N., 2001a. Dynamic contributors to superior shoulder stability. J. Orthop. Res. 19 (2), 206–212.

Halder, A.M., Halder, C.G., Zhao, K.D., O'Driscoll, S.W., Morrey, B.F., An, K.N., 2001b. Dynamic inferior stabilizers of the shoulder joint. Clin. Biomech. 16, 138–143.

Handoll, H.H.G., Al-Maiyah, M.A., 2004. Surgical versus non-surgical treatment for acute anterior shoulder dislocation. Cochrane Database Syst. Rev. (1), Art. No.: CD004325. DOI: 10.1002/14651858.CD004325.pub2.

Handoll, H.H.G., Hanchard, N.C.A., Goodchild, L.M., Feary, J., 2006. Conservative management following closed reduction of traumatic anterior dislocation of the shoulder. Cochrane Database Syst. Rev. (1), Art. No.: CD004962. DOI: 10.1002/14651858.CD004962.pub2.

Hides, J.A., Richardson, C.A., Jull, G.A., 1996. Multifidus muscle recovery is not automatic after resolution of acute first episode low back pain. Spine 21, 2763–2769.

Huijbregts, P.A., 1998. Biomechanics and pathology of the overhead throwing motion: A literature review. J. Man. Manip. Ther. 6, 17–23.

Itoi, E., Sashi, R., Minagawa, H., Shimizu, T., Wakabayashi, I., Sato, K., 2001. Position of immobilization after dislocation of the glenohumeral joint: A study with use of magnetic resonance imaging. J. Bone Joint Surg. 83B, 661–667.

Itoi, E., Hatakeyama, Y., Kido, T., Sato, T., Minagawa, H., Wakabayashi, I., et al., 2003. A new method of immobilization after traumatic anterior dislocation of the shoulder: A preliminary study. J. Shoulder Elbow Surg. 12, 413–415.

Jobe, F.W., Kvitne, R.S., Giangarra, C.E., 1989. Shoulder pain in the overhead or throwing athlete: The relationship of anterior instability and rotator cuff impingement. Orthop. Rev. 18, 963–975.

Kido, T., Ito, E., Lee, S.B., Neale, P.G., An, K.N., 2003. Dynamic stabilizing function of the deltoid muscle in shoulders with anterior instability. Am. J. Sports Med. 31, 399–403.

Kim, S.H., Park, J.S., Jeong, W.K., et al., 2005. The Kim Test: A novel test for postero-inferior labral lesion of the shoulder: a comparison to the jerk test. Am. J. Sports Med. 33, 1188–1192.

Kiss, R.M., Illyés, A., Kiss, J., 2009. Physiotherapy versus capsular shift and physiotherapy in multidirectional shoulder joint instability. J. Electromyogr. Kinesiol. (in press).

Knott, M., Voss, D.E., 1968. Proprioceptive neuromuscular facilitation: Patterns and techniques. Harper and Row, London.

Kralinger, F.S., Golser, K., Wischatta, R., Wambacher, M., Sperner, G., 2002. Predicting recurrence after primary anterior shoulder dislocation. Am. J. Sports Med. 30, 116–120.

Krøner, K., Lind, T., Jensen, J., 1989. The epidemiology of shoulder dislocations. Arch. Orthop. Trauma Surg. 108, 288–290.

Kuhn, J.E., Huston, L.J., Soslowsky, L.J., Shyr, Y., Blasier, R.B., 2005. External rotation of the glenohumeral joint: Ligament restraints and muscle effects in the neutral and abducted positions. J. Shoulder Elbow Surg. 14, (Suppl.): 39S–48S.

Kuhn, J.E., Lindholm, S.R., Huston, L.J., Soslowsky, L.J., Blasier, R.B., 2003. Failure of the biceps superior labral complex: A cadaveric biomechanical investigation comparing the late cocking and early deceleration positions of throwing. Arthroscopy 19, 373–379.

Kuroda, S., Sumiyoshi, T., Moriishi, J., Maruta, K., Ishige, N., 2001. The natural course of atraumatic shoulder instability. J. Shoulder Elbow Surg. 10, 100–104.

Labriola, J., Lee, T., Debski, R., et al., 2005. Stability and instability of the glenohumeral joint: the role of shoulder muscles. J. Shoulder Elbow Surg. 14, 32S–38S.

Lee, D., 1989. The pelvic girdle. Churchill Livingstone, Oxford.

Lee, S.B., Kyu-Jung, K., O'Driscoll, S., et al., 2000. Dynamic glenohumeral stability provided by the rotator cuff muscles in the mid-range and end-range of motion. J. Bone Joint Surg. 82A, 849–857.

Lee, T., Black, A., Tibone, J., et al., 2001. Release of the coracoacromial ligament can lead to glenohumeral laxity: A biomechanical study. J. Shoulder Elbow Surg. 10, 68–72.

Levine, W.M., Flatow, E., 2000. The pathophysiology of shoulder instability. Am. J. Sports Med. 28, 910–917.

Levy, A., Linter, S., Kenter, K., Speer, K., 1999. Intra- and interobserver reproducibility of the shoulder laxity examination. Am. J. Sports Med. 27, 460–463.

Lo, I.K., Nonweiler, B., Woolfrey, M., Litchfield, R., Kirkley, A., 2004. An evaluation of the apprehension, relocation, and surprise tests for anterior shoulder instability. Am. J. Sports Med. 32, 301–307.

Magarey, M., Jones, M., 1992. Clinical diagnosis and management of minor shoulder instability. Aust. J. Physiother. 38, 269–279.

Mallon, W.J., Bassett, F.H., Goldner, R.D., 1990. Luxatio erecta: The inferior glenohumeral dislocation. J. Orthop. Trauma. 4, 19–24.

Marx, R.G., McCarthy, E.C., Montemurno, T.D., Altchek, D.W., Craig, E.V., Warren, R.F., 2002. Development of arthrosis following dislocation of the shoulder: A case-control study. J. Shoulder Elbow Surg. 11, 1–5.

McFarland, E.G., Garzon-Muvdi, J., Jia, X., Desai, P., Petersen, S.A., 2010. Clinical and diagnostic tests for shoulder disorders: a critical review. Br J Sports Med 44, 328–332.

McFarland EG Kim, T.K., Park, H.B., Neira, C.A., Gutierrez, M.I., 2003. The effect of variation in definition on the diagnosis of multidirectional instability of the shoulder. J. Bone Joint Surg. 85A, 2145–2146.

Myers, J.B., Ju, Y.Y., Hwang, J.H., McMahon, P.J., Rodosky, M.W., Lephart, S.M., 2004. Reflexive muscle activation alterations in shoulders with anterior glenohumeral instability. Am. J. Sports Med. 32, 1013–1021.

Naughton, J., Adams, R., Maher, C., 2005. Upper-body wobble board training effects on the post-dislocation shoulder. Phys. Ther. Sport 6, 31–37.

Neer, C.S., Foster, C.R., 1980. Inferior capsular shift for involuntary inferior and multidirectional instability of the shoulder: A preliminary report. J. Bone Joint Surg. 62A, 897–908.

Neer, C.S., Satterlee, C.C., Dalsey, R.M., Flatow, E.L., 1992. The anatomy and potential effects of contracture of the coracohumeral ligament. Clin. Orthop. Relat. Res. 280, 182–185.

O'Connell, P.W., Nuber, G.W., Mileski, R.A., Lautenschlager, E., 1990. The contribution of the glenohumeral ligaments to anterior stability of the shoulder joint. Am. J. Sports Med. 18, 579–584.

Owens, B.D., Dawson, L., Burks, R., Cameron, D.L., 2009. Incidence of shoulder dislocation in the United States military: Considerations from a high-risk population. J. Bone Joint Surg. 91A, 791–796.

Padua, D., Guskiewicz, K., Prentice, W., et al., 2004. The effect of select shoulder exercises on strength, active angle reproduction, single-arm balance, and functional importance. Journal of Sports Rehabilitation 13, 75–95.

Panjabi, M.M., 1992. The stabilizing system of the spine, part II: Neutral zone and instability hypothesis. J. Spinal Disord. 5, 390–396.

Parsons, I.M., Apreleva, M., Fu, F.H., Woo, S.L., 2002. The effect of rotator cuff tears on reaction forces at the glenohumeral joint. J. Orthop. Res. 20, 439–446.

Pulavarti, R.S., Symes, T.H., Rangan, A., 2009. Surgical interventions for anterior shoulder instability in adults. Cochrane Database Syst. Rev. (4), Art. No.: CD005077. DOI: 10.1002/14651858.CD005077.pub2.

Robinson, C.M., Dobson, R., 2004. Anterior instability of the shoulder after trauma. J. Bone Joint Surg. 86B, 469–479.

Sahrmann, S., 2002. Diagnosis and treatment of movement impairment syndromes. Mosby, St. Louis.

Scheibel, M., 2007. Subscapularis dysfunction after open instability repair. Int. J. Shoulder Surg. 1, 16–22.

Schenk, T.J., Brems, J.J., 1998. Multidirectional instability of the shoulder: Pathophysiology, diagnosis, and management. J. Am. Acad. Orthop. Surg. 6, 65–72.

Schmitt, H., Brocal, D., Lukoschek, M., 2004. High prevalence of hip arthrosis in former elite javelin throwers and high jumpers: 41 athletes examined more than 10 year after retirement from competitive sports. Acta Orthop. Scand. 75, 34–39.

Seebauer, L., Keyl, W., 1998. Posterior shoulder joint instability. Classification, pathomechanism, diagnosis, conservative and surgical management. Orthopäde 27, 542–555.

Smith, T.O., 2006. Immobilization following traumatic anterior glenohumeral joint dislocation: A literature review. Injury 37, 228–237.

Sugalski, M., Wiater, J.M., Levine, W., et al., 2005. An anatomic of the humeral insertion of the inferior glenohumeral capsule. J. Shoulder Elbow Surg. 14, 91–95.

Terry, G.C., 1991. The stabilizing function of passive shoulder restraints. Am. J. Sports Med. 19, 26–34.

Te Slaa, R.L., Wijffels, M.P., Brand, R., Marti, R.K., 2004. The prognosis following acute primary glenohumeral dislocation. J. Bone Joint Surg. 86B, 58–64.

Tibone, J., Lee, T., Csintalan, R., et al., 2002. Quantitative assessment of glenohumeral translation. Clin. Orthop. Relat. Res. 400, 93–97.

Turkel, S.J., Panio, M.W., Marshall, J., Girgis, F., 1981. Stabilizing mechanisms preventing anterior dislocation of the glenohumeral joint. J. Bone Joint Surg. 63A, 1208–1217.

Urayama, M., 2001. Function of the 3 portions of the inferior glenohumeral ligament: a cadaveric study. J. Shoulder Elbow Surg. 10, 589–594.

Walton, J., Tzannes, A., Callanan, M., et al., 2002. The unstable shoulder in the adolescent athlete. Am. J. Sports Med. 30, 758–767.

Workman, T.L., Burkhard, T.K., Resnick, D., et al., 1992. Hill-Sachs lesion: Comparison of detection with MR imaging, radiography, and arthroscopy. Radiology 185, 847–852.

Chapter | 18 |

Superior labrum anterior-to-posterior (SLAP) lesions

Janette W Powell, Peter A Huijbregts

INTRODUCTION

Superior labrum anterior-to-posterior (SLAP) lesions have been discussed and investigated since Andrews et al first described this pathology in 1985. SLAP lesions involve the superior glenoid labrum extending anteriorly and posteriorly (Andrews et al 1985, Snyder et al 1990, D'Alessandro et al 2000, Kim et al 2003, Bedi & Allen 2008, Dodson & Altchek 2009). SLAP lesions not only involve the superior glenoid labrum, but can affect the biceps tendon and gleno-humeral ligament attachments as well (D'Alessandro et al 2000, Dessaur & Magarey 2008). SLAP lesions are often complex injuries with a spectrum of locations and varied types of tissue defects in the glenoid labrum and its associated structures (D'Alessandro et al 2000, Lebolt et al 2006, Bedi & Allen 2008).

These variants, in addition to age-related changes in the superior labrum, have thwarted an understanding of the precise epidemiology of SLAP lesions (Bedi & Allen 2008). Their prevalence has been reported in the literature to range between 6% and 76% of all shoulder injuries evaluated arthroscopically but even independent of their large range the relevance of this reported prevalence to primary care settings is unclear (Snyder et al 1990, Liu et al 1996, Mileski & Snyder 1998, D'Alessandro et al 2000, Musgrave & Rodosky 2001, Higgins & Warner 2001, Huijbregts 2001, Kim et al 2002, 2003, Guanche & Jones 2003, Wilk et al 2005, Lebolt et al 2006, Barber et al 2007, Funk & Snow 2007, Bedi & Allen 2008, Walsworth et al 2008, Dodson & Altchek 2009). Without supplying specific quantitative data these lesions have been described as common occurrences in the athletic population, particularly in overhead/throwing athletes (Lebolt et al 2006, Funk & Snow 2007, Bedi & Allen 2008, Dodson & Altchek 2009). A number of authors note the challenge of determining the clinical relevance of a SLAP lesion when there are co-existing lesions in the shoulder (Musgrave & Rodosky 2001, Stetson & Templin 2002, McFarland et al 2002, Kim et al 2003, 2007, Dodson & Altchek 2009). Difficulties associated with investigations of SLAP lesions include the variability of pathological findings, clinical features, and the prevalence, all of which can vary with the population studied (Kim et al 2003).

SLAP lesions have been classified into types on the basis of their morphologic pattern. Snyder et al (1990) classified these pathological variations into four types (Fig 18.1):

- Type I: degenerative fraying with no detachment of the biceps insertion
- Type II: detachment of the biceps insertion
- Type III: a bucket-handle tear of the superior aspect of the labrum with an intact biceps tendon insertion to bone
- Type IV: an intra-substance tear of the biceps tendon with a bucket-handle tear of the superior aspect of the labrum

© 2011 Elsevier Ltd.
DOI: 10.1016/B978-0-7020-3528-9.00018-2

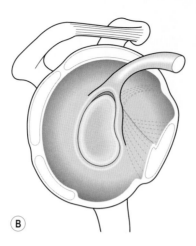

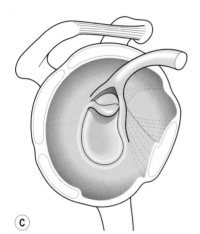

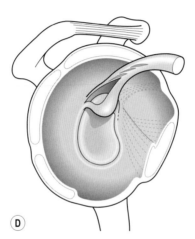

Fig 18.1 Classification of superior glenoid or superior labrum and biceps anchor (SLAP) lesions. (A) Type 1, degenerative fraying of the superior labrum with the edge still firmly attached to the glenoid. (B) Type II, detachment of the superior labrum and biceps tendon from the glenoid with resultant destabilization of the biceps anchor. (C) Type III, bucket-handle tear of superior labrum. The remaining labrum and biceps anchor are stable. (D) Type IV, bucket-handle tear of superior labrum with extension into the biceps tendon.

The Type II SLAP lesions have been further divided into three subtypes (Fig 18.2) depending on whether the detachment of the labrum involved solely the anterior aspect of the labrum, solely the posterior aspect, or both aspects. The above classification system has been expanded to include an additional three types (D'Alessandro et al 2000, Higgins & Warner 2001, Musgrave & Rodosky 2001, Parentis et al 2002, Huijbregts 2001, Kim et al 2003, Nam & Snyder 2003, Wilk et al 2005):

- Type V: a Bankart lesion that extends superiorly to include a Type II SLAP lesion
- Type VI: an unstable flap tear of the labrum in conjunction with a biceps tendon separation
- Type VII: a superior labrum and biceps tendon separation that extends anteriorly, inferior to the middle gleno-humeral ligament

The prevalence of the various types of SLAP lesions as reported in the literature again shows wide ranges: type I 20–74%; type II 21–70%; type III 1–9%; type IV 4–10% (Snyder et al 1995, Kim et al 2003, Kampa & Clasper 2005). The prevalence of associated pathology, other intra-articular lesions, has been reported to range from 62–88% (Snyder et al 1995, Mileski & Snyder 1998, Kim et al 2003).

ANATOMY

The glenoid labrum is a triangular fibrocartilaginous structure that sits on the periphery of the glenoid rim. It is a transitional connective tissue, typically an ovoid circumferential rim, that lies between the articular surface of the glenoid fossa and the fibrous capsule of the glenohumeral joint (D'Alessandro et al 2000, Higgins & Warner 2001, Musgrave & Rodosky 2001, Wilk et al 2005). Musgrave & Rodosky (2001) describe this labral rim as approximately 3 mm high and 4 mm wide. The depth of

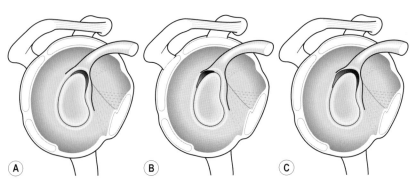

Fig 18.2 Subtypes of type II SLAP lesions. (A) anterior, (B) posterior, (C) combined anterior-posterior.

the glenoid fossa is doubled with the labrum and the surface contact area between the humeral head and the glenoid is greatly enhanced by the labrum (Higgins & Warner 2001, Huijbregts 2001, Musgrave & Rodosky 2001, Wilk et al 2005). The superior labrum is triangular in cross-section, is 'loosely' attached to the glenoid with a free edge and is commonly described as 'meniscal' in its morphology (Huijbregts 2001, Musgrave & Rodosky 2001, Nam & Snyder 2003, Wilk et al 2005, Dessaur & Magarey 2008). The inferior labrum, in contrast, is rounded and firmly attached (Huijbregts 2001, Musgrave & Rodosky 2001, Nam & Snyder 2003, Wilk et al 2005).

The blood supply to the labrum arises mostly from its peripheral attachment to the capsule and is from a combination of the supra-scapular artery, the circumflex scapular branch of the sub-scapular artery and the posterior circumflex humeral arteries (Huijbregts 2001, Nam & Snyder 2003, Wilk et al 2005). The literature on the extent and localization of vascularization of the glenoid labrum is contradictory with some authors describing only vascularization of the peripheral labrum that in addition is more extensive posteriorly and inferiorly than (antero) superiorly (Cooper et al 1992, Huijbregts 2001, Nam & Snyder 2003, Wilk et al 2005, Dessaur & Magarey 2008), whereas other authors have described more global vascularization (Prodromos et al 1990). Whether the superior labrum is indeed a vascular structure has important implications regarding the healing potential of a SLAP lesion (D'Alessandro et al 2000, Dessaur & Magarey 2008). Vascularity of the labrum appears to decrease with increasing age (Huijbregts 2001, Nam & Snyder 2003, Wilk et al 2005).

Other gleno-humeral structures including the superior and middle gleno-humeral ligaments and the biceps tendon are noted to be continuous and intimately related with the superior labrum (D'Alessandro et al 2000, Huijbregts 2001, Musgrave & Rodosky 2001, Parentis et al 2002, Wilk et al 2005, Dessaur & Magarey 2008). The anterosuperior labrum is one of the most variable areas of gleno-humeral anatomy (Fig 18.3). It is important that normal variants of this anatomy are recognized

as non-pathologic (D'Alessandro et al 2000, Higgins & Warner 2001, Huijbregts 2001, Musgrave & Rodosky 2001, Kim et al 2003, Wilk et al 2005). A sublabral recess or foramen has been reported in up to 73% of normal shoulders and consists of an opening or hole between the labrum and glenoid rim (Musgrave & Rodosky 2001). Its size can vary from only a few millimetres to spanning the entire anterosuperior quadrant (Fig. 18.4A) (D'Alessandro et al 2000, Huijbregts 2001, Musgrave & Rodosky 2001, Nam & Snyder 2003, Wilk et al 2005). The Buford complex represents another anatomic variant and is described as a cordlike thickening of the middle gleno-humeral ligament and absence of the antero-superior labrum (Fig 18.4C). This complex is reported to be less common with prevalence ranging between 1.5–5% (Musgrave & Rodosky 2001, Wilk et al 2005, Bents & Skeete 2005). Relevant to accurate diagnosis is that in normal variants, the edges of both the labrum and glenoid can be expected to be smooth without the fraying or hemorrhage that when noted on arthroscopy would be more suggestive of a pathologic detachment (D'Alessandro et al 2000, Higgins & Warner 2001, Huijbregts 2001, Musgrave & Rodosky 2001, Wilk et al 2005).

The anatomy of the origin of the tendon of the long head of biceps (LHB) is noted to be highly variable (Barber A et al 2007, Ghalayini et al 2007, Dierickx et al 2009). Studies have reported between 25% and 60% of LHB tendons originate from the supra-glenoid tubercle with the remainder originating from the superior glenoid labrum (Pal et al 1991, Vangsness et al 1994, Ghalayini et al 2007, Krupp et al 2009). Other variations that have been described include a split tendon from a single origin; a double tendon origin from the capsule, labrum or tuberosity; medial and/or lateral tendon-capsular adhesions; medial and/or lateral tendon-rotator cuff adhesions; or even a complete absence of the LHB tendon (Dierickx et al 2009). It is additionally noted that a greater portion of the LHB attachment to the labrum is to the posterior labrum (Vangsness et al 1994, Dierickx et al 2009). The variable attachment of this biceps anchor may make it difficult to differentiate pathological detachment of the

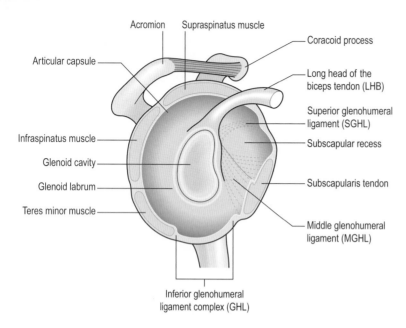

Acromion   Supraspinatus muscle

Coracoid process

Articular capsule

Long head of the
biceps tendon (LHB)

Superior glenohumeral
ligament (SGHL)

Subscapular recess

Infraspinatus muscle

Glenoid cavity

Glenoid labrum

Subscapularis tendon

Teres minor muscle

Middle glenohumeral
ligament (MGHL)

Inferior glenohumeral
ligament complex (GHL)

Fig 18.3 Arthroscopic anatomy of the gleno-humeral joint.

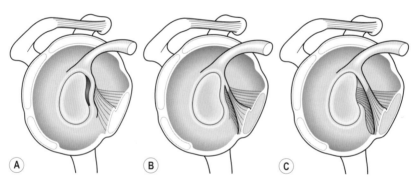

A   B   C

Fig 18.4 Normal anatomic variants of the antero-superior glenoid labrum and gleno-humeral ligaments. (A) Sublabral foramen. (B) Cord-like middle gleno-humeral ligament. (C) Buford complex (cord-like middle gleno-humeral ligament with absence of anterosuperior labral tissue).

biceps anchor from a normal meniscoid labrum with a sublabral recess or a Buford complex (D'Alessandro et al 2000, Higgins & Warner 2001, Huijbregts 2001, Musgrave & Rodosky 2001, Nam & Snyder 2003, Kim et al 2003, Wilk et al 2005, Barber et al 2007).

BIOMECHANICS

The labrum appears to serve as a buttress assisting in controlling gleno-humeral translation, similar to a 'chock-block' (Wilk et al 1997, Huijbregts 2001, Wilk et al 2005). Labral damage disrupts the circular configuration and the hoop stresses rendering this 'chock-block'

mechanism less effective (Howell & Galinat 1989, Huijbregts 2001). Resection of the labrum has been shown to reduce the concavity-compression stabilization of the gleno-humeral joint by 10–20% (Lippitt et al 1993, Wilk et al 1997, Halder et al 2001). The labrum has also been described as functioning like a seal, whereby labral injury results in a loss of negative intra-articular pressure thereby diminishing gleno-humeral joint stability (Huijbregts 2001).

The biceps-labrum complex has been shown to be an important stabilizer of the gleno-humeral joint (Bedi & Allen 2008). Andrews et al (1985) noted that electrical stimulation of the biceps during arthroscopy led to humeral head compression within the glenoid. Increased gleno-humeral translation has been demonstrated when the long head of the biceps tendon has been destabilized (Pagnani et al 1995, Warner & McMahon 1995, Pradhan et al 2001). Warner & McMahon (1995) observed up to 6 mm of superior humeral migration during active abduction in individuals with isolated LHB tendon tears when compared to their intact contralateral shoulders. Kim et al (2001) reported that maximal biceps activity occurred when the shoulder was in the abducted and externally rotated position in patients with anterior instability. SLAP lesions result in significant increase in strain of the anterior band of the gleno-humeral ligament with shoulder abduction and external rotation, suggesting a key role of the superior labrum in gleno-humeral stability (Rodosky et al 1994). Pagnani et al (1995) found that a complete lesion of the superior portion of the labrum was associated with significant increases in gleno-humeral translation and that a simulated SLAP lesion resulted in a 6 mm increase in anterior gleno-humeral translation. Rodosky et al (1994) observed that a SLAP lesion contributed to anterior shoulder instability by decreasing the shoulder's resistance to torsion and placing a greater strain on the inferior gleno-humeral ligament. Panossian et al (2005) demonstrated how a Type II SLAP lesion increased total gleno-humeral range of motion in addition to antero-posterior and inferior translation.

PATHOLOGY

Associated pathology is commonly encountered with SLAP lesions, most notably concomitant rotator cuff tears and other labral pathology (Dodson & Altchek 2009). Andrews et al (1984) noted that 45% of individuals (and 73% of baseball pitchers) with SLAP lesions also had partial-thickness tears of the supraspinatus. Mileski & Snyder (1998) reported that 29% of their individuals with SLAP lesions had partial-thickness rotator cuff tears, 11% complete rotator cuff tears, and 22% Bankart lesions. They also noted that type I lesions were typically associated with rotator cuff pathology, while types III and IV were associated with traumatic instability. Additionally they observed that in patients with type II lesions, older individuals tended to have associated rotator cuff pathology while younger individuals had associated anterior instability.

Dodson & Altchek (2009) explained how recognition of these associated lesions facilitates insight into the biomechanical etiology of SLAP lesions. There are several proposed mechanisms for SLAP lesions. These mechanisms can be divided into acute traumatic events or chronic repetitive injuries that lead to failure (Dodson & Altchek 2009). Acute traumatic events, such as falling onto an outstretched arm, or a direct lateral blow to the shoulder, may result in a SLAP lesion from impaction of the humeral head against the superior labrum and the biceps anchor (D'Alessandro et al 2000, Funk & Snow 2007, Bedi & Allen 2008, Dodson & Altchek 2009). Sudden inferior pull on the arm, as when losing control of a heavy object, anterior traction while water skiing, and superior traction when grasping overhead to stop a fall are traumatic mechanisms of injury described in the literature (Maffet et al 1995, D'Alessandro et al 2000, Barber et al 2007, Bedi & Allen 2008). SLAP lesions in the throwing athlete have also been postulated to be a traction injury of the biceps-labrum complex (Higgins & Warner 2001, Funk & Snow 2007). Andrews et al (1984) theorized that SLAP lesions in overhead throwing athletes were the result of the high eccentric activity of the biceps muscle creating tension on the long head of the biceps tendon during the arm deceleration and follow-through phases of throwing. The sudden tensile load on the biceps was suggested to avulse the biceps-labrum complex (Andrews & Carson 1984, Higgins & Warner 2001). Subsequent research with electrical stimulation applied to the biceps during arthroscopy indeed have noted that biceps activation caused the biceps anchor to separate from the glenoid (Andrews et al 1985). Electromyographic studies showing increased biceps activity after ball release support this theory (Jobe et al 1984, Glousman et al 1988, D'Alessandro et al 2000).

Repetitive overhead activity has been hypothesized as a common mechanism for producing SLAP lesions (Funk & Snow 2007, Dodson & Altchek 2009). The traction injury mechanism described above has also been postulated to result in repetitive micro rather than macro-trauma (avulsion), progressively leading to structural failure of the biceps-labrum complex (D'Alessandro et al 2000). Burkhart & Morgan (1998) hypothesized that a 'peel-back' mechanism may produce a SLAP lesion in the overhead athlete. They theorized that when the shoulder is placed in abduction and maximal external rotation, the rotation causes a torsional force at the base of the biceps. Pradhan et al (2001) measured superior labral strain during each phase of the throwing motion and reported increased superior labral strain during the late cocking phase of throwing, which supports the concept of the 'peel-back' mechanism.

Additional authors (Walch et al 1992, Jobe 1995) have demonstrated contact between the posterior-superior labrum and the rotator cuff when the arm is in an abducted and externally rotated position, which simulates the late cocking phase of throwing. Shepard et al (2004) simulated each of the aforementioned mechanisms in nine pairs of cadaveric shoulders that were loaded to biceps anchor failure in either a position of in-line loading (similar to the deceleration phase of throwing) or in a simulated peel-back mechanism (similar to the late cocking phase of throwing). Their results showed that all of the simulated peel-back group failures resulted in a type II SLAP-lesion, whereas the majority of the simulated in-line-loading group failures occurred in the mid-substance of the biceps tendon. Additionally, the biceps anchor demonstrated a significantly higher strength with in-line loading as opposed to the ultimate strength during the 'peel-back' mechanism. These results support the theory of peel-back as the predominant mechanism but does not exclude a combination of mechanisms in the etiology of SLAP lesions (Dodson & Altchek 2009).

Several authors reported an association between SLAP lesions and gleno-humeral instability (Cordasco et al 1993, Rodosky et al 1994, Pagnani et al 1995, D'Alessandro et al 2000, Higgins & Warner 2001, Kim et al 2001, Pradhan et al 2001, Parentis et al 2002, Panossian et al 2005, Bedi & Allen 2008, Dodson & Altchek 2009). The exact cause-and-effect relationship of instability and SLAP lesions is still unclear (Liu et al 1996, Higgins & Warner 2001, Parentis et al 2002). It may be that instability allows for a pathologic range of motion that facilitates the peel-back mechanism or conversely that SLAP lesions allow for excessive gleno-humeral translation, which then leads to instability (Huijbregts 2001, Parentis et al 2002, Dodson & Altchek 2009).

Internal impingement is another proposed mechanism whereby the superior labrum is subjected to shear and direct contact, in the position of maximal shoulder abduction and external rotation, between the greater tubercle of the humerus and the postero-superior rim of the glenoid (Bedi & Allen 2008, Cools et al 2008, Heyworth & Williams 2009). Recurrent abutment, between the articular side of the rotator cuff, the postero-superior labrum and the glenoid rim, ultimately precipitates articular-sided rotator cuff tears and postero-superior labral lesions (Higgins & Warner 2001, D'Alessandro et al 2000, Bedi & Allen 2008, Heyworth & Williams 2009). A range of theories have been proposed regarding internal impingement and the role it plays in shoulder dysfunction and SLAP lesions (Wilk et al 2005, Heyworth & Williams 2009). A number of clinical findings have been associated with internal impingement including gleno-humeral internal rotation deficit, SICK scapula syndrome, posterior humeral head lesions, posterior glenoid bony injury, and Bankart and inferior gleno-humeral ligament lesions (Heyworth & Williams 2009).

A variety of aetiologic mechanisms have been implicated for SLAP lesions (D'Alessandro et al 2000, Higgins & Warner 2001, Huijbregts 2001, Musgrave & Rodosky 2001, Parentis et al 2002, Burkhart et al 2003, Nam & Snyder 2003, Wilk et al 2005, Bedi & Allen 2008, Heyworth & Williams 2009). Musgrave & Rodosky (2001) suggested that different mechanisms of injury were likely to be operational in the various SLAP-lesion types. It is likely that the varied patho-anatomy and/or pathomechanics of these different types of SLAP lesions significantly alter the clinical presentation (Kim et al 2003,

Wilk et al 2005). Kim et al (2003) note how the rarity of some of the types of SLAP lesions limit the statistical evaluation of some factors that might be important in understanding the pathophysiology of such lesions. Kim et al (2003) and Rao et al (2003) reported a positive association between anterosuperior labral anatomic variants and anterosuperior labral fraying. These authors postulated that anatomic variants influence glenohumeral biomechanics and predispose the shoulder to SLAP lesions (Kim et al 2003, Rao et al 2003, Bedi & Allen 2008). A retrospective review by Bents & Skeete (2005) supported this postulation: they found the presence of a Buford complex correlated with the presence of a SLAP lesion in patients. Additionally, a split biceps tendon has been associated with a displaced superior labrum in a type IV lesion (Parentis et al 2002, Nam & Snyder 2003).

DIAGNOSIS

Clinical diagnosis of the SLAP-lesion is difficult (Musgrave & Rodosky 2001, Dodson & Altchek 2009). The clinical presentation and correct diagnosis, even when using arthroscopy findings as a gold standard, is complicated by the variability of 'normal' anatomy of the superior labrum (D'Alessandro et al 2000, Higgins & Warner 2001, Huijbregts 2001, Musgrave & Rodosky 2001, Kim et al 2003, Nam & Snyder 2003, Wilk et al 2005). Adding to these intrinsic complexities these lesions are often associated with additional concomitant shoulder pathology that influence patient presentation (Mileski & Snyder 1998, Musgrave & Rodosky 2001, Huijbregts 2001, Parentis et al 2002, Kim et al 2003, Wilk et al 2005). A number of authors note the difficulty to clinically differentiate, via examination, a SLAP lesion from concomitant pathology and report that despite efforts seen in literature to find clinical tests for the identification of SLAP lesions a significant number of patients with such lesions are only discovered at arthroscopy (D'Alessandro et al 2000, Kim et al 2003, Wilk et al 2005). Thus, extra and intra-articular shoulder pathology confuse the clinical diagnostic process (Musgrave & Rodosky 2001).

Funk & Snow (2007) noted that the most common presenting clinical symptom with SLAP injuries were mechanical symptoms such as 'locking, catching, popping, or snapping' in the shoulder. Walsworth et al (2008) investigated the diagnostic yield of history findings for glenoid labral tears (including SLAP lesions): a combined patient report of popping or catching and a positive crank (specificity 91%, +LR = 3.0) or anterior slide test (specificity 100%, +LR = ∞) suggested the presence of a labral tear. In the absence of a patient report of popping or clicking, having a negative anterior slide test or a negative crank test suggested absence of a labral tear (−LR = 0.31 and 0.33, respectively). Age as a predictor for such lesions has been investigated by Liu et al (1996) and Walsworth et al (2008) and has not been noted to be of diagnostic utility, yet Liu et al (1996) noted a tendency for younger individuals ($<$ 35 years) to have such lesions.

From a retrospective study Kampa & Clasper (2005) reported that individuals with a history of trauma or symptoms of instability were more likely to have a SLAP lesion than individuals presenting with atraumatic etiologies ($p < 0.0001$). Without providing research data Barber et al (2007) suggested that clinically relevant SLAP injuries are most often found in the dominant arm of a man < 40 years of age, who has participated in high-performance overhead activities for many years, a patient with a specific history of shoulder trauma, or a patient with shoulder instability. Barber et al (2007) additionally noted that a fall on an outstretched hand or a prior motor vehicle accident during which the patient was wearing a shoulder-lap belt was suggestive of a SLAP injury.

As many as 21 different clinical tests have been described and investigated for their value in the diagnosis of SLAP lesions. There exists a large variation in the positions and movements used to reproduce symptoms and many authors report that no clinical test is sensitive and specific enough for the accurate diagnosis of SLAP lesions noting the need for arthroscopic visualization for diagnosis (Mirkovic et al 2005, Powell et al 2008, Bedi & Allen 2008, Dessaur & Magarey 2008, McCaughey et al 2009). In addition, methodological inadequacies have been prevalent in research of SLAP lesion clinical tests (Dessaur & Magarey 2008, Meserve et al 2008, Powell et al 2008, Walsworth et al 2008, Walton & Sadi 2008, Munro & Healy 2009).

It is possible, and maybe even probable, that the varied pathoanatomy and/or pathomechanics of the differing types of SLAP lesions significantly alter the clinical presentation and clinical findings (D'Alessandro et al 2000, Musgrave & Rodosky 2001, Huijbregts 2001, Parentis et al 2002, Nam & Snyder 2003, Wilk et al 2005, Ebinger et al 2008, Dessaur & Magarey 2008, Dodson & Altchek 2009, Kibler et al 2009). Ebinger et al (2008) proposed that the Flexion Resistance Test has high specificity for Type II SLAP lesions. The Speed test and O'Brien test have been reported to be highly specific for anterior Type II SLAP lesions, whereas the modified Jobe relocation test has been reported highly sensitive and highly specific for posterior SLAP lesions (D'Alessandro et al 2000, Burkhart & Morgan 2001, Burkhart et al 2003, Wilk et al 2005). The Anterior Scapular slide test has been reported useful for detecting anterior SLAP lesions (Burkhart & Morgan 2001, Burkhart et al 2003). Huijbregts (2001) reported that the SLAP-prehension test showed greater sensitivity for identifying Types II–IV SLAP lesions and that the Active Compression (O'Brien) test, the provocation test and the biceps load test were useful for distinguishing between stable and unstable SLAP lesions. However, type-specific diagnostic utility statistics have yet to be reported (Powell et al 2008).

The clinical recommendations for the utilization of clinical SLAP lesion tests are varied. There are inconsistencies in the recommendations based on the various reviews available on this topic. Hegedus et al (2008) proposed, with caution, that the Biceps Load II Test appeared diagnostic for SLAP lesions. Cools et al (2008) proposed the inclusion of the Speed Test, the Active Compression Test, and the Biceps Load II test when investigating SLAP lesions. Meserve et al (2008) proposed the Active Compression Test should be utilized to rule out a SLAP lesion and that the Speed Test should be used to rule in a SLAP lesion when the Active Compression Test or Crank Test have positive findings. Meserve et al (2008) reported that a positive sign on all three tests (Active Compression Test, Crank Test, Speed Test) increases the probability that a SLAP lesion is present. Meserve et al (2008) and Pandya et al (2008) claimed the Active Compression Test to be one of the best tests for diagnosing SLAP lesions. Oh et al (2008) concluded from a study of multi-test regimes that combinations of two relatively sensitive clinical tests and one relatively specific clinical test increase the diagnostic efficacy of superior labrum anterior and posterior lesions.

Based on their systematic review of the diagnostic accuracy research the current authors recently recommended the inclusion of the following clinical tests with the following interpretation for the diagnosis of SLAP lesion (with diagnostic accuracy data in Table 18.1):

- A negative finding on the passive compression test (Fig 18.5) to *rule out* a SLAP lesion;
- A positive finding on the anterior apprehension maneuver (Fig 18.6, Guanche & Jones 2003), the anterior slide test (Fig 18.7, Kibler 1995, Powell et al 2008), the Jobe relocation test (Fig 18.8, Cook & Hegedus 2007), the passive compression test, the Speed test, and the Yergason test or on a combination of positive findings on the Jobe relocation test and the active compression test or the Jobe relocation test and the anterior apprehension manoeuvre to *rule in* a SLAP lesion.

The active compression test has been described in Chapter 14 on the acromio-clavicular joint. Rather than pain localized to the top of the shoulder in the internally rotated position relieved in the externally rotated position considered indicative of acromio-clavicular dysfunction, pain 'deep inside the shoulder,' with or without a click, in the first position and eliminated or reduced in the second position is considered indicative of a glenoid labrum tear (O'Brien et al 1998, Powell & Huijbregts 2006). In the context of diagnosis, the greatest value should be placed on a positive finding on the passive compression test due to the strength of its positive likelihood ratio (Powell et al 2008).

Different imaging tests (magnetic resonance imaging (MRI), ultrasonography, or computed tomography) may

Table 18.1 Psychometric data for SLAP-lesion clinical examination tests

	Passive compression	Anterior apprehension	Anterior Slide	Jobe relocation	Speed	Yergason	Active compression
Accuracy	0.84	0.59	0.54–0.86	0.56	0.56–0.57	0.61–0.63	0.54–0.98
Sensitivity	0.82	0.4–0.83	0.05–0.78	0.44–1.0	0.04–0.48	0.09–0.43	0.47–1.0
Specificity	0.86	0.4–0.87	0.81–0.93	0.4–0.87	0.67–1.0	0.79–1.0	0.1–0.98
Positive predictive value	0.87	0.53–0.9	0.05–0.64	0.32–0.91	0.35–1.0	0.46–1.0	0.1–0.94
Negative predictive value	0.8	0.33–0.75	0.56–0.90	0.34–0.71	0.26–0.72	0.25–0.71	0.1–1.0
Positive likelihood ratio	5.72	1.38–3.07	0.50–9.22	1.07–3.39	0.0–1.47	0.0–2.05	0.78–66
Negative likelihood ratio	0.21	0.43–0.72	0.24–1.10	0.63–0.94	0.6–0.94	0.72–1.29	0.0–2.0

From: Kibler 1995; O'Brien et al 1998; Hamner et al 2000; McFarland et al 2002; Stetson & Templin 2002; Guanche & Jones 2003; Holtby & Razmjou 2004; Myers et al 2005; Nakagawa et al 2005; Parentis et al 2006; Kim et al 2007; Powell et al 2008

Fig 18.5 (A) Passive compression test, start position. The clinician rotates the patient's involved arm externally with 30° of abduction and pushes the arm proximally while extending the shoulder, which results in the passive compression of the superior labrum onto the glenoid. (B) End position (from Powell et al 2008, with permission).

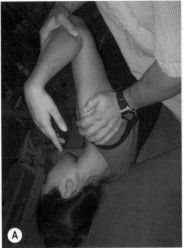
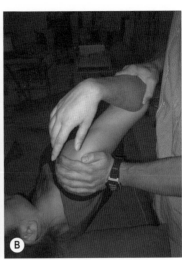

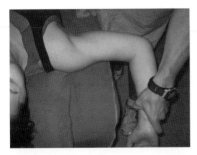

Fig 18.6 Anterior apprehension manoeuvre. The patient is supine and the examiner abducts the arm to 90° with the elbow in 90° of flexion and then progressively externally rotates the involved shoulder. A positive test is indicated by a look or feeling of apprehension or alarm on the patient's face and the patient's resistance to further motion. The patient might also state that the feeling experienced is what it felt like when the shoulder was previously dislocated (from Powell et al 2008, with permission).

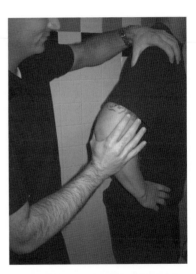

Fig 18.7 Anterior slide test. The patient is examined standing or sitting with hands on hips and the thumbs pointing posteriorly. One of the examiner's hands is positioned at the top of the shoulder from the posterior direction, with the last segment of the index finger extending over the anterior aspect of the acromion at the gleno-humeral joint. The examiner's other hand is placed behind the elbow and a forward and a slightly superiorly directed force is applied to the elbow and upper arm. The patient is asked to push back against the clinician's force. Pain localized to the front of the shoulder under the examiner's hand and/or a pop or click in the same area is considered a positive result. This test is also considered positive if the patient reported this testing manoeuvre reproduces their presenting symptoms as associated with overhead activity (from Powell et al 2008, with permission).

be useful in confirming the presence of a SLAP lesion, but they are reported to have a sensitivity of only 60–90%. The value of imaging studies has been questioned in the orthopaedic literature (Luime et al 2004). Approximately 10–20% of patients with a normal reading on shoulder MRI or ultrasonography may still have a SLAP lesion (Mileski & Snyder 1998, Mimori et al 1999, D'Alessandro et al 2000, Burkhart & Morgan 2001, Parentis et al 2002, Stetson & Templin 2002, Nam & Snyder 2003, Burkhart et al 2003, Holtby & Razmjou 2004, Luime et al 2004, Wilk et al 2005, Mirkovic et al 2005,

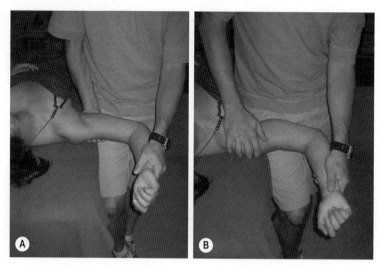

Fig 18.8 Jobe relocation test. (A) The patient is supine and the test performed at 90° of shoulder abduction with the involved shoulder in maximal external rotation. Initially an anterior force is applied to the proximal humerus. (B) A posterior force is applied to the proximal humerus. Pain that occurs with the anterior force and is relieved or diminished pain with the posterior force is considered a positive test finding (from Powell et al 2008, with permission).

Nakagawa et al 2005, Parentis et al 2006, Swearingen et al 2006, Jones & Galluch 2007, Dessaur & Magarey 2008, Calvert et al 2009). Therefore, definitive diagnosis requires arthroscopy (D'Alessandro et al 2000, Burkhart & Morgan 2001, Nam & Snyder 2003, Bedi & Allen 2008).

Standard multiplanar T1- and T2-weighted MRI images can detect supraglenoid cysts, which have been associated with Type II SLAP lesions. These cysts can arise as a result of labral injury with a communication through the capsule (Nam & Snyder, 2003). MR arthrography with gadolinium may offer improved visualization (Nam & Snyder 2003, Clifford 2007, Bedi & Allen 2008, Magee 2009). Bencardino et al (2000) reported 89% sensitivity, 91% specificity, and 90% accuracy for the diagnosis of SLAP lesions with gadolinium-enhanced MR arthrography compared to a gold standard of arthroscopic findings. However, false positive and negative results do occur (Burkhart & Morgan 2001, Parentis et al 2002, Nam & Snyder 2003, Clifford 2007).

SLAP lesions may be visualized on the coronal oblique sequence as a deep cleft between the superior labrum and the glenoid that extends well around and below the biceps anchor (Fig. 18.9). Often the contrast medium will dissipate into the labral fragment causing it to appear ragged/frayed or indistinct. The axial view is sometimes helpful to view the displaced superior labral fragment. Normal labral variants must be kept in mind when viewing these labral images, as these congenital variations of the anterosuperior labrum can be misleading and complicate results (Parentis et al 2002, Clifford 2007). If there is an associated labral split or biceps tear, as seen in a Type III or IV lesion, the displaced fragment may be difficult

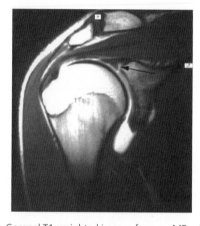

Fig 18.9 Coronal T1-weighted images from an MR arthrogram demonstrate contrast material interposed between the superior labrum and the glenoid (arrows). The labrum is displaced (arrowhead).

to visualize unless the superior labral area is carefully examined.

Standard radiographs (AP, axillary, and outlet views) cannot identify a SLAP lesion, but assessment of the acromial morphology and the acromio-clavicular joint are useful when considering associated disorders (D'Alessandro et al 2000, Bedi & Allen 2008, Dodson & Altchek 2009). Although radiographs are usually normal in isolated SLAP lesions, other potential sources of abnormalities can be evaluated (Wilk et al 2005). With the clinical presentation of SLAP lesions often unclear, radiographic and imaging studies are frequently used to aid in the diagnosis. Imaging options enhance the diagnostic 'picture' by enabling the clinician to determine the presence or absence of common concomitant pathology for SLAP lesions. The clinical value of these diagnostic tools should not be underestimated in the clinically complex SLAP lesions.

MANAGEMENT

Different types of SLAP lesions seem to respond to different types of interventions (D'Alessandro et al 2000, Huijbregts 2001, Parentis et al 2002, Nam & Snyder 2003, Wilk et al 2005, Parentis et al 2006). Some authors (D'Alessandro et al 2000, Bedi & Allen 2008) propose an initial trial of conservative management for SLAP lesions while others (Mileski & Snyder 1998, Wilk et al 2005, Dodson & Altchek 2009) propose that conservative management will be unsuccessful. The natural history of SLAP lesions is unknown and data regarding the efficacy of conservative treatments for SLAP lesions is not available (D'Alessandro et al 2000). Vascularization, and thereby healing potential, is a prerequisite for optimal conservative management (Powell et al 2008, Huijbregts 2001).

Treatment goals for conservative management would include the reduction of pain and mechanical symptoms, restoring and optimizing gleno-humeral and also scapulo-thoracic, acromio-clavicular, sterno-clavicular and thoracic motion, strength, and function. Dodson & Altcheck (2009) describe conservative management as including relative rest from aggravating activities; anti-inflammatory medication; restoration of normal shoulder motion – including addressing gleno-humeral internal rotation deficit, if present; strengthening of the shoulder girdle musculature to restore normal scapulo-thoracic motion; progressing to advanced conditioning activities that includes trunk, core, rotator cuff and scapulo-thoracic musculature and sport/acrobatic/functional skills.

Cordasco et al (1993) stated that SLAP lesions are the result of instability and should not be considered isolated lesions. Shear forces at the gleno-humeral joint have been hypothesized to play a role in producing the labral lesion (Snyder et al 1990, Bey et al 1998). Muscle force has been hypothesized to compress the humeral head into the labrum normally preventing it from rolling up and over the labrum (Howell & Galinat 1989) but in the case of instability imparting excessive shear and compressive forces to the labrum. Addressing gleno-humeral instability would therefore be a treatment priority (Huijbregts 2001). Liu et al (1996) suggested an intensive 3-month programme of activity modification, non-steroidal anti-inflammatory medications, and physical therapy for patients with mild

instability and labral tears. The physical therapy programme they described involves passive range of motion followed by active range of motion of the shoulder; strengthening of the rotator cuff and scapular stabilizers, and finally functional and sport-specific activities. Patients who experience relief are thought to have had pain as a result of the instability. It has been questioned whether the pain individuals with a SLAP lesion complain about is the result of the labral tear or the instability (Liu et al 1996, Huijbregts 2001).

Musgrave & Rodosky (2001) reported that SLAP lesions should be treated based on the type with which an individual presents. They proposed debridement of type I lesions with preservation of the biceps anchor, whereas Wilk et al (2005) suggested conservative management for type I lesions. Type II lesions, due to the disruption of the biceps attachment and consequent gleno-humeral instability, commonly require surgical repair for optimal stabilization and restoration of function (D'Alessandro et al 2000, Musgrave & Rodosky 2001, Parentis et al 2002, Nam & Snyder 2003, Panossian et al 2005, Wilk et al 2005, Parentis et al 2006, Bedi & Allen 2008, Dodson & Altchek 2009). The bucket-handle tear of a type III lesion is typically excised with care taken to avoid destabilization of the middle gleno-humeral ligament, particularly if a cord-like middle gleno-humeral ligament is present (D'Alessandro et al 2000, Higgins & Warner 2001, Musgrave & Rodosky 2001, Bedi & Allen 2008, Dodson & Altchek 2009). Management of type IV lesions is somewhat dependent on the extent of injury to the biceps tendon. When the biceps involvement is less than 30% then the torn tissue is excised and the superior labrum repaired, if the biceps involvement is more extensive then it is either repaired or a tenodesis is performed (Mileski & Snyder 1998, D'Alessandro et al 2000, Higgins & Warner 2001, Musgrave & Rodosky 2001, Parentis et al 2002, Wilk et al 2005, Bedi & Allen 2008, Dodson & Altchek 2009). SLAP-lesion types V, VI, and VII are treated similarly to types I to IV, but there is additional treatment for the associated pathology (type V – Bankart repair and biceps anchor stabilization, type VI – flap debridement and biceps anchor stabilization, type VII – repair of middle gleno-humeral ligament and biceps anchor stabilization) (Musgrave & Rodosky 2001, Parentis et al 2002, Wilk et al 2005, Bedi & Allen 2008). Suture anchor repair is preferred over biodegradable sutureless implants, which have been associated with complications such as synovitis, chondral injury, and mechanical failure (Bedi & Allen 2008).

SLAP lesions that are complex, such as those involving rotator cuff tears, those associated with gleno-humeral joint instability, or those with concomitant biceps tendon pathology, are likely to respond to different management strategies from isolated SLAP lesions (D'Alessandro et al 2000, Kim et al 2003, Nam & Snyder 2003, Panossian et al 2005, Wilk et al 2005). Concomitant shoulder disorders should be addressed and their management may even be critical to ensure a successful outcome (Mileski & Snyder 1998, Higgins & Warner 2001, Dodson & Altchek 2009). SLAP lesions identified at arthroscopy may not be pathologic or clinically significant, but rather part of a constellation of generalized degenerative changes (Lebolt et al 2006, Bedi & Allen 2008).

PROGNOSIS

Information on the natural history of SLAP lesions is lacking. Outcome data, and therefore prognosis, for conservatively managed SLAP lesions is also unknown. Conservative management of SLAP lesions (regardless of type) is often reported to be unsuccessful, but outcome data is not provided (Mileski & Snyder 1998, Wilk et al 2005, Dodson & Altchek 2009). Further, long-term results with simple debridement of lesions is often reported to be poor, but again outcome data is rarely provided (Mileski & Snyder 1998, Wilk et al 2005).

Cordasco et al (1993) reported deterioration of clinical outcomes with longer follow-up (78% pain relief at 1 year, 63% at 2 years) after SLAP lesion debridement with only 45% of individuals returning to preoperative level of function. Abbot et al (2009) reported that in older patients (> 45 years) who presented for management of rotator cuff injury and type II SLAP-lesion, those who had debridement rather than SLAP-repair with concomitant rotator cuff repair had significantly better function, pain relief and range of motion.

The majority of the SLAP lesion surgical outcomes published report that 80–90% of individuals have good or excellent results, at short-term or intermediate follow-up after surgical repair of type II SLAP lesions (D'Alessandro et al 2000, Bedi & Allen 2008, Dodson & Altchek 2009). Dodson & Alcheck (2009) noted a lack of long-term follow-up studies following type II SLAP lesion repairs and suggested that surgical repair of type II SLAP lesions in overhead athletes with a non-traumatic incident may be less successful than other individuals. Bedi & Allen (2008) reported that individuals with traumatic-onset, isolated type II SLAP lesions, who then had surgical repair, reported greater subjective satisfaction than individuals with insidious SLAP injury.

CONCLUSION

In summary, individuals who present with pain or dysfunction of the shoulder may have sustained an injury to the superior labrum. If present, the severity of a SLAP lesion is widely variable and may, or may not, be clinically significant. SLAP lesions are often associated with other intra-articular shoulder injuries, and the examining clinician should have a high index of suspicion for coexisting pathology. SLAP lesions are difficult to identify clinically. There is a paucity of evidence-based guidance for the clinical examination and the optimal management strategy to employ. There is widespread agreement that a traumatic labral injury where the biceps origin is disrupted (types II, IV, V, VI, and VII) needs surgical management, yet long-term outcome studies have not been published to support this. Further studies are needed to gain a better understanding of the causes of SLAP lesions, to improve clinical diagnoses, and to determine the optimal management strategy for such lesions. Areas that are most likely to benefit from more research include:

- Long-Term Prognosis: Studying the sequelae of SLAP injury with validated relevant outcome measures.
- Diagnostic Testing: (i) Study of the diagnostic utility for type-specific clinical tests would allow the clinician to differentiate within SLAP lesions those best managed conservatively and surgically (Huijbregts 2001, Powell et al 2008). (ii) Further diagnostic accuracy investigation into more recently proposed clinical tests for SLAP lesions including the biceps load II, passive compression, and resisted supination external rotation tests (Dessaur & Magarey 2008, Meserve et al 2008). (iii) Study of the combination(s) or clustering of history components and clinical tests for determining the presence or absence of type-specific SLAP lesions (Dessaur & Magarey 2008, Meserve et al 2008, Walsworth et al 2008).
- Conservative Treatment: The comparison of different types of supervised rehabilitation in the management of the varied types of SLAP lesions (Huijbregts 2001).
- Surgical Treatment: Study of the long-term outcomes of surgically managed SLAP lesions.

REFERENCES

Abbot, A.E., Li, X., Busconi, B.D., 2009. Arthroscopic treatment of concomitant superior labral anterior posterior (SLAP) lesions and rotator cuff tears in patients over the age of 45 years. Am. J. Sports Med. 37, 1358–1362.

Andrews, J.R., Carson, W.G., 1984. The arthroscopic treatment of glenoid labrum tears in the throwing athlete. Orthopaedic Transactions 8, 44.

Andrews, J.R., Carson, W.G., McLeod, W.D., 1985. Glenoid labrum tears related to the long head of the biceps. Am. J. Sports Med. 13, 337–341.

Barber, A., Field, L.D., Ryu, R., 2007. Biceps tendon and superior labrum injuries: decision-marking. J. Bone Joint Surg. 89A, 1844–1855.

Bedi, A., Allen, A.A., 2008. Superior labral lesions anterior to posterior-evaluation and arthroscopic management. Clin. Sports Med. 27, 607–630.

Bencardino, J.T., Beltran, J., Rosenberg, Z.S., et al., 2000. Superior labrum anterior-posterior lesions: diagnosis with MR arthrography of the shoulder. Radiology 214, 267–271.

Bents, R.T., Skeete, K.D., 2005. The correlation of the Buford complex and SLAP lesions. J. Shoulder Elbow Surg. 14, 565–569.

Bey, M.J., Elders, G.J., Huston, L.J., et al., 1998. The mechanism of creation of superior labrum, anterior and posterior lesions in a dynamic biomechanical model of the shoulder: The role of inferior subluxation. J. Shoulder Elbow Surg. 7, 397–401.

Burkhart, S.S., Morgan, C., 2001. SLAP lesions in the overhead athlete. Orthop. Clin. North Am. 32, 431–441.

Burkhart, S.S., Morgan, C.D., 1998. The peel-back mechanism: its role in producing and extending posterior type II SLAP lesions and its effect on SLAP repair rehabilitation. Arthroscopy 14, 637–640.

Burkhart, S.S., Morgan, C.D., Kibler, W.B., 2003. The disabled throwing shoulder: spectrum of pathology. Part II: evaluation and treatment of SLAP lesions in throwers. Arthroscopy 19, 531–539.

Calvert, E., Chambers, G.K., Regan, W., et al., 2009. Special physical examination tests for superior labrum anterior posterior shoulder tears are clinically limited and invalid: a diagnostic systematic review. J. Clin. Epidemiol. 62, 558–563.

Clifford, P.D., 2007. Superior labral anterior to posterior (SLAP) tears. Am. J. Orthop. 36, 685–686.

Cook, C., Hegedus, E., 2007. Orthopedic physical examination tests: An evidence-based approach. Prentice Hall, Upper Saddle River, New Jersey.

Cools, A.M., Cambier, D., Witvrouw, E.E., 2008. Screening the athlete's shoulder for impingement symptoms: a clinical reasoning algorithm for early detection of shoulder pathology. Br. J. Sports Med. 42, 628–635.

Cooper, D.E., Arnoczky, S.P., O'Brien, S.J., et al., 1992. Anatomy, histology, and vascularity of the glenoid labrum. J. Bone Joint Surg. 74A, 46–52.

Cordasco, F.A., Steinmann, S., Flatow, E.L., et al., 1993. Arthroscopic treatment of glenoid labral tears. Am. J. Sports Med. 21, 425–430.

D'Alessandro, D.R., Fleischli, J.E., Connor, P.M., 2000. Superior labral lesions: Diagnosis and management. Journal of Athletic Training 35, 286–292.

Dessaur, W.A., Magarey, M.E., 2008. Diagnostic accuracy of clinical tests for superior labral anterior posterior lesions: A systematic review. J. Orthop. Sports Phys. Ther. 38, 341–352.

Dierickx, C., Ceccarelli, E., Conti, M., et al., 2009. Variations of the intra-articular portion of the long head of the biceps tendon: a classification of embryologically explained variations. J. Shoulder Elbow Surg. 18, 556–565.

Dodson, C.C., Altchek, D.W., 2009. SLAP lesions: An update on recognition and treatment. J. Orthop. Sports Phys. Ther. 39, 71–80.

Ebinger, N., Magosch, P., Lichtenberg, S., et al., 2008. A new SLAP test: The supine flexion resistance test. Arthroscopy 24, 500–505.

Funk, L., Snow, M., 2007. SLAP tears of the glenoid labrum in contact athletes. Clin. J. Sport Med. 17, 1–4.

Ghalayini, S.R., Board, T.N., Srinivasan, M.S., 2007. Anatomic variations in the long head of biceps: contribution to shoulder dysfunction. Arthroscopy 23, 1012–1018.

Glousman, R., Jobe, F., Tibone, J., et al., 1988. Dynamic electromyographic analysis of the throwing shoulder with gleno-humeral instability. J. Bone Joint Surg. 70A, 220–226.

Guanche, C.A., Jones, C., 2003. Clinical testing for tears of the glenoid labrum. Arthroscopy 19, 517–523.

Halder, A.M., Kuhl, S.G., Zobitz, M.E., et al., 2001. Effects of the glenoid labrum and gleno-humeral abduction on stability of the shoulder joint through concavity-compression: An in vitro study. J. Bone Joint Surg. 83A, 1062–1069.

Hamner, D.L., Pink, M.M., Jobe, F.W., 2000. A modification of the relocation test: Arthroscopic findings associated with a positive test. J. Shoulder Elbow Surg. 9, 263–267.

Hegedus, E.J., Goode, A., Campbell, S., et al., 2008. Physical examination tests of the shoulder: a systematic review with meta-analysis of individual tests. Br. J. Sports Med. 42, 80–92.

Heyworth, B.E., Williams, R.J., 2009. Internal impingement of the shoulder. Am. J. Sports Med. 37, 1024–1037.

Higgins, L.D., Warner, J.P., 2001. Superior labral lesions: Anatomy, pathology, and treatment. Clin. Orthop. 390, 73–82.

Holtby, R., Razmjou, H., 2004. Accuracy of the Speed's and Yergason's tests in detecting biceps pathology and SLAP lesions: Comparison with arthroscopic findings. Arthroscopy 20, 231–236.

Howell, S.M., Galinat, B.J., 1989. The glenoid-labral socket. Clin. Orthop. 243, 122–125.

Huijbregts, P.A., 2001. SLAP lesions: Structure, function, and physical therapy diagnosis and treatment. J. Man. Manip. Ther. 9, 71–83.

Jobe, C.M., 1995. Posterior superior glenoid impingement: expanded spectrum. Arthroscopy 11, 530–536.

Jobe, F.W., Moynes, D.R., Tibone, J.E., et al., 1984. An EMG analysis of the shoulder in pitching. A second report. Am. J. Sports Med. 12, 218–220.

Jones, G.L., Galluch, D.B., 2007. Clinical assessment of superior glenoid labral lesions. Clin. Orthop. Relat. Res. 455, 45–51.

Kampa, R.J., Clasper, J., 2005. Incidence of SLAP lesions in a military population. J. R. Army Med. Corps. 151, 171–175.

Kibler, W.B., 1995. Specificity and sensitivity of the anterior slide test in throwing athletes with superior glenoid labral tears. Arthroscopy 11, 296–300.

Kibler, W.B., Sciascia, A.D., Hester, P., et al., 2009. Clinical utility of traditional and new tests in the diagnosis of biceps tendon injuries and Superior Labrum Anterior and Posterior Lesions in the shoulder. Am. J. Sports Med. 37 (9), 1840–1847.

Kim, S.H., Ha, K.I., Ahn, J.H., et al., 2001. Biceps load test II: A clinical test for SLAP lesions of the shoulder. Arthroscopy 17, 160–164.

Kim, S.H., Ha, K.I., Kim, S.H., et al., 2002. Results of arthroscopic treatment of superior labral lesions. J. Bone Joint Surg. 84A, 981–985.

Kim, T.K., Queale, W.E., Cosgarea, A.J., et al., 2003. Clinical features of the different types of SLAP lesions: An analysis of one hundred and thirty-nine cases. J. Bone Joint Surg. 85A, 66–71.

Kim, Y.S., Kim, J.M., Ha, K.Y., et al., 2007. The passive compression test: A new clinical test for superior labral tears of the shoulder. Am. J. Sports Med. 35, 1489–1494.

Krupp, R.J., Kevern, M.A., Gaines, M.D., et al., 2009. Long head of the biceps tendon pain: Differential diagnosis and treatment. J. Orthop. Sports Phys. Ther. 39, 55–70.

Lebolt, J.R., Cain, E.L., Andrews, J.R., 2006. SLAP lesions, 2007. Am. J. Orthop. 35, 554–557.

Lippitt, S.B., Vanderhooft, J.E., Harris, S.L., et al., 1993. Gleno-humeral stability from concavity-compression: A quantitative analysis. J. Shoulder Elbow Surg. 2, 27–35.

Liu, S.H., Henry, M.H., Nuccion, S., et al., 1996. Diagnosis of glenoid labral tears. A comparison between magnetic resonance imaging and clinical examinations. Am. J. Sports Med. 24, 149–154.

Liu, S.H., Henry, M.H., Nuccion, S.L., 1996. A prospective evaluation of a new physical examination in predicting glenoid labral tears. Am. J. Sports Med. 24, 721–725.

Luime, J.J., Verhagen, A.P., Miedema, H.S., et al., 2004. Does this patient have an instability of the shoulder or a labrum lesion? J. Am. Med. Assoc. 292, 1989–1999.

Maffet, M.W., Gartsman, G.M., Moseley, B., 1995. Superior labrum-biceps tendon complex lesions of the shoulder. Am. J. Sports Med. 23, 93–98.

Magee, T., 2009. 3-T MRI of the shoulder: is MR arthrography necessary? AJR. Am. J. Roentgenol. 192, 86–92.

McCaughey, R., Green, R.A., Taylor, N.F., 2009. The anatomical basis of the resisted supination external rotation test for superior labral anterior to posterior lesions. Clin. Anat. 22, 665–670.

McFarland, E.G., Kim, T.K., Savino, R.M., 2002. Clinical assessment of three common tests for superior labral anterior-posterior lesions. Am. J. Sports Med. 30, 810–815.

Meserve, B.B., Cleland, J.A., Boucher, T.R., 2008. The anatomical basis of the resisted supination external rotation test for superior labral anterior to posterior lesions. Am J Sp Medicine. 37, 2252–2258.

Mileski, R.A., Snyder, S.J., 1998. Superior labral lesions in the shoulder: Pathoanatomy and surgical management. J. Am. Acad. Orthop, Surg. 6, 121–131.

Mimori, K., Muneta, T., Nakagawa, T., et al., 1999. A new pain provocation test for superior labral tears of the shoulder. Am. J. Sports Med. 27, 137–142.

Mirkovic, M., Green, R., Taylor, N., et al., 2005. Accuracy of clinical tests to diagnose superior labral anterior and posterior (SLAP) lesions. Physical Therapy Reviews 10, 5–14.

Munro, W., Healy, R., 2009. The validity and accuracy of clinical tests used to detect labral pathology of the shoulder – A systematic review. Man. Ther. 14, 119–130.

Musgrave, D.S., Rodosky, M.W., 2001. SLAP lesions: current concepts. Am. J. Orthop. 30, 29–38.

Myers, T.H., Zemanovic, J.R., Andrews, J.R., 2005. The resisted supination external rotation test: A new test for the diagnosis of superior labral anterior posterior lesions. Am. J. Sports Med. 33, 1315–1320.

Nakagawa, S., Yoneda, M., Hayashida, K., et al., 2005. Forced shoulder abduction and elbow flexion test: a new simple clinical test to detect superior labral injury in the throwing shoulder. Arthroscopy 21, 1290–1295.

Nam, E.K., Snyder, S.J., 2003. The diagnosis and treatment of Superior Labrum, Anterior and Posterior (SLAP) lesions. Am. J. Sports Med. 31, 798–810.

O'Brien, S.J., Pagnani, M.J., Fealy, S., et al., 1998. The active compression test: A new and effective test for diagnosing labral tears and acromioclavicular joint abnormality. Am. J. Sports Med. 26, 610–613.

Oh, J.H., Kim, J.Y., Kim, W.S., et al., 2008. The evaluation of various physical examinations for the diagnosis of type II superior labrum anterior and posterior lesion. Am. J. Sports Med. 36, 353–359.

Pagnani, M.J., Deng, X.H., Warren, R.F., et al., 1995. Effect of lesions of the superior portion of the glenoid labrum on gleno-humeral translation. J. Bone Joint Surg. 77A, 1003–1010.

Pal, G.P., Bhatt, R.H., Patel, V.S., 1991. Relationship between the tendon of the long head of biceps brachii and the glenoidal labrum in humans. Anat. Rec. 229, 278–280.

Pandya, N.K., Colton, A., Webner, D., Sennett, B., Huffman, G.R., 2008. Physical examination and magnetic resonance imaging in the diagnosis of superior labrum anterior-posterior lesions of the shoulder: a sensitivity analysis. Arthroscopy 24 (3), 311–317.

Panossian, V.R., Mihata, T., Tibone, J.E., et al., 2005. Biomechanical analysis of isolated type II SLAP lesions and repair. J. Shoulder Elbow Surg. 14, 529–534.

Parentis, M.A., Mohr, K.J., El Attrache, N.S., 2002. Disorders of the superior labrum: review and treatment guidelines. Clin. Orthop. 400, 77–87.

Parentis, M.A., Mohr, K.J., Yocum, L.A., 2006. An evaluation of the provocative tests for Superior Labral Anterior Posterior lesions. Am. J. Sports Med. 34, 265–268.

Powell, J.W., Huijbregts, P.A., 2006. Concurrent criterion-related validity of acromio-clavicular joint physical examination tests: A systematic review. J. Man. Manip. Ther. 14, E19–E29.

Powell, J.W., Huijbregts, P.A., Jensen, R., 2008. Diagnostic utility of clinical tests for SLAP lesions: A systematic literature review. J. Man. Manip. Ther. 16, E58–E79.

Pradhan, R.L., Itoi, E., Hatakeyama, Y., et al., 2001. Superior labral strain during the throwing motion. A cadaveric study. Am. J. Sports Med. 29, 488–492.

Prodromos, C.C., Ferry, J.A., Schiller, A.L., et al., 1990. Histological studies of the glenoid labrum from fetal life to old age. J. Bone Joint Surg. 72A, 1344–1348.

Rao, A.G., Kim, T.K., Chronopoulos, E., et al., 2003. Anatomical variants in the anterosuperior aspect of the glenoid labrum: a statistical analysis of seventy-three cases. J. Bone Joint Surg. 85A, 653–659.

Rodosky, M.W., Harner, C.D., Fu, F.H., 1994. The role of the long head of the biceps muscle and superior glenoid labrum in anterior stability of the shoulder. Am. J. Sports Med. 11, 121–130.

Shepard, M.F., Dugas, J.R., Zeng, N., et al., 2004. Differences in the ultimate strength of the biceps anchor and the generation of type II superior labral anterior posterior lesions in a cadaveric model. Am. J. Sports Med. 32, 1197–1201.

Snyder, S.J., Banas, M.P., Karzel, R.P., 1995. An analysis of 140 injuries to the superior glenoid labrum. J. Shoulder Elbow Surg. 4, 243–248.

Snyder, S.J., Karzel, R.P., Del Pizzo, W., et al., 1990. SLAP lesions of the shoulder. Arthroscopy 6, 274–279.

Stetson, W.B., Templin, K., 2002. The crank test, the O'Brien test, and routine magnetic resonance imaging scans in the diagnosis of labral tears. Am. J. Sports Med. 30, 806–809.

Swearingen, J.C., Mell, A.G., Langenderfer, J., et al., 2006. Electromyographic analysis of physical examination tests for types II superior labrum anterior-posterior lesions. J. Shoulder Elbow Surg. 15, 576–579.

Vangsness, C.T., Jorgenson, S.S., Watson, T., et al., 1994. The origin of the long head of the biceps from the scapula and glenoid labrum. An anatomical study of 100 shoulders. J. Bone Joint Surg. 76B, 951–954.

Walch, G., Boileau, P., Noel, E., et al., 1992. Impingement of the deep surface of the infraspinatus tendon on the posterior glenoid rim. J. Shoulder Elbow Surg. 1, 238–245.

Walsworth, M.K., Doukas, W.C., Murphy, K.P., et al., 2008. Reliability and diagnostic accuracy of history and physical examination for diagnosing glenoid labral tears. Am. J. Sports Med. 36, 162–168.

Walton, D.M., Sadi, J., 2008. Identifying SLAP lesions: a meta-analysis of clinical tests and exercise in clinical reasoning. Phys. Ther. Sport 9, 167–176.

Warner, J.J., McMahon, P.J., 1995. The role of the long head of the biceps brachii in superior stability of the gleno-humeral joint. J. Bone Joint Surg. 77A, 366–372.

Wilk, K.E., Arrigo, C.A., Andrews, J.R., 1997. Current concepts: The stabilizing structures of the gleno-humeral joint. J. Orthop. Sports Phys. Ther. 25, 364–379.

Wilk, K.E., Reinold, M.M., Dugas, J.R., et al., 2005. Current concepts in the recognition and treatment of superior labral (SLAP) lesions. J. Orthop. Sports Phys. Ther. 35, 273–291.

Chapter | 19 |

Frozen shoulder

Carel Bron, Arthur de Gast, Jo L M Franssen

CHAPTER CONTENTS

INTRODUCTION

Frozen shoulder (FS) or adhesive capsulitis is, although known for more than a century, still an enigmatic and poorly defined shoulder disorder. The earliest case report was published in 1872 by the French surgeon Duplay (1872) who used the term 'Peri-arthrite Scapulo-humerale' when he described a disorder similar to the condition we know nowadays as the frozen shoulder. This latter term was introduced several decades later by Codman (1934). Finally, Neviaser (1945), an orthopaedic surgeon also used the term 'Adhesive capsulitis' based on his arthro-graphic and intra-articular findings.

Codman (1934) stated that the frozen shoulder was 'difficult to define, difficult to treat, and difficult to explain from the point of view of pathology'. Obviously, this has not much changed as the years have passed. The three terms 'Frozen shoulder', 'Adhesive capsulitis' and 'Peri-arthrite Scapulo-humerale' (although the one from Duplay is now somewhat outdated) are used to describe a clinical condition of pain and severe (more than 50%) restricted passive range of motion (PROM) of the gleno-humeral joint in all directions (flexion, extension, abduction, adduction, and internal-external rotations). The aetiology of FS is usually unknown. Patients occasionally mention a variety of activities or circumstances that they associate with the start of their complaints. Still, the exact cause of FS has to be established.

It is common use to differentiate between a primary and a secondary frozen shoulder (Lundberg 1969). Primary FS is idiopathic and not related to other diseases, while secondary FS is defined as being related to known systemic pathology, such as diabetes mellitus, thyroid disease, Parkinson's disease, post-surgery, post-trauma or after a period of immobilization. It is difficult to differentiate, but one might suffer from post-surgical shoulder stiffness, which is not the same as secondary post-surgical FS.

In this chapter we will focus on primary FS, which encompasses the following clinical criteria: (1) restriction of shoulder motion without major shoulder injury; (2) global stiffness of the shoulder joint in all directions, without the loss of strength, joint stability, or joint surface integrity; and (3) plain shoulder radiographs demonstrating a normal gleno-humeral joint space and no peri-articular abnormalities, although some osteopoenia of the proximal humerus and glenoid may be seen.

© 2011 Elsevier Ltd.
DOI: 10.1016/B978-0-7020-3528-9.00019-4

INCIDENCE OF FROZEN SHOULDER

FS has an incidence of 3–5% in the general population, and is a common shoulder disorder in orthopaedic practice. In the Netherlands it is calculated that 1 in 105 shoulder patients that consult a general practitioner is diagnosed with primary FS. FS is more common among patients with diabetes, affecting 20% or more (Balci et al 1999, Kordella 2002, Tighe & Oakley 2008).

PATHOLOGY OF FROZEN SHOULDER

Normal functional limits of the gleno-humeral joint are determined by skeletal morphology, articular surface area, and the flexibility of the connection joint capsule, ligaments, musculotendinous units, and integument. In a gleno-humeral joint with smooth articular surfaces, shoulder stiffness occurs as a result of (1) stiffening of the joint capsule, ligaments, or muscle-tendon units, (2) adhesions along the gliding surfaces between the rotator cuff and its surroundings, adhesions in the biceps tendon mechanism and (3) extra-articular adhesions. These restrictions occur independently or in combination. In primary FS the gleno-humeral functional restriction most likely starts in the gleno-humeral joint capsule, and during the course of the disease, stiffness may encompass soft tissue structures outside the joint.

The pathological process in primary FS is not clear, although several authors have tried to elucidate it (Hannafin & Chiaia 2000, Cleland & Durall 2002, Uhthoff & Boileau 2007, Schultheis et al 2008). It is generally accepted that underlying FS is an inflammatory process of the synovial membrane subsequently followed by a fibrotic reaction of the fibrous layer. There is still disagreement whether the underlying pathology is an inflammatory process, but arthroscopy shows a hyperaemic and swollen synovial membrane. The recent discovery of several cytokines in the joint capsule in patients with FS supports the inflammation theory. The synovial reaction (or inflammation) eventually leads to fibrosis of the underlying layer of the gleno-humeral capsule (fibrous membrane). Especially in the area of the coraco-humeral ligament (CHL) and the rotator cuff interval, scar formation and contracture formation is initiated by the expression of vimentin (a cytocontractile protein, usually seen in fibromyocytes), while in the entire joint capsule there is fibroplasia (thickening of the joint capsule) without contraction.

Another important outcome is the need for a distinction between fibroplasia and contracture. Although fibroplasia involves the entire capsule, presence of cytocontractile proteins is limited to the anterior capsular part (Uhthoff & Boileau 2007). Fibroplasia involves the entire joint capsule

to an almost identical degree with no preferential involvement of the anterior capsule. Therefore, it is concluded that the reduced range of motion of the primary FS is foremost attributable to a contracture of anterior capsular structures, particularly the coraco-humeral ligament and the capsule at the rotator interval as seen by the selective expression of the cytocontractile protein vimentin. This finding confirms the clinical experience that surgical division of these structures is usually sufficient to restore the lost range of motion. Yang et al (2009) studied the anatomical relationship of the CHL in 14 normal cadaveric shoulders. In most of the cases (11 of 14) the CHL (Fig 19.1) inserted into the rotator cuff interval and the supraspinatus tendon, while in 4 the tendon of the subscapularis was also involved. The dissimilarity in the insertion of the CHL may be one of the reasons for different clinical pictures with for example more or less limitation of external rotation.

Although it is still controversial whether the CHL is a separate entity or just a thickening of the gleno-humeral capsule, Yang et al (2009) conclude based upon their findings that the CHL position, morphology, and origin are relatively unchanged, but its insertion varies greatly and the CHL is a more capsular than ligamentous structure based on its histologic features. Finally, although Neviaser (1945) was convinced of the formation of intra-articular adhesion between parts of the joint capsule, especially in the axillary recess, and the articular cartilage, there is no scientific evidence that this really exists.

Despite all the scientific work that has been done on primary FS, the question still remains what triggers the

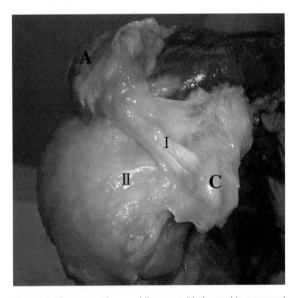

Fig 19.1 The coraco-humeral ligament (II) showed in a normal cadaveric right shoulder. Other visible structures are the coraco-acromial ligament (I), the acromion (A) and the coracoid process (from Yang et al 2009, with permission)

cascade of inflammatory and fibrogenetic processes. There is, however, knowledge on factors that predispose to shoulder stiffness such as (1) age; (2) minor injuries with no detectable structural damage to the gleno-humeral joint; (3) non-shoulder surgery, e.g. cervical neck dissection, thoracotomy, sternotomy and intervention cardiology; (4) immobility; (5) cervical disease such as inter-vertebral disk degeneration in the lower regions of the cervical spine; (6) thyroid disorders; (7) diabetes mellitus; and (8) cardiac and pulmonary disease.

Primary FS seems to be strongly associated to Dupuytren's disease (Bunker & Anthony 1995, Smith et al 2001). Smith et al (2001) confirmed that Dupuytren's disease was commonly seen in patients with frozen shoulder (52%). This finding may suggest that the two conditions may share a common biochemical pathway that leads to contracture. Bunker & Anthony (1995) found that the histological appearances of the tissues excised from primary FS patients and from patients with Dupuytren's contractures of the hand were similar.

Some authors recognize similarities with reflex dystrophy (Sudeck's dystrophy or complex regional pain syndrome type I as it is referred to nowadays) (Hertel 2000, Muller et al 2000).

NATURAL HISTORY AND PROGNOSIS OF FROZEN SHOULDER

Knowledge of the natural history of primary FS is crucial for making treatment decisions. The natural history of FS is not fully understood and remains controversial, since many reports of long-term follow-up concern the evaluation of patient groups who received particular treatment regimens.

Some authors have described FS as a self-limiting disease with an average duration of 1–3 years, but a substantial part of the population presents with substantial limitations in gleno-humeral passive range of motion for up to 10 years after the onset of their FS (Miller et al 1996). Nevertheless, discrepancy may exist between the patient's recognition of functional limitation and the clinically measured objective restrictions of the PROM. This can be explained by the fact that shoulder pain is usually more incapacitating than is restriction of gleno-humeral PROM as such.

To our knowledge, recurrence of primary FS in the same shoulder joint does not occur, although one case report has been published (Cameron et al 2000). In this case the patient fully recovered within 6 weeks, which is very unusual for a FS. Therefore we doubt that this is indeed the first case report of a recurrent FS. Most likely, this case report is an example of mistaking a shoulder complaint for FS, which often happens. In a large (269 shoulders) retrospective study on the long-term (5 years) outcome in primary frozen shoulder Hand et al (2008) report no recurrences. Simultaneous bilateral presentation of FS is rare, but developing a FS over time in the opposite shoulder may occur in about up to 35% of the cases.

FS is classically characterized by three clinical phases: (1) freezing phase; (2) frozen phase, and (3) thawing phase (Neviaser 1945; Box 19.1). Some authors use a classification of four stages, where the first stage is divided in a painful pre-freezing stage and a freezing stage where the PROM gradually decreases (Neviaser & Neviaser 1987, Hannafin & Chiaia 2000, Sheridan & Hannafin 2006, Schultheis et al 2008).

Box 19.1 Stages of Frozen Shoulder

Stage 1: Freezing, synovitis (duration 3–9 months)

There is increasing pain during rest and movement. As the patient is often not able to lie down on the affected side, sleep may be disturbed. When the patient makes a sudden movement (they often call it a wrong movement) it can take several minutes (up to 15) before the pain subsides. The pain is very severe and often scored on a visual analogue scale reaching 9 or 10.

In this phase it might be quite difficult to diagnose the primary FS, because of the absence of PROM limitation. Therefore in this stage patients are often diagnosed with sub-acromial tendinitis or bursitis. At the end of the freezing phase the limitation of PROM becomes progressively worse.

Stage 2: Frozen (duration 4–12 months)

Hypertrophy of the gleno-humeral joint capsule and contracture of the coracohumeral ligament and the rotator cuff interval (Omari & Bunker 2001, Uhthoff & Boileau 2007).

In this phase, pain will diminish gradually, due to the recovery of the inflammatory process. Pain may be completely absent during rest but pain felt at the end of the (significantly limited) range of motion is still present. Sleeping is still disturbed because lying on either side due to the severe restriction of PROM is still not possible (Cleland & Durall 2002). Although there is some muscular atrophy due to inactivity of the shoulder, severe loss of strength will not occur during the course of FS. The PROM is limited by about 50% or even more in all directions.

Stage 3: Thawing (between 12 and 42 months)

This stage is characterized by gradually improving PROM.

PROGNOSIS OF FROZEN SHOULDER

Patient education is one of the important aspects of the treatment. Explaining the benign nature of the primary FS helps to reassure the patient. Although the primary FS is seen as a self-limiting disease, this is probably especially true for the inflammatory processes during the first stages. The PROM restriction occasionally persists for several years and might result in major limitations in daily activities. Therefore it might be useful to instruct patients to perform gentle stretching exercises in the thawing phase. Very few cases will result in a refractory primary frozen shoulder in which more rigorous interventions are needed. According to Tasto & Elias (2007), about 10–15% of the patients continue to suffer from continuous pain and limited motion or need up to 10 years to recover fully. Figure 19.2 shows the natural history of the self-limiting form of primary FS.

DIAGNOSIS OF FROZEN SHOULDER

The diagnosis of a primary FS should be easy. The history is generally clear, physical examination only requires few diagnostic shoulder tests, and even fewer additional diagnostic tools are necessary. Still, FS is chosen as the most frequently misdiagnosed shoulder complaint in patients referred for a second opinion. FS is characterized by three phases, and the practitioner's clinical challenge is formed by the discrimination of the exact phase and appropriate duration of symptoms or signs. For details of these phases see Box 19.1.

History

Patients who present at the clinic are usually aged between 40 and 70 years, and women are more frequently affected than men (Hannafin & Chiaia 2000). Both sides

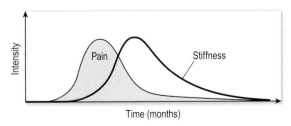

Fig 19.2 The natural history of the self-limiting form of primary frozen shoulder according to Hertel., Orthopäde 2000, 29:845–851.

are equally involved. Even when patients within the typical age group present themselves with a painful and stiff shoulder, the diagnosis of FS seems obvious. Still, other diagnoses, such as neoplasias (Quan et al 2005, Sano et al 2009), gleno-humeral infection, calcific bursitis or tendinitis, rotator cuff lesions, or gleno-humeral osteoarthritis have to be considered.

The pain is usually experienced in the shoulder region, the deltoid insertion and upper arm, but it often radiates to the neck, and more distal regions of the upper extremity. In the freezing phase the pain is felt during rest and intensified during movement and during sleep. The amount of pain strongly depends on the clinical phase of the disease.

Physical examination

Examination starts with both shoulders exposed. The alignment and symmetry of both shoulder girdles and the cervical spine are assessed. The cervical spine is assessed for muscle spasm and local tenderness. Both shoulders are checked for signs of muscle atrophy, former trauma, and pathological swelling. Next, the affected shoulder is palpated. Patients with FS typically demonstrate tenderness in the region of the rotator cuff and sub-acromial bursa, deltoid insertion, and along the course of the biceps tendon. A painful biceps tendon is often confounded with a taut band in the anterior deltoid, which is much more accessible to palpation than the biceps tendon, which lies deep in the biceps groove underneath a tight transverse ligament. Myofascial trigger points (TrPs) may be found in almost all shoulder muscles, but most often in the subscapularis, infraspinatus, teres minor, teres major, deltoid, and trapezius muscle. According to Simons et al (1999) the shoulder becomes more restricted in external rotation (up to 45% or more) when TrPs in the subscapularis muscle become progressively active, while TrPs in the teres major muscle may be responsible for a restriction in abduction. It is unclear whether TrPs in the subscapularis mimic a PFS, or that they initiate the PFS. Simons et al (1999) propose to make a distinction between severely restricted motion due to active TrPs in the shoulder musculature and adhesive capsulitis as a result of true fibrosis (see Chapter 32 for muscle TrPs).

During assessment of the mobility of the shoulder, particular attention should be paid to the contribution of the gleno-humeral joint to the total active and passive range of motion (Fig 19.3). Only then can FS be clinically distinguished from other diseases that limit shoulder mobility.

In the pre-freezing and freezing phase, pain is the most limiting factor and the characteristic global restriction of the gleno-humeral joint may be less clear. In the frozen phase, the characteristic global limitation of PROM of

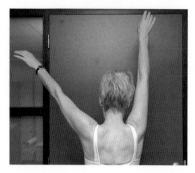

Fig 19.3 Patient with frozen left shoulder during shoulder abduction

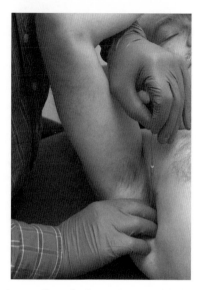

Fig 19.4 Dry needling of subscapularis muscle using a Japanese needle plunger

the gleno-humeral joint is present. In the thawing phase, the global limitation fades out and usually the contracture of the rotator interval causes a marked limitation of external rotation.

Isometric strength testing of the shoulder muscles in a pain-free shoulder position with the arm at the side of the body is usually non-provocative and reveals nearly normal strength.

TREATMENT OF FROZEN SHOULDER

Treatment proposals depend on the stage of the FS. In the pre-freezing (first phase) or freezing phase (second phase), the chief complaint of the patient is the extreme pain. Treatment regimens have to be aimed at pain relief with intra-articular injections of corticosteroids (Buchbinder et al 2003), oral non-steroidal anti-inflammatory drugs (NSAID), supra-scapular nerve block (Harmon & Hearty, 2007) or treating the TrPs in the surrounding shoulder muscles (Simons et al 1999, Jankovic & van Zundert 2006).

The use of corticosteroids did not make any difference in long-term outcome as compared to physiotherapy even if they could provide some pain relief in the early stages (Brue et al 2007). Myofascial TrP may occur in rotator cuff muscles, especially in the subscapularis muscle and in the thoraco-scapular muscles. Manual treatment of the subscapularis muscle may be difficult because the muscle is poorly accessible in severely restricted shoulder joints. Therefore TrP dry needling using a Japanese needle plunger to position the needle deep into the muscle is a good option (Fig 19.4). The other shoulder muscles can be treated manually or by TrP dry needling (see Chapter 34 for TrP dry needling). In some cases application of cold-packs or hot-packs (or hot shower) may be beneficial. The patient can apply this several times a day, as often as necessary.

In this phase it is not useful to perform gleno-humeral joint mobilization, because of the lack of ROM restriction (pre-freezing phase) or because the patient will respond with increasing pain during mobilization and subsequently with increasing joint limitation. It is essential to explain to the patient the nature of the disease and to stop exercising. The patient has to be encouraged to do everything that diminishes the pain. Less pain may lead to diminishing of the inflammation process and subsequently probably to less fibrosis (Hannafin & DiCarlo 1994, Marx et al 2007).

In the frozen phase (third phase) the pain will rapidly decrease as the inflammatory process recedes and anti-inflammatory drugs are no longer indicated. Over-the-counter painkillers may be taken on an irregular basis. There is a great variety in treatment options advised for FS to treat the PROM, indicating the poor consensus of opinions about the best available treatment options. Due to the benign natural course the best choice is to start with conservative, non-surgical interventions. A supervised physical therapy treatment or a gentle home stretching programme may be sufficient. End-range mobilization has shown to be more effective, but the benefits are small (Vermeulen et al 2006). Rigorous mobilization or stretching is not per se more beneficial than gentle mobilization. In the frozen phase one might prefer a milder mobilization technique as it produces less pain during and after the treatment sessions. Occasionally new treatment options are invented. Ruiz (2009) presented a single case report in which he describes positional stretching of the coraco-humeral ligament. The patient regained considerable gleno-humeral range of motion within 4 weeks, which cannot be due to natural recovery alone (Ruiz 2009). Gaspar & Willis (2009) presented in a controlled, cohort study a new intervention, called dynamic splinting. Due to methodological flaws, firm conclusions cannot be made.

In the thawing phase (fourth phase) gentle mobilization may be applied (Diercks & Stevens 2004, Vermeulen et al 2006). In this phase the recovery is mostly due to the natural course of recovery and it is the opinion of the authors that mobilization does not add much benefit (Miller et al 1996, Diercks & Stevens 2004). Recently, Kelley et al (2009) proposed a model for guiding rehabilitation. Because of the lack of evidence to determine which patients may need formal supervised therapy rather than simply a home programme, they propose a patient-centred approach in which the decision is made based on the physician and patient preference, with input from the therapist after initial evaluation (Yang et al 2008).

As range of motion restores gradually the patient will carefully start to use their arm in daily activities. This will help to exercise the shoulder and arm muscles and additional exercises are rarely needed.

RECALCITRANT FROZEN SHOULDERS

Although most of the primary frozen shoulders recover in months, it might be necessary in only a very few cases (especially when the patient or his/her physician or physical therapist is impatient) to use more rigorous treatment options.

These interventions are manipulation under anaesthesia, gleno-humeral joint distension, and arthroscopic capsular release. Closed manipulation under anaesthesia may be effective in terms of joint mobilization; however, the method can cause iatrogenic damage which includes haemarthrosis, rupture of the gleno-humeral capsule, superior labrum anterior-posterior (SLAP), bankart lesions, tendinous or ligamentous ruptures, fractures of the humerus and axillary nerve lesions (Loew et al 2005). Closed manipulation under anaesthesia is contraindicated in patients with significant osteopoenia, recent surgical repair of soft tissue about the shoulder or in the presence of fractures, neurologic injury and instability (Hannafin & Chiaia 2000).

Gleno-humeral joint distension using saline in combination with or without corticosteroids seems to be beneficial only for short term. The technique is often poorly tolerated because of the pain that is experienced during the procedure (Manske & Prohaska 2008).

More recently, arthroscopy has been advocated for confirmation of diagnosis and for selective release of the contracted parts of the capsule (Brue et al 2007). Release of the coraco-humeral ligament and the rotator cuff interval is particularly effective in increasing range of motion in external rotation, abduction and elevation. In cases with a decreased internal rotation and adduction (cross-body adduction) release of the posterior capsule is performed. Arthroscopic release prior to or following a closed manipulation is considered to be an effective and safe procedure and the iatrogenic damage is considered to be of less importance.

PREVENTION OF FROZEN SHOULDER

Patients with severe shoulder complaints are advised to perform mobilizing or stretching exercises to prevent the development of a frozen shoulder. We strongly believe that it is impossible for the patient to succeed in this or even to slow down the development of FS by performing exercises. If doctors or therapists insist on an exercise regime patients will then feel a responsibility for their FS that they should not.

CONCLUSION

The frozen shoulder is still a challenge for physicians, therapists and researchers as there is still controversy on the aetiology, the pathophysiology, the diagnosis and the optimal treatment strategy. Most important is that the prognosis in most cases is good. About 80–90% of all patients will eventually fully recover, although improvement may take up to 10 years. Recurrence of the primary frozen shoulder in the same shoulder does not occur. Patient education about the natural history and good prognosis is an important aspect of the treatment. The treatment is mainly conservative and depends highly on the stage of the frozen shoulder. In the freezing stage the treatment is aimed at inhibiting the pain and diminishing the inflammation, while in the frozen stage it is aimed at regaining range of motion. It is the authors' preferred treatment to search for the least painful approach. Recalcitrant frozen shoulders are very rare and patience has to be maintained before surgery is considered. If necessary, arthroscopic release of carefully selected structures seems to be beneficial in regaining range of motion in refractory frozen shoulder. Recently, new stretching techniques and devices have been published but further research is needed to see if these can be of additional value. The bottom line message for therapists, physicians, and patients should be patience during the course of the primary frozen shoulder.

REFERENCES

Balci, N., Balci, M.K., Tuzuner, S., 1999. Shoulder adhesive capsulitis and shoulder range of motion in type II diabetes mellitus: association with diabetic complications. J. Diabetes Complications 13, 135–140.

Brue, S., Valentin, A., Forssblad, M., Werner, S., Mikkelsen, C., Cerulli, G., et al., 2007. Idiopathic adhesive capsulitis of the shoulder: a review. Knee. Surg. Sports Traumatol. Arthrosc. 15, 1048–1054.

Buchbinder, R., Green, S., Youd, J.M., 2003. Corticosteroid injections for shoulder pain. Cochrane Database Syst. Rev. CD004016.

Bunker, T.D., Anthony, P.P., 1995. The pathology of frozen shoulder: A dupuytrn like disease. J. Bone Joint Surg. Br. 77, 677–683.

Cameron, R.I., McMillan, J., Kelly, I.G., 2000. Recurrence of a 'primary frozen shoulder': a case report. J. Shoulder Elbow Surg. 9, 65–67.

Cleland, J., Durall, C., 2002. Physical therapy for adhesive capsulitis: Systematic review. Physiotherapy 88, 450–457.

Codman, E.A., 1934. The Shoulder. Thomas Odd, Boston.

Diercks, R.L., Stevens, M., 2004. Gentle thawing of the frozen shoulder: a prospective study of supervised neglect versus intensive physical therapy in seventy-seven patients with frozen shoulder syndrome followed up for two years. J. Shoulder Elbow Surg. 13, 499–502.

Duplay, S., 1872. De la periarthrite scapulo-humerale et des raideurs de l'épaule qui en sont la consequence. Arch. Gen. Med. 513–542.

Gaspar, P.D., Willis, F.B., 2009. Adhesive capsulitis and dynamic splinting: a controlled, cohort study. BMC Musculoskelet. Disord. 10, 111.

Hand, C., Clipsham, K., Rees, J.L., Carr, A.J., 2008. Long-term outcome of frozen shoulder. J. Shoulder Elbow Surg. 17, 231–236.

Hannafin, J.A., DiCarlo, E.F., Wickiewicz, T.L., Warren, R.F., 1994. Adhesive capsulitis: Capsular fibroplasia of the glenohumeral joint. J. Shoulder Elbow Surg. 3 (Suppl), 5.

Hannafin, J.A., Chiaia, T.A., 2000. Adhesive capsulitis. A treatment approach. Clin. Orthop. Relat. Res. 1, 95–109.

Harmon, D., Hearty, C., 2007. Ultrasound-guided suprascapular nerve block technique. Pain Physician 10, 743–746.

Hertel, R., 2000. The frozen shoulder. Orthopade 29, 845–851.

Jankovic, D., van Zundert, A., 2006. The frozen shoulder syndrome. Description of a new technique and five case reports using the subscapular nerve block and subscapularis trigger point infiltration. Acta Anaesthesiology Belgica 57, 137–143.

Kelley, M.J., McClure, P.W., Leggin, B.G., 2009. Frozen shoulder: evidence and a proposed model guiding rehabilitation. J. Orthop. Sports Phys. Ther. 39, 135–148.

Kordella, T., 2002. Frozen shoulder & diabetes. Frozen shoulder affects 20 percent of people with diabetes. Proper treatment can help you work through it. Diabetes Forecast 55, 60–64.

Loew, M., Heichel, T.O., Lehner, B., 2005. Intraarticular lesions in primary frozen shoulder after manipulation under general anesthesia. J. Shoulder Elbow Surg. 14, 16–21.

Lundberg, B.J., 1969. The frozen shoulder. Clinical and radiographical observations. The effect of manipulation under general anesthesia. Structure and glycosaminoglycan content of the joint capsule. Local bone metabolism. Acta Orthop. Scand. 119, 1–59.

Manske, R.C., Prohaska, D., 2008. Diagnosis and management of adhesive capsulitis. Current Review in Musculoskeletal Medicine 1, 180–189.

Marx, R.G., Malizia, R.W., Kenter, K., Wickiewicz, T.L., Hannafin, J.A., 2007. Intra-articular corticosteroid injection for the treatment of idiopathic adhesive capsulitis of the shoulder. The Musculoskeletal Journal of Hospital for Special Surgery 3, 202–207.

Miller, M.D., Wirth, M.A., Rockwood, C. A., 1996. Thawing the frozen shoulder: the 'patient' patient. Orthopedics 19, 849–853.

Muller, L.P., Muller, L.A., Happ, J., Kerschbaumer, F., 2000. Frozen shoulder: a sympathetic dystrophy? Arch. Orthop. Trauma Surg. 120, 84–87.

Neviaser, J.S., 1945. Adhesive capsulitis of the shoulder: a study of the pathological findings in periarthritis of the shoulder. J. Bone Joint Surg. Am. 27, 211–222.

Neviaser, R.J., Neviaser, T.J., 1987. The frozen shoulder. Diagnosis and management. Clin. Orthop. Relat. Res. 223, 59–64.

Omari, A., Bunker, T.D., 2001. Open surgical release for frozen shoulder: Surgical findings and results of the release. J. Shoulder Elbow Surg. 10, 353–357.

Quan, G.M., Carr, D., Schlicht, S., Powell, G., Choong, P.F., 2005. Lessons learnt from the painful shoulder; a case series of malignant shoulder girdle tumours misdiagnosed as frozen shoulder. International Seminars in Surgical Oncology 2, 2.

Ruiz, J.O., 2009. Positional stretching of the coracohumeral ligament on a patient with adhesive capsulitis: a case report. J. Man. Manip. Ther. 17, 58–63.

Sano, H., Hatori, M., Mineta, M., Hosaka, M., Itoi, E., 2009. Tumors masked as frozen shoulders: A retrospective analysis. J. Shoulder Elbow Surg. 2010 Mar; 19 (2), 262–266.

Schultheis, A., Reichwein, F., Nebelung, W., 2008. Frozen shoulder: Diagnosis and therapy. Orthopade 37, 1065–1072.

Sheridan, M.A., Hannafin, J.A., 2006. Upper extremity: emphasis on frozen shoulder. Orthop. Clin. North Am. 37, 531–539.

Simons, D.G., Travell, J.G., Simons, L.S., 1999. Myofascial Pain and Dysfunction. The trigger point manual. Upper half of body, second ed., vol. I. Lippincott, Williams and Wilkins, Baltimore, MD.

Smith, S.P., Devaraj, V.S., Bunker, T.D., 2001. The association between frozen shoulder and Dupuytren's disease. J. Shoulder Elbow Surg. 10, 149–151.

Tasto, J.P., Elias, D., 2007. Adhesive capsulitis. Sports Med. Arthrosc. 15, 216–221.

Tighe, C.B., Oakley, W.S., 2008. The prevalence of a diabetic condition and adhesive capsulitis of the shoulder. South Medical Journal 101, 591–595.

Uhthoff, H.K., Boileau, P., 2007. Primary frozen shoulder: Global capsular stiffness versus localized contracture. Clin. Orthop. Relat. Res. 456, 79–84.

Vermeulen, H.M., Rozing, P.M., Obermann, W.R., le Cessie, S., Vliet Vlieland, T.P., 2006. Comparison of high-grade and low-grade mobilization techniques in the management of adhesive capsulitis of the shoulder: randomized controlled trial. Phys. Ther. 86, 355–368.

Yang, H.F., Tang, K.L., Chen, W., et al., 2009. An anatomic and histologic study of the coracohumeral ligament. J. Shoulder Elbow Surg. 18, 305–310.

Yang, J.L., Chang, C.W., Chen, S.Y., Lin, J.J., 2008. Shoulder kinematic features using arm elevation and rotation tests for classifying patients with frozen shoulder syndrome who respond to physical therapy. Man. Ther. 13, 544–551.

Chapter | 20 |

Mobilization with movement of the shoulder joint

Wayne Hing, Jack Miller

INTRODUCTION

The fully functional upper limb is dependent on the optimal pain-free mobility of the shoulder girdle. Shoulder pain and dysfunction limit our ability to utilize the upper limb in activities of daily living resulting in recreational, occupational and societal disabilities. This chapter has been organized to highlight the concept of the restoration of upper limb functional tasks though a continuum of manual therapy interventions to the shoulder joint and shoulder girdle complex. The techniques demonstrated within this chapter are focused on achieving the optimization of upper limb functional activities including overhead elevation, cross body motion and placing the hand behind the back.

The progression of techniques, as determined by key subjective and objective parameters (Hing et al 2003) such as patient irritability, severity of pain, stage of pathology and recovery, the available range of motion and the effect of upper limb load bearing forces, are demonstrated in the multi-panel figures within this chapter.

Manual therapy procedures to restore mobility and function of the shoulder girdle have been developed and described by a variety of authors (Kaltenborn et al 2002, Mulligan 2003, Hengeveld et al 2005). A dispassionate perspective of these apparently diverse approaches reveals that while each may have highly original components, they are invariably progressions of previously established work and form an evolutionary continuum (Miller 1999). While acknowledging the contributions of all those who have added to the body of knowledge of manual therapy, this

© 2011 Elsevier Ltd.
DOI: 10.1016/B978-0-7020-3528-9.00020-0

chapter will highlight manual therapy techniques that have been demonstrated to be safe, effective and are evidence based.

MOBILIZATION INTERVENTIONS

Translatoric accessory joint mobilization techniques are well established and form the basis of much of the curriculum of both entry level and post-graduate manual therapy training programmes. Originally developed by contributors such as Kaltenborn and Evjenth from Norway (Kaltenborn et al 2002), Orthopaedic Manual Therapy (OMT) utilizes a clinical reasoning paradigm based on the manual therapist's perception of joint restriction as revealed by passive movement examination and the application of the concave-convex rule. Passive translatoric accessory mobilizations are performed parallel or perpendicular to the treatment plane as determined by the specific orientation of the joint surfaces. Mobilizations are graded in their range and sustained for specific durations according to their intended therapeutic goal(s) including pain relief and improving joint mobility.

The conceptual model of OMT is that of joint capsule contracture that must be passively elongated through tissue creep affected by sustained passive mobilization techniques into the tissue barrier. Technique repetition and an appropriate self-treatment regime along with consideration of associated peri-articular soft tissue dysfunctions, neurophysiological and motor control factors are proposed to provide short and long-term positive outcomes.

A growing body of recent evidence has demonstrated the value of combining traditional OMT therapy mobilizations concurrently with the patient's pain-limited physiological movements. Termed Mobilizations with Movement (MWM), this concept was developed by Brian Mulligan of New Zealand (Mulligan 2003) and built on the foundations of OMT. Within the Mulligan concept, the management of the patient requires the identification of a comparable sign or client specific outcome measure (CSOM) as a baseline measure, to evaluate treatment effectiveness, often measured as a functionally limited motor activity. This clinically measurable functional deficit becomes the benchmark by which assessment of the efficacy of the intervention(s) is continually re-assessed.

The clinical reasoning paradigm of selection and progression of MWMs rests on the patient's individual response to selected trial mobilizations as measured by pain-free improvement in the identified CSOM. The therapist must continuously monitor the patient's reaction to ensure minimal to no pain is recreated. Utilizing their knowledge of joint arthrology, a well-developed sense of tissue tension and active clinical reasoning, the therapist investigates various combinations of mobilization directions to find the ideal treatment plane and grade of movement. While sustaining the pain-free accessory mobilization, the patient is requested to perform the previously identified pain-restricted CSOM. The CSOM should now be significantly improved i.e. increased range of motion, and a significantly decreased or ideally, absence of the original pain. Failure to improve the CSOM would indicate that the therapist has not found the correct contact point, treatment plane, grade or direction of mobilization, spinal segment or that the technique is not indicated. The previously restricted and/or painful CSOM is repeated by the patient initially as a trial treatment progressing up to sets of 10 while the therapist continues to maintain the appropriate accessory glide. Further gains are expected with repetition during a treatment session typically involving 3 to 4 sets of 10 repetitions. Repetition of the CSOM and pain-free end range loading in the form of passive overpressure appear to be critical to achieve durable results (Miller 1999, Mulligan 2003, Hing et al 2008). As with all manual therapy concepts, a properly structured subjective and objective assessment of the patient and continuous reflective clinical reasoning (Jones & Rivett 2004) are mandatory within the patient's assessment and during treatment sessions.

The theoretical model of the effect of MWMs is that either a positional fault of bony positional malalignment and/or a neuromechanical dysfunction is corrected or affected by the mobilization component of the procedures. In place of the therapist's perception of passive accessory movement restriction and the concave-convex rule, the specific direction and grade of mobilization is determined by the client's reports of an accessory direction of preference of pain abolition and objective improvements in CSOM function (Miller 2006, Hing et al 2009). Self-treatment procedures along with the application of sports adhesive tape are often used to maintain gains achieved in the clinical setting.

OVERHEAD ELEVATION MOBILIZATIONS

Individuals with shoulder dysfunction usually report that regaining a functional range of overhead elevation is often of prime importance. In highly irritable and restricted cases the patient may initially need to be treated in a non-gravity dependent, recumbent position with a graduated progression to upright gravity-dependent postures and resisted load bearing environments. The selection of the appropriate initial procedure and the appropriate progression of loads will always be dependent on the findings at assessment, ongoing re-evaluation and active clinical reasoning.

Posterior glide (Fig 20.1)

This mobilization is indicated to increase the available range of passive posterior glide of the head of the humerus, to reposition the head of the humerus in the optimal glenoid position, and to decrease pain related to

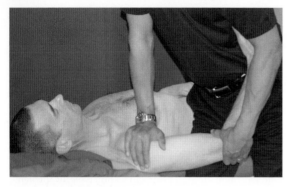

Fig 20.1 Posterior glide of the humeral head.

an anteriorly positioned humeral head. For that purpose, the patient is supine with the arm in neutral internal/external rotation and the cervical spine neutral. The therapist is standing at side of bed. The cephalic hand cups the humeral head with the palm, and the caudal hand supports the upper arm/forearm in a slightly flexed and abducted position. The therapist applies a postero-lateral glide of the humerus along joint plane of glenoid fossa. Clinicians should ensure the glide is translatoric by moving both hands equally in a postero-lateral direction, avoiding contact with the coracoid process.

Mobilization with movement – elevation (Fig 20.2)

This mobilization is indicated to reposition the humeral head in the glenoid fossa while restoring functional range of overhead elevation, and to increase active range of pain-free elevation during a trial treatment. The patient is sitting or standing dependent on the height of the therapist and patient with the cervical spine neutral. The therapist is standing on the contralateral side of the patient. With one hand the therapist makes a manual contact of the anterior humeral head with cup of their hand, and with the other stabilizes the scapula posteriorly. The

technique consists of an application of a posterolateral glide along joint plane of the glenoid fossa at the same time that the patient is asked to perform active shoulder elevation through the scaption plane (30° from frontal plane). It is important to allow normal scapulo-thoracic movement throughout the technique to ensure that the patient elevates the arm fully to achieve end range loading, and progressing to resistance loading with the use of soft weights or elastic tubing as tissue irritability decreases.

Mobilization with movement – elevation, belt assisted (Fig 20.3)

This mobilization is indicated in larger patients requiring a greater mobilization force than available by a manual mobilization technique. The aim of the mobilization is to reposition the humeral head in the glenoid fossa while restoring functional range of overhead elevation and to increase active range of pain-free elevation. The patient is sitting on the chair with their spine fully supported but the scapula exposed and cervical spine in neutral. The therapist is standing posterior to the patient. The mobilization belt is looped around the therapists' buttocks and over the humeral head of the patient. One hand is placed over the scapula, thus stabilizing the scapula to chest wall but allowing normal scapulo-thoracic movement. The technique consists of the application of a posterolateral glide along joint plane of the glenoid fossa, at the same time that the patient is asked to perform active shoulder elevation through the scaption plane (30° from frontal plane). Note: the clinician should ensure the belt is on the humeral head and does not impede elevation of the arm, and ensure the patient elevates the arm fully to achieve end range loading. The mobilization progresses

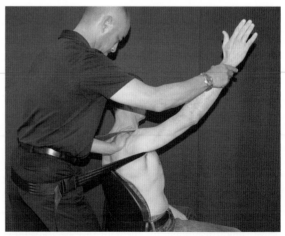

Fig 20.3 Mobilization with movement – elevation, belt assisted.

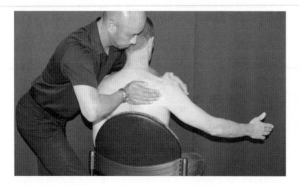

Fig 20.2 Mobilization with movement – elevation.

to resistance loading with the use of soft weights or elastic tubing as tissue irritability decreases.

OVERHEAD ELEVATION: PROGRESSION OF RANGE OF MOTION

During normal arm elevation the humerus undergoes a conjunct external rotation, often referred to as Codman's paradox (Cheng 2006). In order to accomplish full overhead elevation it may be necessary to ensure the recovery of external rotation firstly in neutral, then in varying degrees of elevation culminating in the position originally described by Maitland (Hengeveld et al 2005) as 'the quadrant'. Additionally, in order to achieve full elevation the therapist may need to progress into an inferior glide of the humerus and consider the significant involvement of the full shoulder girdle complex.

Mobilization with movement – end range elevation (external rotation) (Fig 20.4)

This mobilization is indicated where the patient presents with a loss of functional range of external rotation or restriction of elevation due to loss of conjunct external rotation at or above 90° elevation. The patient is lying supine with the shoulder slightly abducted to the comfortable range, with the elbow flexed to 90° and the cervical spine neutral. The therapist is standing at the side of patient. The cephalic hand cups the head of the humerus with the palm, whereas the caudal hand supports the upper arm. The mobilization consists of the application of a posterolateral glide in the treatment plane of the scapula by the cephalic hand. Additional inferior glide can be applied with the caudal hand, allowing the humerus to translate posteriorly. The patient performs passive external rotation using the unaffected hand to passively push the hand of the affected arm laterally with a short stick while the therapist maintains the patient's elbow at their side, creating a 'spin' of the humerus into external rotation. Clinicians should ensure that the posterior mobilization force is maintained until the patient returns to a neutral position. The technique can progress into greater ranges of abduction/elevation (the quadrant position).

Mobilization with movement – end range elevation (inferior glide) (Fig 20.5)

This mobilization is indicated in patients with end range loss of elevation. The patient is lying supine with the scapula supported by the bed surface or a small folded towel. The therapist is standing at the head of the bed. The therapist grips the anterior forearm and posterior humerus in order to control elbow flexion. The technique consists of applying a postero-caudal glide at the end of range elevation. The patient is asked to perform an active arm elevation through scaption. The clinician should ensure that the humerus is in external rotation, and does not allow the elbow to bend/flex.

Mobilization with movement – elevation (shoulder girdle) (Fig 20.6)

This mobilization is indicated in patients with observable winging or dyskinesis of scapulo-humeral rhythm, or those with persistent shoulder pain with active elevation not responding to treatment of the gleno-humeral joint. The patient is sitting on a low back chair with the cervical

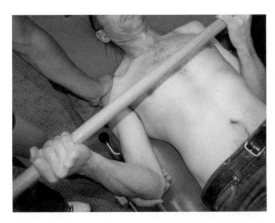

Fig 20.4 Mobilization with movement – end range elevation (external rotation).

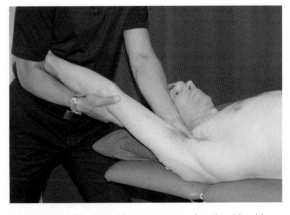

Fig 20.5 Mobilization with movement – elevation (shoulder girdle).

275

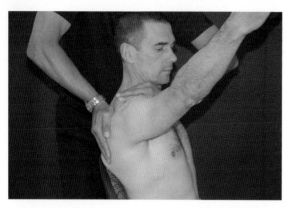

Fig 20.6 Mobilization with movement – end range elevation (inferior glide).

spine in neutral. The therapist is standing on the contra-lateral side of the patient. One hand contacts with the posterior hand on the superior edge of lateral one-third of the spine of the scapula, whereas the anterior hand provides stability to the medial half of the clavicle. The technique consists of gliding the scapula infero-medially, rotating the scapula externally and controlling any winging of the scapula bone. At the same time the patient is asked to perform active arm elevation through scaption. Finally, an assistant may also provide an additional postero-caudal glide of the humerus during elevation. Some important points are: (a) progression of the patient onto a closed chain environment may be accomplished by having them adopting a four-point kneeling stance, (b) having the patient sit back on his heels will recreate controlled weight bearing forces on the shoulder girdle during the application of a mobilization with movement which should now render the activity pain-free.

HAND BEHIND BACK

This movement is a multi-plane movement requiring a combination of shoulder extension, internal rotation and adduction components. Often limited by significant pain, this motion is often avoided by patients with impairments of the shoulder with a resulting loss of function including the ability to effectively dress, reach for a wallet and personal hygiene.

Mobilization with movement – hand behind back (Fig 20.7)

This mobilization is indicated in patients with pain or with a loss of the hand-behind-back movement including adduction, internal rotation, and extension. The patient is standing with the contralateral hip supported by a treatment plinth to counteract the adductory forces. A mobilization belt is draped over the contralateral shoulder, held anteriorly by the free hand and posteriorly by the involved arm hand. The therapist is standing at the side of the patient. A posterior hand is placed high in axilla with the palm facing away from the patient, and the anterior hand is supinated fully to grip the distal humerus with the thumb hooked into the cubital fossa of the patient. For this technique the therapist stabilizes the scapula with the cephalic hand and medially directed force from the posterior hand. The mobilization consists of an inferior glide of the humerus with the thumb of the anterior hand in the cubital fossa. At the same time, the patient moves the hand behind their back via the pull of the belt. Clinicians should ensure the patient does not attempt to lift the hand away from the back and ensure that the posterior hand force in the axilla is adductory and cephalic to stabilize the scapula.

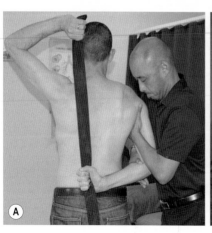
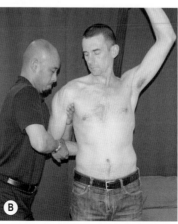

Fig 20.7 (A) Mobilization with movement – hand behind back (posterior view). (B) Mobilization with movement – hand behind back (anterior view).

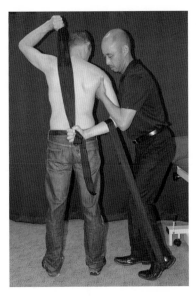

Fig 20.8 Mobilization with movement – hand behind back, belt assisted.

Mobilization with movement – hand behind back, belt assisted (Fig 20.8)

This technique is indicated in larger patients or smaller therapists and in those patients with pain or loss of hand behind back movement. The patient is standing with the contralateral hip supported by a treatment plinth to counteract adductory forces. The mobilization belt is draped over the contralateral shoulder and held anteriorly by the free hand and posteriorly by the involved side hand. Both hands of the therapist are placed high in the axilla with the palms facing away from patient. The mobilization belt is folded in half and hooked into the cubital fossa of the patient, and the toe of one foot in the belt loop with the heel on the floor for control of the belt force. For this technique the therapist stabilizes the scapula with the cephalic hand and a medially directed force from the posterior hand. The mobilization consists of an inferior glide of the humerus by pulling the belt by plantar-flexing the foot. At the same time, the patient moves the hand behind the back via the pull of belt. The clinician should ensure that the patient does not attempt to lift the hand away from the back. Some important points are: (a) to ensure hand force in the axilla is adductory and cephalic to stabilize the scapula; and (b) gentle pressure from the belt with the heel on the floor for control.

HORIZONTAL ADDUCTION MOTION

Reaching across the body to the opposite shoulder is an activity involving multiple articulations in addition to the gleno-humeral joint. Optimal functioning of the acromio-clavicular and sterno-clavicular joints is intimately associated with normal pain-free performance of cross body motion. Spinal mobilizations with arm movement may render shoulder movements pain-free and restore functional mobility when the neck is involved in dysfunction of the upper quadrant.

Mobilization with movement – horizontal adduction (AC/SC joints) (Fig 20.9)

This technique is indicated when there is pain reaching across the body towards the contralateral shoulder in the transverse plane. The patient is seated on a low back chair with the cervical spine neutral. The therapist is standing behind the patient with the hypothenar portion of the hand on the superior surface of the distal clavicle bone. The technique consists of an inferior glide of the clavicle, at the same time that the patient is asked for cross body reaching towards the contralateral shoulder or rib cage. Some important points are the presence of moderate pain-free crepitus is normal and to begin with gentle active movement progressing to more vigorous motion as irritability decreases.

Spinal mobilization with arm movement – horizontal adduction (Fig 20.10)

This technique is indicated when there is pain with cross body movement related to cervical dysfunction. The patient is seated with cervical spine in neutral. The therapist is standing behind the patient, with the side of a

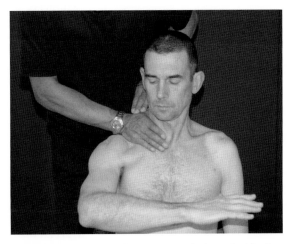

Fig 20.9 Mobilization with movement – horizontal adduction (AC/SC joints).

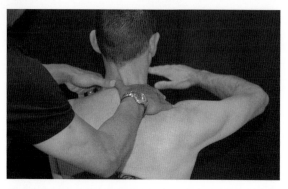

Fig 20.10 Spinal mobilization with arm movement – horizontal adduction.

thumb contacting the lateral slope of the involved cervical vertebrae spinous process. The thumb may be reinforced by the contralateral thumb or index finger tip. The mobilization intervention consists of applying a medial translation/rotation of the cervical vertebrae, at the same time that the patient is asked for cross body movement towards the contralateral shoulder or rib cage. Some important points are that the mobilization force controls but does not block the normal ipsilateral rotation of the cervical vertebrae and spinous process, and to begin with gentle active movement progressing to more vigorous motion as irritability decreases.

CONCLUSIONS

The inclusion of mobilization with movement interventions of the shoulder region into a multimodal approach of patients with neck and arm pain syndromes should be considered in order to improve the function and decrease the disability of the patient. The intensity and progression of the mobilizations should be adapted to the irritability of the tissue of the patient.

REFERENCES

Cheng, P.L., 2006. Simulation of Codman's paradox reveals a general law of motion. J. Biomech. 39, 1201–1207.

Hengeveld, E., Banks, K., Maitland, G.D. (Eds.), 2005. Maitland's peripheral manipulation. fourth ed. Elsevier/ Butterworth Heinemann, Edinburgh.

Hing, W.A., Bigalow, R., Bremner, T., 2008. Mulligan's Mobilisation with Movement: A review of the tenets & prescription of MWMs. New Zealand Journal of Physiotherapy 36, 34–54.

Hing, W.A., Bigalow, R., Bremner, T., 2009. Mulligans Mobilisation with Movement: A Systematic Review. J. Man. Manip. Ther. 17, E39–E66.

Hing, W.A., Reid, D.A., Monaghan, M., 2003. Manipulation of the cervical spine. Man. Ther. 8, 2–9.

Jones, M.A., Rivett, D.A. (Eds.), 2004. Clinical reasoning for manual therapists. first ed. Butterworth Heinemann, Edinburgh.

Kaltenborn, F.M., Evjenth, O., Kaltenborn, T.B., Morgan, D., Vollowitz, E., 2002. Manual Mobilization of the Joints: The Kaltenborn Method of Joint Examination and Treatment: The Extremities, sixth ed. Olaf Norlis Bokhandel, Oslo.

Miller, J., 1999. The Mulligan Concept – the next step in the evolution of manual therapy. Canadian Physiotherapy Association, Orthopaedic Division Review, March/April 9–13.

Miller, J., 2006. The Mulligan Concept: How: Clinical Application, When: Clinical Reasoning, Why: Clinical Research. Canadian Physiotherapy Association, Orthopaedic Division Review May/ June, 22–28.

Mulligan, B.R., 2003. Manual therapy: 'NAGS', 'SNAGS', 'MWMS', etc, third ed. Plane View Services, Wellington.

Chapter | 21 |

Motor control of the shoulder region

Mary E Magarey, Mark A Jones

INTRODUCTION

Motor control around the shoulder, its examination and management, are vast and complex topics. In this chapter, a brief background on motor control theory and the evidence in support of impairments in motor control around the shoulder is provided, together with a summary of the principles of motor learning in the context of shoulder rehabilitation. The focus is on control aspects of the scapulo-thoracic and gleno-humeral joints as directly relevant to shoulder function. While the focus here is on evaluation and management associated with motor control abilities and impairments, evaluation for and management of impairments in pain, range of movement, strength, endurance, power, and technique must also be addressed in a holistic context, with appropriate diagnostic considerations and a thorough bio-psychosocial approach. The influence of the remainder of the kinetic chain on shoulder function and of shoulder girdle influence on arm function should also be acknowledged and considered in both examination and management.

MOTOR CONTROL

Motor control theories proposed to explain possible mechanisms responsible for regulating movement address the roles of sensory systems (particularly vision, audition and proprioception) and central processes underpinning posture, movement and stability (Schmidt & Lee 2005,

© 2011 Elsevier Ltd.
DOI: 10.1016/B978-0-7020-3528-9.00021-2

279

Shumway-Cook & Woollacott 2007). The concept of a motor programme partially explains the infinite movement options available in performing even simple tasks. A motor programme is considered to be a pre-structured generalized code about the order of events, their relative timing and the relative force required across different tasks. For example, the sequencing of muscle activity and joint motion for shoulder elevation is included in a motor programme of elevation, which is supplemented by rules that specify the parameters related to the particular way the programme is executed according to the task, such as speed (Schmidt & Lee 2005). With increased variability of practice, the motor programme rules are strengthened, improving motor learning. Movement arises from the interactions of perceptual, cognitive and motor processes within the individual and interactions between the individual, the task and the environment (Shumway-Cook & Woollacott 2007). This 'systems' theory approach to motor control emphasizes the importance of assessing for impairments in all processes and being alert to their manifestation in different tasks and environments as a guide to commencing and progressing rehabilitation. Similarly, these interactions necessitate systematic reassessment of treatment interventions to reveal potential influences of one process (e.g. perception) on another (e.g. motor control).

Motor control and joint stability

Motor control and joint stability are closely linked and should be considered as a dynamic process of controlling static position while allowing movement with control (Hodges 2004). Panjabi's now familiar model of three inter-related systems responsible for control of the neutral zone (Panjabi 1992a,b, 1996) forms the basis for much recent work in relation to function and differences in behaviour of different types of muscles. As a result, two groups of muscles have been identified that fulfil different roles – 'stabilizers' or 'local system' and 'mobilizers' or 'global system' (Hodges 2004, Magee & Zachazewski 2007). While this categorization is debated (McGill 2007) and further research is needed to clarify this distinction and its clinical efficacy, we find this construct helpful in focussing assessment and treatment procedures, with excellent results.

Based on a review of the effect of musculoskeletal pain on motor activity and control, Sterling et al (2001) proposed a 'neuromuscular activation model' that identifies dysfunction of synergistic muscle control as a specific and important consequence of pain and injury. This model provides explanation for alteration in muscle activation, proprioception, arthrogenous muscle weakness and muscle fibre changes in the presence of pain. Examination is recommended of all components of the neuromuscular system, including dysfunction of synergistic control, timing of muscle activation, patterns of co-contraction and

proprioceptive control in a patient with musculoskeletal pain, especially pain of any duration. This recommendation, built on the hypothesis related to the relationship between afferent nociceptive input and motor control and the principles of motor learning, forms the foundation of our approach to evaluation and management of patients with shoulder dysfunction.

Evidence of altered motor control around the scapula

Alterations to muscle function around the scapula have been demonstrated in the presence of cervical pain or headaches (Nederhand et al 2000, Falla 2004, Szeto et al 2005, 2009, Falla et al 2007, Jull et al 2008). With respect to the shoulder, a consistent recruitment pattern has been demonstrated in asymptomatic shoulders related to active abduction in the scapular plane (Wadsworth & Bullock-Saxton 1997, Moraes et al 2008) or response to sudden release from an abducted position (Cools et al 2002, 2003) and reaching tasks (Roy et al 2008). Upper trapezius is activated first, followed by serratus anterior, middle trapezius and finally lower trapezius muscles. The temporal characteristics are delayed but not changed by fatigue in asymptomatic subjects (Moraes et al 2008).

A reasonably consistent pattern of decreased activity has been demonstrated in both lower trapezius and serratus anterior and increased activity in upper trapezius in patients with shoulder pain or pathology during different tasks (Glousman et al 1988, Scovazzo et al 1991, Pink et al 1993, Ludewig & Cook 2000, Cools et al 2003, 2004, 2005, 2007a, McClure et al 2006, Roy et al 2008). Kibler (1998) observed that inhibition of lower trapezius and serratus anterior appears to be a non-specific response to shoulder pain irrespective of the pathology. Lower trapezius muscle has a predominance of type I fibres whereas upper trapezius has predominantly type II (Simons et al 1999), with the implication that lower trapezius is best suited for postural and stabilizing roles and upper trapezius for phasic activity. Findings of delayed and/or reduced activity in lower trapezius and serratus anterior in response to shoulder pain coupled with increased activity in upper trapezius, while not universally reported, lend support to this hypothesis. These results support findings from other body regions of a neuromuscular impairment associated with pain in an adjacent joint (Cowan et al 2001, 2002, 2003, Hodges 2004, Colné & Thoumie 2006, Hertel & Olmsted-Kramer 2007, Jull et al 2008).

Altered scapular position is common in association with shoulder pain with typical patterns identified and given various names. Very common is the 'Scapular Downwardly Rotated Syndrome' (Sahrmann 2002), also termed 'Type 1 Scapular Dyskinesis' (Kibler et al 2002, Kibler 2003) and SICK scapula (**S**capular mal-position, **I**nferior medial border prominence, **C**oracoid pain and mal-position and dysKinesis of scapular movement) (Burkhart et al 2003). This pattern appears to be associated with insufficiency of the upward rotation force couple and over-activity or increased tone in the antagonist muscles, in particular levator scapulae, rhomboids and pectoralis minor (Kibler 2003).

Serratus anterior and lower trapezius muscles are important components of the scapular upward rotation force couple, particularly above 60° of arm elevation (Bagg & Forrest 1986, 1988). Decreased activity in lower trapezius and serratus anterior associated with arm elevation (Ludewig & Cook 2000, Cools et al 2007a) in patients with sub-acromial pain supports the observation of delayed or reduced upward rotation in the clinical setting. Increased upper trapezius activity under heavier load (Ludewig & Cook 2000) and in the upper ranges of elevation (Cools et al 2007a) possibly reflects a compensation for decreased activity in lower trapezius and serratus anterior and/or an attempt to overcome the increased tone in the antagonists.

A second altered scapular posture, an elevated scapula, is described as Type III scapular dyskinesis (Kibler et al 2002, Kibler 2003). This pattern appears to present in association with either shoulder stiffness into elevation or major rotator cuff dysfunction, such that the deltoid/rotator cuff force couple is disrupted and the humeral head translates superiorly to abut against the undersurface of the acromion. Increased activity in upper trapezius and levator scapulae is dominant.

Not all responses to shoulder pain are consistent (Cools et al 2003, 2004, 2005, 2007a), possibly reflecting the different patterns demonstrated in subgroups within sample populations with the same diagnosis (Graichen et al 2001, Hébert et al 2002, Roy et al 2008). The observation of variations in patterns of muscle activity supports the need to address each patient's impairment during assessment and management.

Altered scapular positioning and scapular plane elevation are frequently associated with increased thoracic kyphosis, cervical flexion or forward head posture (Crawford & Jull 1993, Greenfield et al 1995, Ludewig & Cook 1996, Bullock et al 2005), supporting the kinematic relationship of spinal posture, scapular posture and shoulder elevation. While spinal posture may not be correlated with specific shoulder pathology (Lewis et al 2005a,b), its relationship to shoulder elevation warrants attention in rehabilitation.

Clearly, when considering rehabilitation of the shoulder, attention to the scapular muscle impairments, particularly those related to motor control, is imperative (Ebaugh et al 2005). Equally the shoulder should not be considered in isolation from the cervical and thoracic spine (Jull et al 2008) and the control and movement patterns of the lumbar spine, pelvis and lower limbs (Kibler 1998). While in this chapter the focus is on motor control of the shoulder, the important contributions of these other areas must not be forgotten.

Evidence of altered motor control around the gleno-humeral joint

Evidence related to local stabilizing muscle function around the gleno-humeral joint is less robust, with only two studies reporting on rotator cuff control. David et al (2000) demonstrated that, during isokinetic gleno-humeral rotation, the rotator cuff and biceps brachii when considered as a group, were always activated prior to the superficial muscles, deltoid and pectoralis major, in asymptomatic shoulders and there was always an element of co-contraction, regardless of direction or speed of rotation. The rotator cuff group was also always activated before movement of the isokinetic device's lever arm. This finding supports the hypothesis that the rotator cuff functions in a joint stabilizing role. Delayed activation of the rotator cuff/biceps in individuals with unstable shoulders was also demonstrated in a clinical, but not a research setting.

Hess et al (2005) demonstrated delayed activation of sub-scapularis during a reaction time test into external rotation in throwers with painful shoulders compared to a matched group of asymptomatic volunteers, hypothesizing that sub-scapularis fulfilled a joint stabilization role. However, their testing protocol required use of infraspinatus as a prime mover. Lumbar spine research demonstrates that competing demands on the central nervous system lead to an alteration in muscle use (Hodges 2004) so that when required to function in its primary role, a muscle's secondary stabilizing role is compromised.

Ginn et al (2009) demonstrated from EMG research that the rotator cuff does not function at equal loads through all activities, rather the majority of activation is direction specific. The antagonist cuff muscle was activated at approximately 6% MVC during each of the movements. However, given only 1–3% MVC is required to stiffen a joint (Cholewicki & McGill 1996) their findings do not disprove the stabilization role. There is also a wealth of biomechanical literature that supports a stabilization role for the rotator cuff (Clark & Harryman 1992, Wuelker et al 1995, Burkhart 1996, Kibler 1998, Lee et al 2000), particularly sub-scapularis and infraspinatus/teres minor muscles (Burkhart 1996).

EVALUATION OF MOTOR CONTROL AROUND THE SHOULDER GIRDLE

The assessments described below are used to guide motor control retraining. Impairments in motor control exist within a continuum and manifest as poor postural awareness combined with inability to produce smooth kinematically correct movements through full range without compensation under varying demands of posture, load and speed. While severe impairments will be apparent even in gravity eliminated positions, lesser impairments will often only be evident in certain ranges of movement, loads (Ludewig & Cook 2000, McClure et al 2001, 2006), speeds (Roy et al 2008) and during distracting tasks (Hodges 2004). Equally side to side comparison provides evidence of bilateral movement dysfunction, possibly indicating pre-disposition to impairment (Hébert et al 2002, McClure et al 2006) and/or more central contribution (Sterling et al 2001) and a poorer prognosis to change. With the aim of converting identified motor control impairments into retraining exercises, each assessment evaluates where (range, posture, load, speed) the patient has control and where that control is lost, attending to all components in the kinetic chain (upper and lower trunk, scapula, gleno-humeral). Assessment is varied with respect to position (against gravity versus gravity eliminated or assisted) to identify the position/function in which control is sufficient to initiate retraining.

Postural assessment

Detailed evaluation of posture allows formation of initial hypotheses in relation to potential impairments in motor control. Postural abnormalities may be associated with movement and control impairments, although an association must not be assumed. Such hypotheses must be tested with movement, resistive and palpatory assessment and specific postural impairment correction during provocative active movements to ascertain the effect (Lewis et al 2005a). Static posture should be assessed in positions relevant to the patient's function and symptom production, not just in a standardized starting position. In addition to visual assessment, the scapular slide test (Kibler 1998, 2003) is a validated measure of scapular resting position, although resting position is not necessarily correlated with function and more objective measures of spinal posture are available (Jull et al 2008).

If an apparent postural impairment is identified, its association to the patient's presenting condition should be tested to determine its direct or indirect relevance by assessing whether alteration of the impairment, either passively or actively, influences the patient's symptoms or sense of 'normalcy'. Although not confirmatory, alteration in response to postural correction and the ability to achieve a corrected position provide an indication of the significance of the positional fault to the symptom presentation, level of awareness or control impairment.

Evaluation of movement impairments and awareness

The focus of this movement assessment is not 'diagnostic' of structural sources of symptoms, but rather on impairments of awareness, movement and control, however always with appropriate caution and monitoring of symptom provocation.

All active movements of the shoulder girdle provide an indication of motor control, in addition to movement awareness, dissociation, relative activity within and between force couples, more so than specific strength or endurance. Therefore, all active shoulder movements should be examined as part of an evaluation of motor control. Any movement impairments are evaluated for their relevance to provocation of symptoms. Assistance with active movement, such as the Scapular Assistance Test (SAT) (Kibler et al 2002, 2006, Kibler 2003) (Fig 21.1 and Box 21.1) to facilitate scapular upward rotation or passive posterior translation for an anteriorly placed humeral head will, for example, often improve movement and lessen symptoms.

Active physiological gleno-humeral movements that are most useful from a motor control perspective include:

- Flexion, abduction, scapular plane abduction: all provide an indication of relative scapular to gleno-humeral contribution, timing of movement of each component and a visual impression of activation of the key muscle groups.
- Gleno-humeral rotations, particularly in 90° abduction/flexion: they demonstrate the ability to move the gleno-humeral joint on a stable scapula and an awareness of dissociation of the arm from the scapula.

Traditional manual muscle tests provide an indication of strength of specific movement directions, not individual muscles, as both stabilizer and mobilizer muscles contribute to the generation of force. Observation of relative control of scapula and gleno-humeral joint during maximal strength tests is useful but does not identify specific individual muscle

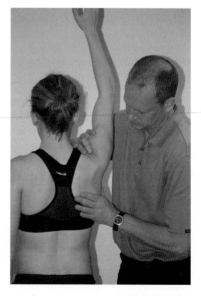

Fig 21.1 Scapular Assistance Test (SAT) (Kibler 2003, Kibler et al 2002, 2006)

Box 21.1 Description / discussion of tests

Figure 21.1

The scapular assistance test involves the therapist providing manual assistance to upward rotation of the scapula during gleno-humeral elevation through flexion, abduction or scapular plane abduction.

Figure 21.2

Strength of rotator cuff muscles is more accurately evaluated when the scapula is supported in a retracted position, such that it provides a stable base from which the rotator cuff can work. The therapist maintains the scapula in a retracted position with manual pressure while providing manual resistance to the arm for the relevant rotator cuff test.

Figure 21.3

A shoulder shrug in standing with the arms by the side demonstrates the patient's ability to elevate the shoulder girdles to full passive range, the pattern of activation associated with the movement and symmetry between sides. Shoulder shrug is frequently accompanied by significant low cervical flexion and upper cervical extension, scapular elevation combined with protraction and apparent gleno-humeral internal rotation, possibly representing a dominance of levator scapulae over upper trapezius, as the forward poking head lengthens the upper component of the muscle, thus allowing it more leverage to complete the movement at its distal end. The accompanying scapular movement is reflective of the dominance of levator scapulae and pectoralis minor. Correction of this movement pattern leads to an inability to raise the scapulae to their full passive range. A tape or ruler can be used to measure vertical distance between the ear lobe and the shoulder girdle to provide an objective outcome measure.

The hypothesized basis for this test is that, in the elevated arm position, upper trapezius is in its maximally shortened position, so if lengthened in its resting posture, as with a downwardly rotated scapula, attaining the same level of shoulder shrug as with the arms by the side will be difficult. Lack of passive flexibility or overactivity in the levator scapulae, rhomboids or latissimus dorsi will limit passive range of shoulder shrug in this position. An equivalent measure may be taken to compare the range in the two positions.

Figure 21.4

Gleno-humeral rotations, particularly in 90 degrees of abduction/flexion, demonstrate the ability to move the gleno-humeral joint on a stable scapula and an awareness of dissociation of the arm from the scapula. Differences in the ability to dissociate in standing and in prone/supine provide indication of the effect of load on the scapular stabilizers and rotator cuff during this task.

This analysis can be made more objective by measuring distance moved by the acromion from its neutral start position during the arm movement. Ideally, movement should be minimal. Excessive scapular movement leads to greater acromial movement from its resting position.

Figure 21.5

Evaluation of awareness of scapular movement can be undertaken using scapular PNF patterns. Given that the movements involved are unfamiliar to the patient, several steps are taken in this evaluation:

- Explain the direction of movement required, using cues such as 'Take the point of your shoulder towards the corner of your eye', while at the same time, touching the corresponding acromial angle and outer corner of the eye and doing the movement with the patient passively, using traditional PNF hand holds and principles. For the opposite direction, 'Take the point of your shoulder blade [while touching it with your fingers] down towards the opposite hip/back pocket' and again, guide the patient in the appropriate movement direction.
- Talk the patient through the movement while performing it passively, ensuring availability of full passive range.
- Ask the patient to assist with the movement, following which unassisted performance determines their ability to replicate it.
- If the patient has difficulty grasping the feel of the movement, further facilitation can be given by means of verbal encouragement, resistance to the movement through range, holds at end of range with slow eccentric contraction and reversals etc (Fig 21.5A).
- In patients with poor awareness or control, the scapula tends to follow a curvilinear path rather than a diagonal, with jerky uncoordinated movement. Frequently, the scapula moves into excessive protraction and anterior tilt when attempting the 'up and forward' direction in particular, as demonstrated in Figure 21.5B. Such an inability to control the movement in a direct diagonal and to the desired end point is an indication that use of PNF as a hands-on facilitation may be indicated in the early stages of rehabilitation.

Figure 21.6

The test is performed in side lying, tested arm uppermost, supported on the therapist's arm in approximately 120° elevation, such that the therapist can apply progressively increased resistance into scapular protraction, gleno-humeral elevation and external rotation with the heel of the other hand against the lateral border of the scapula used to assess and resist scapular upward rotation. The activation can be tested isometrically, isotonically both concentrically and, at higher levels, eccentrically. Poor activation is felt as a sluggish response of the scapula to resistance and/or more 'give' to the movement. The test may be progressed from simply holding the arm while applying resistance to the scapula to resisting protraction and elevation/external rotation on the arm concurrent with upward rotation on the scapula.

Continued

Box 21.1 **Description / discussion of tests—cont'd**

Figure 21.7

Evaluation in four point kneeling

- Initially, spontaneous posture is noted with respect to spinal, scapular, shoulder and hip alignments and the position maintained for an arbitrary period (e.g. 2 minutes) while observing for fatigue. Typical compensation strategies include locking the elbows into full extension; arms into endrange rotation; dropping the trunk forward, leading to a passive scapular retraction and thoracic extension, increased lumbar lordosis, forward head posture and cervical flexion; elevation of the shoulder girdle towards the ears; scapular winging or tremor of the arm and/or shoulder girdle muscles. Asymmetries from neutral are highlighted to the patient and correction facilitated by passive guidance if necessary. In this context neutral refers to normal spinal curves and scapular posture taking account of patient's individual spinal mobility. The patient's abilities and impairments are then recorded.
- The patient is instructed to shift weight onto one hand, initially without lifting the other arm and then, in conjunction with arm elevation so that the pattern of head on neck, trunk, scapular and arm control can be further evaluated. Again, impairments are recorded. This assessment may be taken through further steps to increase the challenge to match relevant sporting requirements. Raising diagonally opposite arm and leg, in a full push-up position, undertaking the assessment with the legs and trunk on an unstable surface, such as a gym ball or the hand balancing on an unstable surface, such as a slide mat, spin disk or ball all provide additional challenge to the system and may highlight impairments. These steps also integrate the whole kinetic chain so impairments more distant to the shoulder may be identified.

Figure 21.8

Evaluation in four point kneeling

- During evaluation of spinal dissociation, a frequent finding is an inability to position the head in neutral without concomitant thoracic and lumbar extension. Instruction to extend the neck frequently leads to a whole spine extension pattern. A request for pelvic neutral may have a similar effect, with the patient unable to isolate lumbar spine movement.
- With pro/retraction of the scapula, the chest 'drops through' the scapulae on retraction and is elevated between them on protraction. Typically, a patient with shoulder pain is unable to perform this movement independent of thoracic flexion/extension. An inability to fully protract (push up plus position) is also often observed. Education about the impairment and facilitation of an improved movement is undertaken to determine how 'fixed' the impairment is in the patient's motor patterning and therefore, how significant it might be in the context of the presenting problem.

Figure 21.9

The therapist palpates the humeral head with one hand, ensuring no restraint of humeral head movement. This hand feels for humeral head translation or altered quality of movement through each stage of the test. The therapist also observes scapular and spinal control and movement and enquires about provocation of symptoms.

- With the patient's arm by the side, elbow flexed to 90°, neutral forearm rotation, manual resistance is applied slowly through the wrist to an isometric contraction. This contraction is repeated in as many positions as appropriate for the particular patient's presentation. Do not stop in the sequence of positions when an impairment is noted as activity regularly performed at higher range, such as throwing, may lead to better function in this range. The movement is repeated from the neutral start position into the opposite rotation.
- In most instances, at least three elevation positions are tested – neutral, 45–60° elevation and an end position relevant to function – for example, 110° elevation in the scapular plane for a thrower or full elevation for a swimmer, mimicking the catch position.
- The test procedures are repeated using an isotonic contraction through the full available range, first in one rotation and then the other, ensuring that the movement is one of pure rotation.
- If no impairment is detected through any part of the test, it is repeated at higher speed, with an eccentric component, quick reversals or with increased load. Occasionally, the resistance of the therapist's hand is sufficient to facilitate co-contraction. Asking the patient to repeat the test movements with a small weight in the hand may lead to altered humeral head control or the patient may be able to feel when control is lost even if the therapist cannot.
- Once a position of impairment is detected, whether isometrically or dynamically, small variations of positions are evaluated until a position of control is found as close to where control is lost as possible. If impairment on the DRST is prioritized for inclusion in a management plan, this would be the position where training is commenced.

Figure 21.10

- The start position is usually sitting with the arm supported in 60–90° scapular plane elevation, neutral rotation. The start position must be painfree, with a relaxed scapula and relatively neutral spinal position. The therapist palpates the axillary aspect of sub-scapularis with the tips of the middle two fingers, usually from a posterior direction, with the pads adjacent to latissimus dorsi on the posterior axillary wall. Concurrently, the therapist places the pad of the thumb vertically along the tendon of infraspinatus/teres minor so that activation of both components of the force couple can be palpated simultaneously. Finding the sub-scapularis tendon may be difficult on some people,

---

Box 21.1 Description / discussion of tests—cont'd

especially those with a superiorly translated humeral head or hypertrophy of either latissimus dorsi or pectoralis major. Confirmation of correct positioning is made by gentle resistance into first one rotation and then the other while feeling for increased tone in the relevant tendon.

- Very gentle traction is applied to the humerus and the patient asked to 'draw the arm into the socket'. The therapist palpates both tendons to evaluate levels of contraction while monitoring unwanted activation in other muscles. Manual facilitation by pressure on the tendons may be useful, reinforced by verbal encouragement and visual imagery. This is an unfamiliar task, so initial assessment should be on the non-affected side.

- If co-contraction can be felt but only in association with superficial muscle activity, training is undertaken to reduce the extraneous activity. If no co-contraction can be facilitated, further tactile stimulation and/or imagery may help. For example, the anteriorly unstable shoulder may respond to instruction to 'draw the arm up and back' in association with a traction force combined with gentle internal rotation, thus biasing the facilitation to the external rotators, while the superiorly placed humeral head may respond better to a suggestion to 'draw in and gently push down on my finger in your armpit' in conjunction with pressure on sub-scapularis, although excessive activation of latissimus dorsi and pectoralis major may be the result of this suggestion. Persistence with facilitation and multiple trials may be needed to achieve success. In the future, biofeedback with real time ultrasound is planned to facilitate training.

- Once the co-contraction can be achieved, a benchmark is established to form the basis for a home programme and further training, during which, the patient must be able to find the sub-scapularis tendon and co-contract without the traction facilitation. An arbitrary 10 repeats

of 10-second hold with slow, smooth build-up and release of contraction is used as a goal before progression. Once this can be achieved, the direction of progression depends on the presentation of the patient. If an athlete whose primary range of poor control is in elevation, progression is quickly made into positions within the DRST where control was lost, whereas the patient with pathology of the rotator cuff or sub-acromial bursa may need much slower and more deliberate co-contraction training before any load is applied to the arm.

Figure 21.11

The patient drives the hands forwards and upwards in a position of elevation, external rotation, elbow extension, thus facilitating the upward rotation component of the movement. Slight tension maintained on a lighter weight theraband into gleno-humeral external rotation ensures that the patient does not drift into internal rotation and scapular position of downward rotation/anterior tilt. The lumbar and cervical spines must be maintained in a neutral position.

Figure 21.12

The theraband is looped over the shoulder and under the opposite foot. The patient catches hold the theraband and steps through the loop. Placing the foot behind in a walk-stand position provides a down & back force on the shoulder, facilitating correct movement of the acromion towards the corner of the eye. Maintenance of chin tuck, arm external rotation and a neutral lumbar spine will all assist correct movement of the scapula.

The reverse 'down & back' pattern can also be trained by placing the theraband over a door and shutting the door while looping the theraband under the axilla. A small towel placed in the axilla makes this more comfortable. The patient stands facing the door so that the theraband pulls the shoulder girdle up and forwards and works the scapula down and back towards the opposite hip.

---

dysfunction, simply a faulty movement pattern under load. Evaluation and possible correction of scapular position, for example with the Scapular Retraction Test (Kibler et al 2006), during manual muscle testing is essential to determine whether the scapula is fulfilling its stabilizing role (Fig 21.2).

Evaluation of specific motor control impairments around the scapula

On the basis of the evidence and clinical experience, we use the following key movement impairment tests to gain

a broad picture of the ability and level of impairment of the axio-scapular muscles. If movement impairment is noted, its significance is evaluated using the principles outlined above. These assessments are by no means exhaustive, but representative of those commonly found useful.

Shoulder shrug (Roberts 2009)

A shoulder shrug in standing with the arms both by the side and overhead demonstrates the patient's ability to elevate the shoulder girdles to full passive range, the

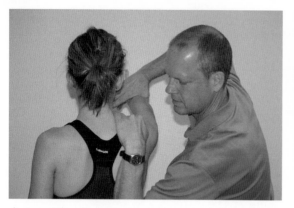

Fig 21.2 Scapular Retraction Test (SRT) (Kibler et al., 2006)

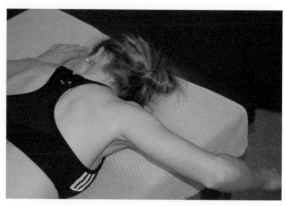

Fig 21.4 Gleno-humeral rotation on a stable scapula.

pattern of activation and movement symmetry and the effect of the altered muscle balance in different arm positions. A tape or ruler can be used to measure vertical distance between the ear lobe and the shoulder girdle to provide an objective outcome measure (Fig 21.3).

Scapular control through gleno-humeral rotations in prone and supine (Sahrmann 2002)

Gleno-humeral rotations in 90° abduction or flexion demonstrate the ability to move the gleno-humeral joint on a stable scapula and an awareness of dissociation between arm and scapular movement (Fig 21.4). Poor awareness leads to excessive scapular elevation, anterior tilt and protraction during internal rotation and the reverse on external rotation, or simply an inability to maintain a stable position. Measurement of acromial movement from neutral start position during the arm movement makes the test more objective.

Scapular PNF patterns (Voss et al 1985)

Awareness of movement of the scapula in isolation from the arm is difficult. Use of the scapular component of the traditional PNF diagonal arm patterns provides useful information on the kinaesthetic awareness of the scapula (Fig 21.5). Given that this is an unfamiliar movement, it is unreasonable to expect a patient to perform it without some facilitation and education. More detailed description of these tests can be found in Magarey & Jones (2003a).

Evaluation of range and control of scapular upward rotation

Scapular upward rotation occurs actively in conjunction with elevation of the arm. Therefore, the optimal position in which to evaluate activity in the upward rotation force couples is with the arm in elevation greater than 90°, with resistance applied through the arm to gleno-humeral elevation and external rotation and

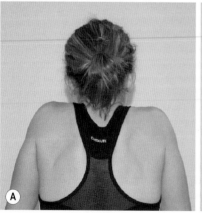

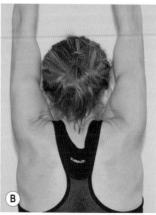

Fig 21.3 (A) Shoulder shrug with arms by the side. (B) Shoulder shrug with arms in full elevation.

(A)

(B)

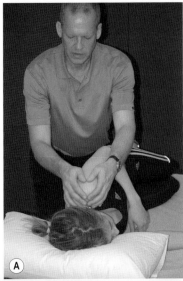

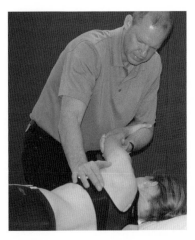

Fig 21.6 Evaluation of scapular upward rotation in gleno-humeral elevation.

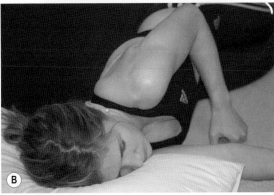

Fig 21.5 Evaluation of scapular movement awareness using scapular PNF patterns. (A) Manual correction and guidance into a more normal movement pattern. (B) Poor movement pattern during scapular movement in an up & forward direction.

position for re-training. Positional and movement impairments of the scapula and humerus are observed and loss of control/position from either identified as the limiting factor.

Steps in the evaluation include observation of spontaneous posture and muscular endurance with a sustained hold, scapular and gleno-humeral control during weight shift from one arm to the other (Fig 21.7), dissociation (the ability to isolate movement of one body part from another) of different regions of the spine and between spine and scapula (Fig 21.8), control of scapular and cervical movements, endurance of pro/retraction while weight-bearing on one or both hands and with trunk movement on a fixed hand. All components can be progressed to more challenging situations, such as with the trunk on a gym ball or hand on an unstable surface, as appropriate for the patient. More detailed

through the lateral border and inferior angle of the scapula against upward rotation (Fig 21.6) The stage of the assessment, the quality of contraction of this important force couple, the load applied through the arm and the number of repetitions are all useful clinical outcome measures.

Evaluation of four point kneeling

Four-point kneeling, while itself not particularly functional, is useful for assessing patients' dissociation and control capabilities. The steps can also be applied in prone on elbows or modified plantigrade (i.e. standing with hands supported on table or wall) with the aim of identifying where the patient has control and where that control is lost thereby providing an effective starting

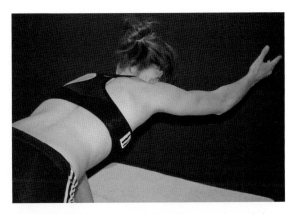

Fig 21.7 Evaluation in four point kneeling: scapular and gleno-humeral control in a single arm loaded position.

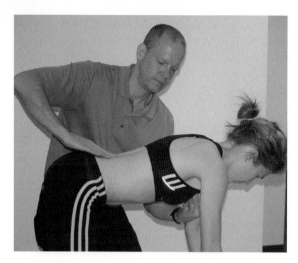

Fig 21.8 Dissociation evaluation in four-point kneeling: scapular protraction in a spinal neutral position.

description of these tests can be found in Magarey & Jones (2003a).

Evaluation of specific thoracic extension and control of scapular retraction

The patient's ability to perform thoracic extension in a relatively segmental fashion provides an indication of the priority for its re-training during rehabilitation. One effective evaluation is facilitated inter-segmental extension from C7 to T7/8 over a gym ball, with the trunk remaining in contact with the ball to reduce the lumbar spine contribution. Once relative segmental thoracic extension is achieved, assessment is progressed by addition of scapular retraction and arm movements.

Evaluation of isolated motor control around the shoulder

Dynamic rotary stability test (DRST) (Magarey & Jones 2003a,b)

The DRST is used to evaluate the rotator cuff's ability to maintain the humeral head centred in the glenoid when loaded through rotation. DRST is predicated on the knowledge that the humeral head should remain centred in the glenoid throughout rotation range in any position of elevation, except at end-range, where coupled translation forces the humeral head to translate (Harryman et al 1990, Terry et al 1991). When dynamic control is lacking, the humeral head is felt to translate anteriorly, posteriorly or superiorly when the rotator cuff is loaded. In more subtle situations, symptom provocation, alteration in the contraction quality, or compensation elsewhere alerts the examiner to dysfunction without the sensation of humeral head translation. The patient's subjective sensation of 'stability' during testing is also informative.

DRST is undertaken in different parts of the elevation range from neutral towards the patient's symptomatic functional position(s) (Fig 21.9). The number of positions in which the test is performed depends on the irritability of the condition, the general physical status of the patient, the clarity with which the patient can identify the symptomatic position(s) and the demands placed on the shoulder by the patient. The aim is to find the position(s) in range where the patient has humeral head control as close as possible to the position at which control is lost when isometric and progressively challenging dynamic load is applied to the arm. The amount of resistance added is light/moderate, as the assessment is one of the ability to stabilize, rather than one of rotation strength. All movements are performed in one direction first rather than alternately as patients find this easier. If lack of control is identified, rehabilitation can be undertaken starting from positions of control to facilitate

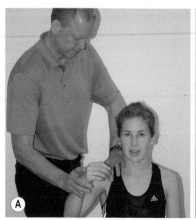
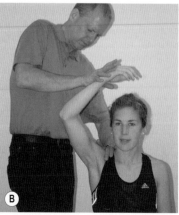

Fig 21.9 Dynamic rotary stability test (Magarey & Jones 2003a,b). (A) Evaluation of humeral head movement during isometric rotation in low range of elevation. (B) Evaluation of humeral head movement during isometric rotation in high range of elevation.

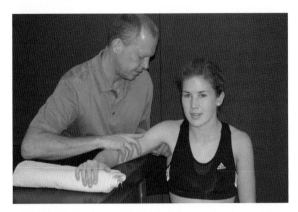

Fig 21.10 Dynamic relocation test (Magarey & Jones 2003a,b)

activation of the rotator cuff with progression to more challenging positions. More detailed description of this test may be found in Magarey & Jones (2003b).

Dynamic relocation test (DRT) (Magarey & Jones 2003a,b)

The DRT is a test of the ability of the rotator cuff, particularly the lower elements, to stabilize the humeral head in the glenoid by means of co-contraction against a de-stabilizing load. Once the ability to isolate the co-contraction has been determined in an optimal position, it can be evaluated in different positions and during different tasks. If a patient is unable to achieve more than the very basic levels of the DRST, assessment should start with the DRT. The principles of testing are similar to those for the cranio-cervical flexion test (Jull et al 2008) and transversus abdominis activation (Hodges 2004).

Patient education about test performance is important as it is an unfamiliar task. Use of diagrams and/or anatomical models is helpful so that the patient understands that the movement required is one of a subtle 'drawing in' of the humeral head to the glenoid via co-contraction of infraspinatus/teres minor and sub-scapularis with minimal involvement of the superficial muscles, in response to a gentle longitudinal movement applied to the arm (Fig 21.10). Occasionally, patients' ability to co-contract is enhanced in a loaded, closed kinetic chain position. More detailed description of this test may be found in Magarey & Jones (2003b).

MANAGEMENT OF MOTOR CONTROL IMPAIRMENTS AROUND THE SHOULDER GIRDLE

Motor learning refers to the processes associated with practice or experience that lead to the acquisition/reacquisition of relatively permanent movement capability

(Schmidt & Lee 2005, Shumway-Cook & Woollacott 2007). Rehabilitation strategies should be tailored to the individual's goals and specific neuromuscular impairments and motor control capabilities that may vary in different body segments and over different tasks.

While the Fitts & Posner (1967) (cognitive, associative, autonomous) model of motor learning is perhaps more familiar, Vereijken et al (1992) described another three-stage (novice, advanced, expert) theory of motor learning that accounts for reductions in body degrees of freedom seen in child development and new skill acquisition in general. Given that much research around disruptions to motor control relates to freezing of degrees of freedom (Cowan et al 2001, 2002, 2003, Hodges 2004, Colné & Thoumie 2006, Hertel & Olmsted-Kramer 2007, Jull et al 2008), we feel this model complements and adds to the useful model of Fitts & Posner (1967). The novice stage involves the learner freezing degrees of freedom by co-contracting agonists and antagonists to constrain a joint to simplify the movement, as with the rigid bracing of the wrist when first learning to use a hammer. Degrees of freedom are progressively released through the advanced and expert stages enabling movement at more joints and more sophisticated muscle synergies across multiple joints until smooth, coordinated movements are performed. This theory offers rationale for the clinical effectiveness of strategic posturing and external support commonly used in early stages of rehabilitation such as re-training co-contraction of sub-scapularis and infraspinatus initially with the arm supported in a stabilized scapular and gleno-humeral neutral position. Decreasing degrees of freedom requirements at the scapula through external support of the table and neutral positioning simplifies the task allowing the patient to focus on the correct activation.

Shoulder complex rehabilitation exercises should be individualized to specific impairments identified from the examination as potential contributors to the patients' activity (e.g. shoulder elevation or throwing) and participation limitations (e.g. activities of daily living or sport) (Graichen et al 2001, Hébert et al 2002, Roy et al 2008). The focus in relation to motor learning theory and research in this chapter is limited to retraining of skills with which patients are already familiar, not learning new skills. While this implies commencing with the associative/advanced stage of motor skill development, pre-existing impairments in posture and movement patterns commonly require that attention is given to the cognitive/novice stage to ensure understanding and correct performance (e.g. retraining shoulder elevation with less scapular protraction). Awareness training is generally started in neutral positions while control training is commenced from neutral or a position close to the position of impairment where the action/hold can be performed correctly.

Patient understanding and motivation, goal setting, practice and feedback (Schmidt & Lee 2005, Shumway-Cook & Woollacott 2007, Sousa 2006) facilitate motor learning. Understanding, where explanations are meaningful to the individual, enhances patient motivation, attention and learning. The more thoroughly information is processed, the deeper the learning and more likely the transfer to new situations outside the therapeutic setting (Sousa 2006). Explanations of assessment findings and management recommendations, linked to research and successful clinical outcomes, use of anatomical pictures and models and opportunities to ask questions and summarize main points all promote deeper learning.

Goal setting also facilitates motivation and learning. Specific, absolute goals of moderate difficulty produce better performance than either vague (e.g. 'do your best') (Kyllo & Landers 1995, Schmidt & Lee 2005) or no goals. Specific goals, both short and long term assist patient focus and facilitate performance while providing a reference for monitoring progress (Kyllo & Landers 1995).

Practice is recognized as the single most important variable influencing learning with large improvements early and smaller improvements later (Schmidt & Lee 2005, Shumway-Cook & Woollacott 2007). While synaptic connections are strengthened through experience and repetition (Spitzer 1999), success during exercise enhances learning necessitating exercises chosen are ones that can be successfully achieved with good kinematic control and no symptom aggravation. Successful exercise performance in one position is progressed to other positions or activities, leading to improved and more generalized learning. The basic premise is that with practice, people develop rules about their motor behaviour, not individual movements, and these rules are more effectively learned for use in other, even novel tasks, if the experience is varied rather than constant.

Augmented feedback regarding performance of a movement or exercise is considered a critical variable to motor learning; second only to practice itself (Schmidt & Lee 2005). Performance feedback can be provided visually, as with video, real-time ultrasound (RTUS) or EMG-based biofeedback or verbally, typically highlighting some aspect of the movement pattern that is difficult to perceive (e.g. recognition of spinal posture/movement during shoulder elevation). Inherent feedback refers to sensory information directly available to the individual during or resulting from the execution of a movement. Understanding when control is lost is essential for home motor control exercises to ensure exercises are not continued past this point potentially reinforcing incorrect movement patterns. For example, while the patient cannot see the loss of scapular control, by drawing their attention to their scapula they can be taught to recognize the local sensation associated with control and loss of control and thereby learn to continue the exercise only to the point when that sensation occurs.

Management of shoulder motor control through patient examples

Two brief patient cases are presented as examples of implementation of the suggestions above and to highlight clinical reasoning and implementation of motor learning principles.

Case 1

- *Tom – 19-year-old, left hand dominant, elite baseball player with a painful shoulder with throwing*

Tom presented with deep, moderately severe superior shoulder pain associated primarily with the late cocking phase of a throw. The onset was gradual through the previous baseball season and he was keen to address it in the off-season. There were no red flag issues to consider, no apparent frank rotator cuff or labral pathology, cervical or neurodynamic involvement.

Tom had good range of movement but poor awareness of dissociation of different regions of his spine and between spine and scapula, leading to poor ability to stabilize scapula or arm. He stood with poor spinal posture, particularly thoracic kyphosis and forward head posture. Active assisted correction was possible but could not be maintained. His scapula was downwardly rotated and anteriorly tilted so that his arm hung in medial rotation. His ability to dissociate in four point kneeling was inadequate as he was unable to sustain good scapular position without fatigue related compensations. Increased 'give' to resistance on the lateral scapular border was evident on upward rotation of his affected side (Fig 21.7). DRST demonstrated poor isometric control of his humeral head in 110° scapular elevation with both rotations, the position relevant to his throwing, and at 90° with slow isotonic rotations. With facilitation, Tom was able to achieve good contraction and control in neutral with the DRT.

Tom's management consisted of education about the relevance of his postural and movement impairments to his throwing pain, followed by spinal and scapular postural correction and dissociation training in both sitting and four-point kneeling, later progressed to standing and positions relevant for throwing. Re-training upward rotation of his scapula, with hands-on facilitation/feedback was followed by a home programme, ensuring maintenance of neutral spine, gleno-humeral external rotation and elbow extension as he drove forwards through his hands (Fig 21.11). As Tom improved, training was progressed to closed kinetic chain activities such as slide board in four point kneeling and push-up position, concentric and eccentric load, always focussing on good positioning.

Isolation training for gleno-humeral stabilization was not warranted as Tom was able to learn the technique quickly and integrate it into the DRST, to which training was directed immediately close to positions of lost control, both isometrically and isotonically, stopping when he felt humeral head translation or lost control of his scapular position, both of which required explicit sensory recognition training for him to recognize. Over time, he increased the speed and range of movement, as required for throwing, and later increased load.

Attention to Tom's throwing technique and the rest of his kinetic chain was an integral part of his management, with strengthening and skill training built around

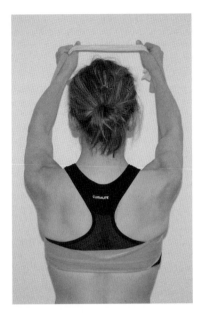

Fig 21.11 Home exercise for re-training scapular upward rotation.

dynamic control. If any given strengthening exercise resulted in loss of control, the task was judged too challenging and modified in position or load. For each task, frequent practice in as many different environments as practical was encouraged to facilitate motor learning (Schmidt & Lee 2005). Over time, lengths of hold, load, and repetitions were increased and other cognitively distracting tasks added to challenge the neuromuscular system further.

Tom was provided with thoracic extension facilitation training over the gym ball, learning inter-segmental thoracic extension and then loaded endurance exercises into extension. As a result of the postural training and maintenance of good cervical posture throughout these exercises, inclusion of formal cranio-cervical flexor training was not necessary. Later progressions were added to further challenge his spinal control and endurance in conjunction with arm movements.

The need to lose co-contraction is part of the autonomous/expert stage of learning associated with skilled activity (Shumway-Cook & Woollacott 2007) such that the task becomes a feed-forward mechanism not a feedback one. As Tom's control of the DRST position improved and he returned to throwing, it is likely that he lost the majority of the co-contraction while refining his technique. Loss of co-contraction in skilled pitchers (Glousman et al 1988) and elite swimmers (Carr et al 1998) compared to untrained controls supports the need to increase degrees of freedom with development of skill (Vereijken et al 1992). However, intermittent but regular co-contraction training is recommended as clinical

experience demonstrates a tendency to lose this ability with the potential to lead to higher risk of injury. Such control is still required for activities requiring high degrees of accuracy (Gribble et al 2003).

Case 2

- *Joan – 59-year-old, right hand dominant, office worker with MRI confirmed full thickness rotator cuff tear involving supraspinatus and a small portion of infraspinatus, coupled with a thickened swollen sub-acromial bursa.*

Joan presented with sharp severe left sub-acromial pain on quick movements, an inability to raise her arm above 90° elevation because 'it won't go' and difficulty sleeping because of pain. Three weeks previously, her dog pulled suddenly on the leash and she felt something 'give' in her shoulder. Joan had a history of 'nuisance value' discomfort in her shoulder and neck pain with prolonged computer use. She had difficulty with hand behind back activities, brushing her hair and reaching to the top cupboard because of painful limitation of movement. However, the pain settled quickly. There were no neurological symptoms, VBI issues or red flags. As a result of painful restricted range, Joan's motor control assessment was limited.

Joan's key postural impairments included increased thoracic kyphosis, forward head posture, elevation of her left acromion compared to right, apparent increased tone in both levator scapulae and upper trapezius, wasting of supraspinatus. Correction of spinal posture was impossible due to low cervical/upper thoracic stiffness on extension. Active shoulder elevation of 80° led to immediate humeral superior translation and scapular elevation, while assistance to scapular upward rotation gained a further 30° before pain increased. Pain and weakness prevented Joan from holding this position.

Joan's movement awareness on scapular PNF patterns was poor, even with facilitation. DRT was taught initially on her right shoulder where she could activate the rotator cuff well; however, she had great difficulty in the left shoulder, eventually able to create only a weak pain-free co-contraction, sustained for 3–4 seconds.

Joan's rotator cuff tear was not large but extended into infraspinatus, such that it disrupted the biomechanics of the shoulder (Burkhart 1996). Therefore, the lower rotator cuff force couple was unable to control superior humeral migration during active elevation. The motor control approach required focus on scapula and rotator cuff concurrently as the movement impairment was so closely linked. Joan's accessory movement of the lower cervical and upper thoracic spine revealed significant stiffness which also contributed to her loss of shoulder elevation.

The priorities for Joan's treatment were very different to those for Tom. Isolated rotator cuff training with the dynamic relocation manoeuvre was appropriate in

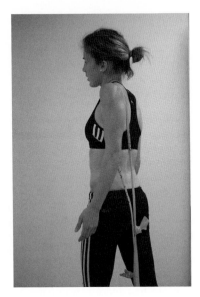

Fig 21.12 Home exercise for re-training scapular movement awareness in the PNF pattern of 'up & forward'.

conjunction with re-training scapular movement patterns. Passive mobilization and mobility exercises improved her spinal range following which awareness and inter-segmental control were facilitated with training. Joan's poor cervical posture and previous cervical pain meant that cranio-cervical flexor evaluation and training were appropriate and integrated (Jull et al 2008).

Scapular PNF patterns were used to facilitate improved scapular awareness and movement. Tactile and verbal stimulation of correct movement was complemented with a home programme (Fig 21.12).

Dynamic relocation training was initiated in a pain-free neutral position, gradually building her capacity to 10 sets of 10-second holds of good quality contraction. Training was then progressed into increased ranges of elevation, always with the arm supported and pain-free. Only when Joan could perform 10 sets of 10 holds in each position was she progressed to taking the weight of her arm. Gradually, she was able to support her arm in each training position and could start to work into functional positions through elevation with controlled scapulo-humeral and gleno-humeral movement.

Once Joan could perform the PNF patterns well, side-lying scapular upward rotation training was instigated in the increased range available, initially with no load through the arm and later, adding a protraction load but upward rotation stimulus only to the lateral scapular border, with progression focussed on increased elevation range rather than load, again with an associated home programme.

Tom's problems were largely a result of poor movement awareness and technique combined with inadequate postural awareness, endurance and explosive power for throwing. Joan's poor movement patterns were much more entrenched and associated with spinal stiffness, pathology within the tissues and provocation of pain. Reduction in pain and increase in range likely resulted at least in part from improved spinal and shoulder girdle movement patterns plus reduced superior humeral translation, reducing the compressive force through the inflamed sub-acromial bursa. As a result of her initial poor ability to control the humeral head position, isolation training of the rotator cuff was warranted, combined with progressive scapular training. Progression was slow whereas for Tom, it was quick.

The training programmes chosen incorporate exercises from or are similar to those recommended by Cools et al (2007b) and Kibler et al (2006). While not exhaustive, this approach to management of poor motor control is effective and applicable across a range of presentations of patients with shoulder pain.

CONCLUSION

Our approach to motor control evaluation and management has not been validated in formal research but is based on strong evidence, sound clinical reasoning and experience. While we readily acknowledge that motor control re-training extends beyond re-gaining control of the neutral zone, for the purposes of this chapter, the main focus has been on the early stages as progressive loading is covered in Chapter 22. Building more functional re-training on the basis of sound motor control enhances the benefits of more advanced training and improves chances of successful management.

REFERENCES

Bagg, S.D., Forrest, W.J., 1986. Electromyographic study of the scapular rotators during arm abduction in the scapular plane. Am. J. Phys. Med. Rehabil. 65, 111–124.

Bagg, S.D., Forrest, W.J., 1988. A biomechanical analysis of scapular rotation during arm abduction in the scapular plane. Am. J. Phys. Med. Rehabil. 67, 238–245.

Bullock, M.P., Foster, N.E., Wright, C.C., 2005. Shoulder impingement: the effect of sitting posture on shoulder pain and range of motion. Man. Ther. 10, 28–37.

Burkhart, S.S., 1996. A unified biomechanical rationale for the treatment of rotator cuff tears: debridement versus repair. In: Burkhead, W.Z. (Ed.), Rotator cuff disorders. Williams and Wilkins, Baltimore, pp. 293–312.

Burkhart, S.S., Morgan, C., Kibler, W.B., 2003. The Disabled Throwing Shoulder: Spectrum of Pathology Part III: The SICK Scapula, Scapular Dyskinesis, the Kinetic Chain, and Rehabilitation. Arthroscopy 19 (6), 641–661.

Carr, A., David, G., Magarey, M.E., Jones, M.A., 1998. Rotator cuff muscle performances during gleno-humeral joint rotations: An isokinetic and electromyographic study of freestyle swimmers. In: Proceedings, Australian Conference of Science & Medicine in Sport. Adelaide.

Cholewicki, J., McGill, S.M., 1996. Mechanical stability of the in vivo lumbar spine: implications for injury and chronic low back pain. Clin. Biomech. (Bristol, Avon) 11, 1–15.

Clark, J.C., Harryman, D.T., 1992. Tendons, ligaments and capsule of the rotator cuff. J. Bone Joint Surg. 74A, 5713–5725.

Colné, P., Thoumie, P., 2006. Muscular compensation and lesion of the anterior cruciate ligament: Contribution of the soleus muscle during recovery from a forward fall. Clin. Biomech. (Bristol, Avon) 21, 849–859.

Cools, A.M., Witvrouw, E.E., Declercq, G.A., et al., 2002. Scapular muscle recruitment pattern: electromyographic response of the trapezius muscle to sudden shoulder movement before and after a fatiguing exercise. J. Orthop. Sports Phys. Ther. 32, 222–229.

Cools, A.M., Witvrouw, E.E., Declercq, G.A., Danneels, L.A., Cambier, D.C., 2003. Scapular muscle recruitment patterns: Trapezius muscle latency with and without impingement symptoms. Am. J. Sports Med. 31, 542.

Cools, A.M., Witvrouw, E.E., Declercq, G.A., Vanderstraeten, G.G., Cambier, D.C., 2004. Evaluation of isokinetic force production and associated muscular activity in the scapular rotators during a protraction-retraction movement in overhead athletes with impingement symptoms. Br. J. Sports Med. 38, 64–68.

Cools, A.M., Witvrouw, E.E., Maheu, N. N., Daneels, L.A., 2005. Isokinetic scapular muscle performance in overhead athletes with and without impingement symptoms. J. Athl. Train. 40, 104–110.

Cools, A.M., Declearcq, G.A., Cambier, D.C., Mahieu, N.N., Witvrouw, E.E., 2007a. Trapezius activity and intramuscular balance during isokinetic exercise in overhead athletes with impingement symptoms. Scand. J. Med. Sci. Sports 17, 25–33.

Cools, A.M., DEwitte, V., Lanszweert, F., et al., 2007b. Rehabilitation of scapular muscle balance: Which exercises to prescribe? Am. J. Sports Med. 35, 1744–1751.

Cowan, S.M., Bennell, K.L., Hodges, P.W., Crossley, K.M., McConnell, J., 2001. Delayed onset of electromyographic activity of vastus medialis obliquus relative to vastus lateralis in subjects with patellofemoral pain syndrome. Arch. Phys. Med. Rehabil. 82, 183–189.

Cowan, S.M., Hodges, P.W., Bennell, K.L., Crossley, K.M., 2002. Altered vastii recruitment when people with patellofemoral pain syndrome complete a postural task. Arch. Phys. Med. Rehabil. 83, 989–995.

Cowan, S.M., Bennell, K.L., Hodges, P.W., Crossley, K.M., McConnell, J., 2003. Simultaneous feedforward recruitment of the vasti in untrained postural tasks can be restored by physical therapy. J. Orthop. Res. 21, 553–558.

Crawford, H.J., Jull, G.A., 1993. The influence of thoracic range and posture on range of arm elevation. Physiother. Theory Pract. 9, 143–148.

David, G., Magarey, M., Jones, M., Türker, K., Sharpe, M., Dvir, Z., et al., 2000. EMG and strength correlates of selected shoulder muscles during rotations of the gleno-humeral joint. Clin. Biomech. (Bristol, Avon) 15, 95–102.

Ebaugh, D.D., McClure, P.W., Karduna, A., 2005. Three dimensional scapulothoracic motion during active and passive arm elevation. Clin. Biomech. (Bristol, Avon) 20, 700–709.

Falla, D., 2004. Unravelling the complexity of muscle impairment in chronic neck pain. Man. Ther. 9, 125–133.

Falla, D., Farina, D., Graven-Neilsen, T., 2007. Experimental muscle pain results in reorganization of coordination among trapezius muscle subdivisions during repetitive shoulder flexion. Exp. Brain Res. 178, 385–393.

Fitts, P.M., Posner, M.I., 1967. Human Performance. Brooks/Cole, Belmont CA.

Ginn, K., Boetcher, C., Cathers, I., 2009. Are rotator cuff muscles functioning to stabilise the shoulder joint during isometric flexion, extension and rotation contractions. In: Proceedings, Sports Physiotherapy Australia Conference. Sydney, Australia.

Glousman, R., Jobe, F., Tibone, J., Moynes, D., Antonelli, D., Perry, J., et al., 1988. Dynamic electromyographic analysis of the throwing shoulder with gleno-humeral instability. J. Bone Joint Surg. 70A, 220–226.

Graichen, H., Stammberger, T., Bonkl, H., Wiedemann, E., Englmeier, K.H., Reiser, M., et al., 2001. Three-dimensional analysis of shoulder girdle and supraspinatus motion patterns in patients with impingement syndrome. J. Orthop. Res. 19, 1192–1198.

Greenfield, B., Catlin, P.A., Coats, P.W., Green, E., McDonald, J.J., North, C., et al., 1995. Posture in patients with shoulder overuse injuries and healthy individuals. J. Orthop. Sports Phys. Ther. 21 (5), 287–295.

Gribble, P.L., Mullin, L.I., Cothros, N., Matter, A., 2003. Role of co-contraction in arm movement accuracy. J. Neurophysiol. 89, 2396–2405.

Harryman, D.T., Sidles, J.A., Matsen, F.A., 1990. The humeral head translates on the glenoid with passive motion. In: Post, M., Morrey, B.F., Hawkins, R.J. (Eds.), Surgery of the shoulder. Mosby Year Book, St Louis, p. 186.

Hébert, L.J., Moffet, H., McFadyen, B.J., Dionne, C.E., 2002. Scapular behaviour in shoulder impingement syndrome. Arch. Phys. Med. Rehabil. 83, 60–69.

Hertel, J., Olmsted-Kramer, L.C., 2007. Deficits of time-to-boundary measures of postural control with chronic ankle instability. Gait Posture 25, 33s–39s.

Hess, S.A., Richardson, C., Darnell, R., Friis, P., Lyle, D., Myers, P., et al., 2005. Timing of rotator cuff activity during shoulder external rotation in throwers with and without shoulder pain. J. Orthop. Sports Phys. Ther. 35, 812–820.

Hodges, P.W., 2004. Lumbopelvic stability: a functional model of the biomechanics and motor control. In: Richardson, C., Hodges, P.W., Hides, J. (Eds.), Therapeutic exercise for lumbo-pelvic stabilization. A motor control approach for the treatment and prevention of low back pain. Churchill Livingstone, Edinburgh, Ch 2, pp. 13–28.

Jull, G.A., Sterling, M., Falla, D., Treleaven, J., O'Leary, S., 2008. Whiplash, headache and neck pain. Churchill Livingstone, Elsevier, Edinburgh.

Kibler, W.B., 1998. The role of the scapula in athletic shoulder function. Am. J. Sports Med. 26, 325–337.

Kibler, W.B., 2003. Management of the scapula in gleno-humeral instability. Techniques in Shoulder & Elbow Surgery 4 (3), 89–98.

Kibler, W.B., Uhl, T.L., Maddux, J.W.Q., Brooks, P.V., Zellar, B., McMullen, J., et al., 2002. Qualitative clinical evaluation of scapular dysfunction: a reliability study. J. Shoulder Elbow. Surg. 11, 550–556.

Kibler, W.B., Sciascia, A., Dome, D., 2006. Evaluation of apparent and absolute supraspinatus strength in patients with shoulder injury using the scapular retraction test. Am. J. Sports Med. 34, 1643–1647.

Kyllo, L.B., Landers, D.M., 1995. Goal setting in sport and exercise: A research synthesis to resolve the controversy. Journal of Sport & Exercise Psychology 17, 117–177.

Lee, B.S.B., Kim, K.J., O'Driscoll, S.W., Morrey, B.F., An, K.N., 2000. Dynamic gleno-humeral stability provided by the rotator cuff muscles in the mid-range and end-range of motion. J. Bone Joint Surg. 82A, 849–857.

Lewis, J.S., Green, A., Wright, C., 2005a. Sub-acromial impingement syndrome: The role of posture and muscle balance. J. Shoulder Elbow. Surg. 14, 385–392.

Lewis, J.S., Wright, C., Green, A., 2005b. Sub-acromial impingement syndrome: The effect of changing posture on shoulder range of movement. J. Orthop. Sports Phys. Ther. 35, 72–87.

Ludewig, P.M., Cook, T.M., 1996. The effect of head position on scapular orientation and muscle activity during shoulder elevation. J. Occup. Rehabil. 6, 147–158.

Ludewig, P.M., Cook, T.M., 2000. Alterations in shoulder kinematics and associated muscle activity in people with symptoms of shoulder impingement. Phys. Ther. 80, 276–291.

Magarey, M.E., Jones, M.A., 2003a. Dynamic evaluation and early management of altered motor control around the shoulder complex. Man. Ther. 8, 195–206.

Magarey, M.E., Jones, M.A., 2003b. Specific evaluation of the function of force couples relevant for the stabilization of the gleno-humeral joint. Man. Ther. 8, 247–253.

Magee, D.J., Zachazewski, J.E., 2007. Principles of stabilization training. In: Magee, D.J., Zachazewski, J.E., Quillen, W.S. (Eds.), Scientific foundations and principles of practice in musculoskeletal rehabilitation. Saunders, Elsevier, St Louis Missouri, pp. 388–431.

McClure, P.W., Michener, L.A., Sennett, B.J., Karduna, A.R., 2001. Direct 3-dimensional measurement of scapular kinematics during dynamic movements in vivo. J. Shoulder Elbow. Surg. 10, 269–277.

McClure, P.W., Michener, L.A., Karduna, A.R., 2006. Shoulder function and 3-dimensional scapular kinematics in people with and without shoulder impingement syndrome. Phys. Ther. 86, 1075–1090.

McGill, S., 2007. Low back disorders. Evidence-based prevention and rehabilitation, second ed. Human Kinetics, Champaign Illinois.

Moraes, G.F.S., Faria, C.D.C.M., Teixeira-Salmela, L.F., 2008. Scapular muscle recruitment patterns and isokinetic strength ratios of the shoulder rotator muscles in individuals with and without impingement syndrome. J. Shoulder Elbow. Surg. 17, 48S–53S.

Nederhand, N.J., Hermens, H.J., Ijzman, M.J., Turk, D.C., Zilvold, G., 2000. Cervical Muscle Dysfunction in Chronic Whiplash-Associated Disorder Grade 2: The Relevance of the Trauma. Spine 27, 1056–1061.

Panjabi, M.M., 1992a. The stabilizing system of the spine. Part I: function, dysfunction, adaptation and enhancement. J. Spinal Disord. 5, 383–389.

Panjabi, M.M., 1992b. The stabilizing system of the spine. Part II. Neutral zone and instability hypothesis. J. Spinal Disord. 5, 390–396.

Panjabi, M.M., 1996. Low back pain and spinal instability. In: Weinstein, J.N., Gordon, S.L. Eds.: Low back pain: a scientific and clinical overview. American Academy of Orthopaedic Surgeons, Rosemont, Ill.

Pink, M., Jobe, F.W., Perry, J., Browne, A., Scovazzo, L., Kerrigan, J., et al., 1993. The painful shoulder during butterfly swimming. An electromyographic and cinematico-graphic analysis of 12 muscles. Clin. Orthop. Relat. Res. 288, 60–72.

Roberts, P.D., 2009. Movement Analysis & Training. Educational lecture notes, Master of Musculoskeletal & Sports Physiotherapy, University of South Australia.

Roy, J.S., Moffet, H., McFadyen, B.J., 2008. Upper limb motor strategies in persons with and without shoulder impingement syndrome across different speeds of movement. Clin. Biomech. (Bristol, Avon) 23, 1227–1236.

Sahrmann, S., 2002. Diagnosis and treatment of movement impairment disorders. Mosby, St Louis Missouri.

Schmidt, R.A.S., Lee, T.D., 2005. Motor Control and Learning: A Behavioral Emphasis, fourth ed. Human Kinetics, Champaign, Illinois.

Scovazzo, M.L., Browne, A., Pink, M., Jobe, F.W., Kerrigan, J., 1991. The painful shoulder during freestyle swimming. An electromyographic and cinematographic analysis of 12 muscles. Am. J. Sports Med. 6, 577–582.

Shumway-Cook, A., Woollacott, M.H., 2007. Motor Control. Translating Research into Clinical Practice, third ed. Lippincott Williams & Wilkins, Philadelphia, Pennsylvania.

Simons, D.G., Travell, J.G., Simons, L.S., 1999. second ed. Travell and Simon's myofascial pain and dysfunction: the trigger point manual, vol. 2. Williams and Wilkins, Baltimore, MD.

Sousa, D., 2006. How the Brain Learns, Chapters 2–4. Corwin Press, Thousand Oaks, California.

Spitzer, M., 1999. Learning. Chapter 3. In: Spitzer, M. (Ed.), The Mind Within the Net: Models of Learning, Thinking and Acting. MIT Press, pp. 39–63.

Sterling, M., Jull, G., Wright, A., 2001. The effect of musculoskeletal pain on motor activity and control. J. Pain 2, 135–145.

Szeto, G.P.R., Straker, L., O'sullivan, P.B., 2005. A comparison of symptomatic and asymptomatic office workers performing monotonous keyboard work 2: Neck and shoulder kinematics. Man. Ther. 10, 281–291.

Szeto, G.P.R., Straker, L.M., O'sullivan, P.B., 2009. Neck-shoulder muscle activity in general and task-specific resting postures of symptomatic computer users with chronic neck pain. Man. Ther. 14, 338–345.

Terry, G.C., Hammon, D., France, P., Norwood, L.A., 1991. The stabilizing function of passive shoulder restraints. Am. J. Sports Med. 19, 26–34.

Vereijken, B., van Emmerik, R.E.A., Whiting, H.T.A., Newell, K.M., 1992. Free (z)ing degrees of freedom in skill acquisition. J. Mot. Behav. 24, 739–749.

Voss, D.E., Ionta, M.K., Myers, B.J., 1985. Proprioceptive Neuromuscular Facilitation. Patterns and Techniques, third ed. Harper & Row, Philadelphia.

Wadsworth, D.J., Bullock-Saxton, J.E., 1997. Recruitment patterns of the scapular-rotator muscle in freestyle swimmers with sub-acromial impingement. Int. J. Sports Med. 18, 618–624.

Wuelker, N., Roetman, B., Roessig, S., 1995. Coracoacromial pressure recordings in a cadaveric model. J. Shoulder Elbow. Surg. 4, 462–467.

Chapter | 22 |

Therapeutic exercises for the shoulder region

Johnson McEvoy, Kieran O'Sullivan, Carel Bron

INTRODUCTION

Therapeutic exercise is a cornerstone of physiotherapy practice and was initially referred to as *medical gymnastics*. The development of medical gymnastics in physical therapy has had many diverse influences including Dr Francis Fuller author of Medicina Gymnasticia (1740), Swedish gymnast Per Henrik Ling (1776–1839) and the Dutch physical education teacher and physician Dr Johann Georg Mezger (1838–1909) (Barclay 1994, Terlouw 2007). More recently Kendall (2002) summed up the role of therapeutic exercise in physical therapy: 'Central to the practice of physical therapy is the prevention of movement dysfunction and the rehabilitation through restoration and maintenance of active movement – in other words, therapeutic exercise in its broadest sense'. The focus of this chapter is to introduce general principles of therapeutic exercise for the shoulder, and to stimulate clinical reasoning and rational rehabilitation. The chapter will briefly discuss posture, stretching and strengthening of a selection of muscles, without focussing on one specific clinical population.

CLINICAL BACKGROUND

Essential to an understanding of therapeutic exercise is an in-depth knowledge of anatomy, physiology and function, specifically related to the neuromuscular and musculoskeletal systems (Kendall 2002). The shoulder is a complex functional system producing movement of the arm on the trunk and allowing the upper limb and hand to be dynamically moved and positioned for function. The shoulder consists of the scapula, clavicle and humerus giving rise to the sterno-clavicular, acromio-clavicular, gleno-humeral and scapulo-thoracic joints and has a close relationship to the neck, thorax and ribs. The shoulder is supported by capsular, ligamentous and muscular systems with complex neuromuscular processing that offers a wide range of motion with a subsequent compromise in joint stability. This trade off in stability makes the shoulder potentially vulnerable to dysfunction and injury, and stability is often the main focus of therapeutic exercise for the shoulder complex. Readers should refer to appropriate chapters of this book and other texts for a comprehensive review of shoulder anatomy, biomechanics, kinesiology and patho-mechanics (Donatelli 2004a, Oatis 2004). Further, knowledge of connective tissue properties, force

© 2011 Elsevier Ltd.
DOI: 10.1016/B978-0-7020-3528-9.00022-4

Box 22.1 Indications for therapeutic shoulder exercises

- Gleno-humeral joint lesions, dysfunctions and instability
- Rotator cuff lesions and dysfunctions
- Sub-acromial impingement syndrome
- Acromio-clavicular joint lesions and dysfunctions
- Sterno-clavicular joint lesions and dysfunctions
- Superior labrum anterior to posterior (SLAP) lesions
- Adhesive capsulitis (Frozen Shoulder)
- Arthropathies: arthrosis, arthritis, rheumatoid arthritis
- Post fracture and trauma
- Soft tissue injuries and syndromes
- Sports injuries
- Myofascial pain and dysfunction from trigger points
- Hypermobility syndromes
- Postural dysfunction
- Movement disorders
- Performance enhancement and performance optimization
- Injury prevention
- Post shoulder surgery and arthroscopy
- Shoulder replacement
- Thoracic surgery with shoulder involvement (e.g. mastectomy)
- Spinal cord injuries and nerve root syndromes
- Peripheral nerve injuries
- Central nervous system disorders e.g. hemiplegia

applications, tissue injury (bone, ligament, tendon, muscle, fascia, nerve, etc.) and tissue healing concepts and timelines (inflammation, proliferation, maturation) is an important precursor to the development of a suitable and safe therapeutic exercise programme (Tippet & Voight 1995, Paris & Loubert 1999, Houglum 2005).

Prior to the development of a rehabilitation programme for the shoulder complex a comprehensive assessment and physical examination should be performed with reference to the principles of physical therapy practice to ascertain pertinent information and physical characteristics of the individual patient. Indications for therapeutic exercise of the shoulder are listed in Box 22.1 and are diverse and include specific and non-specific musculoskeletal, orthopaedic, surgical and neurological conditions and dysfunctions and also include postural, performance enhancement and injury prevention strategy.

SHOULDER EXERCISE: EVIDENCE

A wide variety of shoulder disorders have demonstrated alterations in shoulder range of motion (Hall & Elvey

1999, Vermeulen et al 2002, McClure et al 2006), scapular kinematics (Lukasiewicz et al 1999, Ludewig & Cook 2000, McClure et al 2006, Roy et al 2009, Tate et al 2009), scapular and rotator cuff muscle activation (Ludewig & Cook 2000, Cools et al 2007, Moraes et al 2008, Myers et al 2009), gleno-humeral translation (Chen et al 1999, Ludewig & Cook 2002), repositioning sense (Naughton et al 2005), and shoulder strength (McClure et al 2006, Lombardi et al 2008, Baydar et al 2009, Bigoni et al 2009). Therefore, therapeutic exercises are commonly advocated to address these dysfunctions in mobility, posture, muscle activation, proprioception and strength.

Overall, the evidence that therapeutic exercise is effective for non-specific shoulder pain is mixed (Smidt et al 2005), similar to other approaches including manual therapy (Ho et al 2009) and acupuncture (Green et al 2009). However, exercise appears to be as effective for non-specific shoulder pain as more expensive treatments such as multidisciplinary bio-psychosocial rehabilitation (Karjalainen et al 2001). Furthermore, when specific shoulder disorders are considered there is little evidence that alternative approaches are superior to therapeutic exercise. For example medium and long-term outcomes after therapeutic exercise in adhesive capsulitis are similar to those after other treatments including arthrographic distension (Buchbinder et al 2009a) and corticosteroid injection (Winters et al 1997, 1999, Buchbinder et al 2009b). There is also evidence that combining corticosteroid injection with physiotherapy including therapeutic exercise results in greater improvement than either treatment in isolation (Carette et al 2003).

The use of therapeutic exercise is supported in the management of specific disorders including sub-acromial impingement syndrome (SAIS) and rotator cuff lesions by much research (Bang & Deyle 2000, Desmeules et al 2003, Green et al 2003, Michener et al 2004, Dickens et al 2005, Jonsson et al 2006, Trampas & Kitsios 2006, Senbursa et al 2007, Lombardi et al 2008, Baydar et al 2009, Chen et al 2009, Kuhn 2009, Roy et al 2009). Furthermore, outcomes following conservative treatment (incorporating therapeutic exercise) appear to be similar to outcomes after surgical intervention in SAIS and rotator cuff lesions (Haahr & Andersen 2006, Dorrestijn et al 2009). This key role of therapeutic exercise in shoulder rehabilitation is emphasized by the fact that good clinical outcomes have been associated with normalization of scapular kinematics (Roy et al 2009), and recovery of strength (Nho et al 2009).

PRINCIPLES OF EXERCISE

A clinical assessment should be completed prior to exercise prescription and clinicians should remain cognisant of the various facets of an exercise programme and suit the needs to the individual patient: posture, flexibility and stretching, stability, strengthening, proprioception and functional progression (Tippet & Voight 1995, Lephart & Fu 2000, Alter 2004, Donatelli 2004b & 2006, Kraemer & Ratamess 2004, Weerapong et al 2004, Houglum 2005, Kendall et al 2005, MacIntosh et al 2006). It is important for the clinician to gather information including the subjective history, objective examination, special tests, functional ability, impairment, dysfunctions, diagnosis and any other pertinent information. Two-way communication with other team members (e.g. medical, surgical, psychological, coach, strength and conditioning etc.) is essential to enhance the overall physical therapy plan of care, and set appropriate and safe goals. Clinicians should employ evidence-based practice and clinical reasoning with respect to current research and patient orientated goals as the basis for rational rehabilitation (Cicerone 2005). Safety is of paramount importance and clinicians should ensure that exercises are suitable and safe for individual patients. Furthermore, since painful sensory input may alter motor output during exercise, reducing the pain where possible with appropriate physical, pharmacological and/or psychological strategies is an important part of the rehabilitation process.

There are three phases of a therapeutic exercise programme which are worked through progressively based on the requirements of the individual patient and these include (1) posture, joint range of motion and flexibility, (2) muscle strength and endurance, and (3) functional aspects including proprioception, coordination and agility (Houglum 2005). For example, the exercise prescription and goals of a patient with adhesive capsulitis will differ significantly from a patient with gleno-humeral instability. Principles to guide rehabilitation include avoidance of aggravation, timing of exercise, compliance, individualization, specific sequencing, intensity and total patient approach (Houglum 2005), and are presented in Figure 22.1.

Exercise programmes should be progressive and graded according to the stage of healing and should not aggravate pain, swelling or result in deterioration in other clinical signs such as range of motion, strength and function (Fig 22.1) (Tippet & Voight 1995). The ability to perform exercises with appropriate skill should be monitored closely (Tippet & Voight 1995). These authors referred to the three 'C's (1) carriage – appropriate weight shift, weight acceptance and symmetry of movement, (2) confidence – verbal and non-verbal communication, speed and deliberateness of exercise performed, and (3) control – smooth unrestricted automatic movements with skilled task performance (Tippet & Voight 1995).

Bone and soft tissues adapt according to the stresses placed upon them, highlighting the importance of appropriate loading of tissue in a graded progressive manner to enhance healing, and has been described by Wolff's Law and Davis's Law respectively (Wolff 1986, Tippet & Voight 1995). These principles also apply to the hypertrophy of uninjured tissues and for example, it has been demonstrated that baseball athletes have thicker biceps and supraspinatus tendons when compared to non-athletes (Wang et al 2005). On the other hand, over-loading of bone and soft tissue can result in injury such as bone stress fracture or tendon failure.

The principle of specific adaptations to imposed demands (SAID) refers to the body's ability to change to specific demands placed upon it and therefore has implications for rehabilitation design in that exercises should mimic the expected functional stressors of the individual patient as much as possible (Houglum 2005). Implementing variance of activities and rest phases are important to allow adaptation. An example of the relevance of these principles is when considering the introduction of eccentric strength training into the rehabilitation programme. Eccentric strength training programmes appear to be effective in the management of knee and ankle tendon pathology (Alfredson et al 1998, Young et al 2005). There has been less research on eccentric programmes for rotator cuff tendon pathology, however initial results are encouraging (Jonsson et al 2006). Eccentric programmes are, however, associated with muscle damage (Clarkson & Hubal 2002). Before placing such high stresses on previously injured tissues, basic isometric and isotonic strength programmes should be already in place. Further, the introduction of such eccentric training programmes should be progressed.

Shoulder muscle balance ratios have been reported including ratios between the external and internal rotators of 1.5:1 (66%) for both fast and slow isokinetic torque arm speed in normal subjects (Ivey et al 1985). Ratios have also been presented for professional baseball pitchers (Ellenbecker & Mattalino 1997). Clinicians should consider these ratios in exercise programme design. A discussion of isokinetics is beyond the scope of this chapter but has been reviewed by Ellenbecker & Davies (2000).

The following sections will discuss, posture, stretching and strengthening (isometric and isotonic) and a brief mention of functional exercise. Specific parameters for timing and repetitions of stretching and strengthening will be covered under each appropriate section.

POSTURE

Postural assessment is an important part of the objective evaluation and ideal static postural alignments have been suggested (Kendall et al 2005). However it is important to assess both static and dynamic postures to ascertain the patient's functional movement and ability to self-correct a static habitus. An example of this is in a boxer, who enhances a hyper-kyphotic and rounded shoulder posture to reduce his target size for strategic advantage, but when dynamically tested, may be able to self correct the seemingly poor posture.

Therapeutic exercise programme

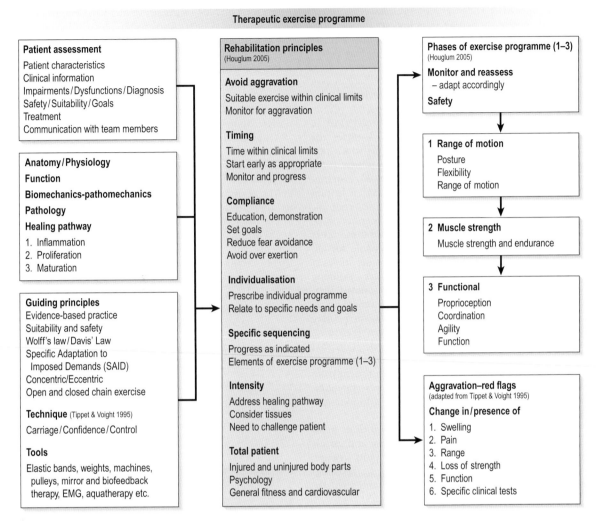

Fig 22.1 Principles of therapeutic exercise.

It is important to assess for muscle length, joint mobility and muscle control. Altered posture may be related to muscle imbalances and altered joint position, which ultimately could result in movement dysfunction and pain. Deviations in normal upright positions may include forward head position, a greater curve in the thoracic kyphosis and rounded shoulders. Deviations in scapular kinematics may present in multiple planes, including changes in scapular elevation, protraction, tilt and rotation, affecting the size of the sub-acromial space (Solem-Bertoft et al 1993), as well as both activation (Roy et al 2009) and mechanical advantage (Kibler et al 2006) of muscular structures. It has been demonstrated that the size of the sub-acromial space is reduced in the presence of thoracic hyperkyphosis (Raine & Twomey 1997, Gumina et al 2008) and shoulder protraction (Solem-Bertoft et al 1993).

It is however, uncertain whether a strong correlation exists between narrowing of the sub-acromial space and shoulder symptoms (Graichen et al 2001, Roberts et al 2002, Hinterwimmer et al 2003, Lewis et al 2005, Mayerhoefer et al 2009). In fact, while it has been assumed that there is a definitive correlation between these postural deviations, a study of 160 asymptomatic subjects found no such correlation (Raine & Twomey 1997). Therefore, although there may be a relationship between posture and sub-acromial space, this is not yet fully understood.

Thoracic kyphosis and forward shoulder position influence the length of the upper back and scapular muscles and place the intervertebral joints in an end-range position (Griegel-Morris et al 1992). The sustained strain on these soft tissues may lead to upper back pain or shoulder pain. In the front of the body the pectoral muscles may shorten (Borstad & Ludewig 2006, Muraki et al 2009). Sustained muscle shortening may lead to the development or activation of myofascial trigger points (Simons et al 1999). Referred pain from the pectorals may be felt in the front of the shoulder and arm (Simons et al 1999) and sometimes even in the upper back region (Dejung et al 2003). See Chapter 32 for a review of these mechanisms and muscle referral patterns.

Sustained contractions impair normal blood flow in skeletal muscles. Optimal posture allows muscles the opportunity to relax in between contractions which permits and facilitates recovery of circulation (Otten 1988, Sjogaard & Sogaard 1998, Palmerud et al 2000). Combining postural exercises with myofeedback / EMG is helpful to teach patients how to use their muscles in an economic and healthy manner (Peper et al 2003, Voerman et al 2006). Though there is a wide range of postures, rather than focusing on an idealized posture suitable for all, clinicians should consider the optimal posture for each patient and individualize exercise programmes. Assuming appropriate upright trunk postures can change muscle activation and modify range of motion and symptoms (Bullock et al 2005). Scapular taping can be used as a temporary means of altering scapular muscle activation (Selkowitz et al 2007). Furthermore, Lucas et al (2004) demonstrated that latent trigger points can alter muscle activation patterns of the shoulder as assessed by EMG and subsequently dry needling and stretch, when compared to placebo ultrasound, was reported to improve the muscle activation patterns significantly and similar to controls.

Treatment for postural dysfunctions may include manual therapies including joint mobilization and manipulation, massage and myofascial trigger point release, myofascial release techniques, trigger point dry needling, biofeedback and EMG, stretching, stability and strengthening and cognitive and behavioural strategies.

STRETCHING

Flexibility and stretching is a broad topic with conflicting opinion in the literature, and a full discussion of this topic is beyond the scope of this chapter. Readers are referred elsewhere for a comprehensive review of stretching (Alter 1996, Weerapong et al 2004). A rehabilitation programme of the shoulder may incorporate a muscle stretching programme and is usually employed for muscle lengthening and associated clinical implications, pain inhibition and potential injury prevention.

It has been reported that alterations in scapular movement are related to changes in myofascial length (Borstad & Ludewig 2005, Borstad 2006). The addition of appropriate manual therapy techniques may increase the effectiveness of therapeutic exercise (Winters et al 1997, Conroy & Hayes 1998, Bang & Deyle 2000, Desmeules et al 2003,

Bergman et al 2004, Michener et al 2004, Senbursa et al 2007, Boyles et al 2009). These techniques may include soft tissue techniques, passive stretching, joint mobilization, and may increase range of motion in subjects with shoulder pain (Vermeulen et al 2006, Johnson et al 2007). Therapeutic exercise alone however may be as effective as adding passive joint mobilizations to therapeutic exercise (Trampas & Kitsios 2006, Chen et al 2009). Different joint mobilizations techniques are described in detail in Chapter 20.

A muscle stretching programme should be based on assessment of muscle length and end feel. Muscles and fascia may present with neuromuscular, viscoelastic or connective tissue alterations (Chaitow & Liebenson 2001). It is important to evaluate muscle length and its influence on the length–tension relationship should not be overlooked (Janda 1993, Sahrmann 2002, Ekstrom & Osborn 2004, Kendall et al 2005). Though individual patients will present with varying degrees of muscle length, certain patterns as outlined by Janda and others are often seen in clinic practice (Chaitow & Liebenson 2001):

- Short muscles and often facilitated: pectoralis major and minor, latissimus dorsi, levator scapula, upper trapezius (at times)
- Long muscles and often inhibited: serratus anterior, lower and middle trapezius

A stretch for the levator scapula and a clinician assisted stretch for the pectorals and latissimus dorsi muscles are presented in Figures 22.2 & 22.3 respectively. Other self stretch exercises for the pectorals and latissimus dorsi may include the doorway stretch and one sided unilateral

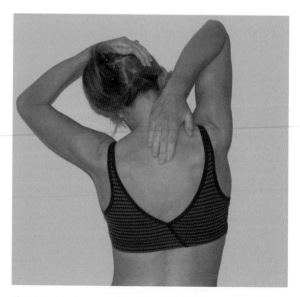

Fig 22.2 Levator scapula stretch. Ipsilateral arm elevated position is proposed to assist in isolating the levator scapula from the upper trapezius.

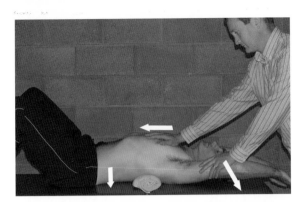

Fig 22.3 Pectoral and latissimus dorsi, clinician assisted stretch. Patient maintains a neutral lumbar spine and a towel can be used to reduce thoracic kyphosis. Clinician applies low grade smooth stretch against soft tissue barrier. For appropriate modesty the patients opposite hand can be placed across the chest and clinicians hand can be placed on top. Contract relax application can also be added to augment stretch.

self stretch of the pectoralis minor, which has been shown to be superior to a supine manual stretch and a sitting manual stretch (Borstad & Ludewig 2006).

Muscle stretching techniques include static, ballistic, dynamic and proprioceptive neuromuscular facilitation (Weerapong et al 2004, Houglum 2005). Other techniques have been described including post-isometric relaxation (PIR) (Lewit & Simons 1984, Lewit 1988, 1999), muscle energy technique (MET) (Greenman 1989, Chaitow & Crenshaw 2006), activated isolated stretching (AIS) (Mattes 1995) and spray and stretch (Travell & Simons 1983, Simons et al 1999, Kostopoulos & Rizopoulos 2008). Stretching has been employed for the treatment of pain especially in relation to the treatment of myofascial trigger points (Simons et al 1999).

The recommendation for duration of static stretching has been varied, but it is reasonable to recommend a 15 to 30 second hold with 3–5 repetitions (Taylor et al 1990, Houglum 2005) repeated daily or several times/day. Good form should be maintained during stretching technique and should be smooth and within the clinical limits of the presenting problem. Longer hold times up to and beyond 5 minutes have been recommended for fascial tissue release (Barnes 1999).

Patients with a history of subluxation, dislocation, hyper-mobility of the shoulder or general hyper-mobility syndrome need to be identified as a stretching programme may be inappropriate and potentially detrimental. The patient history, muscle length tests, joint end feel, passive joint tests and the Beigthon score (Alter 1996) may assist the clinician in identifying hyper-mobility and instability. Up to 11.7% of people have some form of joint hyper-mobility, and it has been reported to be up to three times more prevalent in females than males (Hakim & Grahame 2003, Seckin et al 2005).

The majority of current research does not support the hypothesis that stretching prevents injury (Shrier 1999, Weerapong et al 2004). However there is some evidence to suggest that lower limb stretching can reduce the risk of injury (Hartig & Henderson 1999, Amako et al 2003, Jamtvedt et al 2009), or the rate of return from injury (Malliaropoulos et al 2004). Interestingly, reviewed research on stretching demonstrates a negative effect on muscle strength and functional performance (Weerapong et al 2004). The fact that most research has focussed on the lower extremities raises validity issues on extrapolating the findings to the upper extremity; however clinicians should consider these issues in prescribing flexibility programmes especially in relation to performance athletes and players. More research is required to assist in a better understanding of the role of stretching in injury management and prevention.

External rotation is fundamental for elevation and shoulder function and it is important to restore passive and active external rotation (Donatelli 2004a). External rotation is primarily limited at 0° by the sub-scapularis; at 45° of abduction by the sub-scapularis, middle and inferior gleno-humeral ligament and at 90° of abduction by the inferior gleno-humeral ligament (Turkel et al 1981). Muscle length testing of the sub-scapularis is carried out with the arm in neutral and testing into external rotation (Donatelli 2004b). An auto assisted stretch for sub-scapularis, using a cane, is presented in Figure 22.4. Stretching position for example at 0°, 45°, 90° abduction etc, should be based on any restrictions of the sub-scapularis and gleno-humeral capsule and ligaments identified from the physical

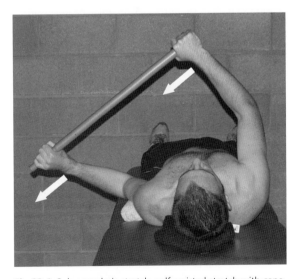

Fig 22.4 Sub-scapularis stretch, self assisted stretch with cane. Supine position offers stability of the scapula while external rotation of the gleno-humeral joint is assisted with self control using the cane. A towel is placed under the elbow to maintain alignment of the humerus.

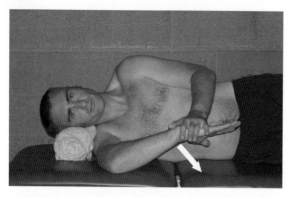

Fig 22.5 Sleeper stretch: 90° position stabilizes the scapula and downward pressure is applied with a self stretch to the opposite hand into internal rotation.

assessment. Contribution of the gleno-humeral joint capsule (and other posterior soft tissue structures including the infraspinatus, teres minor and deltoid) to shoulder movement should not be overlooked and has been proposed to be particularly important in certain shoulder disorders, including SAIS (Donatelli 2004a). Reduced cross-body adduction has been linked to tightness of the posterior capsule, and associated with abnormal gleno-humeral translation (Ludewig & Cook 2002). Cross body adduction and the 'sleeper stretch' (internal rotation of the shoulder in 90° of shoulder flexion) have been recommended as stretches for posterior shoulder capsular tightness (Cooper et al 2004, McClure et al 2007, Laudner et al 2008). The 'sleeper stretch' is presented in Figure 22.5. However modification into less shoulder flexion may be necessary if symptoms are aggravated in this position.

ISOMETRIC EXERCISE OF THE SHOULDER

Isometric exercise is usually utilized in the early phase of rehabilitation to minimize muscle atrophy when movement of the shoulder is limited. Studies have demonstrated up to a 41% decrease in isometric strength after immobilization of the upper extremity for 5 to 6 weeks with significant decreases in muscle fibre area by 33% and 25% for fast and slow twitch fibres respectively (MacDougall et al 1980). During immobilization of the upper limb, strength training with maximal isometric exercise 5 days/week of the free limb may prevent atrophy of the immobilized limb (Farthing et al 2009). Further research has suggested that adding a 0.5 kg weight to the ipsilateral hand during isometric and dynamic shoulder exertions increases shoulder muscle activity by 4% maximum voluntary excitation (Antony & Keir 2010). Static exercises for the shoulder are presented in Figure 22.6,

where a belt is employed to allow multidirectional static exercises, however other options include resistance against a wall. A hand held weight of 0.5 kg is used here to assist in increasing shoulder muscle activity (Antony & Keir 2010). Suggested parameters for isometric exercises include pain-free 5 to 10 second holds with 10 repetitions, graded to maximal contraction and repeated several times per day with progression as indicated (Houglum 2005).

ISOTONIC EXERCISES OF THE SHOULDER

There are a plethora of exercises for the shoulder girdle and research employing EMG has aimed at identifying exercises that target specific shoulder muscles and here we briefly review a selection of exercises that target the rotator cuff, trapezius and serratus anterior muscles. For a further expansion of this, readers are recommended to review other publications (Ekstrom & Osborn 2004, Houglum 2005, Reinold et al 2009). When designing a strengthening programme the clinician should target muscles identified as weak during the evaluation and on the basis of this prescribe suitable exercises. The clinician should prescribe the specific exercise, resistance (or none), repetitions, sets and frequency of the programme. This programme should be monitored, adjusted and advanced progressively. A programme can be initiated with or without weight, as appropriate. Recommendations have been made in relation to exercise repetitions and include 1–6 reps for strength, 6–12 for hypertrophy, 12–15 for endurance (Kraemer & Ratamess 2004). The weight used is appropriate to cause fatigue towards the end of the stated number of repetitions. It has been found that two to six sets per exercise produce significant increases in muscular strength in both trained and untrained individuals (Kraemer & Ratamess 2004).

Other recommendations include 6–15 repetitions of 2 sets where the patient can control the weight and progressing to 20–25 repetitions of 3 sets (Houglum 2005). When this is reached progress the weight accordingly and start the process again with 6–15 repetitions of 2 sets etc. (Houglum 2005). There are various exercise progressions that can be considered including Delorme & Watkins (1948), Oxford Technique (Zinovieff 1951) and Daily Adjusted Progressive Resistive Exercise (Knight 1985, Houglum 2005). The clinician should consider the principles of exercise as outlined in Figure 22.1 when prescribing strength programmes. The rotator cuff muscles are important stabilizers of the gleno-humeral joint and assist in stabilizing the humerus in the glenoid by compression and preventing shear and upward movement of the humeral head during arm movements (Oatis 2004). Other muscles assist in stabilizing the scapulo-thoracic

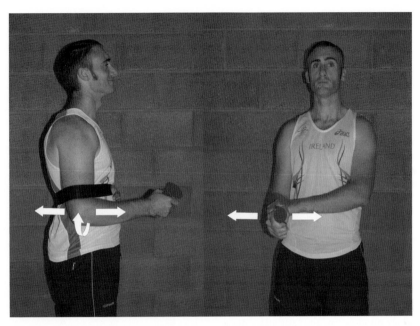

Fig 22.6 Isometric exercises for the shoulder. The use of a belt allows the patient to perform isometric exercise in multi-directions. This can be also done against a wall. Internal and external rotation is performed with self assisted resistance. The use of a hand held weight of 0.5 kg has been shown to assist in increase shoulder muscle EMG by 4%. The arrows indicate direction of force but as an isometric exercise there is no movement.

complex and assist in dynamic stability (Oatis 2004) and these muscle specific exercises are covered below. For muscles, such as deltoid, levator scapulae and rhomboids, and indications for strengthening, readers are recommended to review Reinold et al (2009).

Supraspinatus muscle

The supraspinatus is the most superior of the rotator cuff muscles and lies deep to the sub-acromial bursa and the coraco-acromial ligament within the sub-acromial space (Oatis 2004). The reported actions of this muscle include abduction, external rotation and stabilization of the shoulder (Oatis 2004). Activity of the supraspinatus increases with increased loading during abduction and scaption movements peaking at 30° to 60° of elevation (Reinold et al 2009). Reinold et al (2007) demonstrated EMG activity was similar across three exercises, full can, empty can and prone full can. The full can results in significantly less activity of middle and posterior deltoid, which may reduce harmful shear force on the gleno-humeral joint from deltoid activity (Reinold et al 2007, 2009). In addition, the full can reduces the potential for sub-acromial impingement because of the external rotation component (Ekstrom & Osborn 2004). Moreover, the full can exercise has been recommended by previous research (Kelly et al 1996). The full can exercise in the plane of the scapula with external rotation of the shoulder is presented in Figure 22.7.

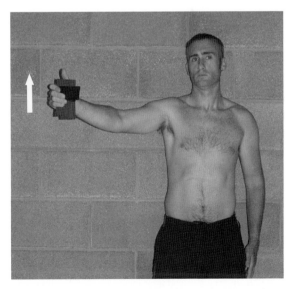

Fig 22.7 Supraspinatus full can strengthen. This is carried out in the plane of the scapula. Slow and controlled with thumb up to ensure a degree of external rotation.

Infraspinatus and teres minor muscles

The actions of infraspinatus and teres minor are primarily external rotation and functionally assisting stability of the gleno-humeral joint during elevation movements (Reinold et al 2009). Stabilization of the shoulder by these muscles is achieved also by opposing superior and anterior humeral head translation (Reinold et al 2009). The infraspinatus has potentially a role in abduction and horizontal abduction with teres minor involved in adduction, apparently due to different moment arms (Oatis 2004). EMG analysis demonstrated best isolation of infraspinatus in 0° abduction with 45° of medial rotation from neutral (Kelly et al 1996) and Reinold et al (2009) suggested incorporating this position as an exercise to any rehabilitation programme when focusing on increasing external rotation strength. Adding a roll support between the arm and the trunk (Fig 22.8) has been shown to increase EMG activity in the infraspinatus and teres minor muscles by up to 25% (Reinold et al 2004, 2009). A second exercise worth considering is standing external rotation in the scapular plane (45° degrees abduction) (Fig 22.9) as this has demonstrated good EMG activation of infraspinatus and teres minor (Reinold et al 2004) and isokinetic external rotational strength values in the plane of the scapula have been reported to be significantly higher than in the frontal plane (Greenfield et al 1990).

Other exercises for external rotation have been recommended that place the shoulder in a more compromised position (e.g. external rotation in 90° abduction) and clinicians should carefully consider the appropriateness of these exercises in the presence of capsulo-labral dysfunction and pathology (Reinold et al 2009).

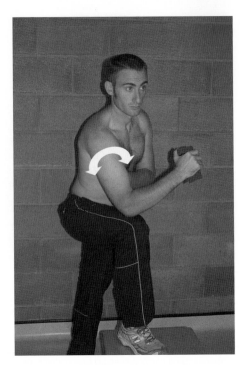

Fig 22.9 External rotation in the plane of the scapula. Shoulder is rotated from internal to external rotation.

Sub-scapularis muscle

Sub-scapularis is the largest of the rotator cuff muscles and acts to internally rotate, flex, extend, abduct, adduct, horizontal adduct and stabilize the shoulder with broad agreement that internal rotation and stabilization are the primary roles (Oatis 2004). Sub-scapularis weakness leads to significant decrease in internal rotation strength and may contribute to anterior instability of the shoulder (Oatis 2004). The lift-off test as described by Gerber (Gerber & Krushell 1991) has been demonstrated to isolate sub-scapularis (Greis et al 1996, Kelly et al 1996). The lift-off exercise for sub-scapularis muscle is presented in Figure 22.10.

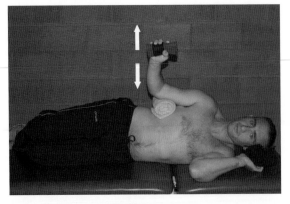

Fig 22.8 Infraspinatus and teres minor muscles strengthening. Side lying, arm is brought from internal into external rotation. Towel positioned between arm and trunk has been shown to increase EMG of the muscles by 25%.

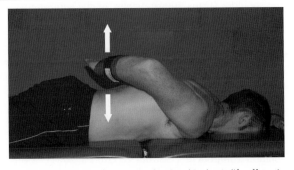

Fig 22.10 Sub-scapularis strengthening (Gerber's lift off test). The hand is raised upwards from the trunk.

Trapezius muscle

The trapezius is an expansive muscle that has three distinct muscle sections; upper, middle and lower, with each having a distinct function and combining to assist in the overall function of the trapezius (Oatis 2004). The actions of the three sections have been reported as follows (Oatis 2004): upper trapezius – elevation of the scapula, adduction and upward rotation of the scapula; middle trapezius – adduction of the scapula; lower trapezius – depression, adduction and upward rotation of the scapula. In particular the upper and lower trapezius form an anatomical force couple that assists in stabilizing the scapula and maintaining a balance between these muscle segments is important for optimum function (Oatis 2004). Further the lower fibres have been reported to play an important role in posterior tilt and upward rotation of the scapula during shoulder elevation (Ludewig et al 1996). Therefore, the lower trapezius and serratus anterior are an important target for rehabilitation and prevention of shoulder dysfunction and impingement syndromes (Ludewig & Cook 2000). In regard to exercises for the upper trapezius the shoulder shrug has been reported to produce the greatest EMG activity (Ekstrom et al 2003). However it has been reported that the shrug exercise also highly activates the levator scapula and if this needs to be avoided, due to the levator scapulae action of scapular downward rotation, the military press may be more appropriate (Ekstrom & Osborn 2004).

For the middle trapezius abduction and external rotation of the shoulder at 90° in prone (Fig 22.11) has been shown to induce good EMG activity and is considered a suitable exercise (Moseley et al 1992, Ekstrom & Osborn 2004, Reinold et al 2009). This exercise has also been recommended for strengthening the trapezius as a whole due to high EMG activity in the upper, middle and lower muscle segments (Ekstrom et al 2003, Ekstrom & Osborn 2004).

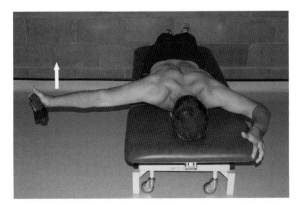

Fig 22.11 Trapezius strengthening. Targets the upper, middle lower sections of the trapezius muscle. Thumb is maintained in an upright position.

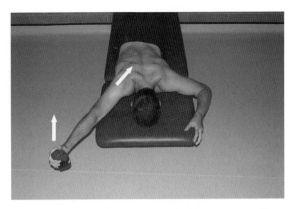

Fig 22.12 Trapezius strengthening. Targets mainly lower fibres of trapezius performed at approximately 120° to 135° of abduction or with the arm positioned in line with the lower fibres of trapezius.

The lower trapezius has been shown to be best activated with the arm raise overhead exercise in the prone position performed at approximately 120° (Reinold et al 2009) to 135° of abduction or with the arm positioned in line with the lower fibres of trapezius (Fig 22.12) (Ekstrom et al 2003, Ekstrom & Osborn 2004).

Serratus anterior muscle

The serratus anterior muscle action has been reported as protraction, abduction, upward rotation and elevation of the scapula, and functions in actions such as pushing a revolving door and weakness may lead to winging of the scapula and difficulty with overhead activities (Oatis 2004). Shoulder abduction in the plane of the scapula above 120° (to avoid painful arc) in the standing position has demonstrated more EMG activity in serratus anterior than straight scapular protraction (Fig 22.13). The increased serratus anterior activation should however be balanced against the increased risk of impingement when exercises are performed in elevation (Roberts et al 2002). Other recommended exercises for serratus anterior include the dynamic hug, push-up with a plus and punch exercises (Decker et al 1999, Reinold et al 2009).

FUNCTIONAL EXERCISES

The daily tasks and movements performed by each individual should be considered when prescribing therapeutic exercise, so that the exercises take into account specific functional demands of each person. Functional

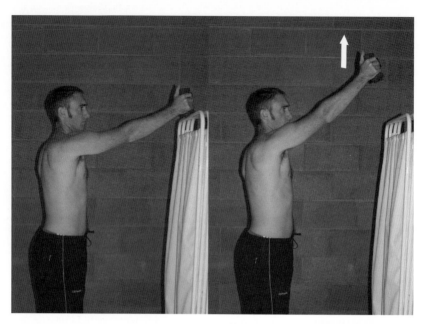

Fig 22.13 Serratus anterior strengthening. Shoulder abduction in the plane of the scapula above 120° (to avoid painful arc) in the standing position.

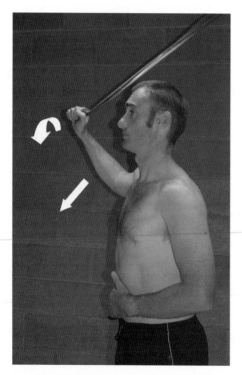

Fig 22.14 Proprioceptive neuromuscular facilitation with elastic band: elastic bands can assist with creating open chain coordinated movements that mimic functional patterns.

progression may include movement from isolated plane to multi-plane strengthening (Fig 22.14) and eventually plyometric exercise (Houglum 2005). Upper limb tasks are commonly open kinetic chain movements. In athlete subjects with recurrent anterior shoulder dislocation, rehabilitation near/in the zone of instability is indicated in late-stage rehabilitation and therefore, tasks which load the rotator cuff in semi-compromised positions may help replicate the stability action required on return to sport. Closed chain and stability exercises (Figs 22.15 & 22.16) for the shoulder girdle are important to assist in motor control and re-education (Houglum 2005) and are discussed in Chapter 21. The shoulder girdle relationship to the kinetic chain should be considered in the overall management of the patient and exercise programmes may incorporate standing balance and eye hand coordination tasks etc. (Donatelli 2006). A common barrier to shoulder rehabilitation is difficulty replicating therapeutic exercise correctly at home, possibly due to reduced position sense (Naughton et al 2005). Tasks which challenge the proprioceptive acuity and load-bearing ability of the shoulder region may help restore position sense awareness (Figs 22.14–22.16). Clinicians can incorporate the use of exercise equipment to assist in functional progression and may include elastic bands, pulleys, theraballs, wobble boards, proprioceptive exercise devices and feedback devices such as mirrors etc.

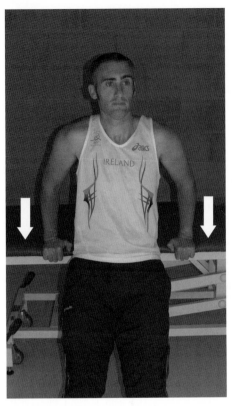

Fig 22.15 Shoulder dip: closed chain kinetic loading and proprioceptive exercise.

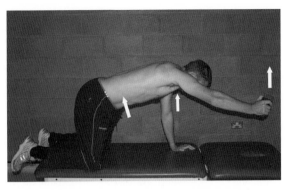

Fig 22.16 Prone kneel, single arm raise: abdominals are primed prior to lift. This offers closed chain exercise for weight bearing shoulder and dynamic open chain exercise for opposite arm. This exercise can be advanced to alternative arm and leg lift for stability.

be indicated in the clinical setting especially in relation to strength of the rotator cuff and stabilizers of the scapula. Clinicians should remain cognisant of the need for a comprehensive assessment and ensure safe and suitable exercise prescription and progression. The nature, intensity and volume of exercise prescribed must be matched to the clinical presentation. Individual therapists may use the principles outlined in this chapter as a guide when prescribing a therapeutic exercise programme that is suitable for the needs of each individual patient or athlete. Further research is required and should focus on identifying exercises to suit the specific patient presentation.

CONCLUSIONS

Therapeutic exercises can play an important role in the management of shoulder pain. This chapter has outlined some basic principles on the type of exercise that may

ACKNOWLEDGEMENT

Thank you to the photographic volunteers: Derek Malone, Irish Paralympic athlete and S.M.

REFERENCES

Alfredson, H., Pietilä, T., Jonshon, P., et al., 1998. Heavy-Load Eccentric Calf Muscle Training For the Treatment of Chronic Achilles Tendinosis. Am. J. Sports Med. 26, 360–366.

Alter, M.J., 1996. Science of flexibility. Human Kinetics, Champaign, IL.

Alter, M.J., 2004. Science of flexibility. Human Kinetics, Champaign, IL.

Amako, M., Oda, T., Masuoka, K., et al., 2003. Effect of static stretching on prevention of injuries for military recruits. Mil. Med. 168, 442–446.

Antony, N.T., Keir, P.J., 2010. Effects of posture, movement and hand load on shoulder muscle activity. J. Electromyogr. Kinesiol. 20, 191–198.

Bang, M., Deyle, G., 2000. Comparison of supervised exercise with and without manual physical therapy for patients with shoulder impingement syndrome. J. Orthop. Sports Phys. Ther. 30, 126–137.

Barclay, J., 1994. In good hands: the history of the Chartered Society of Physiotherapy 1894–1994. Butterworth Heinemann, Oxford.

Barnes, J., 1999. Myofascial Release. Functional soft tissue examination and treatment by manual methods: new perspectives. In: Hammer, W.I. (Ed.), Aspen Publishers, Gaithersburg, Md., x, p. 625.

Baydar, M., Akalin, E., El, O., et al., 2009. The efficacy of conservative treatment in patients with full-thickness rotator cuff tears. Rheumatol. Int. 29, 623–628.

Bergman, G., Winters, J., Groenier, K., et al., 2004. Manipulative therapy in addition to usual medical care for patients with shoulder dysfunction and pain: A Randomized, Controlled Trial. Ann. Intern. Med. 141, 432–439.

Bigoni, M., Gorla, M., Guerraio, S., et al., 2009. Shoulder evaluation with isokinetic strength testing after arthroscopic rotator cuff repairs. J. Shoulder Elbow Surg. 18, 178–183.

Borstad, J., 2006. Resting posture variables at the shoulder: evidence to support a posture-impairment association. Phys. Ther. 86, 549–557.

Borstad, J., Ludewig, P., 2005. The effect of long versus short pectoralis minor resting length on scapular kinematics in healthy individuals. J. Orthop. Sports Phys. Ther. 35, 227–238.

Borstad, J.D., Ludewig, P.M., 2006. Comparison of three stretches for the pectoralis minor muscle. J. Shoulder Elbow Surg. 15, 324–330.

Boyles, R.E., Ritland, B.M., Miracle, B.M., et al., 2009. The short-term effects of thoracic spine thrust manipulation on patients with shoulder impingement syndrome. Man. Ther. 14, 375–380.

Buchbinder, R., Green, S., Youd, J., et al., 2009a. Arthrographic distension for adhesive capsulitis. Cochrane Database Syst. Rev.

Buchbinder, R., Green, S., Youd, J., et al., 2009b. Corticosteroid injections for shoulder pain. Cochrane Database Syst. Rev.

Bullock, M., Foster, N., Wright, C., 2005. Shoulder impingement: the effect of sitting posture on shoulder pain and range of motion. Man. Ther. 10, 28–37.

Carette, S., Moffet, H., Tardif, J., et al., 2003. Intra-articular corticosteroids, supervised physiotherapy, or a combination of the two in the treatment of adhesive capsulitis of the shoulder: A placebo-controlled trial. Arthritis Rheum. 48, 829–838.

Chaitow, L., Crenshaw, K., 2006. Muscle energy techniques: with accompanying DVD. Churchill Livingstone Elsevier, Edinburgh.

Chaitow, L., Liebenson, C., 2001. Muscle energy techniques. Churchill Livingstone, Edinburgh.

Chen, J., Ginn, K.A., Herbert, R., et al., 2009. Passive mobilisation of shoulder region joints plus advice and exercise does not reduce pain and disability more than advice and exercise alone: a randomised trial. Aust. J. Physiother. 55, 17–23.

Chen, S., Simonian, P., Wickiewicz, T., et al., 1999. Radiographic evaluation of gleno-humeral kinematics: A muscle fatigue model. J. Shoulder Elbow Surg. 8, 49–52.

Cicerone, K.D., 2005. Evidence-based practice and the limits of rational rehabilitation. Arch. Phys. Med. Rehabil. 86, 1073–1074.

Clarkson, P.M., Hubal, M.J., 2002. Exercise-induced muscle damage in humans. Am. J. Phys. Med. Rehabil. 81, S52–S69.

Conroy, D., Hayes, K., 1998. The effect of joint mobilisation as a component of comprehensive treatment for primary shoulder impingement syndrome. J. Orthop. Sports Phys. Ther. 28, 3–14.

Cools, A., Witvrouw, E., Declercq, G., et al., 2007. Scapular muscle recruitment patterns: Trapezius muscle latency with and without impingement symptoms. Am. J. Sports Med. 31, 542–549.

Cooper, J., Donley, P., Morgan, C., et al., 2004. Throwing injuries. In: Donatelli, R. (Ed.), Physical therapy of the shoulder. Churchill Livingstone, St. Louis, Mo., pp. 29–78.

Decker, M.J., Hintermeister, R.A., Faber, K.J., et al., 1999. Serratus anterior muscle activity during selected rehabilitation exercises. Am. J. Sports Med. 27, 784–791.

Dejung, B., Gröbli, C., Colla, F., et al., 2003. Triggerpunkttherapie. Hans Huber, Bern.

Delorme, T.L., Watkins, A.L., 1948. Technics of progressive resistance exercise. Arch. Phys. Med. Rehabil. l (29), 263–273.

Desmeules, F., Côté, C.H., Fremont, P., et al., 2003. Therapeutic Exercise and Orthopedic Manual Therapy for Impingement Syndrome: A Systematic Review. Clin. J. Sport Med. 13, 176–182.

Dickens, V., Willimas, J., Bhamra, M., 2005. Role of physiotherapy in the treatment of sub-acromial impingement syndrome: a prospective study. Physiotherapy 91, 159–164.

Donatelli, R., 2004a. Functional anatomy and mechanics. In: Donatelli, R. (Ed.), Physical therapy of the shoulder. Churchill Livingstone, St. Louis, Mo., pp. 11–28.

Donatelli, R., 2004b. Physical therapy of the shoulder. Churchill Livingstone, St. Louis, Mo.

Donatelli, R., 2006. Sports-specific rehabilitation. Elsevier Churchill Livingstone, St. Louis, Mo.

Dorrestijn, O., Stevens, M., Winers, J., et al., 2009. Conservative or surgical treatment for sub-acromial impingement syndrome? A systematic review. J. Shoulder Elbow Surg. 18, 652–660.

Ekstrom, R.A., Donatelli, R.A., Soderberg, G.L., 2003. Surface electromyographic analysis of exercises for the trapezius and serratus anterior muscles. J. Orthop. Sports Phys. Ther. 33, 247–258.

Ekstrom, R., Osborn, R., 2004. Muscle length testing and electromyographic data for manual strength testing and exercises for the shoulder. In: Donatelli, R. (Ed.), Physical Therapy of the Shoulder. Churchill Livingstone, St Louis.

Ellenbecker, T.S., Davies, G.J., 2000. The Application of Isokinetics in Testing and Rehabilitation of the Shoulder Complex. J. Athl. Train. 35, 338–350.

Ellenbecker, T.S., Mattalino, A.J., 1997. Concentric isokinetic shoulder internal and external rotation strength in professional baseball pitchers. J. Orthop. Sports Phys. Ther. 25, 323–328.

Farthing, J.P., Krentz, J.R., Magnus, C.R., 2009. Strength training the free limb attenuates strength loss during unilateral immobilization. J. Appl. Physiol. 106, 830–836.

Gerber, C., Krushell, R.J., 1991. Isolated rupture of the tendon of the sub-scapularis muscle. Clinical features in 16 cases. J. Bone Joint Surg. Br. 73, 389–394.

Graichen, H., Bonel, H., Stammberger, T., et al., 2001. Sex-specific differences of subacromial space width during abduction, with and without muscular activity, and correlation with anthropometric variables. J. Bone Joint Surg. 10, 129–135.

Greenfield, B.H., Donatelli, R., Wooden, M.J., et al., 1990. Isokinetic evaluation of shoulder rotational strength between the plane of scapula and the frontal plane. Am. J. Sports Med. 18, 124–128.

Greenman, P.E., 1989. Principles of manual medicine. Williams & Wilkins, Baltimore.

Green, S., Buchbinder, R., Hetrick, S., 2003. Physiotherapy interventions for shoulder pain. Cochrane Database Syst. Rev. 2.

Green, S., Buchbinder, R., Hetrick, S., 2009. Acupuncture for shoulder pain. Cochrane Database Syst. Rev.

Greis, P.E., Kuhn, J.E., Schultheis, J., et al., 1996. Validation of the lift-off test and analysis of sub-scapularis activity during maximal internal rotation. Am. J. Sports Med. 24, 589–593.

Griegel-Morris, P., Larson, K., Mueller-Klaus, K., et al., 1992. Incidence of common postural abnormalities in the cervical, shoulder, and thoracic regions and their association with pain in two age groups of healthy subjects. Phys. Ther. 72, 425–431.

Gumina, S., Di Giorgio, G., Postacchini, F., et al., 2008. Sub-acromial space in adult patients with thoracic hyperkyphosis and in healthy volunteers. Chir. Organi. Mov. 91, 93–96.

Haahr, J.P., Andersen, J.H., 2006. Exercises may be as efficient as subacromial decompression in patients with subacromial stage II impingement: 4–8-years' follow-up in a prospective, randomized study. Scand. J. Rheumatol. 35, 224–228.

Hakim, A., Grahame, R., 2003. Joint hypermobility. Best Pract. Res. Clin. Rheumatol. 17, 989–1004.

Hall, T., Elvey, R., 1999. Nerve trunk pain: physical diagnosis and treatment. Man. Ther. 4, 63–73.

Hartig, D.E., Henderson, J.M., 1999. Increasing hamstring flexibility decreases lower extremity overuse injuries in military basic trainees. Am. J. Sports Med. 27, 173–176.

Hinterwimmer, S., Von Eisenhart-Rothe, R., Siebert, M., et al., 2003. Influence of adducting and abducting muscle forces on the sub-acromial

space width. Medicine Science in Sports Exercise 35, 2055–2059.

Ho, C., Sole, G., Munn, J., 2009. The effectiveness of manual therapy in the management of musculoskeletal disorders of the shoulder: A systematic review. Man. Ther. 14, 463–474.

Houglum, P.A., 2005. Therapeutic exercise for musculoskeletal injuries. Human Kinetics, Champaign, IL.

Ivey, F.M., Calhoun, J.H., Rusche, K., et al., 1985. Isokinetic testing of shoulder strength: normal values. Arch. Phys. Med. Rehabil. 66, 384–386.

Jamtvedt, G., Herbert, R.D., Flottorp, S., et al., 2010 (epub). A pragmatic randomised trial of stretching before and after physical activity to prevent injury and soreness. Br. J. Sports Med. 44 (14), 1002–1009.

Janda, V., 1993. Muscle strength in relation to muscle length, pain, and muscle imbalance. In: Harms-Ringdahl, K. (Ed.), Muscle Strength. Churchill Livingstone, Edinburgh, pp. 83–91.

Johnson, A., Godges, J., Zimmerman, G., et al., 2007. The effect of anterior versus posterior glide joint mobilization on external rotation range of motion in patients with shoulder adhesive capsulitis. J. Orthop. Sports Phys. Ther. 37, 88–99.

Jonsson, P., Wahlstrom, P., Ohberg, L., et al., 2006. Eccentric training in chronic painful impingement syndrome of the shoulder: results of a pilot study. Knee Surg. Sports Traumatol. Arthrosc. 14, 76–81.

Karjalainen, K., Malmivaara, A., Van Tulder, M., et al., 2001. Multidisciplinary biopsychosocial rehabilitation for neck and shoulder pain among working age adults: a systematic review within the framework of the Cochrane Collaboration Back Review Group. Spine 26, 174–181.

Kelly, B.T., Kadrmas, W.R., Speer, K.P., 1996. The manual muscle examination for rotator cuff strength. An electromyographic investigation. Am. J. Sports Med. 24, 581–588.

Kendall, F., Kendall McCreary, E., Provance, P., et al., 2005. Muscles: testing and function with posture and pain. Lippincott Williams & Wilkins, Baltimore.

Kendall, F.P., 2002. Kendall urges a return to basics. PT Bulletin Online 3.

Kibler, W., Sciascia, A., Dome, D., 2006. Evaluation of apparent and absolute supraspinatus strength in patients with shoulder injury using the scapular retraction test. Am. J. Sports Med. 34, 1643–1647.

Knight, K.L., 1985. Guidelines for rehabilitation of sports injuries. Clinical Sports in Medicine 4, 405–416.

Kostopoulos, D., Rizopoulos, K., 2008. Effect of topical aerosol skin refrigerant (spray and stretch technique) on passive and active stretching. J. Bodyw. Mov. Ther. 12, 96–104.

Kraemer, W.J., Ratamess, N.A., 2004. Fundamentals of resistance training: progression and exercise prescription. Medicine Science in Sports Exercise 36, 674–688.

Kuhn, J.E., 2009. Exercise in the treatment of rotator cuff impingement: A systematic review and a synthesized evidence-based rehabilitation protocol. J. Shoulder Elbow Surg. 18, 138–160.

Laudner, K.G., Sipes, R.C., Wilson, J.T., 2008. The acute effects of sleeper stretches on shoulder range of motion. J. Athl. Train. 43, 359–363.

Lephart, S.M., Fu, F.H., 2000. Proprioception and neuromuscular control in joint stability. Human Kinetics, Champaign, IL.

Lewis, J.S., Green, A., Wright, C., 2005. Subacromial impingement syndrome: the role of posture and muscle imbalance. J. Shoulder Elbow Surg. 14, 385–392.

Lewit, K., 1988. Postisometric relaxation in combination with other methods of muscular facilitation and inhibition. Manuelle Medizin 2, 101–104.

Lewit, K., 1999. Manipulative therapy in rehabilitation of the locomotor system. Butterworth-Heinemann, Oxford.

Lewit, K., Simons, D.G., 1984. Myofascial pain: relief by post-isometric relaxation. Arch. Phys. Med. Rehabil. 65, 452–456.

Lombardi, I.J., Magri, A., Fleury, A., et al., 2008. Progressive resistance training in patients with shoulder impingement syndrome: a randomized controlled trial. Arthritis Rheum. 59, 615–622.

Lucas, K.R., Polus, B.I., Rich, P.S., 2004. Latent myofascial trigger points: their effect on muscle activation and movement efficiency. J. Bodyw. Mov. Ther. 8, 160–166.

Ludewig, P.M., Cook, T., 2000. Alterations in shoulder kinematics and associated muscle activity in people with symptoms of shoulder impingement. Phys. Ther. 80, 276–291.

Ludewig, P.M., Cook, T., 2002. Translations of the humerus in persons with shoulder impingement symptoms. J. Orthop. Sports Phys. Ther. 32, 248–259.

Ludewig, P.M., Cook, T.M., Nawoczenski, D.A., 1996. Three-dimensional scapular orientation and muscle activity at selected positions of humeral elevation. J. Orthop. Sports Phys. Ther. 24, 57–65.

Lukasiewicz, A., McClure, P., Michener, L., et al., 1999. Comparison of 3-dimensional scapular position and orientation between subjects with and without shoulder impingement. J. Orthop. Sports Phys. Ther. 29, 574–583.

MacDougall, J.D., Elder, G.C., Sal, D.G., et al., 1980. Effects of strength training and immobilization on human muscle fibres. Eur. J. Appl. Physiol. Occup. Physiol. 43, 25–34.

MacIntosh, B.R., Gardiner, P.F., McComas, A.J., 2006. Skeletal muscle: form and function. Leeds, Human Kinetics, Champaign, Ill.

Malliaropoulos, N., Papalexandris, S., Papalada, A., et al., 2004. The Role of Stretching in Rehabilitation of Hamstring Injuries: 80 Athletes Follow-Up. Med. Sci. Sports Exerc. 36, 756–759.

Mattes A.L., 1995. Active isolated stretching (A.L. Mattes, Ed.). Sarasota, FL. (2932 Lexington St., Sarasota 34231-6118).

Mayerhoefer, M.E., Breitenseher, M.J., Wurnig, C., et al., 2009. Shoulder impingement: relationship of clinical symptoms and imaging criteria. Clin. J. Sport Med. 19, 83–89.

McClure, P., Balaicuis, J., Heiland, D., et al., 2007. A randomized controlled comparison of stretching procedures for posterior shoulder tightness. J.

Orthop. Sports Phys. Ther. 37, 108–114.

McClure, P.W., Michener, L.A., Karduna, A.R., 2006. Shoulder Function and 3-Dimensional Scapular Kinematics in People With and Without Shoulder Impingement Syndrome. Phys. Ther. 86, 1075–1090.

Michener, L., Walsworth, M., Burnet, E., 2004. Effectiveness of rehabilitation for patients with sub-acromial impingement syndrome: a systematic review. J. Hand Ther. 17, 152–164.

Moraes, G., Faria, C., Teixeira-Salmela, L., 2008. Scapular muscle recruitment patterns and isokinetic strength ratios of the shoulder rotator muscles in individuals with and without impingement syndrome. J. Shoulder Elbow Surg. 17, 48S–53S.

Moseley, J.B., Jobe, F.W., Pink, M., et al., 1992. EMG analysis of the scapular muscles during a shoulder rehabilitation program. Am. J. Sports Med. 20, 128–134.

Muraki, T., Aoki, M., Izumi, T., et al., 2009. Lengthening of the pectoralis minor muscle during passive shoulder motions and stretching techniques: a cadaveric biomechanical study. Phys. Ther. 89, 333–341.

Myers, J.B., Hwang, J.H., Pasquale, M.R., et al., 2009. Rotator cuff coactivation ratios in participants with subacromial impingement syndrome. J. Sci. Med. Sport 12, 603–608.

Naughton, J., Adams, R., Maher, C., 2005. Upper-body wobbleboard training effects on the post-dislocation shoulder. Phys. Ther. Sport 6, 31–37.

Nho, S.J., Brown, B.S., Lyman, S., et al., 2009. Prospective analysis of arthroscopic rotator cuff repair: Prognostic factors affecting clinical and ultrasound outcome. J. Shoulder Elbow Surg. 18, 13–20.

Oatis, C.A., 2004. Kinesiology: the mechanics and pathomechanics of human movement. Lippincott Williams & Wilkins, Philadelphia.

Otten, E., 1988. Concepts and models of functional architecture in skeletal muscle. Exercise Sport Science Review 16, 89–137.

Palmerud, G., Forsman, M., Sporrong, H., et al., 2000.

Intramuscular pressure of the infra- and supraspinatus muscles in relation to hand load and arm posture. Eur. J. Appl. Physiol. 83, 223–230.

Paris, S., Loubert, P., 1999. Foundations of Clinical Orthopaedics. Institute of Physical Therapy, University of St Augustine, St Augustine.

Peper, E., Wilson, V.S., Gibney, K.H., et al., 2003. The integration of electromyography (SEMG) at the workstation: assessment, treatment, and prevention of repetitive strain injury (RSI). Appl. Psychophysiol. Biofeedback 28, 167–182.

Raine, S., Twomey, L.T., 1997. Head and shoulder posture variations in 160 asymptomatic women and men. Arch. Phys. Med. Rehabil. 78, 1215–1223.

Reinold, M.M., Wilk, K.E., Fleisig, G.S., et al., 2004. Electromyographic analysis of the rotator cuff and deltoid musculature during common shoulder external rotation exercises. J. Orthop. Sports Phys. Ther. 34, 385–394.

Reinold, M.M., Macrina, L.C., Wilk, K.E., et al., 2007. Electromyographic analysis of the supraspinatus and deltoid muscles during 3 common rehabilitation exercises. J. Athl. Train. 42, 464–469.

Reinold, M.M., Escamilla, R.F., Wilk, K.E., 2009. Current concepts in the scientific and clinical rationale behind exercises for glenohumeral and scapulothoracic musculature. J. Orthop. Sports Phys. Ther. 39, 105–117.

Roberts, C., Davila, J., Hushek, S., et al., 2002. Magnetic resonance imaging analysis of the subacromial space in the impingement sign positions. J. Shoulder Elbow Surg. 11, 595–599.

Roy, J.S., Moffet, H., Hébert, L.J., et al., 2009. Effect of motor control and strengthening exercises on shoulder function in persons with impingement syndrome: A single-subject study design. Man. Ther. 14, 180–188.

Sahrmann, S., 2002. Diagnosis and treatment of movement impairment syndromes. Mosby, St. Louis, Mo.

Seckin, U., Tur, B.S., Yilmaz, O., et al., 2005. The prevalence of joint hypermobility among high school students. Rheumatol. Int. 25, 260–263.

Selkowitz, D., Chaney, C., Stuckey, S., et al., 2007. The effects of scapular taping on the surface electromyographic signal amplitude of shoulder girdle muscles during upper extremity elevation in individuals with suspected shoulder impingement syndrome. J. Orthop. Sports Phys. Ther. 37, 694–702.

Senbursa, G., Baltacı, G., Atay, A., 2007. Comparison of conservative treatment with and without manual physical therapy for patients with shoulder impingement syndrome: a prospective, randomized clinical trial. Knee Surg. Sports Traumatol. Arthrosc. 15, 915–921.

Shrier, I., 1999. Stretching before exercise does not reduce the risk of local muscle injury: a critical review of the clinical and basic science literature. Clin. J. Sport Med. 9, 221–227.

Simons, D.G., Travell, J.G., Simons, L., 1999. Travell and Simons' myofascial pain and dysfunction; the trigger point manual. Williams & Wilkins, Baltimore.

Sjogaard, G., Sogaard, K., 1998. Muscle injury in repetitive motion disorders. Clin. Orthop. Relat. Res. 351, 21–31.

Smidt, N., De Vet, H., Bouter, L., et al., 2005. Effectiveness of exercise therapy: a best-evidence summary of systematic reviews. Aust. J. Physiother. 51, 71–85.

Solem-Bertoft, E., Thuomas, K.A., Westerberg, C.E., 1993. The influence of scapular retraction and protraction on the width of the subacromial space. An MRI study. Clin. Orthop. Relat. Res. 296, 99–103.

Tate, A., McClure, P., Kareha, S., et al., 2009. A Clinical Method for Identifying Scapular Dyskinesis, Part 2: Validity. J. Athl. Train. 44, 165–173.

Taylor, D.C., Dalton, J.D., Seaber, A.V., et al., 1990. Viscoelastic properties of muscle-tendon units. The biomechanical effects of stretching. Am. J. Sports Med. 18, 300–309.

Terlouw, T.J., 2007. Roots of Physical Medicine, Physical Therapy, and Mechano-therapy in the Netherlands in the 19th Century: A Disputed Area within the Healthcare Domain. J. Man. Manip. Ther. 15, E23–E41.

Tippet, S.R., Voight, M.L., 1995. Functional progression for sports rehabilitation. Human Kinetics.

Trampas, A., Kitsios, A., 2006. Exercise and manual therapy for the treatment of impingement syndrome of the shoulder: a systematic review. Phys. Ther. Rev. 11, 125–142.

Travell, J.G., Simons, D.G., 1983. Myofascial pain and dysfunction; the trigger point manual. Williams & Wilkins, Baltimore.

Turkel, S.J., Panio, M.W., Marshall, J.L., et al., 1981. Stabilizing mechanisms preventing anterior dislocation of the glenohumeral joint. J. Bone Joint Surg. Am. 63, 1208–1217.

Vermeulen, H.M., Stokdijk, M., Eilers, P.H., et al., 2002. Measurement of three dimensional shoulder movement patterns with an electromagnetic tracking device in patients with a frozen shoulder. Ann. Rheum. Dis. 61, 115–120.

Vermeulen, H.M., Rozing, P.M., Obermann, W.R., et al., 2006. Comparison of High-Grade and Low-Grade Mobilization Techniques in the Management of Adhesive Capsulitis of the Shoulder: Randomized Controlled Trial. Phys. Ther. 86, 355–368.

Voerman, G.E., Vollenbroek-Hutten, M. M., Hermens, H.J., 2006. Changes in pain, disability, and muscle activation patterns in chronic whiplash patients after ambulant myofeedback training. Clin. J. Pain 22, 656–663.

Wang, H.K., Lin, J.J., Pan, S.L., et al., 2005. Sonographic evaluations in elite college baseball athletes. Scand. J. Med. Sci. Sports 15, 29–35.

Weerapong, P., Hume, P.A., Kolt, G.S., 2004. Stretching: Mechanisms and Benefits for Sport Performance and Injury Prevention. Phys. Ther. Rev. 9, 189–206.

Winters, J., Sobel, J., Groenier, K., et al., 1997. Comparison of physiotherapy, manipulation and corticosteroid injection for treating shoulder complaints in general practice: randomised, single blind study. Br. Med. J. 314, 1320–1325.

Winters, J., Jorritsma, W., Groenier, K., et al., 1999. Treatment of shoulder complaints in general practice: long-term results of a randomised, single blind study comparing physiotherapy, manipulation, and corticosteroid injection. Br. Med. J. 318, 1395–1396.

Wolff, J., 1986. The law of bone remodelling. Springer-Verlag, Berlin; New York.

Young, M., Cook, J., Purdam, C., et al., 2005. Eccentric decline squat protocol offers superior results at 12 months compared with traditional eccentric protocol for patellar tendinopathy in volleyball players. Br. J. Sports Med. 39, 102–105.

Zinovieff, A.N., 1951. Heavy-resistance exercises the 'Oxford technique. Br. J. Phys. Med. 14, 129–132.

Chapter | 23 |

Elbow tendinopathy: lateral epicondylalgia

Bill Vicenzino

INTRODUCTION

The common tendon of the extensor muscles of the wrist and fingers is the most frequently implicated tendon in elbow tendinopathy and will be the focus of this chapter. There is contention as to the correct nomenclature for the tendinopathy of the extensor muscles of the wrist and fingers. A number of terms are used in reference to this tendinopathy, such as, tennis elbow, lateral epicondylitis, lateral epicondylosis and lateral epicondylalgia. Tennis elbow is frequently used colloquially, but this term confuses many patients, as the condition is also very prevalent in those patients who do not play tennis. Epicondylitis infers inflammation, which has long been shown not to be the case (Nirschl & Pettrone 1979, Regan et al 1992, Potter et al 1995, Kraushaar & Nirschl 1999, Alfredson et al 2000). Epicondylosis or tendinosis connotes a degenerative change, but whilst there has been identified elements of disarray, breakdown or degeneration of collagen fibrils in such tendons (Regan et al 1992, Kraushaar & Nirschl 1999), the relationship to presenting pain symptoms and associated clinical signs is not clear (Khan & Cook 2000).

Lateral epicondylalgia indicates that there is pain over the lateral epicondyle which may be an accurate term to use for the patient presenting with pain over the lateral epicondyle, but it provides little information about the underlying pathology. Recent reports of neovascularization and associated increased concentrations of algogenic mediators such as glutamate, substance P and calcitonin gene-related peptide (Ljung et al 1999, 2004, Alfredson et al 2000, Zeisig et al 2006, du Toit et al 2008) suggests that tendinopathy is far more complex than any of these commonly used terms suggest. For this chapter, the term lateral epicondylalgia will be used to describe the patient who attends the clinic with pain over the lateral epicondyle, as will be highlighted, this may be due to some pathology in the tendon, that is, tendinopathy, but the pain may also be associated with other conditions, which need to be considered to fully rehabilitate the patient.

Although there is no definitive evidence, the incidence of lateral epicondylalgia varies from 1% to 3% in the general population (Allander 1974, Verhaar 1994), which contrasts to reports of prevalence rates as high as 35–64% in occupations requiring repetitive manual tasks (Kivi 1982, Dimberg 1987, Feuerstein et al 1998), where it is one of the most costly of all work-related injuries (Kivi 1982, Dimberg 1987, Feuerstein et al 1998). A survey of United States of America Department of Labor, Office of Worker's Compensation Programs, accepted claims of occupational upper extremity disorders demonstrated that lateral epicondylalgia was responsible for approximately 27% and 48% of all work related claims for upper limb tendinopathies and enthesopathies, respectively (Feuerstein et al 1998). This chapter focuses on the most common tendinopathy about the elbow, lateral epicondylalgia, with specific consideration of the

© 2011 Elsevier Ltd.
DOI: 10.1016/B978-0-7020-3528-9.00023-6

evidence in regards to diagnosis, pathology, conservative management and prognosis.

DIAGNOSTIC CONSIDERATIONS

Lateral epicondylalgia is usually identified or diagnosed on the basis of a clinical examination. Classically, the patient presents with pain over the lateral elbow and may spread into the dorsal forearm as far as the wrist, but no further than the wrist and not proximally to the elbow (see Slater et al (2003, 2005) for patterns of pain maps). Those with pain and symptoms into the hand and fingers or proximal to the elbow should be considered to have concomitant problems (e.g. cervical spine referral, neuropathy) in addition to, or instead of, lateral epicondylalgia. Patients with lateral epicondylalgia will have pain and weakness with tests that challenge the wrist extensor muscles, for example, muscle contraction tasks of gripping, wrist extension, and middle finger extension (clinically described as a test of extensor carpi radialis brevis, largely due to the insertion of that tendon at the wrist). It is commonly reported that stretch of the wrist and finger extensors is present in these patients, though while pain may be reproduced on stretching, it is not an uncommon observation by this author that patients exhibit increased length of these muscles (i.e. increased range of flexion of the wrist and fingers) associated with pain reproduction in those with chronic conditions. The pain reproduction is limited to the lateral epicondyle and at most some spread down into the dorsal forearm. Palpation will identify areas of hyperalgesia in and around the lateral epicondyle, at the site of the common extensor tendon as well as in some cases pain into the dorsal forearm muscles. These palpation findings need to be present with impairment in muscle contraction; otherwise it is more likely that the symptoms could be largely referred from other regions, such as the cervical spine.

Typically patients attending general practice with lateral epicondylalgia will characteristically be in their 4th or 5th decade of life. There is upper limb dominance bias, but not sex. Patients who perform repetitive tasks requiring sustained or repeated gripping of an implement or tool, such as those playing tennis or undertaking manual labour, may be outside of this decade (i.e. younger), but there should be a higher degree of suspicion of an alternative underlying cause and diagnosis. For example, in younger people consideration needs to be given to osteochondritis dissecans of the capitellum and radius in cases with insidious onset, and bursitis, radio-humeral joint synovitis and other soft tissue sprains in more acute onset pain and swelling, whereas in more elderly patients the practitioner will need to consider degenerative conditions of the radio-humeral joint and referral from the cervical spine (Brukner & Khan 2007).

Lateral epicondylalgia is by definition a clinical entity not usually requiring confirmatory diagnostic imaging or other medical pathology tests. Diagnostic imaging is likely more helpful in excluding differential diagnoses. For example, radiographs may be used to identify injuries of bone, such as, fractures, apophysitis and sub-chondral arthritic changes. Ultrasound has taken on a greater role in the direct identification of grey scale hypoechoic lesions, which imply dysfunction in the connective tissues. These grey scale changes are not necessarily linked to pain in the tendon (Cook et al 2001, 2004, du Toit et al 2008) and so they could be legitimately termed tendinopathy, meaning some pathology in the tendon, and is most likely due to degenerative breakdown of collagen fibrils (epicondylosis), though fusiform swelling may be more indicative of cellular and matrix dysfunction (Cook & Purdam 2009). Increasingly, evidence is pointing towards a link between neovessels and symptoms, namely pain (Cook et al 2001, 2004, du Toit et al 2008), with a recent study showing that in a patient with longstanding lateral elbow pain, which has failed to respond to treatment, the lack of neovessels strongly indicates that the pain is not due to tendinopathy, thus prompting the practitioner to consider other diagnoses (du Toit et al 2008). Magnetic resonance imaging may be used to follow up recalcitrant cases where there are no radiographic or ultrasonographic changes present, but these cases will be in the minority.

PATHOLOGIC CONSIDERATIONS

Nirschl & Pettrone (1979) described the underlying pathology of lateral epicondylalgia to be one of angiofibroblastic hyperplasia with the following identified histological changes: (a) proliferation in the number of cells and in ground substance, (b) neovascularization or vascular hyperplasia, (c) higher levels of algogenic substances, as well as (d) disorganized immature collagen (Nirschl & Pettrone 1979, Nirschl 1992, Regan et al 1992, Fredberg et al 2008). In an effort to more adequately explain different clinical presentations, Cook & Purdam (2009) have recently proposed a clinical model of histo-pathological changes across a continuum from: (a) reactive tendinopathy, (b) tendon disrepair to (c) degenerative tendinopathy. A brief summary of this proposed clinical model follows and the reader is referred to their paper for more detail.

Reactive tendinopathy is a non-inflammatory proliferative cellular and matrix response in response to either an acute tensile overload as may occur with a bout of unaccustomed physical activity or from a compressive overload due to a direct contact injury. This is likely to occur in the younger athlete who rapidly increases the intensity or volume of physical activity and is managed well with a short period of absence from the increased loading activities before restoring pain free function. Consequently the classic presentation of lateral epicondylalgia is not likely to fall into this category, though it is important to keep this category in mind for younger athletes such as tennis players or manual labourers, as well as patients who present with pain after an acute traumatic blow to the common extensor origin at the elbow. At the other end of the spectrum the degenerative phase is characterized by angiofibroblastic hyperplasia changes, with considerable breakdown in the collagen framework and neovascularization. This tends to occur with chronic overloading in the older person; hence more appropriately fits that which is likely to be present in a classical presentation of lateral epicondylalgia. There is a sound argument that exercises need to be a fundamental inclusion in the treatment plan for degenerative tendinopathy (Cook & Purdam 2009, Khan & Scott 2009).

PROGNOSTIC CONSIDERATIONS

Lateral epicondylalgia is widely regarded as being self-limiting and resolving within 6 months to 2 years, however this is low-level evidence as the natural history of this condition has not been definitively determined. Notwithstanding this, recently a number of randomized clinical trials that have followed cases over 12 months (Smidt et al 2002, Bisset et al 2006, 2007, Smidt & van der Windt 2006) and provide data that may be used in determining prognosis.

The evidence from two randomized clinical trials (n = 383) (Smidt et al 2002, Bisset et al 2006), which included randomizing a group of patients to following a wait-and-see policy indicates that 87% of patients reported being much improved or completely recovered 12 months after inclusion into the study (Bisset et al 2007). When considering that patients had on average approximately 6 months duration of pain at inclusion into the study (Bisset et al 2007), an approximate indicative natural history of the condition is in the order of 18 months for the majority of sufferers. It is important to keep in mind that the patients allocated to the group following the wait and see policy were given advice on avoiding aggravating activities (e.g. ergonomic advice on how to lift objects and manipulate implements without aggravating pain) as well as being closely monitored in a clinical trial (and thereby prone to the Hawthorne effect), which is not necessarily the same as a person with lateral epicondylalgia not seeking out advice and doing nothing about the condition. Furthermore, Bisset et al (2006) reported that those in the group allocated to wait and see policy were 2.7 times more likely to seek out other treatments than those allocated to a mobilization with movement and exercise group (OR, 95% CI: 4.7, 2.1–10.3), which is

not the same as doing nothing about the lateral epicondylalgia. To the contrary it tends to indicate that despite being recruited into a clinical trial and being closely monitored patients do not feel comfortable in doing nothing about their condition.

Smidt et al (2006) prospectively followed 349 patients from two randomized clinical trials (Hay et al 1999, Smidt et al 2002) over a 12-month period and found that those who had more severe pain of longer duration had greater likelihood of a worse outcome (more severe pain) at 12 months. Another prognostic factor of poor outcome was concomitant neck pain (Smidt et al 2006). This finding is interesting because it indicates that the patient pool recruited in this study had a heterogenic pain presentation, including cases with more complex presentations (e.g. lateral epicondylalgia plus neck pain) and did not consist solely of patients with isolated lateral epicondylalgia.

CONSIDERATIONS IN CONSERVATIVE TREATMENT

A wide range of conservative treatments, such as, medication, electrophysical agents, exercise and manual therapy are advocated for lateral epicondylalgia, which usually is an indication that no one treatment has proven superiority, but also in part a product of an inconclusive understanding of the underlying pathology of the condition.

Corticosteroid injections are the most common conservative medical intervention for lateral epicondylalgia and accordingly they have been studied the most in high quality rigorous clinical trials. There is level 1 evidence from a number of randomized clinical trials of short term efficacy with success rates over 80% in the first 4–6 weeks (Hay et al 1999, Smidt et al 2002, Bisset et al 2006, 2007, Smidt & van der Windt 2006), but this needs to be considered in light of post-6 weeks poorer outcomes in the form of lower success rates compared to the adoption of a wait and see policy (Smidt et al 2002, Bisset et al 2006, 2007, Smidt & van der Windt 2006), higher recurrence rates (70% vs 8%) and greater use of other not per protocol co-interventions (49% vs 21%) than those patients undergoing mobilization with movements and exercise intervention (Bisset et al 2006, 2007). The poorer downstream effects are sufficient to prompt caution in their use and some have advocated against their use in lateral epicondylalgia (Young et al 1954, Osborne 2009, Vicenzino 2009), at least in the first instance without a concerted attempt at other interventions that do not have such a poor longer-term effect on the condition. Others have advocated combining the use of these injections with physiotherapy (Coombes et al 2009a, Olaussen et al 2009), but there has not been the same level of enquiry.

There is a sound level of evidence in support of exercise in treating lateral epicondylalgia, but unlike in lower limb tendinopathy, eccentric exercise is not necessarily better than concentric exercise (Woodley et al 2007). Perhaps the most illustrative evidence comes from a randomized clinical trial comparing an exercise programme versus ultrasound in a group of patients who had recalcitrant lateral epicondylalgia having failed other treatments including corticosteroid injections and other common modalities (Pienimaki et al 1996). Follow up some 3 years later revealed that the exercise group required fewer medical consultations, had less surgery (NNT = 3) and 586 fewer sick days than the group that had ultrasound (Pienimaki et al 1998). The exercise programme was graduated and progressive from isometric to isotonic contractions of the wrist and forearm muscles, culminating in pragmatic exercises that replicated patient's required function. It was supervised two times per week for approximately 8 weeks. A recent study has shown that supervision of the exercise programme returns superior effects to a home based one (Stasinopoulos et al 2009), which should be considered when prescribing exercise.

Electrophysical agents such as LASER, ultrasound, and extracorporeal shock wave therapy (ESWT) have attracted attention. Low level LASER therapy has been shown to be effective in improving pain levels in the short term compared to control, but only at wavelength of 908 nm (Bjordal et al 2008). There appears to be less conclusive evidence and some contention for or against the use of ultrasound and ESWT in the treatment of lateral epicondylalgia, perhaps because of a lack of specification and stratification of dosage parameters.

Elbow orthotics or tennis elbow bands that fit about the proximal forearm are frequently used, often on a self-selection basis by patients. Systematic reviews have been unable to find sufficient high quality clinical trials to support or refute their use (Struijs et al 2001, 2002, 2004).

Joint (high and low velocity) and soft tissue manipulations have been proposed for use in treatment of lateral epicondylalgia (Lee 1986, Vicenzino et al 2007a). The initial effects of elbow mobilizations with movement (Vicenzino 2003) used as a single modality have been shown in a number of studies (Vicenzino et al 1996, 2001, 2007b, Abbott et al 2001, Paungmali et al 2003) and shown to be effective when used in combination with exercise (Kochar & Dogra 2002, Bisset et al 2006). There are conflicting interpretations of the literature regarding the use of Mill's manipulation and friction massage, also referred to as Cyriax physiotherapy (Vicenzino et al 2007a, Kohia et al 2008), which may be in part due to the lack of high quality clinical trials (Bisset et al 2005). There is a randomized clinical trial that has shown that wrist manipulation was efficacious when compared to ultrasound, friction massage and exercise (Struijs et al 2003).

As identified in a prognostic analysis, patients with concomitant neck pain have a poorer outcome (Smidt et al 2006), but the neck was not treated and so it is not possible to determine if it would have been beneficial to have added neck treatment to the elbow treatment. However, there are several other studies that show benefits of adding treatment of the cervical spine to elbow treatment (Gunn & Milbrandt 1976, Cleland et al 2004, 2005). Gunn & Milbrandt (1976) treated 50 recalcitrant cases of lateral epicondylalgia with non-thrust manipulation and traction of the cervical spine and showed an 86% success rate after treatment that persisted at 6 months. In a retrospective case audit of 112 cases, Cleland et al (2004) showed significantly fewer treatments were required for those (n = 51) who received additional manual therapy to the cervical spine in the form of non-thrust oscillatory manipulations, mobilization with movements and/or muscle energy techniques. More recently in a pilot trial of 10 cases, Cleland et al (2005) reported a better result on pain free grip force and the Disability of the Arm, Shoulder and Hand questionnaire. Furthermore, there are a number of studies that show both high and low-velocity manipulations of the cervical spine produce an initial improvement in pain at the elbow (Vicenzino et al 1996, 1998, Fernández-Carnero et al 2008). This evidence provides a basis for the cervical spine to be treated if found to be implicated on physical examination, especially since there have been reported significant differences in pain provocation on manual examination of the cervical spine and significant reductions in sagittal plane motion in patients with lateral epicondylalgia when compared to age-matched controls (Waugh et al 2004, Berglund et al 2008).

The challenge facing the practitioner is how to best select a treatment approach for each individual patient, who is likely to be somewhat different in their individual clinical presentations. The continuum model of presentation of tendinopathy (Cook & Purdam 2009) outlined above along with the proposed integrative model of lateral epicondylalgia (Coombes et al 2009b) may provide some guidance on how the practitioner may wish to select from the many proposed treatments. In brief, Coombes et al (2009b) propose that each patient presents with a different proportional representation of dysfunction in the pain and motor systems as well as in tendon structure and physiology, which could be used to select specific interventions. For example, if a patient presents with relatively greater pain system impediment as would be seen clinically with large deficits in pressure pain thresholds and high pain severity scores, then pain relieving medications, electrophysical agents and manual therapy should be favoured. In contrast, a patient who presented with a progressed stage of degenerative tendinopathy with moderate to low levels of pain would be managed more so with specific exercise (Coombes et al 2009b, Khan & Scott 2009) and possibly injections of medication/materials (Rabago et al 2009) or glyceryl trinitrate transdermal patches (Paoloni et al 2003, 2009, Murrell 2007) that promote collagen synthesis. Further detail regarding the integrative model of lateral epicondylalgia can be found in Coombes et al (2009b).

CONCLUSION

Tendinopathy at the elbow is commonly experienced over the lateral epicondyle. Over the past decade there has been an increase in the knowledge of our understanding of the underlying pathology, conservative management and prognosis of this pain condition. While this has provided more information and data for practitioners to consider when treating patients with lateral epicondylalgia, the challenge still remains to selectively apply specific treatments to individual patients in order to drive optimum outcomes. This chapter provides a synopsis of the recent evidence and some indication of possible means by which to apply such evidence clinically.

REFERENCES

Abbott, J.H., Patla, C.E., Jensen, R.H., 2001. The initial effects of an elbow mobilization with movement technique on grip strength in subjects with lateral epicondylalgia. Man. Ther. 6, 163–169.

Alfredson, H., Ljung, B.O., Thorsen, K., Lorentzon, R., 2000. In vivo investigation of ECRB tendons with microdialysis technique – no signs of inflammation but high amounts of glutamate in tennis elbow. Acta Orthop. Scand. 71, 475–479.

Allander, E., 1974. Prevalence, incidence, and remission rates of some common rheumatic diseases or syndromes. Scand. J. Rheumatol. 3, 145–153.

Berglund, K.M., Persson, B.H., Denison, E., 2008. Prevalence of pain and dysfunction in the cervical and thoracic spine in persons with and without lateral elbow pain. Man. Ther. 13, 295–339.

Bisset, L., Paungmali, A., Vicenzino, B., Beller, E., 2005. A systematic review and meta-analysis of clinical trials on physical interventions for lateral epicondylalgia. Br. J. Sports Med. 39, 411–422.

Bisset, L., Beller, E., Jull, G., Brooks, P., Darnell, R., Vicenzino, B., 2006. Mobilisation with movement and exercise, corticosteroid injection, or wait and see for tennis elbow: randomised trial. BMJ bmj 38961.584653.AE.

Bisset, L., Smidt, N., Van der Windt, D.A., Bouter, L.M., Jull, G., Brooks, P., et al., 2007. Conservative treatments for tennis elbow do subgroups of patients respond differently? Rheumatology (Oxford) 46, 1601–1605.

Bjordal, J.M., Lopes-Martins, R.A., Joensen, J., Couppe, C., Ljunggren, A.E., Stergioulas, A., et al., 2008. A systematic review with procedural assessments and meta-analysis of low level laser therapy in lateral elbow tendinopathy (tennis elbow). BMC Musculoskelet. Disord. 9, 75.

Brukner, P., Khan, K., 2007. Clinical Sports Medicine. McGraw-Hill, Northe Ryde, NSW.

Cleland, J.A., Whitman, J.M., Fritz, J.M., 2004. Effectiveness of manual physical therapy to the cervical spine in the management of lateral epicondylalgia: a retrospective analysis. J. Orthop. Sports Phys. Ther. 34, 713–722 discussion 722–714.

Cleland, J., Flynn, T., Palmer, J., 2005. Incorporation of manual therapy directed at the cervicothoracic spine in patients with lateral epicondylalgia: A pilot clinical trial. J. Man. Manip. Ther. 13, 143–151.

Cook, J.L., Purdam, C.R., 2009. Is tendon pathology a continuum? A pathology model to explain the clinical presentation of load-induced tendinopathy. Br. J. Sports Med. 43, 409–416.

Cook, J.L., Khan, K.M., Kiss, Z.S., Coleman, B.D., Griffiths, L., 2001. Asymptomatic hypoechoic regions on patellar tendon ultrasound: A 4-year clinical and ultrasound follow-up of 46 tendons. Scand. J. Med. Sci. Sports 11, 321–327.

Cook, J.L., Malliaras, P., De Luca, J., Ptasznik, R., Morris, M.E., Goldie, P., 2004. Neovascularization and pain in abnormal patellar tendons of active jumping athletes. Clin. J. Sport Med. 14, 296–299.

Coombes, B., Bisset, L., Connelly, L., Brooks, P., Vicenzino, B., 2009a. Optimising corticosteroid injection for lateral epicondylalgia with the addition of physiotherapy: A protocol for a randomised control trial with placebo comparison. BMC Musculoskelet. Disord. 10, 76.

Coombes, B., Bisset, L., Vicenzino, B., 2009b. An integrative model of lateral epicondylalgia. Br. J. Sports Med. 43, 252–258.

Dimberg, L., 1987. The prevalence and causation of tennis elbow (lateral humeral epicondylitis) in a population of workers in an engineering industry. Ergonomics 30, 573–580.

Du Toit, C., Stieler, M., Saunders, R., Bisset, L., Vicenzino, B., 2008. Diagnostic accuracy of power-Doppler Ultrasound In Patients With Chronic Tennis Elbow. Br. J. Sports Med. 42, 572–666.

Fernández-Carnero, J., Fernández-de-las-Peñas, C., Cleland, J.A., 2008. Immediate hypoalgesic and motor effects after a single cervical spine manipulation in subjects with lateral epicondylalgia. J. Manipulative Physiol. Ther. 31, 675–681.

Feuerstein, M., Miller, V.L., Burrell, L.M., Berger, R., 1998. Occupational upper extremity disorders in the federal workforce: Prevalence, health care expenditures, and patterns of work disability. J. Occup. Environ. Med. 40, 546–555.

Fredberg, U., Bolvig, L., Andersen, N.T., 2008. Prophylactic training in asymptomatic soccer players with ultrasonographic abnormalities in Achilles and patellar tendons: the Danish Super League Study. Am. J. Sports Med. 36, 451–460.

Gunn, C.C., Milbrandt, W.E., 1976. Tennis elbow and the cervical spine. Can. Med. Assoc. J. 114, 803–809.

Hay, E.M., Paterson, S.M., Lewis, M., Hosie, G., Croft, P., 1999. Pragmatic randomised controlled trial of local corticosteroid injection and naproxen for treatment of lateral epicondylitis of elbow in primary care. Br. Med. J. 319, 964–968.

Khan, K.M., Cook, J.L., 2000. Overuse tendon injuries: Where does the pain come from? Sports Med. Arthrosc. 8, 17–31.

Khan, K., Scott, A., 2009. Mechanotherapy: How physical therapists' prescription of exercise affects tissue repair. Br. J. Sports Med. 43, 247–252.

Kivi, P., 1982. The etiology and conservative treatment of humeral epicondylitis. Scand. J. Rehabil. Med. 15, 37–41.

Kochar, M., Dogra, A., 2002. Effectiveness of a specific physiotherapy regimen on patients with tennis elbow. Physiotherapy 88, 333–341.

Kohia, M., Brackle, J., Byrd, K., Jennings, A., Murray, W., Wilfong, E., 2008. Effectiveness of physical therapy treatments on lateral epicondylitis. Journal of Sport Rehabilitation 17, 119–136.

Kraushaar, B.S., Nirschl, R.P., 1999. Tendinosis of the elbow (tennis elbow). Clinical features and findings of histological, immunohistochemical, and electron microscopy studies. J. Bone Joint Surg. Am. 81, 259–278.

Lee, D., 1986. Tennis elbow: A manual therapist's perspective. J. Orthop. Sports Phys. Ther. 8, 134–142.

Ljung, B.O., Forsgren, S., Friden, J., 1999. Substance P and calcitonin gene-related peptide expression at the extensor carpi radialis brevis muscle origin: Implications for the etiology of tennis elbow. J. Orthop. Res. 17, 554–559.

Ljung, B.O., Alfredson, H., Forsgren, S., 2004. Neurokinin 1-receptors and sensory neuropeptides in tendon insertions at the medial and lateral epicondyles of the humerus: Studies on tennis elbow and medial epicondylalgia. J. Orthop. Res. 22, 321–327.

Murrell, G.A.C., 2007. Using nitric oxide to treat tendinopathy. Br. J. Sports Med. 41, 227–231.

Nirschl, R.P., 1992. Elbow tendinosis/tennis elbow. Clin. Sports Med. 11, 851–870.

Nirschl, R., Pettrone, F., 1979a. Tennis Elbow: The surgical treatment of lateral epicondylitis. J. Bone Surg. 61, 832–839.

Olaussen, M., Holmedal, O., Lindbaek, M., Brage, S., 2009. Physiotherapy alone or in combination with corticosteroid injection for acute lateral epicondylitis in general practice: A protocol for a randomised, placebo-controlled study. BMC Musculoskelet. Disord. 10, 152.

Osborne, H., 2010. Stop injecting corticosteroid into patients with tennis elbow, they are much more likely to get better by themselves!. J. Sports Sci. Med. 13 (4), 380–381.

Paoloni, J.A., Appleyard, R.C., Nelson, J., Murrell, G.A., 2003. Topical nitric oxide application in the treatment of chronic extensor tendinosis at the elbow: a randomized, double-blinded, placebo-controlled clinical trial. Am. J. Sports Med. 31, 915–920.

Paoloni, J.A., Murrell, G.A., Burch, R., Ang, R., 2009. Randomised, double blind, placebo controlled, multicentre dose-ranging clinical trial of a new topical Glyceryl Trinitrate patch for chronic lateral epicondylosis. Br. J. Sports Med. 43, 299–302.

Paungmali, A., O'Leary, S., Souvlis, T., Vicenzino, B., 2003. Hypoalgesic and sympathoexcitatory effects of mobilization with movement for lateral epicondylalgia. Phys. Ther. 83, 374–383.

Pienimaki, T., Tarvainen, T., Siira, P., Vanharanta, H., 1996. Progressive strengthening and stretching exercises and ultrasound for chronic lateral epicondylitis. Physiotherapy 82, 522–530.

Pienimaki, T., Karinen, P., Kemila, T., Koivukangas, P., Vanharanta, H., 1998. Long-term follow-up of conservatively treated chronic tennis elbow patients. A prospective and retrospective analysis. Scand. J. Rehabil. Med. 30, 159–166.

Potter, H.G., Hannafin, J.A., Morwessel, R.M., DiCarlo, E.F., O'Brien, S.J., Altchek, D.W., 1995. Lateral epicondylitis: correlation of MR imaging, surgical, and histopathologic findings. Radiology 196, 43–46.

Rabago, D., Best, T.M., Zgierska, A.E., Zeisig, E., Ryan, M., Crane, D., 2009. A systematic review of four injection therapies for lateral epicondylosis: prolotherapy, polidocanol, whole blood and platelet-rich plasma. Br. J. Sports Med. 43, 471–481.

Regan, W., Wold, L.E., Coonrad, R., Morrey, B.F., 1992. Microscopic histopathology of chronic refractory lateral epicondylitis. Am. J. Sports Med. 20, 746–749.

Slater, H., Arendt-Nielsen, L., Wright, A., Graven-Nielsen, T., 2003. Experimental deep tissue pain in wrist extensors – a model of lateral epicondylalgia. Eur. J. Pain 7, 277–288.

Slater, H., Arendt-Nielsen, L., Wright, A., Graven-Nielsen, T., 2005. Sensory and motor effects of experimental muscle pain in patients with lateral epicondylalgia and controls with delayed onset muscle soreness. Pain 114, 118–130.

Smidt, N., van der Windt, D.A.W.M., 2006. Tennis elbow in primary care. Br. Med. J. 333, 927–928.

Smidt, N., van der Windt, D., Assendelft, W.J.J., Deville, W., Korthals-de Bos, I.B.C., Bouter, L.M., 2002. Corticosteroid injections, physiotherapy, or a wait-and-see policy for lateral epicondylitis: a randomised controlled trial. Lancet 359, 657–662.

Smidt, N., Lewis, M., DA, V.D.W., Hay, E.M., Bouter, L.M., Croft, P., 2006. Lateral epicondylitis in general practice: course and prognostic indicators of outcome. J. Rheumatol. 33, 2053–2059.

Stasinopoulos, D., Stasinopoulou, K., Stasinopoulos, I., Manias, P., 2010. Comparison of effects of a home exercise programme and a supervised exercise programme for the management of lateral elbow tendinopathy. Br. J. Sports Med. 44 (8), 579–583.

Struijs, P.A.A., Smidt, N., Arola, H., van Dijk, C.N., Buchbinder, R., Assendelft, W.J.J., 2001. Orthotic devices for tennis elbow: a systematic review. Br. J. Gen. Pract. 51, 924–929.

Struijs, P.A.A., Smidt, N., Arola, H., van Dijk, C.N., Buchbinder, R., Assendelft, W.J.J., 2002. Orthotic devices for the treatment of tennis elbow (Cochrane Review). In: The Cochrane Library. Update Software, Oxford Issue 4.

Struijs, P.A.A., Damen, P.J., Bakker, E.W. P., Blankevoort, L., Assendelft, W.J.J., van Dijk, C.N., 2003. Manipulation of the wrist for management of lateral epicondylitis: A randomized pilot study. Phys. Ther. 83, 608–616.

Struijs, P.A.A., Kerkhoffs, G., Assendelft, W.J.J., van Dijk, C.N., 2004. Conservative treatment of lateral epicondylitis – Brace versus physical therapy or a combination of both: A randomized clinical trial. Am. J. Sports Med. 32, 462–469.

Verhaar, J.A., 1994. Tennis elbow. Anatomical, epidemiological and therapeutic aspects. Int. Orthop. 18, 263–267.

Vicenzino, B., 2003. Lateral epicondylalgia: A musculoskeletal physiotherapy perspective. Man. Ther. 8, 66–79.

Vicenzino, B., 2009. Time for a re-think on the role of corticosteroid injections? Rapid Response to: Cohen SP et al, Comparison of fluoroscopically guided and blind corticosteroid injections for greater trochanteric pain syndrome: multicentre randomised controlled trial. Br. Med. J. 338, doi:10.1136/bmj.b1088.

Vicenzino, B., Collins, D., Wright, A., 1996. The initial effects of a cervical spine manipulative physiotherapy treatment on the pain and dysfunction of lateral epicondylalgia. Pain 68, 69–74.

Vicenzino, B., Collins, D., Benson, H., Wright, A., 1998. An investigation of the interrelationship between manipulative therapy induced hypoalgesia and sympathoexcitation. J. Manipulative Physiol. Ther. 21, 448–453.

Vicenzino, B., Paungmali, A., Buratowski, S., Wright, A., 2001. Specific manipulative therapy treatment for chronic lateral epicondylalgia produces uniquely characteristic hypoalgesia. Man. Ther. 6, 205–212.

Vicenzino, B., Cleland, J., Bisset, L., 2007a. Joint manipulation in the management of lateral epicondylalgia: Clinical Commentary. J. Man. Manip. Ther. 15, 50–56.

Vicenzino, B., Paungmali, A., Teys, P., 2007b. Mulligan's mobilization-with-movement, positional faults and pain relief: current concepts from a critical review of literature. Man. Ther. 12, 98–108.

Waugh, E.J., Jaglal, S.B., Davis, A.M., Tomlinson, G., Verrier, M.C., 2004. Factors associated with prognosis of lateral epicondylitis after 8 weeks of physical therapy. Arch. Phys. Med. Rehabil. 85, 308–318.

Woodley, B.L., Newsham-West, R.J., Baxter, G.D., Kjaer, M., Koehle, M.S., 2007. Chronic tendinopathy: effectiveness of eccentric exercise. Br. J. Sports Med. 41, 188–198.

Young, H.H., Ward, L.E., Henderson, E.D., 1954. The use of hydrocortisone acetate (compound F acetate) in the treatment of some common orthopaedic conditions. J. Bone Joint Surg. Am 36, 602–609.

Zeisig, E., Ohberg, L., Alfredson, H., 2006. Extensor origin vascularity related to pain in patients with tennis elbow. Knee Surg. Sports Traumatol. Arthrosc. 14, 659–663.

Chapter | 24 |

Other elbow disorders: elbow instability, arthritic conditions

Chris A Sebelski

INTRODUCTION

This chapter will present two specific conditions of the elbow: elbow instability and arthritic conditions. Each section presents a short introduction with incidence/prevalence, relevant anatomy, clinical examination information and, finally, non-operative treatment. The reader is encouraged to remember that elbow dysfunction rarely occurs in isolation (Royle 1991, Walker-Bone et al 2004). When approaching a clinical case involving elbow pathology, the clinician must determine the underlying primary aetiology, the potential secondary aetiologies, the associated impairments and finally the role of regional interdependence for determination of the appropriate plan of care.

ELBOW INSTABILITY

Overall, the elbow is the second most common dislocated joint in adults, with posterior dislocation being the most common (Royle 1991). It is the most commonly dislocated joint in the paediatric age group (Kuhn & Ross 2008). In the young or with advanced age associated injuries such as fractures occur, while non-complex dislocations most commonly occur within the younger, athletic populations (Mehta & Bain 2004). There are five criteria (O'Driscoll et al 2001a) to assist in classifying elbow instability:

- the involved articulation(s)
- the direction of displacement
- the degree of displacement
- the duration (acute, chronic or recurrent)
- the presence/absence of associated fractures.

Injury progression is represented through the circle of Horii where the injury progresses from lateral to medial through soft tissue, bone or both. Due to the energy absorption by a fracture, one may see ligament sparing with a fracture of the radius or the coronoid. In the progression of stages, stage I would demonstrate disruption of the lateral collateral ligament (LCL) with a presentation of postero-lateral instability; stage II signifies disruption of the capsule with anterior and posterior instability and stage III demonstrates disruption of the portions of the medial collateral ligament. Stage III is further divided into subparts A, B and C (O'Driscoll et al 2001a).

Anatomy review for elbow instability

There are three primary constraints for elbow stability: the ulno-humeral joint, the medial collateral ligament and the lateral ulnar collateral ligament. Though O'Driscoll (2000) originally named the lateral ulnar collateral ligament as a primary constraint, there is controversy regarding its importance. Cadaver studies have demonstrated elbow posterolateral rotatory instability (PLRI) when artificially induced sectioning at various parts throughout the LCL complex (Olsen et al 1996, Singleton & Conway 2004). Secondary constraints include: the radial head, the common flexor origin, the common extensor origin, and the joint capsule. Dynamic constraints produce compressive forces at the joint including the biceps brachii, triceps, and anconeus (O'Driscoll 2000).

General treatment planning guidelines for elbow instability

Treatment varies according to the severity of the injury. With an acute dislocation without an associated elbow fracture, the treatment recommended is a closed reduction followed by bracing for a short period of time. The patient is typically directed to use the upper extremity for daily function within symptom tolerance following weaning of the brace. Simple elbow dislocations have a good prognosis with up to 95% of the persons affected returning to their previous level of activity (Hildebrand et al 1999). However, if symptoms persist, then the intervention plan must be adapted dependent upon the injury and the symptoms reported. The presence of fractures with a dislocation/subluxation changes the course of treatment as typically there is surgical intervention for the fracture. If an acute ligament injury is sustained in conjunction with a fracture of the radius or the coronoid, then a repair of that ligament is necessary to assist with the stability of the joint (O'Driscoll et al 2001a). In the sections which follow, elbow instability is further discussed by injury to the lateral or medial ligament structures.

Lateral elbow instability

Anatomy review for lateral elbow instability

The lateral collateral ligament (LCL) complex originates from the humerus at the trochlea and capitellum and continues distally to blend with the annular ligament inserting at the proximal ulna (Cohen & Bruno 2001). This complex consists of up to four structures: the annular ligament, the ulnar portion of the LCL, the radial portion of the LCL and the inconsistently present accessory LCL. The lateral ligament complex is taut throughout elbow flexion and extension. Ligament tension is increased with the forearm positioned in supination.

Incidence/prevalence of lateral elbow instability

Postero-lateral rotatory elbow instability (PLRI), an injury to the lateral collateral ligament and the soft tissue stabilizers, is the most common type of chronic instability at the elbow. In contrast, isolated varus instability from the laxity of the LCL is not as common as an isolated medial collateral ligament injury (Charalambous & Stanley 2008).

Pathology/patho-anatomy of lateral elbow instability

There are three typical scenarios that may lead to lateral collateral ligament injury: elbow dislocation, varus stress insufficiency/chronic attenuation or iatrogenic causes (Singleton & Conway 2004). Typically, elbow dislocation is an acute occurrence, O'Driscoll et al. (1992) proposed that elbow posterolateral rotatory instability (PLRI) may be the initial step towards elbow laxity. PLRI may present as an independent pathology or it may be part of a continuum leading to dislocation (Smith et al 2001). PLRI has also been cited as the most common cause of recurrent symptoms following dislocation (O'Driscoll et al 2001a). Chronic attenuation and/or varus insufficiency may occur with overuse such as in the cases of patients with significant weight bearing activities on the upper extremities such as crutch ambulation or those persons with generalized ligament laxity. A causal relationship of cubitus varus and recurrent elbow instability in the form of PLRI has been reported by several authors, with symptoms which may not appear until more than two decades post injury (O'Driscoll et al 2001a,b, Arrigoni & Kamineni 2009). It has been theorized that these symptoms may be secondary to the attenuation of the ligament from the repetitive torque on the LCL and the inappropriate pull of secondary stabilizers. Iatrogenic cause to the integrity of the LCL may be from surgical approaches which involve the lateral elbow structures such as a lateral epicondylar release procedure or an approach to access the radial head (O'Driscoll 2000). Surgical approaches at the lateral elbow structures or to access the radial head may endanger the integrity of the LCL (O'Driscoll 2000).

PLRI affects the articulation between the ulna and the humerus while the proximal radio-ulnar joint remains intact. This differs from a simple posterior dislocation of the radial head where the ulno-humeral joint remains intact and the proximal radio-ulnar joint is disrupted. With postero lateral rotatory instability (PLRI), the forearm externally rotates (supinates) away from the humerus, effectively 'pivoting' on the intact medial collateral ligaments allowing the radial head to subluxate in a posterior direction.

These mechanics provide support for special attention to the position of the forearm during orthopaedic testing. Traditionally, varus stress testing is utilized when examining a patient with probable disruption of the lateral ligaments of the elbow. Valgus stress testing is to determine the laxity of the medial collateral ligament. Indications of probable medial collateral ligament laxity would be the presence of laxity/apprehension with the forearm in pronation and application of a valgus stress. The pronated forearm position and medially directed stress tensions the medial collateral ligament. During forearm pronation, the lateral structures of the elbow are tensioned, stabilizing the radial head. However; if the forearm is positioned in supination and a valgus stress is applied, the lateral structures are unable to appropriately stabilize the radial head. Therefore, if the patient demonstrates laxity or appears apprehensive when the forearm is supinated and tensioned in the valgus direction, PLRI should be suspected (Smith et al 2001).

Diagnosis of lateral elbow instability

In a search for lateral collateral laxity, history taking should include inquiring about the three potential mechanisms including both acute dislocations and a history of dislocation if a patient report is suspicious for chronic recurring instability. Questioning should include positions of the upper extremity that place the elbow at risk of chronic attenuation including history of elbow fracture as a youth. Additionally, medical history which may contribute to generalized ligament laxity should be explored.

Patient concerns may include 'vague' aching about the elbow joint, pain, clicking, snapping or clunking that is worse with a supinated position of the forearm. Patients may comment of 'something not right' when extending their arm with the forearm in supination (Lee & Rosenwasser 1999, O'Driscoll 2000). Unless there is an associated traumatic event, rarely will the patient be able to isolate the onset of the symptoms.

Physical exam measures include observation for a cubitus varus deformity, range of motion and special orthopaedic testing (Table 24.1) that may be passive and/or active. Reporting of the statistical evidence for orthopaedic tests is limited and due to the supportive roles of the secondary soft tissue constraints, the passive exam techniques are

Table 24.1 Orthopaedic examination techniques for lateral elbow instability		
Name of test	**Physical exam technique**	**Outcome to indicate a positive test for pathology**
Varus stress test	Application of a laterally directed force applied in both full extension and at approximately 30° of elbow flexion to allow the olecranon to move out of the olecranon fossa. It is recommended to perform this test with the humerus fully internally rotated (O'Driscoll et al 2001b)	Greater laxity is felt by therapist in comparison to contralateral side.
Lateral pivot shift test	Patient lies supine with the shoulder passively flexed past 90°. With the elbow in extension, the examiner applies axial compression through the ulna and radius towards the humerus with a supination and valgus force causing the elbow to subluxate at ~40–70° of elbow flexion. If the patient allows the passive examination to continue, then an observable clunk occurs with continued flexion as the elbow reduces (O'Driscoll et al 1991, 1992, O'Driscoll, 2000)	Postero-lateral displacement of radius occurs followed by reduction as elbow flexion progresses to 90° (O'Driscoll et al 1991) The apprehension test would have the patient report apprehension prior to the subluxation.

Continued

Table 24.1 Orthopaedic examination techniques for lateral elbow instability—cont'd

Name of test	Physical exam technique	Outcome to indicate a positive test for pathology
Posterolateral instability test	The examiner flexes the elbow to 40°, with the forearm in external rotation: an antero-posterior force is applied to the ulna and radius (O'Driscoll et al 2001b)	Subluxation of the forearm away from the humerus.
Push up sign (from floor) (Arvind & Hargreaves 2006)	Patient pushes up from the floor with shoulders in abduction, forearms supinated.	Apprehension and voluntary/involuntary guarding as involved elbow moves towards terminal extension
Tabletop relocation test (Arvind & Hargreaves 2006)	3-step test: 1. Patient performs a press up from a table top with forearm in supination. 2. With onset of symptoms (approximately 40° of flexion) examiner applies a force through their thumb at the patient's radial head 3. Then the examiner removes the force at the radial head.	First outcome: pain and apprehension. Second outcome: pain and apprehension are reduced. Third outcome: pain/apprehension returns.

often recommended to be completed with the patient under anaesthesia for best results (O'Driscoll et al 2001b). In the case of a varus directed stress test, a false negative may be reported as the ulno-humeral articulation is the main constraint to varus movements (Charalambous & Stanley 2008). As indicated earlier, the examination technique for medial collateral laxity via the valgus stress test may give the examiner clues to a potential PLRI pathology if completed with the forearm in supination (Olsen et al 1998). However, for detection of PLRI the most utilized examination technique is the postero-lateral rotatory instability test. Changing the positive response of the postero-lateral rotatory instability test to be patient apprehension instead of a visible 'clunk' has also been advocated (Charalambous & Stanley 2008). Suggested imaging includes: stress radiographs, arthrogram or for PLRI, MRI imaging can be used though a specific pulse sequence is described (Potter et al 1997).

Prognosis and treatment planning for patients with lateral elbow instability

Despite its high prevalence for dislocation, the elbow is considered to be one of the most stable joints in the body. The philosophy of treatment of elbow instability with associated fractures is to first stabilize the osseous-articular injuries. With the achievement of the osseous stabilization, the next step is to address liagmentous injury. With more complex injuries, the prognosis for full functional return declines. Intervention and management of a dislocation without fracture has demonstrated good outcomes overall (O'Driscoll et al 2001b, Kuhn & Ross 2008).

In general, non-operative care for patients who demonstrate symptom producing recurrent instability such as that found with PLRI or varus insufficiency is not common. However; bracing to assist in avoidance of forearm supination with valgus loading may be advocated for those patients with a low level of symptoms. In cases of recurrent symptoms, operative management may be undertaken via direct repair or reattachment of the ligament or to reconstruct the lateral ligament complex with a tendon graft reconstruction. The results following surgical reconstruction, though limited, are promising (Nestor et al 1992, Lee & Teo 2003) with resolution of symptoms, full range of motion and a return to activity. Operative care may also be advocated for correction of cubitus varus with those patients who demonstrate positive physical exam signs for PLRI (O'Driscoll et al 2001a).

Medial elbow instability

Anatomy review for medial elbow instability

There are three ligaments of the medial collateral ligament (MCL) complex, namely the anterior oblique/bundle, the posterior oblique/band, and the transverse ligament/band. The origin of the MCL is slightly posterior to the elbow joint, demonstrating greater tension with increasing flexion. The anterior bundle of the MCL is the strongest of the three and attaches from the medial epicondyle to the medial coronoid process. Histologically, the anterior bundle may be further divided into anterior and posterior bands (Safran & Baillargeon 2005). The anterior band is primarily taut from full extension to 60° of flexion. The posterior band of the anterior bundle is taut from 60° to 120° of flexion (Cohen & Bruno 2001, Safran 2004, Safran & Baillargeon 2005). The posterior oblique portion of the MCL complex is a thickening of the capsule that has the greatest restraint at 90° of elbow flexion. It arises from the medial epicondyle and inserts onto the medial side of the semilunar notch. The third portion of the MCL is the transverse ligament arising from the medial olecranon and the inferior medial coronoid process. It has limited impact, is variably present, and is often indistinguishable from the capsule (Cohen & Bruno 2001, Safran & Baillargeon 2005).

Additional stabilizers of the elbow include the radio-capitellar joint and the regional muscles. The radio-capitellar joint contributes up to 30% of the stability against valgus stress. The regional muscles of the pronator and the flexors may also have a role, however; the significance of their contribution is not yet completely understood (Cohen & Bruno 2001, Safran 2004).

Incidence/prevalence of medial elbow instability

Injury to the MCL is more common in the overhead athlete population than the non-thrower population. In the throwing athlete, consequences of such instability may include the inability to compete at the desired level. In the general population, it rarely affects activities of daily living (Grace & Field 2008) unless there is a specified job task within the work environment. Bennett et al (1992) provide one example with industrial workers who demonstrated symptoms of chronic medial ligament instability during specific work tasks eventually requiring surgical intervention for return to work.

Pathology/patho-anatomy of medial elbow instability

There are two mechanisms for MCL laxity: acute or spontaneous and chronic attenuation. The symptoms that the patient will report may differ between the two incidences. A 'pop' may be heard in the more acute cases whereas there may be a report of vague elbow discomfort that becomes more prevalent over a length of time in a mechanism which involves chronic attenuation.

The mechanics of throwing have been studied to determine the contribution to medial collateral laxity. Of note, the MCL (primarily the anterior bundle) provides up to 54% of the varus torque to resist the valgus strain in the elbow during the late cocking and early deceleration phases of throwing (Fleisig et al 1995). The ultimate failure load of the MCL is calculated to be less (34 Nm) than the loads that it is exposed to during the majority of overhead sports (52–120 Nm) (Fleisig et al 1995). Therefore, it is hypothesized that there is a significant influence from the proximal segments and core of the upper extremity to generate secondary constraints for control of these forces

(Kibler & Sciascia 2004). It is suggested that an imbalance of the contribution from the local structures and/or inadequate contribution from the proximal segments and core would create an environment of excessive strain which would result in attenuation over time.

Typically with a chronic condition, the MCL laxity may represent only one aspect of a constellation of injuries that contribute to the medial elbow pain. For example, the ligament injury may be a part of valgus extension overload syndrome which involves the compression of the olecranon of the ulna against the humerus with a valgus stress. Associated injuries may include: capitellar wear, posteromedial osteophytes, ulnar neuritis, and degenerative or traumatic arthritis of the elbow. Furthermore, due to the dynamic nature of the population this pathology is often associated with, it is important to consider the influence of the kinetic chain. In two different reports, findings indicated that professional baseball players presenting with both medial elbow symptoms of insufficiency and significant gleno-humeral internal rotation deficits, demonstrate a kinetic chain relationship where impairments outside of the local region may have a causal relationship to the symptoms reported at the elbow (Kibler & Sciascia 2004, Dines et al 2009).

Diagnosis of medial elbow instability

Patient history should not only include location, duration of symptoms and the mechanism of injury but also the details of a throwing or overhead movement history if the patient is an athlete (Safran 2004). The patient presentation may be complicated with the complaints from the secondary structures involved in the overload mechanism including muscular strain, inflammation, or tendinosis that may be associated with the underlying instability.

Physical exam includes palpation, observation for a cubitus varus deformity, range of motion and special orthopedic testing that may be passive or active (Table 24.2). With palpation, the clinician may find tenderness approximately 2 cm distal from the medial epicondyle at the ulnar insertion of MCL. This tenderness has been reported in as many as 80% of those patients undergoing MCL reconstruction. Range of motion limitations may often include a flexion contracture (Thompson et al 2001).

For specific physical exam measures such as the valgus stress test and the milking manoeuvre statistical evidence is limited. Similar to the special testing of the lateral ligaments of the elbow, consideration must be paid to the supportive roles of the secondary soft tissue constraints. For example, during the valgus stress test, it has been stated that the position of supination for the forearm should provide a greater bias of the MCL over the contribution from the LCL (Smith et al 2001). However, in a cadaveric study by Safran et al (2005) where both the anterior and posterior bands of the anterior bundle of the MCL were sectioned and tested at various angles of

Table 24.2 Orthopaedic examination techniques for medial elbow instability

Name of test	Physical exam technique	Outcome to indicate a positive test for pathology
Valgus stress test	Application of a medial directed force applied at the elbow in both full extension and between 30–40° elbow flexion to allow the olecranon to move out of the olecranon fossa. The humeral position is suggested to be in external rotation.	Greater laxity is felt by therapist in comparison to contra-lateral side.
Milking test (Grace & Field 2008)	A valgus force is applied by the patient with the elbow flexed. This is done by the patient holding the thumb on the involved side with the contralateral upper extremity. The contralateral upper extremity must reach under the elbow of the involved side to grasp the thumb.	Medial elbow pain with this manoeuvre indicates a positive result
Moving valgus stress test (O'Driscoll et al 2005)	Therapist passively moves the involved elbow through range of motion flexion to extension while simultaneously applying a valgus force.	The test is positive if the medial elbow pain is reproduced at the medial collateral ligament. Maximum symptoms should be felt between 120° and 70° during flexion and extension.

flexion and forearm position, the neutral position of the forearm in relationship to the horizontal, regardless of the degree of elbow flexion, assessed the integrity of the MCL more clearly than any other position. It should be noted, that this alteration in the procedure of the valgus stress test has not been tested in humans, therefore the information must be viewed cautiously.

For detection of medial ligament instability such as commonly seen with partial tearing or attenuation in the throwing athlete, the moving valgus stress test as described by O'Driscoll et al (2005) is the most widely used with supportive statistical evidence of sensitivity of 1.0 and specificity of 0.75. Imaging techniques such as static imaging, stress radiographs, MRI, CT scan and arthroscopic valgus stress testing have all been utilized with varying degrees of success (O'Driscoll et al 2005).

Prognosis and treatment planning for patients with medial elbow instability

Treatment of non-throwers and the general population is via a non-operative rehabilitation programme with reported successful return to the activities of daily living without symptoms (Grace & Field 2008). For that subset of patients wishing to return to high demand throwing, non-operative therapy is attempted initially and with a failure to return, operative management is considered.

In a single study by Rettig et al (2001) throwers with chronic medial instability were treated non-operatively. They achieved a 42% success rate in returning the athlete to sport within an average of 24.5 weeks. The rehabilitation was divided into two phases. The first phase involved a rest from throwing for up to three months, resolution of

inflammation including brace wear and achievement of full range of motion. The second phase included a progressive strengthening programme and stepwise progression towards a return to throwing.

Information gained from cadaveric studies can provide cues for rehabilitation. Armstrong et al (2000) studied the MCL in cadaveric elbow and concluded that active mobilization of the elbow in the vertical position with either a fully supinated or pronated forearm position is safe for decreased stress at the ligament. With tension in the medial structures, one might construct a rehabilitation programme which incorporates limited humeral external rotation in combination with neutral forearm positioning and avoidance of valgus stresses especially during 70–120 degrees of elbow flexion. In a cadaveric study by Bernas et al (2009) the immediate post rehabilitative phase was concluded to be an appropriate time to introduce isometric flexion and extension below 90° of flexion and to limit motion from full extension to 50° of flexion to protect the MCL.

ARTHRITIC CONDITIONS

Anatomy review for arthritic conditions of the elbow

The elbow is comprised of three articulations: the ulna articulating with the humerus, the ulna articulating with the radius and the radius articulating with the humerus. There are two degrees of freedom in the elbow joint: flexion/extension and pronation/supination. The functional arc of motion of the elbow is 30–130°. A total range of less than 100° degrees in the sagittal plane or the transverse plane will generate significant functional limitations (Morrey et al 1981).

Incidence/prevalence of arthritic conditions of the elbow

Arthritis of the elbow is relatively uncommon. It typically falls into three categories: rheumatoid arthritis (RA), post traumatic arthritis or primary degenerative osteoarthritis (OA). In the patient population with RA, it has been found that 25–66% of the patients may have the presence of disease in one or both elbows (Porter et al 1974, Lehtinen et al 2001). Primary degenerative arthritis of the elbow has been reported to affect less than 2% of the population (Antuna et al 2002). Though the theory remains somewhat controversial, it is generally accepted that primary OA of the elbow affects males with a history of 'heavy use of the upper extremity' such as industrial labour, weight lifting etc. (Gramstad & Galatz 2006, Kokkalis et al 2009). These patients are typically not less than 40 years of age (Gramstad & Galatz 2006).

Pathology/patho-anatomy of arthritic conditions of the elbow

Rheumatoid arthritis is an inflammatory disease process that affects multiple joints. It is characterized by symmetric joint narrowing, disuse osteopenia and peri-articular erosions which will be seen on radiographic imaging (Kokkalis et al 2009). The course and natural history of the osteoarthritis is not well understood, however; it is typically characterized by destruction of the articular cartilage (Gramstad & Galatz 2006). Primary osteoarthritis of the elbow demonstrates unique features such as sparing of the articular surfaces with preservation of the joint spaces and hypertrophic formation of osteophytes and capsular constriction (Cheung et al 2008). Osteoarthritis begins on the lateral aspect of the joint at the radio-capitellar joint (Goodfellow & Bullough 1967). In the younger population with a presentation of elbow stiffness, post traumatic arthritis should be suspected. Associated disorders to this pathology include: trauma, osteochondritis dissecans, synovial chondromatosis and valgus extension overload syndrome (Gramstad & Galatz 2006).

Diagnosis of arthritic conditions of the elbow

Generally, the patient reports pain, stiffness and potential weakness. Functionally, they often have symptoms with attempts at carrying a weighted object next to the body when the elbow is extended. Dependent on the underlying cause of the arthritis, the patient reports may vary. For example, a patient with elbow pain secondary to RA may complain of pain throughout the range of motion (Soojian & Kwon 2007). A patient with osteoarthritis may have concerns of 'pinching' or 'sharp pain' with terminal flexion or extension during the earlier stages of the disease (Cheung et al 2008), whereas, patients with a diagnosis of post-traumatic arthritis may be younger and healthier than those with RA or OA with less involvement of other body regions. These patients may also possess an expectation of higher demand of the elbow (Amirfeyz & Blewitt 2009). In Table 24.3, specific features of each of the most common pathologies associated with elbow arthritis are highlighted.

A detailed interview of the patient to note the onset of symptoms, course of associated disease process or prior surgical/traumatic history is necessary. Prior treatment for either the arthritic disease or specifically to the elbow should be inquired of including pharmacologic therapies.

Table 24.3 Patient presentation with arthritic conditions of the elbow

Underlying disease	Patient report	Comments
Rheumatoid arthritis	Pain throughout the range of motion	Loss of rotation Excessive motion in the coronal plane (Soojian & Kwon 2007) Possible underlying instability
Post-traumatic arthritis	Stiffness and pain with inadequate end ROM	History of trauma, surgery to joint Possible underlying instability
Primary degenerative OA	Initially, pain only at the terminal ROM In later stages, pain throughout the ROM Catching/locking may be reported	Need to monitor progression of disease as this impacts treatment

Radiographs are the standard to determine the phase of the disease process and the potential plan of care. Of special note, one should recognize potential differential diagnoses which may produce similar patient concerns including septic arthritis, crystalline arthropathy, haemophilia and ochronosis (Soojian & Kwon 2007).

Prognosis and treatment planning for patients with arthritic conditions of the elbow

The underlying aetiology, functional limitations including the current range of motion of the elbow and the age of the patient significantly influence treatment course. The current standard is non-operative treatment which may include pharmacologic management, corticosteroid injections, dynamic splinting, and physical therapy (Gramstad & Galatz 2006, Kokkalis et al 2009). With the advent of improved and more aggressive treatment of RA, one report stated that early management has the potential for complete resolution of symptoms in 10% of patients treated (Brasington 2009). For patients with primary OA at the elbow, activity modification is typically suggested with varying results.

With failure of such non-operative measures to resolve the patient's functional limitations or symptoms, there is a wide variety of surgical options including arthroscopy and arthroplasty. The best results for management of OA and post-traumatic OA within the younger patient population has been reported via arthroscopy for a capsular release and clearing of osteophytes (Gramstad & Galatz 2006). The total elbow arthroplasty is typically reserved for the population that is greater than 60 years of age, has lower physical demands and who are more likely to comply with the post operative rehabilitative and long term physical restrictions (Moro & King 2000).

CONCLUSION

In recent years, there has been a significant gain in understanding of the anatomy and pathologies of the elbow which cause instability and stiffness. With the discovery of this information more research needs to be completed to develop rehabilitation guidelines which produce successful outcomes.

REFERENCES

Amirfeyz, R., Blewitt, N., 2009. Mid-term outcome of GSB-III total elbow arthroplasty in patients with rheumatoid arthritis and patients with post-traumatic arthritis. Arch. Orthop. Trauma Surg. August 17, 2009, 1–6.

Antuna, S.A., Morrey, B.F., Adams, R.A., O'Driscoll, S.W., 2002. Ulnohumeral arthroplasty for primary degenerative arthritis of the elbow: long-term outcome and complications. J. Bone Joint Surg. Am. 84A, 2168–2173.

Armstrong, A.D., Dunning, C.E., Faber, K.J., Duck, T.R., Johnson, J.A., King, G.J., 2000. Rehabilitation of the medial collateral ligament-deficient elbow: an in vitro biomechanical study. J. Hand Surg.Am. 25, 1051–1057.

Arrigoni, P., Kamineni, S., 2009. Uncovered posterolateral rotatory elbow instability with cubitus varus deformity correction. Orthopedics 32, 130.

Arvind, C.H., Hargreaves, D.G., 2006. Table top relocation test – New clinical test for posterolateral rotatory instability of the elbow. J. Shoulder Elbow Surg. 15, 500–501.

Bennett, J.B., Green, M.S., Tullos, H.S., 1992. Surgical management of chronic medial elbow instability. Clin. Orthop. Relat. Res. 278, 62–68.

Bernas, G.A., Ruberte Thiele, R., Kinnaman, K.A., Hughes, R.E., Miller, B.S., Carpenter, J.E., 2009. Defining safe rehabilitation for ulnar collateral ligament reconstruction of the elbow: A biomechanical study. Am. J. Sports Med. August 14, 2009, 1–9.

Brasington, R., 2009. TNF-alpha antagonists and other recombinant proteins for the treatment of rheumatoid arthritis. J. Hand Surg. Am. 34, 349–350.

Charalambous, C.P., Stanley, J.K., 2008. Posterolateral rotatory instability of the elbow. J. Bone Joint Surg.Br. 90, 272–279.

Cheung, E.V., Adams, R., Morrey, B.F., 2008. Primary osteoarthritis of the elbow: current treatment options. J. Am. Acad. Orthop. Surg. 16, 77–87.

Cohen, M.S., Bruno, R.J., 2001. The collateral ligaments of the elbow: anatomy and clinical correlation. Clin. Orthop. Relat. Res. 383, 123–130.

Dines, J.S., Frank, J.B., Akerman, M., Yocum, L.A., 2009. Glenohumeral internal rotation deficits in baseball players with ulnar collateral ligament insufficiency. Am. J. Sports Med. 37, 566–570.

Fleisig, G.S., Andrews, J.R., Dillman, C.J., Escamilla, R.F., 1995. Kinetics of baseball pitching with implications about injury mechanisms. Am. J. Sports Med. 23, 233–239.

Goodfellow, J.W., Bullough, P.G., 1967. The pattern of ageing of the articular cartilage of the elbow joint. J. Bone Joint Surg.Br. 49, 175–181.

Grace, S.P., Field, L.D., 2008. Chronic medial elbow instability. Orthop. Clin. North Am. 39, 213–219.

Gramstad, G.D., Galatz, L.M., 2006. Management of elbow osteoarthritis. J. Bone Joint Surg. Am. 88, 421–430.

Hildebrand, K.A., Patterson, S.D., King, G.J., 1999. Acute elbow dislocations: simple and complex. Orthop. Clin. North Am. 30, 63–79.

Kibler, B.W., Sciascia, A., 2004. Kinetic chain contributions to elbow function and dysfunction in sports. Clin. Sports Med. 23, 545–552.

Kokkalis, Z.T., Schmidt, C.C., Sotereanos, D.G., 2009. Elbow arthritis: current concepts. J. Hand Surg. Am. 34, 761–768.

Kuhn, M.A., Ross, G., 2008. Acute elbow dislocations. Orthop. Clin. North Am. 39, 155–161.

Lee, B.P., Teo, L.H., 2003. Surgical reconstruction for posterolateral rotatory instability of the elbow. J. Shoulder Elbow Surg. 12, 476–479.

Lee, M.L., Rosenwasser, M.P., 1999. Chronic elbow instability. Orthop. Clin. North Am. 30, 81–89.

Lehtinen, J.T., Kaarela, K., Ikavalko, M., et al., 2001. Incidence of elbow involvement in rheumatoid arthritis. A 15 year endpoint study. J. Rheumatol. 28, 70–74.

Mehta, J.A., Bain, G.I., 2004. Posterolateral rotatory instability of the elbow. J. Am. Acad. Orthop. Surg. 12, 405–415.

Moro, J.K., King, G.J., 2000. Total elbow arthroplasty in the treatment of posttraumatic conditions of the elbow. Clin. Orthop. Relat. Res. 370, 102–114.

Morrey, B.F., Askew, L.J., Chao, E.Y., 1981. A biomechanical study of normal functional elbow motion. J. Bone Joint Surg. Am. 63, 872–877.

Nestor, B.J., O'Driscoll, S.W., Morrey, B.F., 1992. Ligamentous reconstruction for posterolateral rotatory instability of the elbow. J. Bone Joint Surg. Am. 74, 1235–1241.

O'Driscoll, S.W., 2000. Classification and evaluation of recurrent instability of the elbow. Clin. Orthop. Relat. Res. 370, 34–43.

O'Driscoll, S.W., Bell, D.F., Morrey, B.F., 1991. Posterolateral rotatory instability of the elbow. J. Bone Joint Surg. Am. 73, 440–446.

O'Driscoll, S.W., Morrey, B.F., Korinek, S., An, K.N., 1992. Elbow sub-luxation and dislocation. A spectrum of instability. Clin. Orthop. Relat. Res. 280, 186–197.

O'Driscoll, S.W., Jupiter, J.B., King, G.J., Hotchkiss, R.N., Morrey, B.F., 2001a. The unstable elbow. Instr. Course Lect. 50, 89–102.

O'Driscoll, S.W., Spinner, R.J., McKee, M.D., et al., 2001b. Tardy posterolateral rotatory instability of the elbow due to cubitus varus. J. Bone Joint Surg. Am. 83A, 1358–1369.

O'Driscoll, S.W., Lawton, R.L., Smith, A.M., 2005. The 'moving valgus stress test' for medial collateral ligament tears of the elbow. Am. J. Sports Med. 33, 231–239.

Olsen, B.S., Sojbjerg, J.O., Dalstra, M., Sneppen, O., 1996. Kinematics of the lateral ligamentous constraints of the elbow joint. J. Shoulder Elbow Surg. 5, 333–341.

Olsen, B.S., Sojbjerg, J.O., Nielsen, K.K., Vaesel, M.T., Dalstra, M., Sneppen, O., 1998. Posterolateral elbow joint instability: the basic kinematics. J. Shoulder Elbow Surg. 7, 19–29.

Porter, B.B., Richardson, C., Vainio, K., 1974. Rheumatoid arthritis of the elbow: The results of synovectomy. J. Bone Joint Surg.Br. 56B, 427–437.

Potter, H.G., Weiland, A.J., Schatz, J.A., Paletta, G.A., Hotchkiss, R.N., 1997. Posterolateral rotatory instability of the elbow: usefulness of MR imaging in diagnosis. Radiology 204 (1), 185–189.

Rettig, A.C., Sherrill, C., Snead, D.S., Mendler, J.C., Mieling, P., 2001. Nonoperative treatment of ulnar collateral ligament injuries in throwing athletes. Am. J. Sports Med. 29, 15–17.

Royle, S.G., 1991. Posterior dislocation of the elbow. Clin. Orthop. Relat. Res. 269, 201–204.

Safran, M.R., 2004. Ulnar collateral ligament injury in the overhead athlete: diagnosis and treatment. Clin. Sports Med. 23, 643–663.

Safran, M.R., Baillargeon, D., 2005. Soft-tissue stabilizers of the elbow. J. Shoulder Elbow Surg. 14, 179S–185S.

Safran, M.R., McGarry, M.H., Shin, S., Han, S., Lee, T.Q., 2005. Effects of elbow flexion and forearm rotation on valgus laxity of the elbow. J. Bone Joint Surg. Am. 87, 2065–2074.

Singleton, S.B., Conway, J.E., 2004. PLRI: posterolateral rotatory instability of the elbow. Clin. Sports Med. 23, 629–642.

Smith 3rd, J.P., Savoie, F.H., Field, L.D., 2001. Posterolateral rotatory instability of the elbow. Clin. Sports Med. 20, 47–58.

Soojian, M.G., Kwon, Y.W., 2007. Elbow arthritis. Bulletin of the New York University Hospital for Joint Diseases 65, 61–71.

Thompson, W.H., Jobe, F.W., Yocum, L.A., Pink, M.M., 2001. Ulnar collateral ligament reconstruction in athletes: muscle-splitting approach without transposition of the ulnar nerve. J. Shoulder Elbow Surg. 10, 152–157.

Walker-Bone, K., Reading, I., Coggon, D., Cooper, C., Palmer, K.T., 2004. The anatomical pattern and determinants of pain in the neck and upper limbs: an epidemiologic study. Pain 109, 45–51.

Chapter | 25 |

Joint mobilization and manipulation of the elbow

Helen Slater, César Fernández de las Peñas

INTRODUCTION

Mobilization and manipulation interventions of the elbow joint are frequently used in clinical practice, and although the evidence for their use is as yet insufficient, it is growing (Vicenzino et al 2007). Systematic reviews in relation to the elbow refer mainly to specific elbow conditions such as lateral epicondylalgia (Smidt et al 2003, Assendelft et al 2004, Vicenzino et al 2007). Despite the large number of studies, there is still insufficient evidence for most physiotherapy interventions due to contradicting results, insufficient statistical power, and the low number of studies per intervention (Smidt et al 2003). More recent high quality studies

provide evidence that joint manipulation/mobilization directed at the elbow and wrist results in beneficial alterations in pain and the motor system (Vicenzino et al 2007). A meta-analysis of two randomized controlled trials showed that elbow mobilization improved pain-free grip strength and pressure pain threshold in comparison with placebo at short-term follow-up (Bisset et al 2005). A few cases reporting the use of specific mobilization interventions for elbow disorders have also been published, including a patient with ulnar tunnel syndrome (Lawrence & Humphreys 1997) and a patient with lateral epicondylalgia (Kaufman 2000). Given the low level of evidence for single case studies, clinicians are cautioned against making any conclusions from case studies alone.

EVIDENCE-BASED DECISION-MAKING

In choosing joint mobilization as part of multimodal management, consideration must be given to interpreting the clinical (patient) manifestations of peripheral and central sensitization processes involved in musculoskeletal disorders. For example, in patients with unilateral lateral epicondylalgia, evidence of bilateral manifestations of deep tissue hyperalgesia indicates that peripheral sensitization alone is unlikely to explain the clinical presentation (Slater et al 2005, Fernandez-Carnero et al 2008, 2009). In the Slater et al (2005) study, evidence of widespread pain, referred pain and changes in somatosensory sensitivity raises the index of suspicion that patients with lateral epicondylalgia demonstrate alterations in the way in which the nervous system processes nociceptive and non-nociceptive information. Therefore, clinical management of patients with lateral epicondylalgia may need to extend beyond local tissue-based pathology, to incorporate

© 2011 Elsevier Ltd.
DOI: 10.1016/B978-0-7020-3528-9.00025-X

strategies directed at normalizing nervous system sensitivity. Changes in somatosensory function, manifested clinically by persistent musculoskeletal pain (Graven-Nielsen 2006), also impacts motor systems with changes in the drive to muscle and altered motor control (Arendt-Nielsen & Graven-Nielsen 2008). Management cannot therefore focus on the simple biomechanics of joint mobilization, but must incorporate the more recent findings on sensory–motor interactions in persistent musculoskeletal pain disorders.

In considering the choice of joint mobilization as an intervention, clinicians should also consider the potential neurophysiologic and tissue mechanisms underlying the effects (positive and negative) of mobilization. Multiple interacting tissue and pain mechanisms are likely to contribute to pain modulatory effects of mobilization (Slater et al 2006, Vicenzino et al 2007). For a comprehensive review of putative mechanisms underlying the effects of mobilization readers are referred to Paungmali et al (2003), Bisset et al (2006), Vicenzino et al (2007) and Chapter 23 of this textbook.

Where a patient's elbow disorder appears mediated primarily by peripheral nociceptive mechanisms (dominantly peripheral sensitization), early and appropriate physiologic movements and functional activity should be encouraged. In such cases, while joint mobilization may offer benefits in terms of pain relief and restoration of joint mobility, the ultimate aim of such techniques is the restoration of function limiting the chance of sustained central nervous system facilitation (central sensitization). Seldom in clinical practice would a unimodal approach, using mobilization alone, be considered appropriate for the management of elbow disorders. More commonly, mobilization would be incorporated into a multimodal approach. For example, depending on the chronicity of the disorder and the associated level of impairment and disability, patients would be educated on optimizing normal functional movements and undertaking active and specific exercises to maintain gains in pain-free joint ranges. The use of appropriate soft tissues techniques to address soft tissue contributions at the elbow may also be explored (Chapters 32–36). If required, help may be sought through the patient's doctor in regard to appropriate analgesics, the primary purpose of analgesia (acetoaminophen, non-steroidal anti-inflammatories) being to provide a therapeutic window for regaining function.

Additional considerations may also be required when the elbow condition is compromised by contributing factors such as a loss of the normal dynamic control of the shoulder joint (Chapters 17, 18 and 21), or a compromise of wrist stability (Chapter 27). Such contributing factors need to be addressed in the overall management of the patient with elbow disorders if an optimal outcome is to be achieved. Equally, the possibility of intra-articular pathologies including loose bodies, osteochrondritis,

and other conditions such as osteoarthritis, valgus instability with ulnar nerve trauma in patients involved in throwing sports, or a covert postero-lateral pathology following a fall onto an outstretched hand, should all be given due consideration prior to any decision that manual techniques are indicated in management (Chapter 24).

For all patients, reassessment of the outcome of any intervention, including joint mobilization should include a subjective inquiry as to the treatment effects (positive and negative), re-examination of key initial physical findings (for example, loss of joint range and associated pain provocation, mechanical hyperalgesia) and functional limitations. Where possible, the parallel use of relevant outcome measures to assess the response to treatment is consistent with current best clinical practice. Examples of outcome measures that could be used for elbow disorders include the Patient-Specific Functional Scale (PSFS) or the Disability of Arm, Shoulder and Hand (DASH) tool.

DEFINITIONS AND CLINICAL APPLICATIONS

Joint mobilization is usually defined as low velocity, high amplitude passive motion inducing intra-capsular movement at different amplitudes (Hengeveld et al 2005, Takei 2005), whereas joint manipulation is defined as a high velocity, low amplitude thrust motion. Maitland (1986) described different grades of mobilization according to the amplitude of the motion and resistance offered by the surrounding tissues (Hengeveld et al 2005). Maitland (1986) previously described four different standard oscillatory grades of movement. The differentiation between oscillations relates to amplitude with grade I and IV referring to small amplitude oscillation, while II and III indicate large amplitude oscillation. Conventionally, mobilizations with grades I–II are usually used for patients where the pain is the dominant symptom and a patient's disorder is considered irritable in nature. In contrast, grades III–IV are usually used in patients where the main symptom response relates to limitation of elbow joint range and this restriction is associated with some pain provocation. Grade V refers to high velocity manipulation.

In order to regain range, joint mobilization is provided at the limit of range, and the therapist expects a pain response, which should settle immediately or within seconds of the mobilization being completed. In current clinical practice, the use of a grade I mobilization is rare. More commonly, acute nociceptive elbow pain is managed using a combination of simple analgesia if required and appropriate early active movement to regain function and minimize prolonged sensitization. If passive movement is indicated in such a presentation, then large amplitude mobilization performed short of pain provocation (grade II or III⁻) offers the patient the advantage of increasing range and reducing pain. Patients are encouraged to continue with appropriate analgesia and maintain gains in range with active movements. Where patients present with persistent elbow pain (for example, tendinopathy or osteoarthritis), management will require a combined approach with joint mobilization offering only limited benefit when used as a unimodal intervention. Treatment 'dose' (how long and how many) is decided based on the clinical presentation with 30–60 seconds followed by reassessment typical for more acute disorders (2–3 repetitions) and 60–180 seconds (4–5 repetitions) for more chronic hypomobility disorders.

When choosing to mobilize the elbow joint, a skilled therapist typically uses a clinically reasoned process rather than a doctrinal or didactic approach. For example, the grade of a technique is typically guided by the patient's clinical presentation, with due consideration of irritability (severity of disorder; nature of associated pathology or systemic disease if appropriate; the acute, subacute or chronic stage of the disorder; how easy it is to trigger symptoms; how long these symptoms then take to resolve or reduce to baseline; and any precautions or contraindications to manual interventions such as postero-lateral joint instability or significant neuropathic pain).

Typically, symptoms that are localized, mechanically patterned (nociceptive) and with clearly identifiable aggravating factors and easing factors, appear most amenable to mobilization techniques. In such presentations, the choice of the technique is made by considering which articulation of the elbow joint is problematic (radio-humeral, radio-ulnar or humero-ulnar) and at which point in the joint range the symptoms occur. Most commonly mobilization will be used at the point in range where a loss of mobility occurs. Where an elbow disorder is more acute and hypomobility is evident through a large part of the joint range, physiological mobilization may be useful when performed throughout larger amplitudes of joint range. A good clinical example is the uncomplicated post fracture (out of cast) elbow, where large amplitude physiological joint mobilization helps to encourage joint mobility without compromising the fracture or exacerbating pain. Conversely, where joint mobility is lost at terminal extension or flexion or into abduction or adduction at terminal elbow extension, passive accessory joint mobilization performed at the point in range of restriction is most likely to be beneficial in restoring function. In summary, the use of clinical reasoning and current neurobiology of musculoskeletal pain to problem solve and assist in decision-making should lie central to clinical practice. For a comprehensive review of clinical reasoning in physiotherapy practice see Jones et al (2004).

In the following part of the chapter, we describe some of the more commonly performed elbow mobilization/manipulation interventions. For each technique, the optimal positions for patient relaxation and for the therapist are described, however as with all manual techniques, appropriate positional modifications are to be considered and applied as required. For convenience, all technique descriptions relate to the right elbow. The combining of mobilization techniques with active movement (an approach described by Mulligan in 1989 as 'Mobilization-with-Movement') may also offer alternatives or progressions of the basic techniques described here.

The techniques outlined are not exhaustive. As with any technique, modifications and variations are worthy of consideration if a logical and scientific rationale can be provided. Additionally, given the bony configuration of the elbow joint, most clinical presentations where joint mobilization is indicated as part of management, involve pain provocation associated with hypomobility towards the end of joint ranges. These restrictions typically occur at terminal extension associated with a restriction of abduction and adduction, terminal extension with limitation of end range supination or pronation, and flexion limitation with restriction of pronation and supination. Often these patterns of restriction are associated with soft tissue limitations or heightened deep tissue sensitivity or trigger points (Chapter 32). For example, in patients with lateral epicondylalgia, terminal extension and adduction/abduction can be provocative for pain however, supination performed in extension is also frequently limited.

Careful examination may reveal a loss of tissue extensibility of the flexor and pronator muscle group and trigger points may exist in these tissues as well as in the extensor muscles. Techniques directed at normalizing this soft tissue limitation or heightened sensitivity should assist in restoring supination in extension (Chapters 32–36). Given the intimate anatomical and functional relationships in the upper limb kinetic chain, the techniques described in this chapter are complemented by techniques described in Chapters 20, 23 and 30.

MOBILIZATION AND MANIPULATION TECHNIQUES

Mobilization in extension combined with adduction (varus mobilization)

The aim of this mobilization technique is to improve the lateral glide of the elbow region, particularly of the radio-humeral joint, where pain or restriction is associated with active extension. Therefore, the clinical presentation would require limitation of terminal elbow extension and adduction and pain provocation in this position is likely and probably most evident at the lateral elbow, although medial joint pain can also be elicited.

For this technique, the patient is lying supine with their elbow extended (Fig 25.1). To maximize stabilization, the therapist's left elbow contacts the anterior part of the

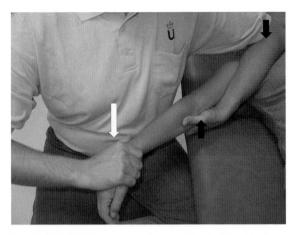

Fig 25.1 Mobilization in extension combined with adduction (varus mobilization). Black arrows show the stabilizations at the shoulder and the elbow of the patient and the white arrow shows the direction of the mobilization force.

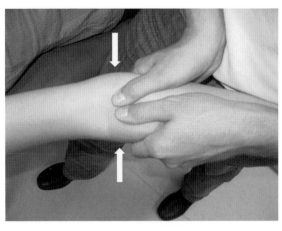

Fig 25.2 Mobilization in adduction and abduction (varus to valgus mobilization). White arrows show the direction of the medial or lateral mobilization force.

patient's shoulder. Medial rotation of the whole arm allows the use of a gravity-assisted medial (varus) mobilization. The therapist's left hand supports the patient's elbow immediately proximal and medial to the elbow joint. The therapist's right hand grasps the patient's wrist with the therapist's fingers placed over the dorsum of the hand. The technique consists of applying an appropriately graded oscillatory mobilisation into adduction (varus). The technique would be performed at the point in range prior to the onset of pain (acute, grade II or III$^-$) or at the limitation of range (chronic, III–IV). Symptoms should be monitored and the grade of movement adjusted if required.

Mobilization in adduction and abduction (varus to valgus mobilization)

The aim of this mobilization technique is to improve the lateral glide of the elbow region, specifically the radio-humeral and humero-ulnar joints, at the limitation of extension range. Therefore, the clinical patient presentation would require limitation of terminal elbow extension and abduction. Pain provocation in this position is likely and probably most evident at the medial elbow, although lateral joint symptoms may also occur.

For this technique, the patient is lying supine with their elbow extended (Fig 25.2). The hands of the therapist grasp the forearm of the patient in close proximity to the elbow, with stabilization provided medially and laterally at the elbow. The tips of both thumbs are placed against the radial head anteriorly, whereas the remaining fingers spread medially/laterally around the patient's forearm. The technique consists of applying a graded oscillatory lateral mobilization into abduction (valgus) or

adduction (varus). The technique would be performed at the point in range prior to the onset of pain (acute, grade II or III$^-$) or at the limitation of range (chronic, III–IV). Symptoms should be monitored as the grade of movement adjusted if required.

Mobilization in pronation/supination combined with flexion

The aim of this mobilization technique is to improve the pronation/supination rotational glide/spin of the radio-humeral joint where the limitation occurs in a flexion position. Therefore, the clinical presentation would require limitation of elbow flexion and pronation, functionally one of the most important positions to be able to attain. Pain provocation in this position is likely and probably most evident at the radio-humeral joint laterally or at the anterior joint line (common post fracture).

For this technique, the patient is supine with the right elbow flexed and the forearm pronated. The therapist's left hand is positioned with the dorsum of the fingers lying proximal to the elbow joint and the thumb distal to the elbow and making contact with the radial head. The proximal contact helps control the internal rotation of the patient's humerus that occurs with forearm pronation. The therapist's right hand grasps the patient's right wrist at the dorsum of the distal radio-ulnar joint. The technique consists of applying an oscillatory mobilization force combining pronation and flexion (Fig 25.3). This technique may be also performed with the forearm in supination and at the limitation of flexion (Fig 25.4), although this is less commonly used in clinical practice. Symptoms should be monitored and the grade of movement adjusted if required.

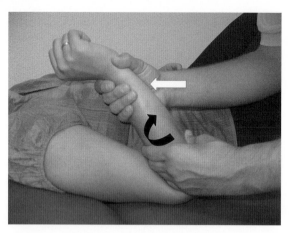

Fig 25.3 Mobilization in pronation combined with flexion. The white arrow shows the direction of the flexion force. A rotational mobilization in pronation of the forearm is applied with the other hand placed over the radio-humeral joint.

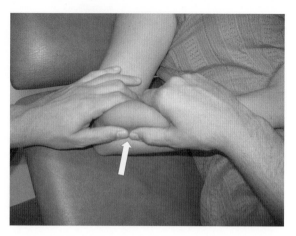

Fig 25.5 Mobilization of the radio-humeral Joint. The white arrow shows the postero-anterior glide applied over the radial head laterally.

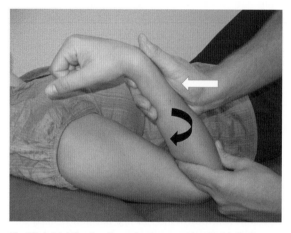

Fig 25.4 Mobilization in supination combined with flexion. The white arrow shows the direction of the flexion force. A rotational mobilization in supination of the forearm is applied with the other hand over the radio-humeral joint.

Mobilization of the radio-humeral joint

The aim of this technique is to improve the anterior glide of the radio-humeral joint (Edmond 2006) where there is associated joint restriction and pain provocation. Radio-ulnar joint mobilization in the posterior-anterior medial direction can be performed effectively at 60° through 90° of flexion.

For this technique, the patient is supine with the right elbow flexed to the point of restriction (Fig 25.5). The forearm may be supinated or pronated at the point in range where there is pain provocation or joint hypomobility. The pads of both thumbs are placed against the radial head posteriorly whereas the remaining fingers spread comfortably proximally and distally around the patient's forearm. The technique consists of applying oscillatory posterior-anterior glides of the radial head using an appropriate grade of movement. Symptoms should be monitored and the grade of movement adjusted if required.

Lateral glide mobilization-with-movement (MWM)

Despite the findings of human and animal studies, the specific mechanisms underlying the effects associated with the mobilization/manipulation techniques remain largely putative. The beneficial effects associated with the specific lateral glide-MWM are likely to relate to multiple and potentially interacting mechanisms and these are discussed in more detail elsewhere (Slater et al 2006, Vicenzino et al 2007). For a detailed description of this technique, see Chapter 23.

Manipulation in lateral glide of the elbow (varus thrust manipulation)

The patient is supine or seated with the elbow extended. For patients where no contraindications exist, joint manipulation can be an effective treatment progression. As with any manipulative technique, due care must be taken to exclude any contraindication to high velocity thrust. Screening questions that contraindicate joint manipulation include evidence of, or suspicion of, intra articular pathologies, fracture, compromised bone density, prolonged use of corticosteroids or anti-coagulant medication, pain dominant disorders and young children

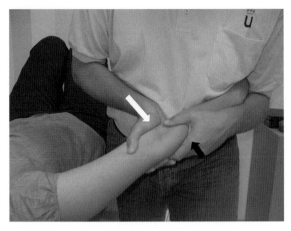

Fig 25.6 Manipulation in lateral glide of the elbow (varus thrust manipulation). The black arrow shows the therapist's lateral stabilizing hand placed distal to the radio-humeral joint. The white arrow shows the varus direction of the high-velocity low-amplitude thrust.

where bone maturity is incomplete. Once the decision is made to proceed to manipulation, clear succinct information should be provided to the patient with risks and benefits discussed. As a minimum, verbal consent and a record in the patient notes indicating agreement to proceed with manipulation is recommended.

The therapist's left hand is placed just distal to the patient's right radio-humeral joint extending over the lateral part of the elbow joint (Fig 25.6). The therapist's right hand grasps the patient's forearm medially at the

elbow. Slight external rotation of the patient's whole arm allows a gravity-assisted thrust. Ensure that the elbow joint is not locked in full extension, but approximately 5° short of full extension as this avoids a painful and unsuccessful thrust. Examine the position of restriction to establish the direction that is restricted by gently guiding the joint laterally (varus force). It is important that the therapist's right (thrusting) arm is placed perpendicular to the patient's elbow joint. Inform the patient to soften their arm and relax. Inform your patient that you will now provide a rapid thrust and this may be associated with an audible clicking or popping sound. Reassurance that this popping sound is expected and simply indicates a joint cavitation, is helpful advice for patients. The technique then consists of applying a high-velocity low-amplitude thrust (grade V) force directed in a medio-lateral direction. Post manipulation, joint range and pain provocation should be reassessed.

CONCLUSION

There is increasing evidence that when used appropriately, joint mobilization and manipulation techniques can help to alleviate pain and assist in restoring function in patients with musculoskeletal elbow disorders. Clinicians need to understand the putative neurophysiologic and tissue mechanisms underlying elbow joint mobilization (including placebo analgesia) and recognize that these techniques typically contribute only a small part of a more comprehensive evidence-based management approach.

REFERENCES

Arendt-Nielsen, L., Graven-Nielsen, T., 2008. Muscle pain: sensory implications and interaction with motor control. Clin. J. Pain 24, 291–298.

Assendelft, W., Green, S., Buchbinder, R., Struijs, P., Smidt, N., 2004. Tennis elbow. Clin. Evid. 11, 1633–1644.

Bisset, L., Paungmali, A., Vicenzino, B., Beller, E., 2005. A systematic review and meta-analysis of clinical trials on physical interventions for lateral epicondylalgia. Br. J. Sports Med. 39, 411–422.

Bisset, L., Beller, E., Jull, G., et al., 2006. Mobilisation with movement and exercise, corticosteroid injection, or wait and see for tennis elbow: randomised trial. BMJ 333, 939.

Edmond, S.L., 2006. Joint mobilization/ manipulation. 2nd ed. Mosby Elsevier, London, pp. 86–87.

Fernandez-Carnero, J., Fernandez-de-las-Peñas, C., de la Llave-Rincon, A.I., Ge, H.Y., Arendt-Nielsen, L., 2008. Bilateral myofascial trigger points in the forearm muscles in patients with chronic unilateral lateral epicondylalgia: a blinded, controlled study. Clin. J. Pain 24, 802–807.

Fernandez-Carnero, J., Fernandez-de-Las-Penas, C., de la Llave-Rincon, A.I., Ge, H.Y., Arendt-Nielsen, L., 2009. Widespread mechanical pain hypersensitivity as sign of central sensitization in unilateral epicondylalgia: a blinded, controlled study. Clin. J. Pain 25, 555–561.

Graven-Nielsen, T., 2006. Fundamentals of muscle pain, referred pain, and deep tissue hyperalgesia. Scand. J. Rheumatol. 122, 1–43.

Hengeveld, E., Banks, K., Wells, P., 2005. Maitland's peripheral manipulation, fourth ed. Elsevier Health Sciences, London.

Jones, M.A., Rivett, D.A., Twomey, L., 2004. Clinical Reasoning for Manual Therapists. Elsevier Science Ltd, Butterworth-Heinemann, London.

Kaufman, R.L., 2000. Conservative chiropractic care of lateral epicondylitis. J. Manipulative Physiol. Ther. 23, 619–622.

Lawrence, D.J., Humphreys, C.R., 1997. Cubital tunnel syndrome: a case report. Chiropractic Techniques 9, 27–31.

Maitland, G.D., 1986. Vertebral manipulation, fifth ed. Butterworth-Heinemann, London.

Mulligan, B., 1989. Manual Therapy 'NAGS', 'SNAGS', 'MWMs' etc. Plane View Services, Wellington, New Zealand.

Paungmali, A., Vicenzino, B., Smith, M., 2003. Hypoalgesia induced by elbow manipulation in lateral epicondylalgia does not exhibit tolerance. J. Pain 4, 448–454.

Slater, H., Arendt-Nielsen, L., Wright, A., Graven-Nielsen, T., 2005. Sensory and motor effects of experimental muscle pain in patients with lateral epicondylalgia and controls with delayed onset muscle soreness. Pain 114, 118–130.

Slater, H., Arendt-Nielsen, L., Wright, A., Graven-Nielsen, T., 2006. Effects of a manual therapy technique in experimental lateral epicondylalgia. Man. Ther. 11, 107–117.

Smidt, N., Assendelft, W.J., Arola, H., et al., 2003. Effectiveness of physiotherapy for lateral epicondylitis: a systematic review. Ann. Med. 35, 51–62.

Takei, H., 2005. Joint mobilization for bone and joint disease. Phys. Ther. Sci. 20, 219–225.

Vicenzino, B., Cleland, J.A., Bisset, L., 2007. Joint manipulation in the management of lateral epicondylalgia: a clinical commentary. J. Man. Manip. Ther. 15, 50–56.

Chapter | 26 |

Tendinopathies of the wrist and hand

C Joseph Yelvington, Ellen J Pong

INTRODUCTION

A large proportion of hand and wrist tendinopathies occur in individuals who perform highly repetitive and forceful jobs (Elder & Harvey 2005). The Department of Labor, Bureau of Labor Statistics (1999), reported incidence of hand and wrist tendinitis (tendinopathy not

© 2011 Elsevier Ltd.
DOI: 10.1016/B978-0-7020-3528-9.00026-1

specified) as 3.66% of upper extremity workplace injuries recorded in 1999, resulting in a mean of 6 lost work days for all hand/wrist injuries.

Patients and practitioners had discovered that once tendinopathy is established resolving symptoms can be difficult. Treatment typically consists of resting in a splint, modifying activities for ergonomic correction, taking non-steroidal anti-inflammatory medications (NSAIDs), and receiving corticosteroid injections; often with positive results (Fredberg & Stengaard-Pedersen 2008). Deep tissue friction massage (DTFM), effleurage, connective tissue release and Rolfing have been utilized on tendons with the premise that it will release scar tissue restrictions and allow improved collagen alignment. However, studies do not reliably confirm the positive benefit of these conservative treatments (Brousseau et al 2002). This demonstrates a typical problem: randomized clinical trials of manual therapy to the tendons of the hand and wrist are scarcely, if at all, available.

Investigators have continued to look more closely at tendons, discovering processes that may explain why outcomes are not more positive. Adequate animal models for in vivo studies have only recently been developed (Soslowsky et al 2000). Tendinopathy has been classified and redefined. Current studies attempt to explain why repetitive motion and strain cause tendon pathologies (Backman et al 2005). This developing knowledge of tendon pathology has shed new light on treatment rationale (Khan et al 2000).

This chapter follows the trend of current studies and expanding knowledge, including a review of the tendinopathy process from a molecular level. This review provides a knowledge base for the ensuing discussion of examination, diagnosis, categorization of tendinopathy, and treatment.

DEFINITION OF TENDINOPATHY

The lack of more positive results with conservative treatment may be due to mislabeling tendinosis as tendinitis (Khan et al 2000). Tendinitis must be qualified. Studies are now consistently showing what was normally diagnosed as *tendonitis* may represent only one classification of *tendinopathy* (Futami & Itoman 1995). Tendinopathy represents histological findings that differ significantly from the generally accepted condition of tendonitis. This is due primarily to the lack of evidence of inflammatory precursors and cells in the tendon itself (Gabel et al 1994, Yuan et al 2003, Curwin 2005, Fredberg & Stengaard-Pedersen 2008). Khan et al (2006) supported Bonar's classification of tendinopathy, which defined four classifications, each with distinct histological findings. Clinicians have yet to apply this knowledge to support specific conservative treatment use (Cannon 2001). A fourth edition

manual of upper extremity rehabilitation printed in 2001 did not use the words *tendinosis* or *tendinopathy*, but used the terms *tendinitis* and *paratendinitis* for all related conditions of upper extremity pain caused by tendon pathology (Cannon 2001).

One reason for the continued consideration of tendon pathologies as tendonitis may be the initially positive outcomes with corticosteroids in symptomatic tendons (Fredberg & Stengaard-Pedersen 2008). The presence of an -*itis* or inflammation in the form of neurogenic inflammation may also support persistence of the old terminology. Fredberg & Stengaard-Pedersen (2008) concluded that some combination of classic inflammation and neurogenic inflammation does mean that tendonitis is not a complete misnomer. It is the histological difference in tendinopathies stemming from tendinitis, tendinosis, and paratendinitis that may dictate different treatments; particularly in manual therapy.

There continue to be areas of needed research into this subject. Findings from animal studies and from tendon studies performed on other areas of the body will be used in this chapter to provide data which may be extrapolated to apply to the hand and wrist, despite differences between weight bearing versus positional tendons (Smith et al 1997).

AETIOLOGY

Researchers report that knowledge of the aetiology of tendinopathy is evolving (Sharma & Maffulli 2005, Fredberg & Stengaard-Pedersen 2008). Many factors contribute to tendinopathy, both intrinsic and extrinsic (Riley 2004). Renstrom & Hach (2005) summarized extrinsic factors as: malalignments, reduced flexibility, muscle weakness or imbalance, overuse and excessive body weight. Hart et al (2005) added genetics, gender, and fitness level, while Hammer (2007a) reported biomechanical faults. Intrinsic factors that affect apoptosis can lead to tendon degeneration. This process of programmed cell death can be exacerbated by intrinsic oxidative or mechanical stresses (Yuan et al 2003, Sharma & Maffulli 2005). Theories on tendon rupture have been separated into two categories: vascular and mechanical (Riley 2004). The reader is encouraged to read the work of Riley (2004) to explore this topic further.

ANATOMY OF THE TENDON

Basic components

The tendon is the attachment site of a muscle to bone. It is designed to transfer tension from the muscle to the bone, thereby causing motion to take place (Kannus 2000).

The basic building block of the tendon, *tropocollagen*, is formed by fibroblasts (O'Brien 2005). These are assembled into *fibrils* which are arranged into *fibres*, which are organized into *fascicles* and bound together with a loose connective tissue called *endotendon* (endotenon) (Kannus 2000, Sharma & Maffulli 2005). The endotendon is the pathway for blood vessels, nerves, and lymphatics (Riley 2004). Bundles of fascicles are bound together by another layer of connective tissue called the *epitendon* (epitenon) which is continuous with the endotendon (Kannus 2000) (Fig 26.1).

Synovial tendon sheaths, also called *paratendon* (paratenon), are found in areas subjected to increased mechanical stress, such as the tendons of the hands and feet, where efficient lubrication is required (Sharma & Maffulli 2005). Fibre bundles are predominantly aligned with the long axis of the tendon and these are responsible for the tensile strength of the tendon (Riley 2004). A small proportion of fibres run transversely, and there are even spirals and plait-like formations (Kannus 2000). This complex ultrastructure provides resistance against transverse, shear, and rotational forces acting on the tendon (Riley 2004).

Blood and nerve supply

Tendon vascular support comes from three sources: at the myotendinous junction, the osteotendinous junction, and the extrinsic system through the paratendon (Benjamin & Ralphs 1996, Sharma & Maffulli 2005, Scott et al 2007). Innervation accompanies vascular pathways through the paratenon (Hart et al 2005). The nerve receptors that supply tendons can terminate in the vicinity of mast cells, where neuropeptides are involved in normal tendon regulatory control (Hart et al 2005).

Patho-anatomy

Tenocytes and *tenoblasts* are the cells involved in tendon healing (Sharma & Maffulli 2005, 2006). Tenocytes are sparse in tendon tissue but have extensions that create an extensive network inside the matrix (O'Brien 2005). They are responsible for maintenance of matrix and collagen (Harley & Bergman 2008). Tenocytes are crucially responsive to environmental conditions. Mechanical demands placed on tendon tissue will promote changes in the microarchitecture of the tissue (Magra et al 2007). Strain applied to a tendon can change its structure; these changes can be damaging or they can be reparative if appropriately and purposefully applied in treatment.

Scott's research (Scott 2007) evidenced that it is stimulation of the tenocyte that is associated with tendinosis, rather than intrinsic inflammation. Alterations in cell activity lead to tendon changes from mechanical stress rather than the converse (Riley 2004). The local stimulation of tenocytes, which is a load-driven cellular response, rather than inflammation or apoptosis, is the true mechanism in tendinosis (Scott et al 2007). Apoptosis plays a role later in the tendinopathic process (Scott et al 2007). Localized hypoxia from vigorous exercise can lead to tenocyte death (Sharma & Maffulli 2005) and tendinopathic changes.

Tenocyte metabolism is regulated partly by mechanical stimulation (Maeda et al 2009). Maeda et al (2009) showed that cyclic strain will change gene expression in tendon cells. Force applied to a tendon changes cellular process via mechano-transduction, the process in which a cell converts biomechanical stimuli into chemical signals (Maffuli & Longo 2008). Mechano-transduction utilizes gap junctions, stretch activated channels (Wall & Banes 2005), voltage operated calcium channels (VOCC) and tandem pore domain potassium channels (TPDPC)

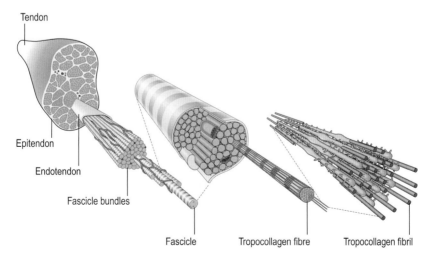

Fig 26.1 Basic tendon structure.

Tendon

Epitendon

Endotendon

Fascicle bundles

Fascicle

Tropocollagen fibre

Tropocollagen fibril

to communicate with adjoining tenocytes (Wall & Banes 2005, Magra et al 2007). Tension on surface proteins, called *integrins*, embedded in the cell membrane is transmitted to the cell's cytoskeleton. This force is transmitted via the intracellular network to the nucleus of the cell and can alter protein expression (Chiquet 1999). Huang et al (2004) observed that mechanical loading is essential for homeostasis of the bone, cartilage, and skin. Additionally, external forces are capable of producing changes in intracellular reactions. Tenocytes are responsible for changing structure in response to demand by altering, 'gene expression patterns, protein synthesis and cell phenotype' (Maffulli & Longo 2008). This alteration is suspected of being the link to overuse and tendinopathic changes (Scott et al 2007). Importantly from a manual therapy perspective, Maffulli & Longo (2008) supported that an alteration of mechanical forces may augment the healing process. Conversely, understimulation can cause tendinopathic changes (Arnoczky et al 2006).

The tendon matrix is responsible for maintenance of the tendon. Its damage, according to Riley (2004), is the leading event in tendinopathy. The ground substance of the extracellular matrix network surrounding the collagen and the tenocytes contains proteoglycans, glycosaminoglycans, glycoproteins, as well as several other small molecules (O'Brien 2005). Water makes up 60–80% of the ground substance (O'Brien 2005). Proteoglycans are strongly hydrophilic, enabling rapid diffusion of water-soluble molecules and the migration of cells (Sharma & Maffulli 2005). They, along with glycoproteins, have a role in organization of collagen into fibrils and fibres (O'Brien 2005). When repetitive damage becomes extensive it overwhelms the ability to heal (Riley 2004). Arnoczky et al (2007) credited extracellular matrix degeneration as a precursor of tendon weakness. Riley (2004) described the possibility that changes in cellular activity in the matrix due to mechanical strain can influence the structural properties of tendons.

Tendon injury

Riley summarized overuse tendinopathy as the phenomenon caused by repeated strains below the failure threshold that outstrips the cell's ability to heal (Riley 2004). Tissue injury from repetitive strain is thought to be a cellular event (Arnoczky et al 2006). Recent studies in animal modeling have produced results of tendinopathy that correspond those found in non-experimental tendinopathies in humans. Soslowky's model of repetitive motion identified tendinopathic changes in supraspinatus tendons in rats (Soslowky et al 2000). These changes mimic what has been found in idiopathic tendinopathies in humans, including reduced mechanical properties (Lavagnino et al 2006, Arnoczky et al 2007). Glazebrook et al (2007) found similar changes in rats after overuse

induced by repetitive running. Backman et al (2005) produced similar results with rabbits.

Post-injury disuse of a tendon, through immobilization or compensation, can also have detrimental effects. The concept of stress shielding can be applied to tendons. An example of this in terms of bone is application of Wolff's law with reduced bone density following fracture immobilization. Woo et al (1981) observed that after fracture healing, reapplied weight bearing will increase bone density. Kannus & Jozsa (1991) showed that under-stimulation of tendon cells post-injury produced degenerative findings in investigation of tendinopathy. DeBoer et al (2007) supported this with his demonstration of tendon protein synthesis rates decreasing progressively through 10 days of immobilization. Lavagnino et al (2006) induced mechanical injury in rat tail tendons, followed by immobilization, which revealed an upregulation of collagenase mRNA and protein synthesis in this damaged area. Even undamaged fascicles showed similar upregulation during the immobilization portion of this study. In an earlier study they found that these adverse effects could be controlled, in vitro, with cyclic stretching (Lavagnino et al 2003). Screen et al (2005) reported similar results with cyclic stretching in non-injured tendon fascicles. In regard to treatment of tendinopathy, attempting to immobilize a tendinosis via splinting or casting thus appears to be detrimental.

Tendon healing

The phases of tendon healing following injury resemble that of other connective tissues in the body. The phases are: (1) acute inflammatory, lasting 1–2 days; (2) repair-regeneration or proliferative phase, lasting up to 6 weeks; and (3) maturation or remodelling phase, lasting 3 weeks to a year (Leadbetter 1992, Sharma & Maffulli 2005). Each of these phases in tendinopathy has unique cellular progression that should be considered when preparing a treatment plan. Tenocytes begin new collagen synthesis around day 5 post-injury and continue synthesis for 5 weeks (Maffulli & Moller 2005). Intrinsic tenocytes begin proliferating at week 4 and are involved in remodelling through week 8 (Maffulli & Moller 2005). Applying standard but specific treatments in a global fashion to all tendinopathies without addressing the stage of healing could be ineffective. Cook & Purdam (2009) recommended that interventions should be tailored to the suspected pathology.

TENDINOPATHY CLASSIFICATION

Tendinopathy actually represents several different, mixed and sometimes overlapping degenerative processes. Histologically there are mixed findings. Absence of inflammatory cells, increased ground substance, increased vascularity and cellularity with collagen disorganization, are evidenced (Khan et al 2006). Each of these can disrupt some tendon fibres and weaken the remaining fibres (Maffulli & Moller 2005). The role of the tenocyte in tendon changes has already been discussed. Murrell (2002) stated that apoptosis, or programmed cell death, may have a roll in tendinopathy. Oystein et al (2007) showed apoptosis was enhanced in patellar tendinopathy biopsies compared to controls.

Inflammation is partially controlled by a neurogenic process. Substance P and calcitonin-related gene peptide (CRGP) are sensory neuropeptides (Hart et al 2005). These, among other substances, are found in symptomatic tendons (Andersson et al 2008) and directly stimulate nociceptor endings (Ueda 1999). Hart et al (2005) hypothesized that neuropeptides are involved via mast cells in tissue in normal tendon regulatory control; also, a dysfunctional regulatory loop produces an inadequate repair response. This differs from classic inflammation. Riley (2004) observed, '...nerve endings and mast cells may function as units to modulate tendon homeostasis and mediate adaptive responses to mechanical strain. He also stated that 'excessive stimulation as a result of overuse may result in pathological changes to the tendon matrix' (Riley 2004, p 137). There is a growing body of evidence that pain associated with tendinopathy may be neurogenic.

Tendinopathy severity is graded according to histological features distinguished under light microscopy (Maffulli et al 2008). Various scales have been proposed. Two early scales were originally developed for lower extremity research. The Movar scale and the Bonar scale have since development each been applied successfully to research of the upper extremity (Maffulli et al 2008). Each scale considers the microscopic appearance of five to seven factors; each factor is given a grade ranging from lowest number (normal tendon), to highest number (markedly abnormal tendon). The sample is graded cumulatively with combined scores from each factor (Maffulli et al 2008). Scott et al (2007) used a modified Bonar scale to specifically assess tendinosis. The modified scale considers five histological changes: (1) tenocyte morphology; (2) tenocyte proliferation; (3) collagen changes; (4) glycosaminoglycans (GAG), and (5) neovascularization (Scott et al 2007).

A lack of common description of these histological tissue changes which vary from scale to scale to modified scale has limited a clear classification and understanding of tendinopathy with its underlying causes. Kahn et al (2006) cited Clancy as having initially made a classification of tendinopathy types that was later modified by Bonar and now includes: *tendinosis, tendinitis* (tendonitis) *or partial rupture, paratenonitis* (paratendonitis/paratendinitis/tenosynovitis/tenovaginitis) and *paratenonitis with tendinosis*. The following sections provide details.

Tendinosis

Tendinosis is defined by Maffulli et al (2003a) as intra-tendinous degeneration typical with aging or devascularization. It is characterized by fibre disorientation, hypercellularity, and focal necrosis and calcification (Maffulli et al 2003a). Kraushaar & Nirschl (1999) defined the three findings in tendinosis as fibroblastic hyperplasia, hypervascularity, and abnormal collagen production with the former being the first response. Kannus & Jozsa (1991) examined 891 spontaneously ruptured tendons in the upper and lower extremity. Histopathologic examination showed that 97% of these had degenerative changes. These were sub-classified into hypoxic degeneration (44%), mucoid degeneration (21%), tendolipomatosis (8%), and calcific tendinopathy (5%) (Kannus & Jozsa 1991) There is multiple cell/tissue involvement and this may be difficult to discern from other classifications.

Tendinitis

Tendinitis and partial rupture are grouped together in this classification. An active inflammatory response, symptomatic degeneration and true vascular disruption are characteristic findings (Kahn et al 2006). Lymphocytes and neutrophils are seen (Kraushaar & Nirschl 1999). It has similar characteristics to tendinosis but histopathologically will also demonstrate fibroblastic proliferation, haemorrhage and granulation tissue (Maffulli et al 2003a). Hammer (2007a) stated that isolated active inflammation is not common but is usually associated with some degree of rupture, which implies that this classification is falsely over-diagnosed.

Paratendinitis

Paratendinitis, also termed *tenosynovitis*, is evidenced as frank inflammation of the outer layer of the tendon (Kahn et al 2006). Microscopically this will reveal infiltrate possibly including fibrin deposition, exudate, and areolar tissue degeneration which could explain the palpable crepitation at certain stages of its progression (Kahn et al 2000, Maffulli et al 2003a).

Combined paratendinitis and tendinosis

This fourth classification (Kahn et al 2006), originally described by Clancy, includes characteristics of both tendinosis with an overlying paratendinitis as described above. Most clinicians, including primary care physicians, would not be able to differentiate which of these were most prominent in a patient presenting with general hand/wrist pain, as the signs and symptoms are similar to isolated paratendinitis.

Of the above categories, only tendinitis and paratendinitis have an inflammatory component and would conceivably respond to an anti-inflammatory regimen, and likewise would logically not respond to deep tissue friction massage.

EXAMINATION AND DIAGNOSIS

A comprehensive assessment is the most important step to determining appropriate treatment of most musculoskeletal disorders. History, clinical tests, and imaging will contribute to a differential diagnosis. The reader is referred to Chapters 2–4 for discussion of history taking, physical examination, and pertinent imaging. Clinical testing for tendinopathy can include palpation, selective tissue testing, and provocation testing. It is theorized that clinical tests will help to differentiate the structure involved, yet reliability and validity are still in research. Indeed, this is only one part of the diagnostic equation. Identifying the type of tendon involvement and stage of pathology is another factor of greater difficulty.

The diagnosis of tendinopathy will be the result from a comprehensive examination, but distinguishing between tendinosis and tendinitis can be difficult (Khan et al 2000). Maffulli et al (2003a) identified tendinopathy clinically as localized tendon swelling and pain with impaired function. Curwin (2005) stated that we must assume the level of tendon involvement can be correlated with the level of dysfunction and pain. Per Curwin (2005), the degree of injury cannot be ascertained acutely. Elder & Harvey (2005) maintained that acutely the specific area is usually easy to isolate. Leadbetter (1992) defined acute injury as having a sudden specific onset followed by gradually decreasing pain. Identifying an acute onset during history taking should help differentiate a current stage of acute or subacute inflammatory process from a chronic stage when inhibiting pain occurs during activity or afterward (Leadbetter 1992), and will help guide treatment.

One complicating factor in isolating a specific involved structure is that most tendons to be identified will have anatomic variations or supernumerary insertions. These vary too much for inclusion here. Another complication is the possibility that a trigger point is responsible for all or a portion of the symptoms. Trigger points in the upper quarter can refer pain to the wrist area. The subscapularis, biceps brachii and brachialis are some of the muscles that can refer pain to the wrist (Finando & Finando 2005). Lack of clearing these points/areas of potential contribution will delay appropriate treatment. It cannot be overemphasized that suspected trigger points should be cleared as part of the initial examination. The reader is referred to Chapter 32 of this text for additional information on referred pain from muscle/myofascial trigger points (TrPs) in arm pain syndromes.

Clinical tests

Regarding general palpation, oedema and hyperaemia of the paratenon may be evidenced clinically. A fibrinous exudate accumulates within the tendon sheath, and crepitus may be felt on clinical examination (Kahn et al 2000, Sharma & Maffulli 2005). This may be important in differentiating paratendinitis from tendinopathy; however, the presence of crepitis to palpation does not prove that paratendinitis is present (Kahn et al 2000, Sharma & Maffulli 2005).

Palpation for tenderness is a common tool for clinical diagnosis and differential testing in tendinopathy. Cook et al (2001) assessed the value of palpation to identify patellar tendinopathy in a group of 326 young athletes. Intra-rater reliability was good at 82%. Palpation of tendons in patients with symptoms resulted in sensitivity of 68% and specificity of 9% (Cook et al 2001). However, applicability to the wrist is limited since the patellar tendon is larger than those of the hand/wrist.

Maffulli et al (2003b) found a high positive predictive value in palpation, when combined with the Royal London Hospital test and a painful arc sign to determine Achilles tendinopathy. The painful arc sign is theorized to differentiate pathology within the tendon itself versus pathology of the paratendon. If the pathology is confined to the tendon structure, a palpable area of thickness and tenderness will move with the tendon as the ankle is moved; if the painful, thickened area stays in a fixed position regardless of ankle movement then the pathology is within the paratendon (Easley & Le 2009). The sensitivity and specificity of this test was 52% and 83% (Maffulli et al 2003b). The Royal London Hospital test identifies tendinopathy by eliciting local tenderness with palpation of the tendon in neutral or slightly on slack. The test is positive if the tenderness decreased significantly or disappears with the tendon on stretch. The sensitivity and specificity of this test was 54% and 91%. The sensitivity and specificity of direct palpation was 58% and 74%. When the three tests were combined, sensitivity was 58% and specificity was 83% (Maffulli et al 2003b). There is a dearth of evidence-based research application of these clinical tests to tendons of the wrist and hand.

Cyriax supported selective tissue tension testing (STT) (Hammer 2007b). Selective tissue tension testing is utilized to compare non-contractile to contractile tissue involvement (Hammer 2007b). The tendon is isolated as much as possible based on planes of motion performed, either isolated or overlapped with other tendons. The examiner attempts to administer a minimal isometric force to the tendon/muscle while the patient resists. Elicitation of pain is a positive test (Hammer 2007b). Hanchard et al (2005) found agreement (0.71–0.79, kappa and 95% confidence interval) among Cyriax-trained assessors using STT combined with clinical history when assessing tendinopathy of the rotator cuff. Reliability has yet to be established for any upper extremity tendon application (Stasinopoulos & Johnson 2007).

Provocation tests (special tests) are used with varying evidence-based support of reliability, sensitivity, and specificity. These tests are included, as available and relevant, in the outlined discussion of tendinopathies unique to specific tendons of the wrist and hand following diagnostic imaging and invasive testing.

Diagnostic imaging and invasive testing

Due to the difficulty in reliably diagnosing tendinopathy, Fredberg & Stengaard-Pedersen (2008) recommended ultrasound (US) or magnetic resonance imaging (MRI) if there is no response to conservative treatment or if radicular pain is present. Fredberg & Stengaard-Pedersen (2008) described the efficacy of ultrasound versus MRI. These include more detailed visualization of tendon microstructure, better tendon border definition, and its interactive nature. A focal thickening, visualized with ultrasound, is associated with tendonitis in tendons without sheaths. This may correspond to angiofibroblastic areas associated with micro-ruptures (Daenen et al 2003). Furthermore, the tendon or tendon sheath, as viewed via ultrasound, will be thickened on more chronically involved tendons (Daenen et al 2003). Ultrasound can be performed directly over the subjectively painful area and even during range of motion (Fredberg & Stengaard-Pedersen 2008). McNee & Teh (2007) considered ultrasound the 'investigation of choice' in tendon pathology. Beddi & Bagga (2007) stated that ultrasound is the gold standard for tendon examination.

Isolated identification of the involved structure can be assessed by removing sensation from specific areas, continuing until the patient's symptoms are resolved. Selective anaesthetic injections, usually with lidocaine, are supported by Elder & Harvey (2005) as 'the best diagnostic test' for tendinopathy of the hand and wrist, but they offer no studies to back up this recommendation.

TENDINOPATHIC ENTITIES OF THE HAND AND WRIST

This section will describe common areas of tendon pain in the wrist. Areas of rare involvement are not included.

Flexor carpi ulnaris

Pathology of the flexor carpi ulnaris (FCU) muscle (Fig 26.2) may include tendinitis, tendinosis, or a combination of these two. This is the most common wrist flexor tendinopathy (Elder & Harvey 2005) and often occurs in those who play racquet sports and golf (Rettig 2001). The FCU inserts into the pisiform, the hook of the

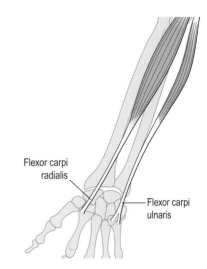

Fig 26.2 Tendiopathic entities: flexor tendons.

hamate, and the fifth metacarpal (Moore 1992). It is not held in place by the flexor retinaculum, but instead relies on its own tendon sheath (Elder & Harvey 2005).

Testing

- Characterized by painful palpation of the pisiform and the FCU tendon, presence of angiofibroblastic hyperplasia is often evidenced by palpable swelling and thickening in symptomatic FCU tendons (Budoff et al 2005)
- Pain with resisted wrist flexion and ulnar deviation
- Shuck test if pisotriquetral involvement is suspected (Rettig 2001)
- Passive wrist extension and radial deviation will provoke symptoms (Elder & Harvey 2005)

Differential diagnosis

Rettig (2001) recommended the pisotriquetral grind test to implicate the pisotriquetral joint pain over a FCU tendinopathy. Campbell (2001) and Burke (1996) describe the test as grasping the pisiform and compressing it onto the triquetrum and rotating the pisiform under pressure. Palpation alone may implicate the tendon with pain and crepitus, whereas pain with compression implicates the pisotriquetral joint. Pisotriquetral compression syndrome (Rettig 2001), arthritis, calcific tendonitis and ulnar neuritis, pisiform ligament complex syndrome, pisotriquetral arthrosis (Rayan 2005), and Guyon's canal syndrome (Elder & Harvey 2005) are additional differential diagnoses.

Extensor carpi ulnaris

Tendinopathy of the extensor carpi ulnaris (ECU) (Fig 26.3) may commonly include a tendinitis, tendinosis, or

341

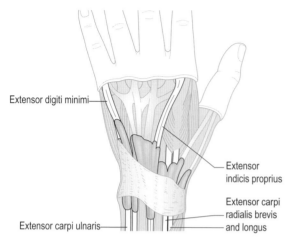

Extensor digiti minimi

Extensor indicis proprius

Extensor carpi radialis brevis and longus

Extensor carpi ulnaris

Fig 26.3 Tendiopathic entities: extensor tendons.

these in combination. It is also subject to subluxation (Elder & Harvey 2005). Activities such as racquet sports and baseball batting will cause rapid and repetitive supination, flexion, and ulnar deviation, which have been cited as promoting factors (Elder & Harvey 2005, Hammer 2007c). Rettig (2001) noted that ECU tendinopathy often involved the non-dominant hand in tennis players who used a two-handed backhand stroke. Futami & Itoman (1995) found that of 155 patients with dorsal wrist pain, 53 had pain possibly caused by tenovaginitis (paratendinitis) of the ECU induced by overuse. Bencardino & Rosenburg (2006) associated sub-luxations of the ECU with tenosynovitis and recommended testing supination and volar flexion for ulnar sub-luxation of the tendon. Montalvan et al (2007) studied 28 clinical cases of ECU related pain with three clinical patterns described: (a) acute traumatic instability of the ECU in the fibro-osseus groove (12 cases); (b) tendinopathy (14 cases); and (c) complete ECU rupture (4 cases).

Testing

- Symptoms are provoked by combined active supination and wrist extension (Elder & Harvey 2005) and combined resisted ulnar deviation and extension (Elder & Harvey 2005, Young et al 2007)
- Dislocation can be reproduced by a clicking on supination and extension actively, not passively (Elder & Harvey 2005)
- Tenderness to palpation over sixth dorsal compartment (Rettig 2001) at the ECU tendon and ulnar head (Elder & Harvey 2005)

Differential diagnosis

Rupture, sub-luxation, dislocation, triangular fibro-cartilage complex (TFCC) pain, triquetrum-lunate ligament lesion,

pisiform-lunate joint pain, and fractures of the lunate, triquetrum and pisiform are differential diagnoses (Futami & Itoman 1995). Additional diagnoses to be excluded are extensor digiti minimi tenosynovitis, TFCC tears (Elder & Harvey 2005), and stenosing tenosynovitis in the ulnar wrist (Rettig 2001).

Extensor carpi radialis longus and brevis (distal tendons)

A common combined pathology of the extensor carpi radialis longus (ECRL) and brevis (ECRB) tendons (Fig 26.3) distally is known as intersection syndrome. This is also termed *peritendinitis crepitans* (Young et al 2007), *crossover tendinitis*, and *squeaker's wrist* (Rettig 2001). The syndrome may include tendinitis, tendinosis, and/or bursitis. It is common among racquet players, weight lifters, and canoeists (Hammer 2007c). Ski pole and hammer usage can also provoke this particular syndrome (Elder & Harvey 2005).

Intersection syndrome is associated with friction from the crossing of the first dorsal compartment abductor pollicis longus (APL) and the extensor pollicis brevis (EPB) over the second dorsal compartment (ECRL and ECRB) (Young et al 2007). It is a paratendinitis (tenosynovitis) that can result in stenosis of the affected tendons.

Cvitanic (2007) noted a natural foramen between the extensor pollicis longus (EPL) and ECRB in cadavers at the site of the intersection. This could explain the areas of multiple symptoms in the dorsal forearm and could make differential diagnoses more complicated. Inflammatory conditions of the ECRB and ECRL at their insertions may be associated with bony protuberances at the capitate, second or third metacarpals, or trapezoid (Daenen et al 2003).

Testing

- Pain to palpation and visible swelling may be evidenced in the tendons proximal to the first compartment (Plancher et al 1996, Benicardino & Rosenburg 2006)
- Thickening and interstitial fluid collection around both tendons approximately 4 to 6 to 8 cm proximal to Lister's tubercle will show on MRI (Benicardino & Rosenburg 2006, Plancher et al 1996)
- Crepitation between the APL/EPB and ECRL/ECRB with wrist flexion or extension may be palpable (Elder & Harvey 2005)

Differential diagnosis

Finkelstein's test will be positive but in a more proximal region of the dorsal forearm than would be the case in

DeQuervain's tenosynovitis (Elder & Harvey 2005, Young et al 2007).

Extensor indicis proprius

Pain and swelling over the fourth dorsal compartment is the most common finding in extensor indicis proprius (EIP) (Fig 26.3) syndrome (Plancher et al 1996). This syndrome involves an irritation of the tenosynovium near the extensor retinaculum (Elder & Harvey 2005). Plancher et al (1996) attributed symptoms of EIP tendinopathy to overuse hypertrophy, or to synovitis secondary to overuse. The former could lead to the latter if symptoms were not addressed in a timely fashion. Anatomic variations (75%) are common, complicating the exact structure involved (Plancher et al 1996, Soejima et al 2002).

Testing

- Pain and swelling are evidenced in fourth dorsal compartment distal to ulnar head with supination (Plancher et al 1996)
- Resisted index extension (Hammer 2007c) with wrist fully flexed (Elder & Harvey 2005) provokes symptoms

Differential diagnosis

Extensor digitorum communis (EDC) or extensor pollicis longus (EPL) tenosynovitis, dorsoradial ganglion, Klebock's disease, extensor digitorum communis tendinopathy, and fourth-compartment syndrome are diagnoses to be excluded (Elder & Harvey 2005).

Extensor digiti minimi

The extensor digiti minimi (EDM) (Fig 26.3) occupies the fifth dorsal compartment. The pathology most often occurring here is a tenosynovitis (Elder & Harvey 2005). Duplication of the tendon is common complicating implication of the proper structure (Young et al 2007). Elder & Harvey (2005) stated that continuous hand usage such as handwriting will provoke symptoms. Hammer (2007c) reported a lack of pain with resisted testing, which is unusual for tendinopathy, but no reason for this phenomenon was given.

Testing

- Grip is painful (Elder & Harvey 2005)
- Limitation in fifth digit extension is seen (Elder & Harvey 2005)
- Wrist flexion after fist closure or flexing a fist is painful (Elder & Harvey 2005)
- Tenderness to palpation is present just distal to ulnar head (Plancher et al 1996)

Differential diagnosis

Extensor carpi ulnaris (ECU) tenosynovitis, TFCC pathology, ulnar impaction should be ruled out (Elder & Harvey 2005).

Abductor pollicis longus and extensor pollicis brevis

Together the abductor pollicis longus (APL) and extensor pollicis brevis (EPB) (Fig 26.4) contribute to De Quervain's tenosynovitis. These tendons normally pass together through a single fibro-osseous tunnel to insert on the first metacarpal and first proximal phalanx respectively (Plancher et al 1996). De Quervain's tenosynovitis often results from excessive pinching or radial deviation (Hammer 2007c). This syndrome is a common occurrence in golf, racquet sports and fishing (Rettig 2001).

Testing

- Finkelstein's test (Fig 26.5A). Ahuja & Chung (2004) detailed the true test and variations, as the test is misrepresented vigorously in the literature. The original test Finkelstein (1930) described was completely passive: the clinician grasps the patient's thumb and quickly pulls the wrist into ulnar deviation via the thumb. A positive result is reproduction of pain at the ulnar styloid. The surgeon Eichhoff described a test for de Quervain's disease that is often mistaken for Finkelstein's test (Fig 26.5B). His test consisted of the patient actively placing the thumb into the palm and folding the fingers down, holding the thumb in place while the clinician passively moves the wrist into ulnar deviation. A positive test is the same as described for Finkelstein's test. This test, which many believe to be the Finkelstein test, has been criticized as giving false-positive results. Brunelli described a test in 2003 that he claimed was more accurate than the true Finkelstein's test. Brunelli criticized Finkelstein's test for false-positive results due to the

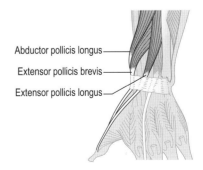

Fig 26.4 Tendiopathic entities: thumb tendons.

Abductor pollicis longus

Extensor pollicis brevis

Extensor pollicis longus

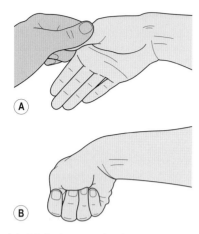

Fig 26.5 (A) Finkelstein's test: The clinician grasps the patient's thumb, uses it to quickly and passively place the wrist into ulnar deviation, causing pain at the radial styloid process. (B) Eichhoff test: The patient actively grips the thumb in the fist and then the clinician passively places the wrist into ulnar deviation, which causes pain at the radial styloid process (after Ahuja & Chung 2004).

stretch of the radial collateral ligament, the scaphotrapezial ligament, or the thumb carpometacarpal ligament caused by the APL and EPB tendons being moved away from the pulley. Brunelli described a test in which the wrist is held in radial deviation while forcibly abducting the thumb (Ahuja & Chung 2004). Psychometric properties of these tests have not been established (Elder & Harvey 2005).

- The EPB entrapment test identifies separate compartments and resulting stenosis; this test was reported to have sensitivity of 81% and specificity of 50% (Alexander et al 2002)
- Tenderness on palpation and swelling over the radial styloid (Elder & Harvey 2005) and first dorsal compartment (Rettig 2001) are present
- Resisted thumb extension is painful (Elder & Harvey 2005)

Differential diagnosis

Intersection syndrome (Elder & Harvey 2005), scaphoid fracture, flexor carpi radialis (FCR) tendinopathy, first carpometacarpal (CMC) joint arthritis, and Wartenburg's syndrome (Plancher et al 1996) are differential diagnoses.

Extensor pollicis longus

The extensor pollicis longus (Fig 26.4) often exhibits a tenosynovitis common to racquet sports players. History of repetitive trauma like racquet sports, pain, crepitus, and swelling around Lister's tubercle will narrow the list

of suspected diagnoses (Plancher et al 1996). Triggering of the thumb may be seen in severe cases.

Testing

- Pain, swelling, and crepitus along the EPL tendon at the third dorsal compartment (Plancher et al 1996), and at Listers tubercle (Elder & Harvey 2005) are evidenced
- Pain is elicited with resisted thumb extension or passive flexion (Elder & Harvey 2005)
- Passive interphalangeal joint flexion can reproduce the pain (Elder & Harvey 2005)

Differential diagnosis

Differential diagnoses have not been established as necessary for this tendon pathology.

Flexor carpi radialis

Flexor carpi radialis (FCR) (Fig 26.2) tendinopathy is common in people who play racquet sports, golf and baseball (Rettig 2001). Elder & Harvey (2005) reported an often insidious onset without known trauma. A primary symptom is pain near the proximal aspect of the trapezium (Gabel et al 1994). This is often a result of overuse with repeated flexion of the wrist, of complication after scaphoid fracture or distal radius fracture, or of other direct trauma (Gabel et al 1994). The FCR is subject to traumatic injury due to its position. The FCR lies in direct contact with the roughened surface of the trapezium. Its insertion onto the trapezium is only 20% of the entire insertion. Additional insertions include the second and third metacarpals (Bishop et al 1994) and the joint capsule of the trapezio-scaphoid joint itself (Schmidt 1987). The tendon occupies 90% of the fibro-osseous tunnel, making it vulnerable to compression (Bishop et al 1994, Elder & Harvey 2005). FCR tendinopathy is also associated with scaphotrapezial joint osteoarthritis, malunion of the trapezium, or scaphoid cyst (Soejima et al 2002).

Testing

- Symptoms are exacerbated by resisted flexion and radial deviation of the wrist (Elder & Harvey 2005, Rayan 2005) and with resisted flexion (Rettig 2001); wrist hyper-extension or resisted wrist flexion with radial deviation can reproduce symptoms (Young et al 2007)
- Pain and notable swelling are evidenced at the level of the distal wrist crease along its course (Elder & Harvey 2005) and near the fibro-osseous tunnel (Young et al 2007).

Differential diagnosis

Differential diagnoses include osteoarthritis of the first CMC joint, scaphoid cysts, fractures, ganglion cysts,

DeQuervain's syndrome, and Lindburg's syndrome (Elder & Harvey 2005).

TREATMENT AND PROGNOSIS

Conservative treatment

Conservative treatment for tendinopathy includes modalities such as ultrasound, electric stimulation, ice, and laser (Curwin 2005); as well as injections and splinting (Plancher et al 1996). Konijnenberg et al (2001) attempted a meta-analysis of outcomes of repetitive strain injuries. Many body areas were included in the analysis. They found no strong evidence for any conservative treatment option (Konijnenberg et al 2001). Conservative treatments included physiotherapy involving multiple types of interventions, but none included the hand or wrist.

Manual therapy, in particular deep tissue friction massage (DTFM), is a conservative treatment for tendinopathy that is utilized by some clinicians; however efficacy has not been proven. This could be due at least in part to study design. DTFM for tendon pain was first popularized by James Cyriax. Cyriax did not perform outcome studies, but studies done by Stasinopoulos & Johnson (2007) concluded that effectiveness of DTFM for lateral epicondylitis could not be assessed from the studies they reviewed. Stasinopoulos did not study outcomes of the wrist.

Cyriax techniques of DTFM for treatment of soft tissue lesions are performed with direct pressure on the painful area. The clinician's finger rubs firmly transversely to the fibres of the tissue, which includes tendon. Recommended duration and frequency are 20-minute sessions for 6–12 treatments with at least 48 hours between treatments (Cyriax 1983). Cyriax (1983) theorized that the treatment eroded scar tissue between muscle fibres via abrasive contact; in tenosynovitis the rolling was theorized to smooth roughened synovial surfaces. More recent work has specified the optimal time of application for tendon strain based on the previously discussed stage of pathology. Research by Zeichen et al (2000) subjected fibroblasts to strain for varying times, monitoring for proliferation of fibroblasts as a response to a biaxial strain over subsequent hours. The results showed that 15 minutes of strain resulted in increased proliferation over controls at 6 and 24 hours (Zeichen et al 2000).

The 48 hours of recommended minimum accepted time frame between treatments roughly equals the ending of the acute stage of inflammation, when remodelling begins (Leadbetter 1992). The harder pressure, as recommended by Cyriax (1983) may be justified by a Gehlsen et al study (1999) showing that firmer pressure had more positive effects.

Hammer (2007d) applied soft tissue mobilization with greater precision regarding stage of tendon pathology. While he generally concurred with treatment in the 5–15

minute duration twice/week lasting 2 weeks to 2 months, Hammer (2007d) recommended no manual treatment until the proliferative phase, which was described as 7–14 days after original injury. Treatment during acute phase when rest is recommended should be light, 'aiding fibroblastic proliferation and breaking down of immature collagen'. The maturation phase could be treated more vigorously to reduce fibrosis (Hammer 2007c).

Kahn (2009) and Kraushaar & Nirschl (1999) theorized that mechanical disruption may transform a failed intrinsic healing into a therapeutic extrinsic healing mechanism. Brousseau et al's (2002) research on DTFM and tendinitis (not tendinosis) considered cross friction treatment as only cross friction and not other techniques, including a stroke along the muscle. This could be one explanation for the lack of more positive outcomes: improper or non-uniform direction of force. Another reason could be lack of proper selection of subcategory of tendinopathy as classified earlier in this section. Some classifications, such as acute inflammation, theoretically cannot be affected by manipulation.

Despite the lack of randomized controlled trials of tendon pain and DTFM, other research is emerging. These studies provide, on a small scale, a patho-anatomic link between manual therapy and reversal of tendinopathic changes. Meltzer & Standley (2007) demonstrated that a modelled indirect osteopathic manipulative technique (IOMT) significantly reduced pro-inflammatory secretions compared to controls 24 h after application, concluding that the modelled IOMT can reverse some of the effects of repetitive strain (Meltzer & Standley 2007). Standley & Meltzer (2008) studied the effect of modelled manual therapy on cellular response. Improved range of motion, reduced analgesic requirements and decreased oedema post-myofascial release was theorized as a result of anti-inflammatory cytokines from strain inducement of myofascial release (Standley & Meltzer 2008).

Eccentric exercise is a more recently applied form of conservative treatment with the theory of reversing degeneration via specific load application. This treatment has shown positive outcomes (Ohberg et al 2004). Eccentric exercise involves contraction of a muscle to control or decelerate a load while the muscle and tendon are lengthening or in a lengthened position. Eccentric exercises have been proven effective at changing ultrasonic findings on involved Achilles tendons within 12 weeks (Ohberg et al 2004). Follow-up showed reduction in tendon diameter and return of normal tendon structure in a majority (19 of 26) of tendons. The unchanged tendons had undefined residual defects (Ohberg et al 2004).

Woodley et al (2006) reviewed 11 studies of eccentric exercises that met inclusion criteria of methodological quality and levels of evidence. They covered both upper and lower extremity tendinopathies. Eccentric exercise was more effective than other treatments that included frictions, stretching, splinting and ultrasound in treating tendon pain and improving patient satisfaction and return to work outcomes (Woodley et al 2006).

Curwin (2005) outlined an eccentric programme that consisted of warm up activities, stretching, 3 sets of 10 eccentric exercises, repeated stretching, and icing. This was continued for 6 weeks unless symptoms resolved first. The protocol was performed by 200 patients with chronic tendinopathy that failed conservative therapy. Marked or complete relief of symptoms was reported in 90% of patients who completed the programme. Despite the large sample size there was no control group or randomization (Curwin 2005).

Knobloch (2008) supported eccentric training on the wrist as equally effective as that on the Achilles tendon in decreasing abnormal capillary tendon flow (angiogenesis) seen in tendinopathy. Kahn et al (2009) promoted the theory that effects of eccentric muscle contraction on the tendon appear to stimulate tissue healing.

The research by Kannus & Josza (1991) illuminated how stress reduction can lead to degenerative changes in tendon including reduction in mechanical properties. That may be why eccentric exercises are effective in some cases in reducing the effects of immobilization. Soft tissue mobilization along the tendon could also reduce the effects of immobilization, but only to a localized portion of that tendon. Any force, including eccentrics, will not affect the tendon equally. Undamaged fascicles will accept and transmit that force normally, while damaged fascicles, according to Arnoczky et al (2007), will not transfer that force to all fascicles, which leads to degeneration of the involved fascicles. This will be a necessary subject of future studies. An algorithm (Fig 26.6) outlines a

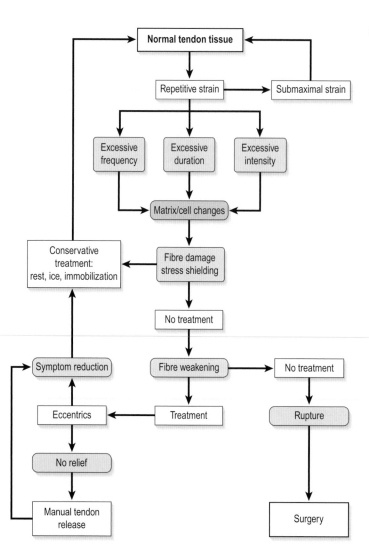

Fig 26.6 Selected treatment algorithm.

proposed pathway of manual treatment and eccentrics in tendinopathy.

Non-conservative treatment

Reviewing the recent literature on surgeries for wrist tendinopathy reveals a consistent use of the terms tendinitis and tenosynovitis in surgical cases. This use is therefore continued in the report of surgical interventions.

DeQuervain's tenosynovitis that does not respond to conservative therapy may undergo surgery. This involves decompression of the first dorsal compartment and is not without risks (Plancher et al 1996). Rettig (2001) reported that after 7–10 days of splinting, return to sports can be expected in 6–9 weeks.

Flexor carpi ulnaris surgery often involves excision of the pisiform (Rettig 2001). The expected return to sports averages 8 weeks (Rettig 2001).

As the flexor carpi radialis occupies 90% of the available space in its synovial tunnel, surgery here involves decompression of the tunnel (Plancher et al 1996).

Plancher et al (1996) stated that extensor carpi ulnaris sub-luxation does not always respond to conservative care. The sixth dorsal compartment is released in extensor carpi ulnaris tendinitis. Due to chance of sub-luxation some authors recommend release of the fibro-osseus tunnel it occupies (Plancher et al 1996). Rettig (2001) reported that after 4–6 weeks of casting return to sports required a minimum of 8 weeks.

Surgery for intersection syndrome, according to Plancher et al (1996), involves release of the second compartment with synovectomy. Rettig (2001) mentioned bursectomy between the involved tendons. Release of the third dorsal compartment is also performed on non-responsive cases of extensor pollicis longus tendinitis.

Prognosis

Prognosis with conservative treatment for specific tendinopathies or syndromes is not widely available in evidence-based studies. Regarding conservative treatment for DeQuervain's tenosynovitis, Harvey et al (1990) reported 80% resolution of symptoms with injections alone. Lane et al (2001) concluded that classifying these patients before conservative treatment was initiated improved outcomes; 17 of 18 patients with classified mild symptoms improved with splinting and non-steroidal anti-inflammatory medications. Patients with symptoms classified as moderate to severe responded most favourably to injections (76%) (Lane et al 2001). Richie & Briner (2003) reviewed seven descriptive studies comparing conservative treatments for DeQuervain's tenosynovitis. They reported an overall cure rate of 83% for injection alone, 61% for injection and splint, 14% for splint alone, and 0% for treatments that consisted solely of non-steroidal anti-inflammatory medications and rest. Tendinopathies of the other structures of the wrist have not been as widely studied.

CONCLUSION

While much more is now known about tenocyte and matrix dysfunction, successful application of these concepts for treatment of tendinopathy in the wrist and hand has not been proven. Studies continued to be hampered by sample size, lack of meaningful outcomes, small population selection, and lack of randomization. Adequate studies regarding conservative treatment of non-inflammatory tendinopathies do not appear to exist currently.

Eccentrics show promise for treating tendinopathy in a majority of weight bearing tendons. Successful application of this into tendinopathies of the upper extremity has yet to be accomplished.

Manual therapy's place in treatment of wrist tendinopathy has not been established. If the efficacy of manual applied eccentrics or what some authors call 'active release' could be likewise established in the upper extremity, they could easily be performed adapting Curwin's (2005) guidelines for eccentric exercises. A study that reveals the effects of manual therapy on tendinopathy will require the following: (1) selection of appropriate tendon pathology, which will pose its own difficulties; (2) soft tissue mobilization such as 'active release' along the tendon fibres; (3) continued self-range of motion routinely for 48 hours, to reduce the effect of immobilization; and (4) the repetition of criteria (2) every 48 hours for up to 6 weeks until function has returned. A design incorporating these factors may be able to discern the true worth of DTFM in tendinopathy.

REFERENCES

Ahuja, N.K., Chung, K.C., 2004. Fritz de Quervain, MD (1868–1940): Stenosing tendovaginitis at the radial styloid process. J. Hand Surg. 29A, 1164–1170.

Alexander, R., Catalano, L., Barron, O., Glickel, S., 2002. Extensor pollicis brevis entrapment test in the treatment of DeQuervain's disease. J. Hand Surg. 27, 813–816.

Andersson, G., Danielson, P., Alfredson, H., Forsgren, S., 2008. Presence of substance P and the neurokinin-1 receptor in tenocytes of the human Achilles tendon. Regul. Pept. 150, 81–87.

Arnoczky, S., Tian, T., Lavagnino, M., et al., 2006. Activation of stress-activated protein kinases (SAPK) in tendon cells following cyclic strain: the effects of strain frequency, strain magnitude and cytosolic calcium. J. Orthop. Res. 20, 947–952.

Arnoczky, S., Lavagnino, M., Egerbacher, M., 2007. The mechanobiological aetiopathogenesis of tendinopathy: is it the over-stimulation or understimulation of tendon cells? International Journal of Exploratory Pathology 88, 217–226.

Backman, C., Boquist, L., Frid'en, J., et al., 2005. Chronic Achilles paratendonitis and tendinosis: an experimental model in the rabbit. J. Orthop. Res. 8, 541–547.

Beddi, T.H., Bagga, R.N., 2007. Ultrasound in rheumatology. Musculoskeletal Ultrasound Symposium 17, 299–305.

Bencardino, J., Rosenburg, Z., 2006. Sports related injuries to the wrist: An approach to MRI interpretation. Clin. Sports Med. 25, 409–432.

Benjamin, M., Ralphs, J., 1996. Tendons in health and disease. Man. Ther. 1, 186–191.

Bishop, A., Gabel, G., Carmichael, S., 1994. Flexor carpi radialis tendonitis I, operative anatomy. J. Bone Joint Surg. 76, 1009–1014.

Brousseau, L., Casimiro, L., Milne, S., et al., 2002. Deep transverse friction massage for treating tendinitis. Cochrane Database Syst. Rev. 2002 4, CD 003528.

Budoff, J., Kraushaar, B., Ayala, G., 2005. Flexor carpi ulnaris tendinopathy. J. Hand Surg. 30, 125–129.

Burke, F.D., 1996. Pisotriquetral pathology: a differential diagnosis. In: Buchler, U. (Ed.), Wrist Instability. Mosby, United Kingdom, pp. 213–217.

Campbell, D.A., 2001. How I examine the wrist. Current Orthopedics 14, 342–346.

Cannon, N., 2001. Diagnosis and treatment manual for physicians and therapists: upper extremity rehabilitation, fourth ed. Hand Rehabilitation Center of Indiana, USA.

Chiquet, M., 1999. Regulation of extracellular matrix gene expression by mechanical stress. Matrix Biol. 18, 417–426. Abstract.

Cook, J., Purdam, C., 2009. Is tendon pathology a continuum? A pathology model to explain the clinical presentation of load-induced tendinopathy. Br. J. Sports Med. 43, 409–416.

Cook, J., Khan, K., Kiss, Z., 2001. Reproducibility and clinical utility of tendon palpation to detect patellar tendinopathy in young basketball players. Br. J. Sports Med. 35, 65–69.

Curwin, S.L., 2005. Rehabilitation after tendon injuries. In: Maffulli, N., Renstrom, P., Leadbetter, W. (Eds.), Tendon Injuries: Basic science and clinical medicine. Springer-Verlag, London, pp. 242–266.

Cvitanic, O.A., 2007. Communicating foramen between tendon sheaths of the extensor carpi radialis brevis and extensor pollicis longus muscles: Imaging of cadaver and patients. AJR. Am. J. Roentgenol. 189, 1190–1197.

Cyriax, J., 1983. Illustrated Manual of Orthopaedic Medicine. Butterworth's, London.

Daenen, B., Houben, G., Bauduin, E., et al., 2003. Sonography in wrist pathology. J. Clin. Ultrasound 32, 462–469.

De Boer, M., Selby, A., Atherton, P., et al., 2007. The temporal responses of protein synthesis, gene expression and cell signaling in human quadriceps muscle and patellar tendon to disuse. J. Physiol. 585, 241–251.

Department of Labor, 1999. Illnesses, Injuries and Fatalities Bureau of Labor Statistics. United States Department of Labor. 1999 Online: Available http://www.bls.gov./iff/home.htm (accessed 29.08.09.).

Easley, M., Le, I., 2009. Non-Insertional Achilles Tendinopathy. In: Nunley, J. (Ed.), The Achilles Tendon: Treatment and Rehabilitation. Springer Science, Durham NC, pp. 145–168.

Elder, G., Harvey, E., 2005. Hand and wrist tendinopathies. In: Maffuli, N., Renstrom, P., Leadbetter, W. (Eds.), Tendon injuries basic science and clinical medicine. Springer-Verlag, London, pp. 137–149.

Finando, D., Finando, S., 2005. Trigger point therapy for myofascial pain. Healing Arts Press, Vermont.

Finkelstein, H., 1930. Stenosing tendovaginitis at the radial styloid process. J. Bone Joint Surg. 12, 509–540.

Fredberg, U., Stengaard-Pedersen, K., 2008. Chronic tendinopathy tissue pathology, pain mechanisms and etiology with a special focus on inflammation. Scandinavian Journal of Sports Medicine 18, 3–15.

Futami, T., Itoman, M., 1995. Extensor carpi ulnaris syndrome: findings in 43 patients. Acta Orthop. Scand. 66, 538–539.

Gabel, G., Bishop, A.T., Wood, M.B., 1994. Flexor carpi radialis tendonitis II, results of operative treatment. J. Bone Joint Surg. 76, 1015–1018.

Gehlsen, G., Ganion, L., Helfst, R., 1999. Fibroblast responses to variation in soft tissue mobilization pressure. Med. Sci. Sports Exerc. 31, 531–555.

Glazebrook, M., Wright, J., Langman, M., et al., 2007. Histological analysis of Achilles tendon in an overuse rat model. J. Orthop. Res. 26, 840–846.

Hammer, W., 2007a. Manual treatment methods. In: Hammer, W. (Ed.), Functional Soft Tissue Examination. Jones and Bartlett, Boston, pp. 475–479.

Hammer, W., 2007b. Basics of soft tissue examination. In: Hammer, W. (Ed.), Functional Soft Tissue Examination. Jones and Bartlett, Boston, pp. 3–14.

Hammer, W., 2007c. Wrist and Hand. In: Hammer, W. (Ed.), Functional Soft Tissue Examination. Jones and Bartlett, Boston, pp. 213–225.

Hammer, W., 2007d. Combining friction massage with neuromuscular reeducation. In: Hammer, W. (Ed.), Functional soft tissue examination and treatment by manual methods. Jones and Bartlett, Boston, pp. 563–589.

Hanchard, N., Howe, T., Gilbert, M., 2005. Diagnosis of shoulder pain by history and selective tissue tension: agreement between assessors. J. Orthop. Sports Phys. Ther. 35, 147–153.

Harley, B., Bergman, J., 2008. Tendon and ligament anatomy, biology and biomechanics. In: Toretta, P.,

Einhorn, T. (Eds.), Oncology and basic science. Lippincott, Williams and Wilkins, Philadelphia, pp. 463–473.

Hart, D., Cyrli, B., Frank, S., et al., 2005. Neurogenic, mast cell, and gender variables in tendon biology: potential role in chronic tendinopathy. In: Maffulli, N., Renstrom, P., Leadbetter, W. (Eds.), Tendon Injuries: Basic Science and Clinical Medicine. Springer-Verlag, London, pp. 40–48.

Harvey, F., Harvey, P., Horsley, M., 1990. DeQuervain's disease: surgical or nonsurgical treatment. J. Hand Surg. Am. 15, 83–87.

Huang, H., Kamm, R., Lee, R.T., 2004. Cell mechanics and mechanotransduction: pathways, probes, and physiology. Am. J. Physiol. Cell Physiol. 287, C1–C11.

Kannus, P., 2000. Structure of the Tendon Connective Tissue. Scand. J. Med. Sci. Sports 10, 312–320.

Kannus, P., Jozsa, L., 1991. Histopathologic changes preceding spontaneous rupture of a tendon. J. Bone Joint Surg. 73, 1507–1525.

Khan, K., 2009. Mechanotherapy: how physical therapists prescription of exercise promotes tissue repair. Br. J. Sports Med. 43, 247–252.

Khan, K., Cook, J., Taunton, J., et al., 2000. Overuse tendinosis not tendinitis: Part 1: a new paradigm for a difficult clinical problem. Phys. Sportsmed. 28 (5), Online. Available: http://www.massagebyjoel.com/downloads/OveruseTendinosis-PhySptsmed.pdf (accessed 12.03.09.).

Khan, K., Cook, J., Bonar, F., et al., 2006. Histopathology of common tendinopathies: Update and implications for clinical management. In: Khan, K., Bruckner, P. (Eds.), Clinical Sports Medicine. third ed. McGraw-Hill, Australia, Online. Available: http://www.clinicalsportsmedicine.com/articles/common_tendinopathies.htm (accessed 26.08.09.).

Knobloch, K., 2008. The Role of Tendon Micrfocirculation in Achilles and Patellar Tendinopahty. J. Orth. Surg. Online. Available at http://www.pubmedcentral.nih.gov/articlerender.fogi artid=2397381.

Konijnenberg, H., deWilde, N., Gerritsen, A., et al., 2001. Conservative treatment for repetitive strain. Scand. J. Work Environ. Health 27, 299–310.

Kraushaar, B., Nirschl, R., 1999. Tendinosis of the elbow. Clinical features and findings of histological, immunohistochemical, and electron microscopy studies. J. Bone Joint Surg. 81, 259–278.

Lane, L.B., Boretz, R.S., Stuchin, S.A., 2001. Treatment of DeQuervain's: role of conservative management. Journal of Hand Surgery (Europe) 26, 258–260.

Lavagnino, M., Arnoczky, S., Tian, T., et al., 2003. Effect of amplitude and frequency of cyclic tensile strain on the inhibition of MMP1 mRNA expression in tendon cells: an in vitro study. Connect. Tissue Res. 44, 181–187.

Lavagnino, M., Arnoczky, S.P., Egrebacher, M., et al., 2006. Isolated fibular damage in tendons stimulates local collagenase mRNA expression and protein synthesis. J. Biomech. 39, 2355–2362.

Leadbetter, W., 1992. Cell-matrix response in tendon injury. Clin. Sports Med. 11, 433–577.

McNee, P.A., Teh, J., 2007. Imaging of the wrist. Imaging 19, 208–219.

Maeda, E., Shelton, J.C., Bader, D.L., et al., 2009. Differential regulation of gene expression in isolated tendon fascicles exposed to cyclic strain in vivo. J. Appl. Physiol. 106, 506–512. (Abstract).

Maffulli, N., Longo, U.G., 2008. How do eccentrics work in tendinopathy. Rheumatology 47, 1444–1445.

Maffulli, N., Moller, H., 2005. Optimization of tendon healing. In: Maffulli, N., Renstrom, P., Leadbetter, W. (Eds.), Tendon Injuries: Basic science and clinical medicine. Springer-Verlag, London, pp. 204–206.

Maffulli, N., Wong, J., Almekinders, L.C., 2003a. Types and epidemiology of tendinopathy. Clin. Sports Med. 22, 675–692.

Maffulli, N., Kenward, M., Testa, V., et al., 2003b. Clinical diagnosis of Achilles tendinopathy with tendinosis. Clin. J. Sports Med. 13, 11–15. Abstract.

Maffulli, N., Longo, U.G., Franceschi, F., 2008. Movin and Bonar scores assess the same characteristics of tendon histology. Clin. Orthop. Relat. Res. 466, 1605–1611.

Magra, M., Hughes, S., El Haj, A.J., et al., 2007. VOCC and TREK-1 ion channel expression in human tenocytes. Am. J. Physiol. Cell Physiol. 292, C1053–C1060.

Meltzer, K., Standley, P., 2007. Modeled repetitive motion strain and indirect osteopathic manipulative techniques in regulation of human fibroblast proliferation and interleukin secretion. J. Am. Osteopath. Assoc. 107, 527–536.

Montalvan, B., Parier, J., Brasseur, J., 2007. Extensor carpi ulnaris injuries in tennis players: A study of 28 cases. Br. J. Sports Med. 40, 424–429.

Moore, K., 1992. Clinically Oriented Anatomy, third ed. Williams and Wilkins, Baltimore, p. 566.

Murrell, G., 2002. Understanding tendinopathies. Br. J. Sports Med. 36, 392.

O'Brien, M., 2005. Anatomy of tendons. In: Maffulli, N., Renstrom, P., Leadbetter, W. (Eds.), Tendon Injuries: basic science and clinical medicine. Springer-Verlag, London, pp. 3–11.

Ohberg, L., Lorentzon, R., Alfredson, H., 2004. Eccentric training in patients with chronic Achilles tendinosis: normalized tendons structure and decreased thickness at follow up. Br. J. Sports Med. 38, 8–11.

Oystein, L., Scott, A., Engebretson, L., 2007. Excessive apoptosis in patellar tendon in athletes. Am. J. Sports Med. 35, 605–611. (April).

Plancher, K.D., Peterson, R.K., Steichen, J.B., 1996. Compressive neuropathies and tendinopathies in athletic elbow and wrist. Clin. Sports Med. 15, 331–371.

Rayan, G., 2005. Pisiform ligament complex syndrome and pisotriquetral arthrosis. Hand. Clin. 21, 507–517.

Renstrom, P., Hach, T., 2005. Insertional tendinopathy in sports. In: Maffulli, N., Renstrom, P., Leadbetter, W. (Eds.), Tendon Injuries: Basic science and clinical medicine. Springer-Verlag, London, pp. 70–85.

Rettig, A., 2001. Wrist and hand overuse syndromes. Clin. Sports Med. 20, 591–611.

Richie, C., Briner, W., 2003. Corticosteroid injection for treatment of DeQuervain's tenosynovitis: a pooled quantitative literature evaluation. J. Am. Board Fam. Pract. 16, 102–106. (abstract).

Riley, G., 2004. The pathogenesis of tendinopathy a molecular perspective. Rheumatology 43, 131–142.

Schmidt, H., 1987. Clinical anatomy of flexor carpi radialis tendon sheath. Acta Morphol. Neerl. Scand. 25, 17–28.

Scott, A., Cook, J., Hart, D., et al., 2007. Tenocyte response to mechanical load in vivo: a role for local insulin-like growth factor1 signaling in early tendinosis in rats. Arthritis Rheum. 56, 871–881.

Screen, H., Shelton, J., Bader, D., 2005. Cyclic tensile strain upregulates collagen synthesis in isolated tendon fascicles. Biochem. Biophys. Res. Commun. 336, 424–429.

Sharma, P., Maffulli, N., 2005. Tendon injury and tendinopathy: healing and repair. J. Bone Joint Surg. 87A, 187–202.

Sharma, P., Maffulli, N., 2006. Biology of tendon injury: healing, modeling and remodeling. J. Musculoskelet. Neuronal Interact. 6, 181–190.

Smith, R., Zunino, L., Webbon, P., et al., 1997. The distribution of cartilage oligomeric matrix protein (COMP) in tendon and its variation with tendon site, age and load. Matrix Biol. 16, 255–271.

Soejima, O., Iida, H., Naito, M., 2002. Flexor carpi radialis tendonitis caused by malunited trapezial ridge fracture in a professional baseball player. J. Orthop. Sci. 7, 151–153.

Soslowsky, L., Thomopoulos, S., Tun, S., et al., 2000. Overuse activity injuries in the supraspinatus tendon in an animal model: a histopathologic and biomechanical study. J. Shoulder Elbow Surg. 9, 79–84.

Standley, P., Melzter, K., 2008. In vitro modeling of repetitive motion strain and manual medicine treatments: Potential roles for pro- and anti-inflammatory cytokines. J. Bodyw. Mov. Ther. 12, 201–203.

Stasinopoulos, S., Johnson, M., 2007. It may be time to modify Cyriax's treatment for lateral epicondylitis. J. Bodyw. Mov. Ther. 11, 64–67.

Ueda, H., 1999. In vivo molecular signal transduction of peripheral mechanisms of pain. Jpn. J. Pharmacol. 79, 263–268.

Wall, M.E., Banes, A.J., 2005. Early responses to mechanical load in tendon: role for calcium signaling, gap junctions and intracellular communication. J. Musculoskelet. Neuronal Interact. 5, 70–84.

Woo, S.L., Kuei, S.C., Amiel, D., et al., 1981. The effect of prolonged physical training on the properties of long bone. J. Bone Joint Surg. 63, 780–787.

Woodley, B., Newsham-West, R., Baxter, G.D., 2006. Chronic tendinopathy: effectiveness of eccentric exercise. Br. J. Sports Med. 41, 188–198. Abstract.

Young, D., Papp, S., Biachino, A., 2007. Physical exam of the wrist. Orthop. Clin. North Am. 38, 149–165.

Yuan, J., Wang, M.X., Murrel, G., 2003. Cell death and tendinopathy. Clin. Sports Med. 22, 693–701.

Zeichen, J., Griensven, M., Bosch, U., 2000. The proliferative response of isolated human tendon fibroblasts to cyclic biaxial mechanical strain. Am. J. Sports Med. 28, 888–892.

Chapter | 27 |

Wrist instability

Ellen J Pong

INTRODUCTION TO WRIST INSTABILITY

Functional stability

The human wrist is a necessary link between the power of the forearm and the precision of the hand. It has been proposed that there was a survival advantage in human evolution to having a carpus whose stability as a stationary platform enhanced precise use of instruments, weapons, and tools (Wolfe et al 2006). Simple grasp of an object relies on at least four mechanisms of carpal stabilization. They include the proximal carpal row, the distal carpal row, the mid-carpal joint, and the radio-carpal joint (Garcia-Elias 1997a). While stability of the radial side is clearly a necessary component of opposable thumb use, stability of the distal radio-ulnar joint is just as important for provision of the rotational forearm in tool use and carrying (Dobbs 2003).

Defining wrist instability

Linscheid and associates are credited as the first to define carpal instability in 1972 (Schmitt et al 2006), but references to conditions of instability are recorded as early as 1923 (Linscheid et al 1972, Lichtman & Wroten 2006). Linscheid & Dobyns (2002) set forth specific concepts in defining types of instability as well as providing an overall definition; however, this definition has continued to evolve with time (Carlsen & Shin 2008).

© 2011 Elsevier Ltd.
DOI: 10.1016/B978-0-7020-3528-9.00027-3

There is disagreement among researchers regarding aetiology and patho-mechanics, resulting in various accepted views of terminology and treatment for instability of the wrist and its specific joints (Lichtman & Wroten 2006). Linscheid & Dobyns (2002) defined wrist instability as a wrist having altered kinematics and/or being unable to support physiological loads. Taking this further, De Filippo et al (2006) specified: carpal instability occurs from all untreated dislocations and displaced or malunited fractures; integrity of inter-osseous ligaments and joint capsule determine stability; congenital ligamentous laxity (such as Ehlers–Danlos syndrome) is not considered pathological wrist/carpal instability; and pain may not be present as a diagnostic symptom in the initial stages of some carpal instabilities.

Four joints are grossly considered in presentation of wrist instability: carpo-metacarpal joint, mid-carpal joint, radio-carpal joint and distal radio-ulnar joint (DRUJ), with DRUJ stability influenced by stability of the associated triangular fibro-cartilage complex (TFCC) (Dumontier 1996). This chapter will focus on mid-carpal, radio-carpal, and DRUJ instability.

Incidence and aetiology of carpal instability

Exact figures of carpal instability incidence and economic impact are difficult to obtain, primarily because many instabilities are not diagnosed early or revealed for treatment at all due to lack of pain in some cases and poor recognition and follow-up in others (Perron et al 2001, Dias & Garcia-Elias 2006).

The most widely recognized cause of carpal instability is trauma, with wrist hyperextension and various forearm rotations; however, the exact combination of joint position varies along with the resulting instability location (De Filippo et al 2006, Garcia-Elias 2006, Schmitt et al 2006). Linscheid et al (1972) found that instability was a complication in 10% of all reported carpal injuries. The most common carpal instability (up to 19% of wrist injuries) is within the mid-carpal joint, between the scaphoid and lunate (Bozentka 1999, Surdziel & Lubiatowski 2006).

The mal-united distal radius fracture is recognized as a cause of carpal malalignment, developing during the period of immobilization and worsening gradually after fracture healing due to continued stress and loading of the wrist (Gupta et al 2002). The incidence of carpal instability from this type of injury is possibly as high as 30% (Tang 1992). Rheumatoid arthritis and calcium pyrophosphate deposition disease (CPPD) are additional causes of wrist instability in the inter-carpal, distal ulna, and radio-carpal joints (Resnick & Niwayama 1977, Schmitt et al 2006). Avascular osteonecrosis, neurologic disorders, neoplastic disease, and specific congenital malformations are attributed causes as well (De Filippo et al 2006, Schmitt et al 2006).

ANATOMY AND BIOMECHANICS

Anatomy

This review is pertinent to wrist instability. The reader is encouraged to utilize other resources to revisit the basic anatomy of the distal forearm, wrist, and hand if needed.

Osseous anatomy

The osseous anatomy is important in considering carpal and wrist stability. Pathologies such as inflammatory arthritis, infection, and fracture can change the shape of the carpal bones sufficiently to alter bony balance and produce instability (Garcia-Elias 2006). Yet even after ligamentous injury, the bony anatomic features of the distal radius and proximal scaphoid have some ability to stabilize the carpus. Werner et al (2007) demonstrated this concept of bony geometry providing scapholunate stability in the presence of a torn scapholunate interosseous ligament.

Discussion begins with the distal radius and ulna. The radius widens distally to form a large articular surface for the scaphoid and lunate, creating the radio-carpal joint (Wadsworth 1988). The distal ends of the radius and ulna form between them the distal radio-ulnar joint. The distal ulna has an articular surface with the distal radius and another with the TFCC (Dobbs 2003). The articular surfaces of the DRUJ are incongruous and therefore vulnerable to translational dorsal and volar instability (Kleinman 2007).

The bones of the proximal carpal row are the scaphoid, lunate, triquetrum, and pisiform. These carpals move with greater degrees of rotation to each other than do the carpals of the distal row. The lunate, coronally wedge-shaped, has a tendency to dislocate into the dorsal direction from the scaphoid; additionally, it is the most frequently dislocated carpal (Wadsworth 1988, Schmitt et al 2006).

The distal carpal row consists of the trapezium, trapezoid, capitate and hamate. This is a more solid functional unit than the proximal row, with less inter-carpal movement. Distal and proximal carpal rows articulate through the mid-carpal joint. The mid-carpal joint is a combination of three joints: the scaphotrapezoid-trapezial (STT) with scaphocapitate components in the lateral compartment; the capitatolunate central compartment; and the hamato-triquetral medial compartment (Schmitt et al 2006). Carlsen & Shin (2008) described the anatomy of the mid-carpal joint somewhat differently in the scaphocapitate/lunocapitate central articulation and the triquetrohamate medial articulation. This mid-carpal joint, as a whole, is compared to a ball and socket joint with the capitate often intruding into the scapholunate gap (Schmitt et al 2006).

Ligamentous anatomy and stabilization

Ligaments of the wrist are classified as intra-articular or intra-capsular. Intra-capsular ligaments are integrated in the capsular sheaths and are either intrinsic or extrinsic to the carpus (Schmitt et al 2006). Schmitt et al (2006) wrote that the inter-osseous scapholunate ligament (SLL, SLIL), inter-osseous lunotriquetral ligament (LTL), and mid-carpal ligaments are intra-articular. Carlsen & Shin (2008), however, stated that all wrist ligaments are intra-capsular with the exception of the transverse carpal ligament, the pisohamate ligament, and the pisometacarpal ligament. They based this description on the intra-capsular ligaments being contained in 'loose connective tissue and fat' (Carlsen & Shin 2008) which was previously poorly visualized with open surgical inspection.

The SLL (Fig 27.1) is considered the most important and is most often injured. Each of the three SLL segments performs different biomechanical functions. It is centrally composed of fibrocartilage that merges with the articular cartilage of the scaphoid and the lunate (Linscheid & Dobyns 2002). The fibro-cartilage section, or middle segment, lacks stabilizing function and is prone to degenerative injury (Ozcelik et al 2005, Schmitt et al 2006). It is the dorsal segment that is vital to scapholunate compartment stability. Rotary subluxation of the scaphoid and symptomatic scapholunate dissociation develops with the rupture of this segment (Schmitt et al 2006).

The LTL (Fig 27.1) plays a role to the stability of the lunotriquetral compartment similar to that of the SLL to the scapholunate compartment. It is smaller but similarly shaped to the SLL, and the central or middle segment, also prone to degeneration, has no stabilizing function. It is the volar segment, however, rather than the dorsal segment that maintains functional stability of the lunotriquetral compartment (Schmitt et al 2006).

While the SLL and the LTL are intrinsic stabilizers of the proximal carpal row, three short extrinsic inter-osseous ligaments stabilize the scaphoid and lunate. The radioscapholunate ligament (RSLL) (Fig 27.1) is unique in that it is proposed to carry an anterior inter-osseous nerve and artery to the proximal pole of the scaphoid (Schmitt et al 2006). These inter-osseous ligaments are deep and transverse while a superficial and oblique complex is termed the *V-ligament* system (Schmitt et al 2006). This system includes the important volar support band or radioscaphocapitate ligament (RSCL) (Fig 27.1), which helps to stabilize the radio-carpal joint with an oblique orientation that prevents carpus translocation (Schmitt et al 2006). Disruption of the RSCL is a primary cause of scapholunate and capitolunate dissociation (Ozcelik et al 2005). The triquetrocapitatoscaphoid ligament (TCSL) (Fig 27.1) has a loose triquetrocapitate section that is called the *ulnar link* and a tight capitoscaphoid portion. This is an important stabilizer of the mid-carpal joint. The RSCL and TCSL with others that make up the volar V-shaped complex are stronger and more supportive than the dorsal complex (Schmitt et al 2006). In the proximal portion of the volar V-ligament, disruption of the radiolunotriquetral ligament will result in lunotriquetral dissociation (Ozcelik et al 2005).

Prevention of axial (columnar) instability is the task of the transverse inter-carpal ligaments and the flexor retinaculum (Schmitt et al 2006). These make up the support of the distal carpal row.

Stability of the DRUJ is minimally supported extrinsically by the inter-osseous mid-forearm ligament. The TFCC intrinsic radio-ulna dorsal and palmer ligaments provide effective ligamentous stability (Kleinman 2007).

Muscular anatomy

The most relevant contribution of the muscular anatomy to stability of the carpus concerns the finding that both wrist flexors and extensors generate their maximum forces with the wrist fully extended (Lieber & Friden 1998). Indeed, there is a 'nearly constant ratio of flexor to extensor torque over the wrist range of motion' (Lieber & Friden 1998). This is possible despite the flexors having a larger physiological cross-section area because of the superior extensor moment over the flexor moment. Thus the wrist is most stable in extension and its design is biased toward balance and control instead of maximum torque (Lieber & Friden 1998).

Kleinman (2007) additionally described the tension of the extensor carpi ulnaris tendon across the ulna distal head with the superficial and deep heads of the pronator quadratus as important to dynamic stability of the DRUJ.

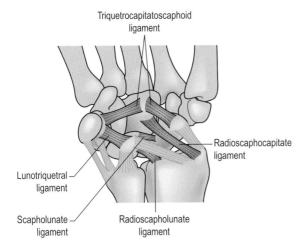

Triquetrocapitatoscaphoid ligament

Radioscaphocapite ligament

Lunotriquetral ligament

Scapholunate ligament

Radioscapholunate ligament

Fig 27.1 Critical volar stabilizing ligaments (right hand).

Biomechanics

An important consideration in understanding forces across the wrist is that there are no tendons attaching directly to the carpal bones, excluding the pisiform. The pisiform is a sesamoid bone within the tendon of the flexor carpi ulnaris, and this relationship is not considered to be significant in carpal stability (Bednar & Osterman 1993). The forces are summed across the carpus as the movement of the wrist begins distally with tendons inserted at the base of the metacarpals. The motion of the carpus is initiated at the distal row with forces proceeding from the distal to the proximal carpal row. The forces at the scaphoid-lunate-capitate compartment are 60%, with the remainder distributing at the radius-lunate joint and ulno-carpal compartment, according to Schmitt et al (2006). Thus movement of the proximal carpal row depends on the compressive forces of the distal row as well as the support of the ligamentous attachments (Bozentka 1999).

Flexion-extension and radial-ulnar deviation are the two planes of motion produced by the carpal joints. Flexion-extension total movement is an average of 121–150° (Bednar & Osterman 1993, De Filippo et al 2006). This motion is split between the radio-carpal and mid-carpal joints. Radial-ulnar deviation total movement is an average of 45–50° with distribution of 60% at the mid-carpal joint and 40% at the radio-carpal joint (Bednar & Osterman 1993, De Filippo et al 2006).

The scaphoid and lunate move dorsally and radially during wrist extension. Volar and ulnar movement of the scaphoid and lunate occur with wrist flexion. This scapholunate movement is three times greater than lunotriquetral movement. With the scaphoid having the widest arc of rotation, wrist flexion and extension produce a spatial change among the carpus elements. This intricate and specific mechanism must be intact to ensure carpal stability (De Filippo et al 2006).

The TFCC central articular disc reportedly bears the burden of load transmission from the medial carpus to the forearm when the wrist is ulnarly deviated (Kleinman 2007). With the forearm in neutral radio-ulnar deviation, the load passes from the mid-carpus to the distal radius interfossal ridge with 84% to the radius and 16% to the TFCC disc (Kleinman 2007). The reader is referred to the work of Kleinman (2007) for an extensive discussion of DRUJ biomechanics.

AETIO-PATHOGENESIS

An understanding of patterns and classification of instability in the wrist is necessary to discussion of aetio-pathogenesis. Each advance in the evolving project of instability classification is accompanied by further knowledge of common cause and effect on specific tissue or structure.

Patterns and classification

Recognized patterns and areas of carpal and wrist instability

There are three basic patterns of instability to consider, although each of these patterns has additional classification to be delineated next in this section. The patterns are based on radiologic appearance. *Pre-dynamic instability* refers to a clinical diagnosis without support of abnormalities seen on a radiograph. *Dynamic instability* has a clinical diagnosis plus altered kinematics viewed on special but not standard radiographs. It occurs when the carpals are loaded under certain conditions, but inconsistently. *Static instability* is supported by clinical diagnosis and altered kinematics appearing on conventional radiographs. The malalignment is evident with any amount of load applied (Garcia-Elias 1997b, Van Rooyen 2005).

Classification of carpal and wrist instability

Linscheid et al (1972) are credited with the first classification for carpal instability. Their work identified two general types, dorsal and volar (Linscheid et al 1972). *Dorsal intercalary segment instability* (DISI) is the more common of the two. De Filippo et al (2006) attributed DISI to scaphotrapezoidal ligament injury, a non-union or badly healed trans-scaphoid fracture, or by scapholunate ligament injury. DISI is detected with a lateral view plain film in which a dorsal tilt of the lunate is seen, along with aberrant capitolunate and scapholunate angles (De Filippo et al 2006). With the same plain film view, a *volar intercalary segment* (VISI) malalignment is evident with a volar tilt to the lunate (Garcia-Elias 1997a). VISI is described as caused by dissociation of the lunotriquetral, radiotriquetral, or scaphotriquetral joints as well as by badly healed and/or displaced fractures of these carpals (De Filippo et al 2006).

The Mayo Clinic system is currently the most widely known and used classification (Carlsen & Shin 2008). This system groups instabilities according to pattern: *carpal instability dissociative* (CID), *carpal instability non-dissociative* (CIND), *carpal instability combined* (CIC), and *adaptive carpal instability* (CIA).

Instability between individual carpals in the same row and involving the intrinsic ligaments is CID. An example of this is scapholunate dissociation. Progressive scapholunate dissociation (CID) becomes DISI before ending in severe degenerative arthritis, described as scapholunate advanced collapse (SLAC) (Bozentka 1999).

Instability that causes aberration of the entire proximal row at radio-carpal and mid-carpal joints and involves the extrinsic ligaments is CIND (Garcia-Elias 1997b, Van Rooyen 2005). Perilunate instability results in CIND due to the complex pathology at radio-carpal and inter-carpal levels.

Instability with combined involvement of intrinsic and extrinsic ligaments, intra-row and inter-row, is CIC. De Filippo et al (2006) listed lunate dislocation as a typical example of CIC. CIA is best described as instability of the carpals caused by pathology either distal or proximal to the carpals, not within the wrist. An example of this is pathology at the distal radius from either mal-united fracture or Madelung's deformity (Van Rooyen 2005, Schmitt et al 2006, Carlsen & Shin 2008).

Discussion of distal radio-ulnar joint (DRUJ) instability functionally includes the triangular fibro-cartilage complex (TFCC). TFCC tears are classified by the Mayo Clinic system as traumatic tears and degenerative tears. Traumatic tears are: (I) radial rim detachment; (II) central tears; (III) ulnar tears; and (IV) palmar tears. Degenerative tears are: (I) central tears; (II) central tear with ulno-carpal impingement; (III) central tear, impingement, and lunotriquetral ligament tear; and (IV) central tear, impingement, and lunotriquetral arthritis (Van Rooyen 2005). TFCC pathology can result from degenerative changes without causing DRUJ instability, however (Van Rooyen 2005).

Additional reading is recommended for evolving classifications as knowledge of carpal biomechanics expands, to include the views of Lichtman (Van Rooyen 2005, Lichtman & Wroten 2006), and Amadio (De Filippo et al 2006). Carlsen & Shin (2008) describe the Mayo system in greater detail, including subdivisions.

Pathogenesis

Destruction of the wrist ligaments, through trauma or degeneration, and alteration of the bony articular surfaces are responsible for wrist instability. Two frequent types of instability due to malunited distal radius fractures are noted, mid-carpal and radio-carpal. Adaptive mid-carpal malalignments occur with the body's attempt to realign the hand to the malunion. Carpal ligaments and radio-carpal capsule are not disrupted. Pathologic radio-carpal malalignments occur from injury to the radio-carpal ligaments and joint capsule during the fracture incident and result in instability of the radio-lunate joint (Gupta et al 2002).

Pathological abnormalities of intra-articular ligaments in rheumatoid arthritis occur due to pannus invasion and destruction, while these abnormalities in calcium pyrophosphate deposition disease occur due to calcific deposition and cystic degeneration (Resnick & Niwayama 1977).

An additional cause of wrist instability at the scapholunate interval was reported by Mehdian & McKee (2005) as excision of a dorsal wrist ganglion. One reason postulated was that manipulation under anaesthesia of the wrist to recover from the ganglion-induced stiffness evoked the instability (Mehdian & McKee 2005).

EXAMINATION AND DIAGNOSIS

Diagnostic considerations

Cooney et al (1990) described an algorithm for diagnosis that included clinical examination, report of the patient's symptoms, and use of provocative stress testing that would together determine, in absence of pathological standard radiographic examination results, an appropriate portal of entry for additional tests, e.g. arthrogram or arthroscopy. The reader is referred to Part 1 of this text for the basic initial examination and history taking.

Clinical tests

General mid-carpal tests

The mid-carpal shift test was described by Feinstein et al (1999) as a valid and useful clinical diagnostic test for indicating mid-carpal non-dissociative carpal instability. The examiner stabilizes the patient's forearm in pronation with one hand. With the other hand, the examiner places a thumb over the patient's dorsal distal capitate. The thumb directs a palmar force via the capitate, allowing translation to occur. Maintaining this pressure, the examiner provides passive ulnar deviation to the patient's wrist. A positive test consists of a degree of clunking and/or laxity during the ulnar deviation. Dysfunction of stabilizing ligaments is thought to cause a loss of normal joint reaction forces between the proximal and distal carpal rows, resulting in loss of smooth translation (Feinstein et al 1999). The test was reviewed under video-fluoroscopy, showing that the proximal carpal row maintained a flexed volar position rather than moving smoothly from flexion to extension as the wrist was moved into ulnar deviation. Instead, the proximal row suddenly snapped into extension once the ulnar deviation was achieved, hence the 'clunk' (Lichtman & Wroten 2006).

Scapholunate, second and third carpometacarpal joints, and capitolunate tests

The scaphoid stress test (scaphoid shift test, Watson's test, SST, modified scaphoid shear test) is the most common used clinical test for detection of scapholunate instability (Christodoulou & Bainbridge 1999). Rodner & Weiss (2008) noted that the test may not be performed as well initially due to swelling and pain. The examiner places a thumb on the scaphoid tubercle, applying pressure volar to dorsal, and passively moves the patient's wrist from ulnar deviation and slight extension into radial deviation with slight flexion (Fig 27.2). The scaphoid will become prominent under the examiner's thumb with the movement to radial deviation. When the thumb pressure is

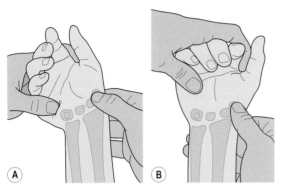

(A) (B)

Fig 27.2 Scaphoid stress test. (A) Examiner applies pressure to scaphoid with wrist in ulnar deviation and extension. (B) Examiner maintains pressure while performing radial deviation and flexion of the wrist, noting *clunk* or pain.

removed, a positive test will demonstrate the scaphoid returning to position with an often painful and palpable 'clunk'. The clunk is thought to occur when, due to laxity or pathology, the proximal pole of the scaphoid shifts onto the dorsal rim of the radius with thumb pressure; then it returns with a clunk when the pressure is removed (Skirven 1996). The test is also meaningful when it reproduces pain over the scapholunate interval (Rodner & Weiss 2008). According to LaStayo & Howell (1995), this test has sensitivity of 69%, specificity of 66%, a positive predictive value of 48% and a negative predictive value of 78% relative to arthroscopic findings in 50 painful wrists.

Watson described the wrist-flexion finger-extension manoeuvre as an additional test of scapholunate instability (Skirven 1996). Truong et al (1994) included this test in their screening criteria that in combination had a sensitivity of 88.5% and a specificity of 84%. The patient's wrist is positioned in flexion while the examiner applies resistance against finger extension, causing pain in the scapholunate region with a positive test (Truong et al 1994).

The synovial irritation sign of the scaphoid has high sensitivity but low specificity for detecting scaphoid instability. Van Buul et al (1993) found that a positive synovial irritation sign test had significantly higher incidence in patients with suspected carpal instability. A positive test consists of pain elicited by the examiner providing pressure on the scaphoid through the anatomical snuffbox (Van Buul et al 1993).

Still assessing the radial wrist, the Linscheid test produces pain in the second and third carpo-metacarpal joints when positive (Skirven 1996). The examiner supports the patient's metacarpal shafts while pressing into the distal metacarpal heads in both dorsal and volar directions (Skirven 1996).

The dorsal capitate-displacement test was found to clinically successfully reproduce dorsal subluxation of the capitolunate or the capitolunate and radiolunate

joints (Lichtman & Wroten 2006). A capitolunate instability pattern was described and tested in this way by Louis et al (1984) under video-fluoroscopy in a series of 11 patients (Lichtman & Wroten 2006). The examiner applied pressure to the scaphoid tuberosity in a dorsal direction while simultaneously performing longitudinal traction and passive flexion to the patient's wrist. This produced nearly complete dorsal subluxation of the capitate from the lunate and reproduced the patient's pain in that area (Louis et al 1984). Instability was credited to dynamic laxity of the radiolunate ligaments and extrinsic scaphoid stabilizers, along with laxity of the dorsal capitolunate ligament complex (Louis et al 1984).

Lunotriquetral tests

The lunotriquetral (LT) ballottement test (Reagan's test) indicates LT instability with production of pain and/or excessive motion as the examiner translates the pisiform and triquetrum (together) volarly and dorsally relative to the stabilized lunate (Rodner & Weiss 2008). The test is performed with the examiner using the thumb and index finger of one hand to hold the patient's lunate while holding the triquetrum in the contralateral hand and providing simultaneous movement of these bones against one another (Dobbs 2003) (Fig 27.3). A positive result is reproduction of pain, crepitus, or excessive laxity. Sensitivity of 64%, specificity of 44%, a positive predictive value of 24% and a negative predictive value of 81% were reported by LaStayo & Howell (1995) for the LT Ballottement test. Dobbs (2003) later described inconsistent sensitivity of 33–100% (Dobbs 2003). Kleinman's shear test described below does not stabilize the lunate but does apply similar dorsal translation to the pisiform and concurrent volar translation to the lunate for symptoms indicating LT instability.

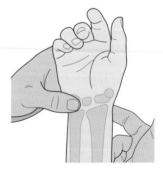

Fig 27.3 Lunotriquetral (LT) ballottement test. Examiner uses the thumb (not shown) and index finger of one hand to hold the patient's lunate while holding the triquetrum in the contralateral hand and providing simultaneous movement of these bones against one another, looking for pain, crepitus, or excessive laxity.

Kleinman's Shear Test is one of three clinical tests that have been reported as specific to lunotriquetral injury (Dobbs 2003). The examiner places several fingers dorsal to the patient's lunate with a thumb on the patient's piso-triquetral joint (Skirven 1996). Other authors have described the use of the examiner's thumb on the lunate with the contralateral thumb on the piso-triquetral joint (Dobbs 2003). While the lunate is stabilized, the thumb provides a volar to dorsal direction of force that creates a shear across the lunotriquetral joint. The examiner then deviates the wrist first in ulnar then radial directions. Pain or clicking demonstrates a positive test (Skirven 1996).

Dobbs (2003) described the ulnar snuffbox compression test (Linscheid's Test, lunotriquetral compression test) as poorly specific for lunotriquetral instability. The test is positive with pain reproduction as the examiner pushes the patient's triquetrum into the lunate from the ulnar wrist, specifically in the sulcus, or snuffbox, formed by the extensor carpi ulnaris and flexor carpi ulnaris tendons (Skirven 1996, Rodner & Weiss 2008).

Distal radio-ulnar joint and triangular fibrocartilage complex tests

The piano-key test is a variation of the piano-key sign, and is used to assess for distal radio-ulnar joint (DRUJ) instability. The examiner stabilizes the radius with one hand while the other hand grasps the patient's distal ulna and moves it in dorsal and volar directions with the forearm positioned in various degrees of pronation and supination. A positive test includes reproduction of pain, tenderness, and hyper-mobility compared to the uninvolved side (Skirven 1996).

As mentioned earlier, the triangular fibro-cartilage complex (TFCC) contributes to DRUJ stability, but it is not known if clinical tests for DRUJ instability accurately demonstrate instability caused from tears of the triangular ligament of the TFCC (Moriya et al 2009). The biomechanical study of Moriya et al (2009), while limited, supported the DRUJ ballottement test but not the piano-key test or the ulno-carpal abutment test as having a statistically significant degree of accuracy demonstrating this concept.

LaStayo & Howell (1995) examined the ulnomenisco-triquetral (UMT) dorsal glide test for pathology of the TFCC. The technique for this test has the patient's elbow resting on a table with forearm in neutral and vertical position. The patient's distal radius is stabilized by a golfer's grip of the examiner's hand. With the other hand, the examiner places his index finger (digit 2) curled such that the radial side of the proximal interphalangeal joint contacts the patient's volar piso-triquetral complex. With this finger providing dorsal pressure, the examiner simultaneously uses the thumb to apply volar pressure against the dorsal distal ulna, producing a dorsal glide of the piso-triquetral complex on the distal ulnar head. A positive test results in reproduction of the patient's pain and/or laxity in the UMT area (Hertling & Kessler 1996). LaStayo & Howell (1995) reported sensitivity of 66%, specificity of 64%, positive predictive value of 58%, and negative predictive value of 69% for this test.

Radiological tests, diagnostic dynamic ultrasound, and arthroscopy

Radiographic examination of the wrist ranges from standard static views to special dynamic positions and loading conditions as well as complex films such as video-fluoroscopy and arthrogram (Garcia-Elias 2006). While additional reading on this topic in Chapter 4 of this text is recommended, it can be summarized here to state that the ultimate radiographic goal is to display the gap between dissociated bones. Toms et al (2009), in a small but relevant study, indicated that dynamic ultrasound may confirm mid-carpal instability via a triquetral catch-up clunk.

Wrist arthroscopy is becoming the gold standard, although clinical tests are widely used to regionalize the pertinent area (Reynolds et al 1998, Garcia-Elias 2006). Arthroscopy versus open arthrotomy avoids suspension of the wrist under traction, enabling otherwise occult differences in ligament appearance to be revealed (Cooney et al 1990).

TREATMENT AND PROGNOSIS

Conservative treatment and prognosis

Additional research is needed to determine true efficacy of conservative treatment, including manual therapy of soft tissue and joint, for wrist instability. Most available information for manual therapy treatment of the wrist has focused on treatment of carpal tunnel syndrome with positive outcomes noted (Burke et al 2007, O'Conner et al 2003).

The literature supports carpal manipulation for wrist instability as a diagnostic rather than treatment tool. Manipulation is used to evoke signs and palpation is used to evoke symptoms during physical examination of the wrist (Dobbs 2003, Young et al 2007). Conservative treatment described in the literature has emphasized patient education, splinting, and exercises (Hofmeister et al 2006, Lichtman & Wroten 2006, Prosser et al 2007).

Hofmeister et al (2006) reported temporary pain relief at best with conservative treatments including immobilization, splinting, non-steroidal medications, and intra-articular injections. Most splinting consists of general immobilization after acute injury such as sprain or dislocation. Splints are often custom made for best fit, and are dorsal or volar, thumb free or protected, depending on location of injured structure (Coppard & Lohman 2001).

Weiss et al (2000) recommended taping, splinting, and anti-inflammatory medications for the athlete with a

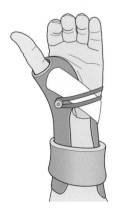

Fig 27.4 DISI Custom Splint.

partial or complete membranous central tear of the luno-triquetral ligament (no VISI). The splint should be carefully moulded with a pad under the pisiform to attempt optimal alignment (Shin et al 2000). Patients with this type of injury and protocol are estimated to require 3 to 6 months for recovery (Weiss et al 2000).

Lichtman & Wroten (2006) supported a trial of conservative treatment as useful in only one of four instability types, that of dorsal mid-carpal instability. Garcia-Elias (1997a) concurred, with the additional specification of a dorsal mid-carpal type termed the 'capitate lunate instability pattern' (CLIP), usually due to congenital laxity. A custom dorsal splint with a dynamic component, termed *DISI splint* or *Lichtman splint* (Fig 27.4) is the only orthotic specifically supported for this application (S Kamal, personal communication, 2009).

Specific statistics for prognosis following conservative treatment are unavailable. The literature does agree, however, that prognosis has an increased chance of being favourable (not requiring surgery for restoration of function) if the injury is conservatively treated acutely (Israeli et al 1981, Bednar & Osterman 1993, Garcia-Elias 1997a, Shin et al 2000, Lichtman & Wroten 2006). Conservative treatment is not recommended for chronic wrist instability.

Surgical treatment and prognosis

Surgical interventions are performed when pain is intractable and affects quality of life. Carlsen & Shin (2008) listed primary considerations that determine course of treatment as: arthritic changes, injury onset (chronicity), probability of the tissues, based on quality, to withstand surgical repair; and the ability of the surgeon to reduce the deformity. An ideal candidate for surgical repair would have an acute injury with reducible deformity and tissues of good quality (Carlsen & Shin 2008).

Decisions for choices of surgical procedure, such as Kirshner wire (K-wire), bone-ligament-bone graft, partial carpal fusion or arthrodesis, mid-carpal or four corner fusion, and proximal row carpectomy are based on the previously listed considerations as well as degree and location of injury (Garcia-Elias 2006). Other surgical options are arthroscopic or open debridement including ligament and synovectomy, capsulodesis, and ligament repair or reconstruction; also anterior and posterior interosseous neurectomy (Hofmeister et al 2006, Johnston et al 2009). Prognosis is as widely varied as are the factors of cause, specific pathology, technique and skill of the surgeon.

CONCLUSION

Wrist instability is only now becoming accurately and successfully identified, classified, and treated, due to recent improvements in technology and a development of knowledge base in the last 25 years. Arthroscopy has allowed a relatively undisturbed view of anatomy, biomechanics and pathology of the wrist that has been incorporated into the body of classifications, clinical tests, formal diagnoses, and treatments.

The literature supports manual interventions by the clinician for clinical tests and not for conservative treatment. Conservative treatment consisting primarily of patient education, splinting, and exercises is most efficacious when applied acutely.

Additional research is necessary to improve the reliability and validity of clinical tests as the aforementioned knowledge base of wrist anatomy and biomechanics improves. Specificity of splint application to pathologic and functional need will likely improve conservative treatment outcomes, but this must be diligently pursued and recorded in the evolution of evidence-based treatment.

REFERENCES

Bednar, J.M., Ostermann, A.L., 1993. Carpal instability: Evaluation and treatment. J. Am. Acad. Orthop. Surg. 1, 10–17.

Bozentka, D.J., 1999. Scapholunate instability. The University of Pennsylvania Orthopaedic Journal 12, 27–32.

Burke, J., Buchberger, D.J., Carey-Loghmani, M.T., et al., 2007. A pilot study comparing two manual therapy interventions for carpal tunnel syndrome. J. Manipulative Physiol. Ther. 30, 50–61.

Carlsen, B.T., Shin, A.Y., 2008. Wrist instability. Scand. J. Surg. 97, 324–332.

Christodoulou, L., Bainbridge, L.C., 1999. Clinical diagnosis of triquetrolunate ligament injuries. J. Hand Surg. [Br.] 24B, 598–600.

Cooney, W.P., Dobyns, J.H., Linscheid, R.L., 1990. Arthroscopy of the wrist: Anatomy and classification of carpal instability. Arthroscopy 6, 133–140.

Coppard, B.M., Lohman, H., 2001. Introduction to Splinting. A Clinical-Reasoning and Problem-Solving Approach. second ed. Mosby, St. Louis, pp. 139–241.

De Filippo, M., Sudberry, J.J., Lombardo, E., et al., 2006. Pathogenesis and evolution of carpal instability: imaging and topography. Acta Biomed. 77, 168–180.

Dias, J.J., Garcia-Elias, M., 2006. Hand injury costs. Injury 37, 1071–1077.

Dobbs, A., 2003. The ulnar side of the wrist. The North American Institute of Orthopaedic Manual Therapy 8, 1–5.

Dumontier, C., 1996. Physical examination of wrist instabilities. Maitrise Orthopedique 49, Online Orthopedic Journal. Available at: http://www.maitrise-orthop.com/viewPage_us.do?id=153 (accessed 10.06.09.).

Feinstein, W.K., Lichtman, D.M., Noble, P.C., et al., 1999. Quantitative assessment of the midcarpal shift test. J. Hand. Surg. [Am.] 24, 977–983.

Garcia-Elias, M., 1997a. The treatment of wrist instability. J. Bone Joint Surg. 79-B (4), 684–690.

Garcia-Elias, M., 1997b. Kinetic analysis of carpal stability during grip. Hand Clin. 13, 151–158.

Garcia-Elias, M., 2006. Treatment of scapholunate instability. Ortop. Traumatol. Rehabil. 2, 160–168.

Gupta, A., Batra, S., Jain, P., et al., 2002. Carpal alignment in distal radius fractures. BMC Musculoskelet. Disord. 3, 14.

Hertling, D., Kessler, R.M., 1996. Management of Common Musculoskeletal Disorders: Physical Therapy Principals and Methods. third ed. Lippincott-Raven Publishers, Philadelphia, p. 278.

Hofmeister, E.P., Moran, S.L., Shin, A.Y., 2006. Anterior and posterior interosseous neurectomy for the treatment of chronic dynamic instability of the wrist. Hand 1, 63–70.

Israeli, A., Ganel, A., Engel, J., 1981. Post traumatic ligamentous instability of the wrist. Br. J. Sports Med. 15, 17–19.

Johnston, K., Durand, D., Hildebrand, K.A., et al., 2009. Chronic volar distal radioulnar joint instability: joint capsular placation to restore function. Can. J. Surg. 52, 112–118.

Kleinman, W.B., 2007. Stability of the distal radioulnar joint: biomechanics, pathophysiology, physical diagnosis, and restoration of function what we have learned in 25 years. J. Hand Surg. 32A, 1086–1106.

LaStayo, P., Howell, J., 1995. Clinical provocative tests used in evaluating wrist pain: a descriptive study. J. Hand Ther. 8, 10–17.

Lichtman, D.M., Wroten, E.S., 2006. Understanding midcarpal instability. J. Hand Surg. 31A, 491–498.

Lieber, R.L., Friden, J., 1998. Musculoskeletal balance of the human wrist elucidated using intraoperative laser diffraction. J. Electromyogr. Kinesiol. 8, 93–100.

Linscheid, R.L., Dobyns, J.H., Beabout, J.W., et al., 1972. Traumatic instability of the wrist: Diagnosis, classification and pathomechanics. J. Bone Joint Surg. Am. 54, 1612–1632.

Linscheid, R.L., Dobyns, J.H., 2002. Dynamic carpal stability. Keio J. Med. 51, 140–147.

Louis, D.S., Hankin, F.M., Greene, T.L., et al., 1984. Central carpal instability – capitate lunate instability pattern: diagnosis by dynamic displacement. Orthopedics 7, 1693–1696.

Mehdian, H., McKee, D., 2005. Scapholunate instability following dorsal wrist ganglion excision: A case report. Iowa Orthop. J. 25, 203–206.

Moriya, T., Aoki, M., Iba, K., et al., 2009. Effect of triangular ligament tears on distal radioulnar joint instability and evaluation of three clinical tests: a biomechanical study. The Journal of Hand Surgery. European 34E, 219–223.

O'Conner, D., Marshall, S.C., Massey-Westropp, N., 2003. Non-surgical treatment (other than steroid injection) for carpal tunnel syndrome. Cochrane Database of Syst. Rev. (1), Art. No. CD0033219. DOI: 10.1002/14651858.CD003219.

Ozcelik, A., Gunal, I., Kose, N., et al., 2005. Wrist ligaments: their significance in carpal instability. TJTES 11, 115–120.

Perron, A.D., Brady, W.J., Keats, T.E., et al., 2001. Orthopedic pitfalls in the ED: Lunate and perilunate injuries. Am. J. Emerg. Med. 19, 157–162.

Prosser, R., Herbert, R., LaStayo, P.C., 2007. Current practice in the diagnosis and treatment of carpal instability – results of a survey of Australian hand therapists. J. Hand Ther. 20, 239–242.

Resnick, D., Niwayama, G., 1977. Carpal instability in rheumatoid arthritis and calcium pyrophosphate deposition disease. Pathogenesis and roentgen appearance. Ann. Rheum. Dis. 36, 311–318.

Reynolds, R.A.K., Johnston, G.H.F., Friedman, L., et al., 1998. The carpal stretch test. Can. J. Surg. 41, 119–126.

Rodner, C.M., Weiss, A.P.C., 2008. Acute scapholunate and lunotriquetral dissociation. (PDF) Fractures of the Upper Extremity: A Master Skills Publication. American Society for Surgery of the Hand, Chapter 10, pp. 155–171.

Schmitt, R., Froehner, S., Coblenz, G., et al., 2006. Carpal instability. Eur. Radiol. 16, 2161–2178.

Shin, A.Y., Battaglia, M.J., Bishop, A.T., 2000. Lunotriquetral instability: Diagnosis and treatment. J. Am. Acad. Orthop. Surg. 8, 170–179.

Skirven, T., 1996. Clinical examination of the wrist. J. Hand Ther. 9, 96–107.

Surdziel, P., Lubiatowski, P., 2006. Scapholunate instability: Natural history, diagnostics and therapeutic algorithm. Ortop. Traumatol. Rehabil. 8, 115–121.

Tang, J.B., 1992. Carpal instability associated with fracture of the distal radius. Incidence, influencing factors and pathomechanics. Chin. Med. J. 105, 758–765.

Toms, A., Chojnowski, A., Cahir, J., 2009. Midcarpal instability: A diagnostic role for dynamic ultrasound? Ultraschall Med. 30, 286–290.

Truong, N.P., Mann, F.A., Gilula, L.A., et al., 1994. Wrist instability series: increased yield with clinical-radiologic screening criteria. Radiology 192, 481–484.

van Buul, M.M., Bos, K.E., Dijkstra, P.F., et al., 1993. Carpal instability, the missed diagnosis in patients with clinically suspected scaphoid fracture. Injury 24, 257–262.

Van Rooyen, C., 2005. Radiologic evaluation of the hand and wrist. In: McKinnis, L.N. (Ed.), Fundamentals of Musculoskeletal Imaging, second ed. FA Davis, Philadelphia, pp. 509–521.

Wadsworth, C., 1988. Manual Examination and Treatment of the Spine and Extremities. Williams and Wilkins, Philadelphia, p. 154.

Weiss, L.E., Taras, J.S., Sweet, S., et al., 2000. Lunotriquetral injuries in the athlete. Hand Clin. 16, 433–438.

Werner, F.W., Short, W.H., Green, J.K., et al., 2007. Severity of scapholunate instability is related to joint anatomy and congruency. J. Hand Surg. [Am.] 32, 55–60.

Wolfe, S.W., Crisco, J.J., Orr, C.M., et al., 2006. Clinical perspective: The dart-throwing motion of the wrist: Is it unique to humans? J. Hand Surg. 31A, 1429–1437.

Young, D., Papp, S., Giachino, A., 2007. Physical examination of the wrist. Orthop. Clin. North Am. Apr 38, 149–165.

Chapter | 28 |

Carpal tunnel syndrome

Luca Padua, Costanza Pazzaglia, Ana Isabel-de-la-Llave-Rincón

INTRODUCTION

Carpal tunnel syndrome (CTS) is characterized by a compression of the median nerve in the carpal tunnel. It is a common pathology affecting an estimated 10% of the population according to the American Academy of Neurology (AAN 1993a,b, Olney 2001). It is considered the most common nerve compression disorder of the arm, with reported prevalence rates of 3.8% (95% CI, 3.1–4.6%) for women and 2.7% (95% CI, 2.1–3.4%) for men (Atroshi et al 1999). Bland et al (2003) found an annual incidence of 139.4 cases per 100,000 females and 67.2 cases per 100,000 males, with a female:male ratio of 2.1. Bongers et al (2007) have recently reported an incidence rate of CTS of 1.8/1000 (95% CI, 1.7–2.0). In females the incidence was 2.8 (95% CI, 2.6–3.1) and in males 0.9 (95% CI, 0.8–1.0) showing a female:male ratio of 3:1 (Bongers et al 2007). Further, this study showed that in 2001 the incidence of CTS was calculated to be 1.5 times higher than in 1987 (this difference disappeared after subdividing patients by age and sex) (Bongers et al 2007). It has been estimated that in the USA around one million people require care for CTS, around 200,000 surgical interventions are needed and that the social costs are in the millions of dollars range (Tanaka et al 1995).

Analysis of the literature raises the difficulty of accurately estimating the incidence and prevalence of CTS due to the fact that it is a very common pathology and, as we discuss below, can be associated with manual work. This last controversial association means that incidence and prevalence of CTS are often calculated in a specific work-population. Moreover, another confounding factor could be the method used to diagnose CTS, as Atroshi et al (1999) reported. In Atroshi et al's (1999) study, the combination of clinical and neurophysiological evaluations contributed to diagnosing CTS in 1 in 5 symptomatic subjects in the general population.

ANATOMY

In the carpal tunnel the median nerve is surrounded by bones on three sides with the transverse carpal ligament on the top. The nerve lies within the nine flexor tendons of the hand, and supplies function, feeling and movement to first digit of the hand and one-half of the ring finger (Fig 28.1).

© 2011 Elsevier Ltd.
DOI: 10.1016/B978-0-7020-3528-9.00028-5

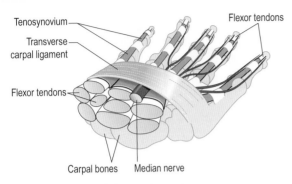

Fig 28.1 Anatomy of the carpal tunnel.

The median branches for finger and wrist flexors originate in the forearm, while motor branches, that control the thumb flexor and adductor muscles, and sensory branches, that provide over half the hand with the sense of touch, usually originate at the end of the tunnel.

Compression of the nerve can be due to a decrease in the size of the canal, an increase of the size of tendons, or both. For further information, readers are referred to Heidelberg (1989).

PATHO-BIOMECHANISM OF CARPAL TUNNEL SYNDROME

In most case CTS is idiopathic (Sternbach 1999) but sometimes it is associated with trauma, pregnancy, hypothyroidism, multiple myeloma, amyloidosis, rheumatoid arthritis, or acromegaly (Stevens et al 1992). As discussed above, in this pathology the changes occurring in the carpal tunnel are responsible for the median compression. For example:

- Rheumatoid arthritis causes inflammation of the flexor tendons determining median nerve compression.
- Pregnancy and hypothyroidism cause fluid retention in tissues, which swells the tenosynovium (we discuss the role of pregnancy in more detail later in this chapter).
- Acromegaly causes the compression of the nerve because of the abnormal growth of bones around the hand and wrist.
- Tumours (usually benign), such as a ganglion or a lipoma, can protrude into the carpal tunnel, reducing the amount of space. This is exceedingly rare (< 1%). Carpal tunnel tumours can mimic CTS (Padua et al 2006) and in these cases the use of ultrasound evaluation has been crucial. This topic will be discussed below (Granata et al 2008).
- Obesity also increases the risk of CTS; a BMI > 29 (obese individuals) increases the risk by 2.5 compared

to a BMI < 20 (slender individuals) (Werner et al 1994).

- Double crush syndrome is a speculative and debated theory which postulates that when there is compression or irritation of nerve branches contributing to the median nerve in the neck or anywhere above the wrist, this increases the liability of the nerve to compression in the wrist. Pierre-Jerome & Bekkelund (2005) reported that patients with CTS experienced a higher incidence of narrowing of the cervical foramen when compared to controls. These authors hypothesized that the compromised neural foramen could potentially lead to nerve compression and possibly a double crush syndrome in patients with CTS. However, there is little evidence that this syndrome really exists in CTS (Wilbourn & Gilliatt 1997, Russell 2008).
- There is a great number of traumas can cause CTS (Colles' fracture, dislocation of one of the carpal bones of the wrist, haematoma forming inside the wrist, etc.).
- The role of manual activities and CTS is still a matter of debate. A number of authors found that there is strong relation between hand positions and increased pressure on the carpal tunnel (Keir et al 1998, Luchetti et al 1998) and strongly supports the hypothesis that forceful use of the hands, repetitive use of the hands, and hand-arm vibration may cause or contribute to CTS. But other studies do not support the relationship between manual activity and CTS (Chiang et al 1993, Moore & Garg 1994). Despite researchers' efforts, the debate is still far from concluded.

Readers are referred to other texts for a greater understanding of these mechanisms (Werner 2006, Van Rijn et al 2009).

SENSITIZATION MECHANISMS IN CARPAL TUNNEL SYNDROME

Although the aetiology of CTS is not completely understood, there is some evidence involving the whole nociceptive system. Previous studies have investigated the function of nociceptive thermo-receptive fibres in CTS patients. Different studies found elevated thermal pain thresholds in the fingers and the palm within the affected hand in patients (Arendt-Nielsen et al 1991, Westerman & Delaney 1991, Goadsby & Burke 1994). Lang et al (1995) suggested that pain intensity in CTS depends on alterations of peripheral and central nervous function.

More recent studies reported that 45% of CTS patients also reported spreading proximal symptoms, which might be related to central nervous system mechanisms (Zannete et al 2006, 2007). Chow et al (2005) found that neck pain was present in 14% of patients with CTS. Tucker et al

(2007) found bilateral generalized increase in vibration thresholds in patients with CTS which suggests a generalized disturbance of somato-sensory functions rather than the existence of an isolated peripheral neuropathy. In fact, two image studies have shown cortical remapping in the primary somato-sensory cortex (S1) in patients with CTS supporting a possible role of central mechanisms in CTS (Tecchio et al 2002, Napadow et al 2006).

Additionally, recent clinical studies also support the presence of peripheral and central sensitization mechanisms in patients with moderate CTS. Fernández-de-las-Peñas et al (2009a) found bilateral widespread decrease in pressure pain thresholds in patients with unilateral CTS (clinically and neurophysiological) when compared to healthy controls. This study reported bilateral lower pressure pain thresholds (PPT) over the median, radial and ulnar nerve, the carpal tunnel, the C5–C6 zygapophyseal joint and the tibialis anterior muscle. A significant decrease in PPT over C5–C6 zygapophyseal joint may represent the existence of segmental sensitization of the nociceptive system in CTS, whereas a bilateral decrease in PPT over the tibialis anterior muscle indicate multi-segmental sensory sensitization or sensitization of the central nervous system in patients with CTS (Fernández-de-las-Peñas et al 2009a). De-la-Llave Rincón et al (2009) reported that patients with unilateral CTS also show a bilaterally thermal hyperalgesia (lower heat pain thresholds and reduced cold pain threshold), but not hypoaesthesia (normal thermal detection threshold) as compared to healthy subjects. Again, bilateral changes in patients with unilateral diagnosis (clinical and neurophysiological) of CTS reflect central sensitization mechanisms. These clinical findings are supported by animal studies where peripheral neural pathology in one local area can cause widespread effects, including effects in apparently uninvolved limbs (Koltzenburg et al 1999, Kleinschnitz et al 2005).

A recent study investigating impairments in fine motor control and ability skills also showed bilateral deficits in fine motor control ability and pinch grip force in unilateral CTS (Fernández-de-las-Peñas et al 2009b). The authors of this study hypothesized that bilateral motor control impairment and pinch grip force deficit can reflect a reorganization of the motor control strategy of the central nervous system as a consequence of the pain in CTS, which was supported by Tamburin et al (2008).

Finally, these studies also showed that bilateral sensory and motor deficits were associated to the intensity and duration of pain symptoms, supporting a role of the peripheral drive to initiate and maintain central widespread sensitization (De-la-Llave-Rincón et al 2009, Fernández-de-las-Peñas et al 2009a,b). Gracely et al (1992) proposed a model of neuropathic pain in which ongoing nociceptive afferent input from a peripheral nociceptive focus dynamically maintains altered central processing. In such instances, it can be suggested the painful condition, that is the ischaemia of the *nervi nervorum* (Watkins & Maier 2004) (the nerves innervating the

connective tissue layers of the nerve itself) sensitized by the compression of the median nerve in the carpal tunnel (Hall & Elvey 1999), may as such act as a trigger for gradual sensitization of nociceptive pathways in CTS patients. New studies should investigate the role of these sensitization mechanisms in the evolution of CTS.

DIAGNOSIS OF CARPAL TUNNEL SYNDROME

Clinical examination

The gold standard for the diagnosis of CTS is considered the clinical picture, according to the AAN (1993a,b) diagnostic criteria: paraesthesia, pain, swelling, weakness or clumsiness of the hand provoked or worsened by sleep, sustained hand or arm position, repetitive action of the hand or wrist that is mitigated by changing posture or by shaking of the hand, sensory deficits in the median innervated region of the hand and motor deficit or hypotrophy of the median innervated thenar muscles. Wainner et al (2005) developed a clinical prediction rule for the diagnosis of CTS. The rule identified consisted of 1 question (shaking hands for symptom relief), wrist-ratio index > 0.67, symptom severity scale score > 1.9, reduced median sensory field of digit 1, and age > 45 years (LR = 18.3).

Recent studies have evidenced the relationship between the distribution of sensory symptoms and the severity of CTS, according to the neurophysiological classification. Patients with lower severity of pathology complain of sensory symptoms with a glove distribution, while patients with higher severity of pathology complain of sensory symptoms with the 'classical' median distribution (Caliandro et al 2006).

The patient history is extremely important for the differential diagnosis, especially as CTS can be secondary to endocrine and metabolic pathologies; therapy for the primary pathology can remit the CTS. For clinical examination, in addition it is possible to use a historic and objective scale (Hi-Ob) of CTS that includes two measures (Giannini et al 2002). The first has clinical history and objective sub-scores: (1) nocturnal paraesthesia only; (2) nocturnal and diurnal paraesthesia; (3) sensory deficit; (4) hypotrophy or motor deficit of the median innervated thenar muscles; (5) plegia of median thenar eminence muscles. The second evaluates, by patient-oriented measurement, the presence or absence of pain with a forced-choice answer ('yes' or 'no'). Therefore, the Hi-Ob score is composed of a number (Hi-Ob) with or without the pain variable (Giannini et al 2002).

The physical examination includes the Phalen test (Fig 28.2), performed by a prolonged (1-minute) passive forced flexion of the wrist; the Tinel test that consists

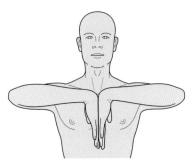

Fig 28.2 The Phalen test.

of a percussion of the median nerve trophism of the thenar eminence; motor function of the median innervated muscles; and sensory function (cotton wool is used as a standard material for skin stimulation).

Questionnaires

As doctors want to help patients, the assessment of patients' perspective is also useful in the comprehensive evaluation of CTS. The most common used questionnaire is the Boston Carpal Tunnel Questionnaire (BCTQ) (Levine et al 1993). The BCTQ evaluates two domains of CTS: 'symptoms' (SYMPT = patient-oriented symptom) assessed on an 11-step scale; and 'functional status' (FUNCT = patient-oriented function) assessed on a 8-step scale. Each item includes five possible responses, and the score for each section (SYMPT or FUNCT) is calculated as the mean of the responses to the individual items. The use of this questionnaire in several multi-centric studies on CTS showed interesting results; while function has a linear significant correlation when assessed both by physicians and patients, symptoms do not have a clear linear correlation (Padua et al 2002). Patients with mild-to-moderate CTS seemed to function well, although severe symptoms may be reported by the patient. However, when nerve impairment becomes severe, the patient's hand function is extremely impaired although symptoms may be milder. The data show that the patient's point of view is reliable (Padua et al 2002).

Electrodiagnostic evaluation

Electrodiagnostic evaluation is very important to define the impairment of the median nerve. It is now accepted that, in order to increase the sensitivity of conventional nerve conduction studies (sensory digit-wrist and motor wrist-thenar), segmentary and/or comparative tests should be used (see below) as stated in AAN and AAEM recommendations (AAN 1993a,b). When the standard tests yield normal results ('standard negative' hands), the following studies increase the electrodiagnostic sensitivity:

1. Segmental motor or sensory conduction tests in palm-wrist segment.
2. Comparative studies (median-ulnar or median radial)
3. Segmental/comparative studies (as disto-proximal ratio)

A study conducted on CTS patients showed that the sensitivity of standard tests can reach 83.5%, comparative/segmental tests can disclose abnormal findings in a further 11.4% of cases, providing CTS electro-diagnosis in about 7 of 10 'standard negative' cases. The overall sensitivity of protocol thus reaches 94.9% (Padua et al 1999). The severity of neurophysiologic CTS impairment can be assessed and scored according to a published neurophysiologic classification (Padua et al 1997a,b).

ULTRASOUND ASSESSMENT

Thanks to the advances in technology (refinement of high-frequency broadband linear-array transducers, and sensitive colour and power Doppler technology), the low cost, the wide availability, and the ease of use, ultrasound (US) has recently been applied to the study of tendons and nerves.

In tendon and nerve imaging, US can assess a great number of pathologies such as dislocations, degenerative changes, extrinsic or intrinsic focal compression. Moreover US can support clinical and electrophysiological testing and in most cases, a focused US examination can be performed more rapidly and efficiently than MR imaging (Martinoli et al 2002).

From a technical point of view, although tendons and nerves share similar characteristics (dimensions, tubular conformation, and striated appearance) US can easily differentiate them. Tendons have a fibrillar pattern of parallel hyperechoic lines in the longitudinal plane because of collagen bundles and endotendineum septa with a hyperechoic round to ovoid image containing bright dots (Fornage & Rifkin 1988, Martinoli et al 1993); nerves have a fascicular pattern due to hypoechoic parallel linear, the neuronal fascicles, separated by hyperechoic bands (the interfascicular epineurium) (Graif et al 1991, Silvestri et al 1995). On transverse scans, nerves assume a honeycomb-like appearance with hypoechoic dots surrounded by a hyperechoic background (Fig 28.3).

Ultrasound has been mainly tested in the evaluation of CTS because of the complementary perspective it provides (Beekman & Visser 2003, Hobson-Webb & Padua 2009, Karadağ et al 2010, Smith et al 2009). CTS can be assessed by using the following measures: cross-sectional area (CSA), swelling ratio, retinacular bowing, retinacular thickness, flattening ratio. Several studies have shown that the most useful diagnostic criterion is the CSA, which is the area of median nerve calculated at the wrist, both by using the ellipse formula or by manual tracing; the best cut off value is CSA of ≥ 9.875 mm^2 at the pisiform level (Wang et al 2008).

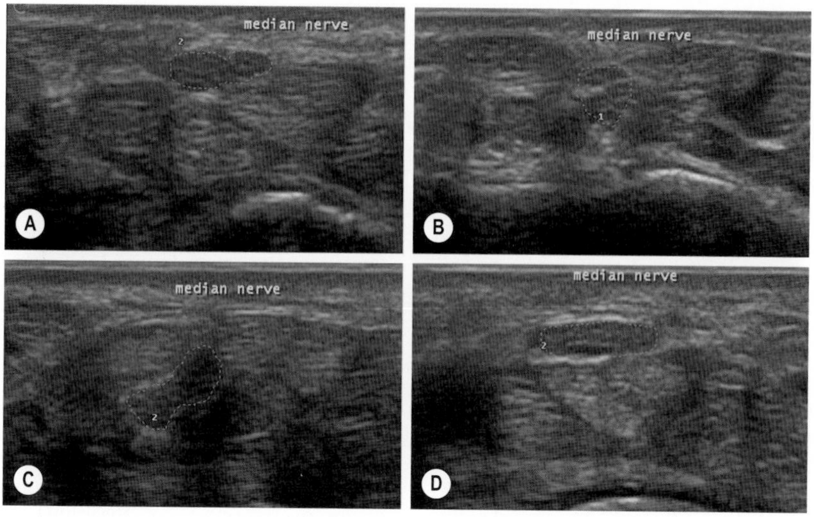

Fig 28.3 The median nerve at the wrist (in the carpal tunnel): note the change in shape and position among the nerve and the tendons in relation to the different wrist angle A= neutral position, B= 45° wrist flexion, C= 90° wrist flexion and D= maximal wrist extension.

Moreover, more sensitive tests have been developed in order to obtain the best sensitivity and specificity. For example, the wrist-to-forearm ratio (WFR) of median nerve area can be considered more sensitive than measure of median nerve area at the wrist alone (Hobson-Webb et al 2008). The sensitivity of the combination of US and neurophysiology is higher than that of neurophysiology or US alone. US is hence a useful complementary tool for CTS assessment, with a positive correlation between US findings and conventional measures of CTS severity (clinical, neurophysiological and patient-oriented) (Padua et al 2008).

In conclusion, there is increasing evidence that US is a useful complement in a neurophysiology laboratory, it greatly increases the diagnostic power and therapeutic work-up of patients with mononeuropathies (Padua et al 2007) and the morphological evaluation of nerves helps in avoiding severe misdiagnoses (e.g. a median nerve tumour that may mimic CTS), especially in cases with atypical neurophysiological findings (Padua & Martinoli 2008).

PROGNOSIS

Prognosis of untreated carpal tunnel syndrome

The knowledge of evolution of untreated CTS is very important in order to administer the best therapeutic approach. Only a few studies have evaluated this topic (Padua et al 1998, 2001, Resende et al 2003, Ortiz-Corredor et al 2008) and all authors agreed that many patients improved spontaneously. When the evolution is analyzed according to the initial picture, it is observed that CTS hands with initial low severity tend to get worse while CTS hands with initial high severe impairment tend to improve (this is observed in all CTS measurements, either patient-oriented or neurophysiologic).

Moreover, the factor that is most predictive of untreated CTS evolution is the duration of symptoms. In particular, a long duration of symptoms is a negative prognostic factor according to all patient-oriented measurements. Conversely a long duration of symptoms is not significantly associated with a bad neurophysiological or clinical examination outcome. With regard to the positive prognostic value of hand stress at the baseline, note that this value is probably due to the interruption of the stress. In this sense it is interesting to note that in the entrapment syndrome the 'natural history' can be influenced by the physicians with an explanation of the patho-physiology of CTS. If doctors, while giving the patients the diagnosis, also provide practical information about the hand positions to be avoided, they can alter the natural course of the pathology.

Therapy

With regard to the conservative options of CTS therapy a review by Piazzini et al (2007), including 33 randomized controlled trials, showed that there is a strong evidence (level 1) on efficacy of local and oral steroids; moderate evidence (level 2) that vitamin B6 is ineffective and that splints are effective, and limited or conflicting evidence that NSAIDs, diuretics, yoga, laser and ultrasound are effective whereas exercise therapy and botulinum toxin B injection are ineffective. A recent systematic review focused on neural mobilization interventions for the management of CTS included six studies and found weak to strong effects of neural gliding exercises with benefits seen across different outcome measures (Medina McKeon & Yancosek 2008). Nevertheless, these authors proposed that the benefit of neural gliding may be best identified within a specific subpopulation of CTS patients. It is possible that neural gliding may be more effective in a population with less advanced CTS. A clinical prediction rule identifying CTS patients who will benefit from neural mobilization interventions is urgently needed.

Regarding the surgical approach, a Cochrane review of 2003 concluded that surgical treatment relieves symptoms significantly better than splinting but further research is needed to discover whether this conclusion applies to people with mild symptoms and whether surgical treatment is better than steroid injection (Verdugo et al 2003).

Analyzing the factors that influence the surgical results in different populations, a number of studies have been performed, e.g. the results of surgical decompression were similar in men and women (Mondelli et al 2004a). On the other hand elderly patients showed less improvement with respect to younger patients, presumably due to greater preoperative damage and less repair capacity of the compressed nerve, but this aspect was not a contraindication for surgical release in elderly patients (Mondelli et al 2004b). Also the presence of comorbidity has been investigated, e.g. patients with diabetes have the same probability of positive surgical outcome as patients with idiopathic CTS (Mondelli et al 2004a).

In the same trend, the analysis of cost-effectiveness of non-surgical versus surgical treatment showed that surgery, rather than non-surgical care, should be considered as the initial form of treatment when patients are diagnosed with CTS (confirmed by nerve conduction studies), as this provides symptom resolution with a favourable cost analysis (Pomerance et al 2009).

CARPAL TUNNEL SYNDROME AND PREGNANCY

Because CTS is frequent during pregnancy (PRCTS) it can be considered a distinct entity. Studies have shown that PRCTS does not disappear after delivery (it may improve but on the contrary it may remain and the prolonged compression may result in median nerve defect) so CTS symptoms must be accurately assessed in pregnant women, and when present they must be monitored either clinically or neuro-physiologically (the role of ultrasound in PRCTS is not well known and must be assessed as it could be a non-invasive monitoring tool).

In cases of early appearance (before the last trimester) the median compression must be well assessed as it may result in acute or disabling CTS and improvement is less frequent. In case of severe CTS with early onset the surgical decompression during pregnancy may prevent nerve damage and a negative psychological influence after delivery.

Appearance of CTS symptoms in the last trimester is the more usual condition and has a higher probability of improvement after delivery; but around half of women may complain of CTS symptoms for a long time post partum, so clinical and neurophysiological monitoring is suggested. Note that despite improvement of symptoms, the distal sensory conduction velocity of the median nerve improved but remained delayed in 84% of women long after delivery (Mondelli et al 2007).

Apart from acute CTS, which may be an emergency (with the need for rapid surgical decompression), the first line in approaching PRCTS should be conservative therapy. But in absence of improvement and the presence of severe neurophysiological CTS (disappearance of sensory or motor responses) or disabling symptoms, surgical decompression before delivery must be considered in order to prevent not only nerve damage but also deterioration of quality of life due to difficulty and anxiety in handling the baby.

CONCLUSION

Although CTS has been defined as "complex issues with a 'simple' condition" (Olney 2001), and this is confirmed by the high number of publications concerning all aspects of CTS, in recent years efforts have been conducted to improve knowledge of this condition. Tools imported from other fields, such as ultrasound, have been commonly accepted in improving the diagnostic sensibility, although the gold standard remains the clinical picture. The natural history of the pathology shows that some untreated CTS patients can improve, but this is probably due to the doctor explaining to the patient how to avoid wrong hand postures and thus reducing the stresses on the hand. Conservative therapies have been used and were demonstrated to be effective, but surgical decompression, also used in elderly or diabetic patients, remains the definite cure and is efficient from the cost effectiveness point of view.

The opinion of the authors concerning surgical decompression, based on clinical experience and on unpublished data on the natural history of CTS, is that surgery is suggested in severe cases (either neuro-physiologically or clinically) with duration of symptoms longer than 1 year and in patients over 50 years old. A brief period of conservative therapy can be tried in cases of acute CTS, but any case in which we suspect an acute CTS that is not secondary to a particularly stressing event – a very rare but very severe condition – urgent decompression must be considered together with a comprehensive assessment of a possible primary subclinical cause.

REFERENCES

AAN, 1993a. American Academy of Neurology, American Association of Electrodiagnostic Medicine, American Academy of Physical Medicine and Rehabilitation. Practice parameter for electrodiagnostic studies in carpal tunnel syndrome (summary statement). Neurology 43, 2404–2405.

AAN, 1993b. American Academy of Neurology, American Association of Electrodiagnostic Medicine, American Academy of Physical Medicine and Rehabilitation. Practice parameter for carpal tunnel syndrome (summary statement). Neurology 43, 2406–2409.

Arendt-Nielsen, L., Gregersen, H., Toft, E., Bjerring, P., 1991. Involvement of thin afferents in carpal tunnel syndrome: evaluated quantitatively by argon laser stimulation. Muscle Nerve 14, 508–514.

Atroshi, I., Gummesson, C., Johnsson, R., et al., 1999. Prevalence of carpal tunnel syndrome in a general population. JAMA 282, 153–158.

Beekman, R., Visser, L.H., 2003. Sonography in the diagnosis of carpal tunnel syndrome: a critical review of the literature. Muscle Nerve 27, 26–33.

Bland, J.D., Rudolfer, S.M., 2003. Clinical surveillance of carpal tunnel syndrome in two areas of the United Kingdom, 1991–2001. J. Neurol. Neurosurg. Psychiatry 74, 1674–1679.

Bongers, F.J., Schellevis, F.G., van den Bosch, W.J., et al., 2007. Carpal tunnel syndrome in general practice (1987 and 2001): incidence and the role of occupational and non-occupational factors. British Journal of Genealogy Practice 57, 36–39.

Caliandro, P., La Torre, G., Aprile, I., et al., 2006. Distribution of paresthesias in Carpal Tunnel Syndrome reflects the degree of nerve damage at wrist. Clin. Neurophysiol. 117, 228–231.

Chiang, H.C., Ko, Y.C., Chen, S.S., et al., 1993. Prevalence of shoulder and upper-limb disorders among workers in the fish-processing industry. Scand. J. Work Environ. Health 19, 126–131.

Chow, C.S., Hung, L.K., Chiu, C.P., et al., 2005. Is symptomatology useful in distinguishing between carpal tunnel syndrome and cervical spondylosis? Hand Surg. 10, 1–5.

De-la-Llave-Rincón, A.I., Fernández-de-las-Peñas, C., Fernández-Carnero, J., Padua, L., Arendt-Nielsen, L., Pareja, J.A., et al., 2009. Bilateral hand/wrist head and cold hyperalgesia, but not hypoesthesia, in unilateral carpal tunnel syndrome. Exp. Brain Res. 198, 455–463.

Fernández-de-las-Peñas, C., De-la-Llave-Rincón, A.I., Fernández-Carnero, J., Cuadrado, M., Arendt-Nielsen, L., Pareja, J., et al., 2009a. Bilateral widespread mechanical pain sensitivity in carpal tunnel syndrome: Evidence of central processing in unilateral neuropathy. Brain 132, 1472–1479.

Fernández-de-las-Peñas, C., Pérez-de-Heredia, M., Martínez-Piédrola, R., De-la-Llave-Rincón, A.I., Cleland, J.A., et al., 2009b. Bilateral deficits in fine motor control and pinch grip force in patients with unilateral carpal tunnel syndrome. Exp. Brain Res. 194, 29–37.

Fornage, B.D, Rifkin, M., 1988. Ultrasound examination of tendons. Radiol. Clin. North Am. 6, 87–107.

Giannini, F., Cioni, R., Mondelli, M., et al., 2002. A new clinical scale of carpal tunnel syndrome: validation of the measurement and clinical-neurophysiological assessment. Clin. Neurophysiol. 113, 71–77.

Goadsby, P., Burke, D., 1994. Deficit in the function of small and large afferent fibres in confirmed cases of carpal tunnel syndrome. Muscle Nerve 17, 614–622.

Gracely, R.H., Lynch, S.A., Bennett, G.J., 1992. Painful neuropathy: altered central processing maintained dynamically by peripheral input. Pain 51, 175–194.

Graif, M., Seton, A., Nerubali, J., et al., 1991. Sciatic nerve: sonographic evaluation and anatomic–pathologic considerations. Radiology 18, 405–408.

Granata, G., Martinoli, C., Pazzaglia, C., et al., 2008. Letter to Editor: Carpal tunnel syndrome due to an atypical deep soft tissue leiomyoma: the risk of misdiagnosis and mismanagement. World J. Surg. Oncol. 6, 22.

Hall, T.M., Elvey, R.L., 1999. Nerve trunk pain: physical diagnosis and treatment. Man. Ther. 4, 63–73.

Heidelberg, A., 1989. Anatomy of the carpal tunnel, carpal tunnel syndrome, Part 1. Springer, Berlin.

Hobson-Webb, L.D., Padua, L., 2009. Median nerve ultrasonography in carpal tunnel syndrome: findings from two laboratories. Muscle Nerve 40, 94–97.

Hobson-Webb, L.D., Massey, J.M., Juel, V.C., et al., 2008. The ultrasonographic wrist-to-forearm median nerve area ratio in carpal tunnel syndrome. Clin. Neurophysiol. 119, 1353–1357.

Karadağ, Y.S., Karadağ, O., Ciçekli, E., et al., 2010. Severity of carpal tunnel syndrome assessed with high frequency ultrasonography. Rheumatol. Int. 30 (6), 761–765.

Keir, P.J., Bach, J.M., Rempel, D.M., 1998. Effects of finger posture on carpal tunnel pressure during wrist motion. J. Hand Surg. [Am.] 23, 1004–1009.

Kleinschnitz, C., Brinkhoff, J., Sommer, C., Stoll, G., 2005. Contra-lateral cytokine gene induction after peripheral nerve lesions: dependence on the mode of injury and NMDA receptor signalling. Molecular Brain Research 136, 23–28.

Koltzenburg, M., Wall, P.D., McMahon, S.B., 1999. Does the right side know what the left is doing? Trends Neurosci. 22, 122–127.

Lang, E., Claus, D., Neundörfer, B., Handwerker, H., 1995. Parameters of thick and thin nerve-fibres functions as predictors of pain in carpal tunnel syndrome. Pain 60, 295–302.

Levine, D.W., Simmons, B.P., Koris, M.J., et al., 1993. A self-administered questionnaire for the assessment of severity of symptoms and functional status in carpal tunnel syndrome. J. Bone Joint Surg. Am. 75, 1585–1592.

Luchetti, R., Schoenhuber, R., Nathan, P., 1998. Correlation of segmental carpal tunnel pressures with changes in hand and wrist positions in patients with carpal tunnel syndrome and controls. J. Hand Surg. 23, 598–602.

Martinoli, C., Derchi, L.E., Pastorino, C., et al., 1993. Analysis of echotexture of tendons with US. Radiology 186, 839–843.

Martinoli, C., Bianchi, S., Dahmane, M., et al., 2002. Ultrasound of tendons and nerves. Eur. Radiol. 12, 44–55.

Medina McKeon, J.M., Yancosek, K.E., 2008. Neural gliding techniques for the treatment of carpal tunnel syndrome: a systematic review. Journal of Sports Rehabilitation 17, 324–341.

Mondelli, M., Padua, L., Reale, F., et al., 2004a. Outcome of surgical release among diabetics with carpal tunnel syndrome. Arch. Phys. Med. Rehabil. 85, 7–13.

Mondelli, M., Padua, L., Reale, F., 2004b. Carpal tunnel syndrome in elderly patients: results of surgical decompression. J. Peripher. Nerv. Syst. 9, 168–176.

Mondelli, M., Rossi, S., Monti, E., et al., 2007. Long term follow-up of carpal tunnel syndrome during pregnancy: a cohort study and review of the literature. Electromyogr. Clin. Neurophysiol. 6, 259–271.

Moore, J.S., Garg, A., 1994. Upper extremity disorders in a pork processing plant: relationships between job risk factors and morbidity. Am. Ind. Hyg. Assoc. J. 55, 703–715.

Napadow, V., Kettner, N., Ryan, A., Kwong, K.K., Audette, J., Hui, K.K., 2006. Somatosensory cortical plasticity in carpal tunnel syndrome: a cross-sectional fMRI evaluation. Neuroimage 31, 520–530.

Olney, R.K., 2001. Carpal tunnel syndrome. Complex issues with a 'simple' condition. Neurology 56, 1431–1432.

Ortiz-Corredor, F., Enríquez, F., Díaz-Ruíz, J., Calambas, N., 2008. Natural evolution of carpal tunnel syndrome in untreated patients. Clin. Neurophysiol. 119, 1373–1378.

Padua, L., Martinoli, C., 2008. From square to cube: ultrasound as a natural complement of neurophysiology. Clin. Neurophysiol. 119, 1217–1218.

Padua, L., Lo Monaco, M., Padua, R., et al., 1997a. Neurophysiological classification of carpal tunnel syndrome: assessment of 600 symptomatic hands. Ital. J. Neurol. Sci. 18, 145–150.

Padua, L., Lo Monaco, M., Gregori, B., et al., 1997b. Neurophysiological classification and sensitivity in 500 carpal tunnel syndrome hands. Acta Neurol. Scand. 96, 211–217.

Padua, L., Padua, R., Lo Monaco, M., et al., 1998. Natural history of carpal tunnel syndrome according to the neurophysiological classification. Ital. J. Neurol. Sci. 19, 357–361.

Padua, L., Giannini, F., Girlanda, P., et al., 1999. Usefulness of segmental and comparative tests in the electrodiagnosis of carpal tunnel syndrome: the Italian multicenter study. Italian CTS Study Group. Ital. J. Neurol. Sci. 20, 315–320.

Padua, L., Padua, R., Aprile, I., et al., 2001. Italian CTS Study Group. Carpal tunnel syndrome. Multi-perspective follow-up of untreated carpal tunnel syndrome: a multicenter study. Neurology 56, 1459–1466.

Padua, L., Padua, R., Aprile, I., et al., 2002. Carpal tunnel syndrome: relationship between clinical and patient-oriented assessment. Clin. Orthop. Relat. Res. 395, 128–134.

Padua, L., Pazzaglia, C., Insola, A., et al., 2006. Schwannoma of the median nerve (even outside the wrist) may mimic carpal tunnel syndrome. Neurol. Sci. 26, 430–434.

Padua, L., Aprile, I., Pazzaglia, C., et al., 2007. Contribution of ultrasound in a neurophysiological lab in diagnosing nerve impairment: A one-year systematic assessment. Clin. Neurophysiol. 118, 1410–1416.

Padua, L., Pazzaglia, C., Caliandro, P., et al., 2008. Carpal tunnel syndrome: ultrasound, neurophysiology, clinical and patient-oriented assessment. Clin. Neurophysiol. 119, 2064–2069.

Piazzini, D.B., Aprile, I., Ferrara, P.E., et al., 2007. A systematic review of conservative treatment of carpal

tunnel syndrome. Clin. Rehabil. 21, 299–314.

Pierre-Jerome, C., Bekkelund, S.I., 2005. Magnetic resonance assessment of the double-crush phenomenon in patients with carpal tunnel syndrome: a bilateral quantitative study. Scand. J. Plast. Reconstr. Surg. Hand Surg. 37, 46–53.

Pomerance, J., Zurakowski, D., Fine, I., 2009. The cost-effectiveness of nonsurgical versus surgical treatment for carpal tunnel syndrome. J. Hand Surgery [Am.] 7, 1193–1200.

Resende, L.A., Tahara, A., Fonseca, R.G., et al., 2003. The natural history of carpal tunnel syndrome. A study of 20 hands evaluated 4 to 9 years after initial diagnosis. Electromyogr. Clin. Neurophysiol. 43, 301–304.

Russell, B.S., 2008. Carpal tunnel syndrome and the 'double crush' hypothesis: a review and implications for chiropractic. Chiropr. Osteopat. 16, 2.

Silvestri, E., Martinoli, C., Derchi, L.E., et al., 1995. Echotexture of peripheral nerves: correlation between US and histologic findings and criteria to differentiate tendons. Radiology 197, 291–296.

Smith, C., O'Neill, J., Parasu, N., Finlay, K., 2009. The role of ultrasonography in the assessment of carpal tunnel syndrome. Can. Assoc. Radiol. J. 60, 279–280.

Sternbach, G., 1999. The carpal tunnel syndrome. J. Emerg. Med. 17, 519–523.

Stevens, J.C., Beard, C.M., O'Fallon, W.M., Kurland, L.T., 1992. Conditions associated with carpal tunnel syndrome. Mayo Clin. Proc. 67, 541–548.

Tamburin, S., Cacciatori, C., Marani, S., Zanette, G., 2008. Pain and motor function in carpal tunnel syndrome: A clinical, neurophysiological and psychophysical study. J. Neurol. 255, 1636–1643.

Tanaka, S., Wild, D.K., Seligman, P.J., et al., 1995. The U.S. prevalence of self-reported carpal tunnel syndrome: 1988 national health interview survey data. American Journal of Indirect Medicine 27, 451–470.

Tecchio, F., Padua, L., Aprile, I., Rossini, P.M., 2002. Carpal tunnel syndrome modifies sensory hand cortical somatotopy: a MEG study. Hum. Brain Mapp. 17, 28–36.

Tucker, A.T., White, P.D., Kosek, E., et al., 2007. Comparison of vibration perception thresholds in individuals with diffuse upper limb pain and carpal tunnel syndrome. Pain 127, 263–269.

van Rijn, R.M., Huisstede, B.M., Koes, B. W., Burdorf, A., 2009. Associations between work-related factors and the carpal tunnel syndrome: a systematic review. Scand. J. Work Environ. Health 35, 19–36.

Verdugo, R.J., Salinas, R.A., Castillo, J.L., Cea, J.G., 2003. Surgical versus non-surgical treatment for carpal tunnel syndrome. Cochrane Database Syst. Rev. (3). CD001552.

Wainner, R.S., Fritz, J.M., Irrgang, J.J., Delitto, A., Allison, S., Boninger, M.L., 2005. Development of a clinical prediction rule for the diagnosis of carpal tunnel syndrome. Arch. Phys. Med. Rehabil. 86, 609–618.

Wang, L.Y., Leong, C.P., Huang, Y.C., et al., 2008. Best diagnostic criterion in high-resolution ultrasonography for carpal tunnel syndrome. Chang Gung Med. J. 31, 469–476.

Watkins, L., Maier, S., 2004. Neuropathic pain: the immune connection. Pain Clinical Updated 13, 1–4.

Werner, R.A., 2006. Evaluation of work-related carpal tunnel syndrome. J. Occup. Rehabil. 16, 207–222.

Werner, R.A., Albers, J.W., Franzblau, A., Armstrong, T.J., 1994. The relationship between body mass index and the diagnosis of carpal tunnel syndrome. Muscle Nerve 17, 632–636.

Westerman, R.A., Delaney, C.A., 1991. Palmar cold threshold test and median nerve electromyography in carpal tunnel compression neuropathy. Clin. Exp. Neur. 28, 154–167.

Wilbourn, A.J., Gilliatt, R.W., 1997. Double-crush syndrome: a critical analysis. Neurology 1, 21–27.

Zanette, G., Marani, S., Tamburin, S., 2006. Extra-median spread of sensory symptoms in carpal tunnel syndrome suggests the presence of pain-related mechanisms. Pain 2122, 264–270.

Zanette, G., Marani, S., Tamburin, S., 2007. Proximal pain in patients with carpal tunnel syndrome: a clinical neuro-physiological study. J. Peripher. Nerv. Syst. 12, 91–97.

Chapter | 29 |

Nerve compression syndromes of the forearm

Joy C MacDermid, David M Walton

EPIDEMIOLOGY

Compression neuropathy can exist anywhere along the course of a nerve, although all reported sites are uncommon compared to the carpal tunnel. The second most common site of upper extremity compression involves the ulnar nerve at the cubital tunnel (Mondelli et al 2005). The ulnar nerve may also be compromised at Guyon's canal. The annual incidence of cubital tunnel in workers performing repetitive work has been estimated at 0.8% per person-year (Descatha et al 2004). A single large study suggested that the rate of electrophysiological abnormality in the median nerve at the upper extremity is twice that of the ulnar (Pascarelli & Hsu, 2001) nerve, with affected median nerves being twice as likely to be symptomatic, thus resulting in a 4:1 ratio in carpal to cubital tunnel syndromes.(Seror & Nathan 1993).

Entrapment of the median nerve in the proximal forearm is relatively uncommon, but is an important component of differential diagnosis and a potential explanation for failed treatment of carpal tunnel syndrome. The most reported compression syndromes are pronator teres syndrome or anterior interosseous nerve (Kiloh–Nevin) syndrome. In a large series these contributed 1% of the compression syndromes of the upper limb.

The radial nerve has multiple sites of compression in the forearm, with 'radial tunnel' the most common. Since there is little agreement on diagnostic approaches or criteria for radial nerve compressions of the forearm, incidence/prevalence rates have not been clearly defined. In a large series of patients with work-related upper extremity disorders, 7% were diagnosed as having radial tunnel syndrome (Pascarelli & Hsu 2001).

Risk factors for developing nerve compression in the forearm are related to both activity and the individual. 'Holding a tool in position' was predictive of risk for cubital tunnel (odds ratio (OR: 4.1). Obesity (OR: 4.3) had a similar risk, and the presence of concomitant upper extremity tendinosis also increased the risk (Descatha et al 2004). A gender effect has been established for cubital tunnel syndrome with males at greater risk (Richardson et al 2001). A recent systematic review examined the exposure-response relationships between work-related physical and psychosocial factors including cubital

© 2011 Elsevier Ltd.
DOI: 10.1016/B978-0-7020-3528-9.00029-7

tunnel syndrome and radial tunnel syndrome in occupational populations. The occurrence of cubital tunnel syndrome was associated with the factor 'holding a tool in position' (OR: 3.5), handling loads > 1 kg (OR: 9), static work of the hand during the majority of the cycle time (OR: 5.9) and full extension (0–45°) of the elbow (OR: 4.9) were associated with radial tunnel syndrome. Roquelaure et al (2000) found similar risk factors: Exertion of force of over 1 kg (OR: 9.1), Prolonged static loading of the hand (OR: 6), or working with the elbow extended (OR: 5) (Roquelaure et al 2000).

ANATOMY

Ulnar nerve

The ulnar nerve is vulnerable by its location, its path through the forearm and the effects of position and movement. The C8 and T1 nerve roots give rise to the medial cord of the brachial plexus which branches into the ulnar nerve and the medial component of the median nerve. The ulnar nerve travels on the medial side of the brachial artery in the upper arm, and at mid upper arm pierces the inter-muscular septum to continue on the medial head of the triceps. At the elbow, it passes through the cubital tunnel, a groove between the medial humeral epicondyle and the olecranon. The nerve then travels between the two heads of the flexor carpi ulnaris and down the forearm between the deep and superficial finger flexors. Just below the elbow, it sends branches to the *flexor carpi ulnaris* and the ulnar half of the *flexor digitorum profundus*. There are five potential entrapment sites:

1. The arcade of Struthers, a fibrous band from the medial head of the triceps to the medial intermuscular septum (the fibrous band only occurs in 70% of people)
2. The medial inter-muscular septum
3. The cubital tunnel (most common site) where the medial collateral ligament of the elbow forms the floor and the arcuate ligament (cubital tunnel retinaculum) the roof
4. The aponeurosis between the two heads of the flexor carpi ulnaris (Osborne band)
5. The aponeurotic covering between the flexors digitorum profundus and superficialis is occasionally a site of compression. Anatomic variants are commonly reported in case studies as unusual causes of nerve compression.

An average of 5 mm of ulnar nerve excursion is required at the elbow to accommodate shoulder motion from 30° to 110° of abduction or elbow motion from 10° to 90°. When the wrist is moved from 60° of extension to 65° of flexion, 14 mm excursion of the ulnar nerve is required at the wrist. When all the motions of the wrist, fingers, elbow, and shoulder are combined, 22 mm of ulnar nerve excursion is required at the elbow and 23 mm at the wrist. Ulnar nerve strain of 15% or greater occurs at the elbow with elbow flexion and at the wrist with wrist extension and radial deviation (Wright et al 2001). Ultrasonography of 200 normal individuals revealed that the ulnar nerve changes its course at the fibrous band region 11.5 mm distal to the medial epicondyle. Dynamic studies showed that during elbow flexion, the nerve moved to the tip of the epicondyle in 27% of individuals whereas it dislocated anteriorly in 20% (Okamoto et al 2000). Some believe that subluxation of the nerve during movement can contribute to cubital tunnel syndrome.

At the wrist, the ulnar nerve runs above the flexor retinaculum lateral to the flexor carpi ulnaris tendon and medial to the ulnar artery. At the proximal carpal bones, it courses between the pisiform and the hook of the hamate at the entrance to the Guyon canal (the roof of the canal is formed by an extension of the *transverse carpal ligament* that links these two bones). Three zones of the ulnar nerve within the distal ulnar tunnel have been defined as follows:

- Zone 1 – Ulnar nerve proximal to the bifurcation
- Zone 2 – The deep branch
- Zone 3 – The superficial branch or branches.

The deep (motor) branch supplies the abductor digiti minimi (ADM), then crosses under one head of the flexor digiti minimi (FDM), supplies this muscle, and crosses over to supply the opponens digiti minimi (ODM) before rounding the hook of the hamate bone to enter the mid palmar space and supply other hand muscles. These anatomic zones correlate with clinical symptomatology. After Zone 1 nerve bifurcates into superficial and deep branches. These *terminal branches* include the superficial cutaneous branch to the ulnar portion of palm & volar surfaces of ulnar 1½ fingers, the deep motor branch that passes adjacent to hook of hamate bone, and the deep branch that innervates the hypothenar muscles, 3rd and 4th lumbricales, adductor pollicis, all interossei, and deep head of *flexor pollicis brevis*. Depending on the exact site of compression within the Guyon canal, the ADM or both the ADM and the FDM may be spared. The ODM is always affected, together with the interossei, lumbricals 3 and 4, and the adductor pollicis. Patients with zone 1 compression can present with motor, sensory or mixed lesions; those with zone 2, motor lesions, and zone 3, sensory only. Compression of the deep branch is the most common and usually occurs at the level of the fibrous arch of the hypothenar muscles. The distal canal is also the common site for ganglions arising from the wrist.

Radial nerve

The radial nerve is the largest branch of the brachial plexus (posterior cord) and receives fibres from C6, C7 and C8 (sometimes T1). Its crosses the latissimus dorsi deep to the axillary artery, passes the inferior border of the teres major, winds around the humerus, and then enters the triceps muscle between the long and medial heads. It progresses along the spiral groove of the humerus to pierce the lateral inter-muscular septum and runs between the brachialis and brachioradialis to lie anterior to the lateral condyle of the humerus. Branches to the brachioradialis and extensor carpi radialis longus are given off just proximal to the elbow. The anconeus receives a branch, and the nerve then divides into a superficial branch and a deep branch. The extensor carpi radialis brevis (ECRB) receives its innervation either from the radial nerve proper or from the posterior interosseous nerve. The superficial branch, which is purely sensory, runs under cover of the brachioradialis in the forearm. Eight centimetres proximal to the tip of the radial styloid, the nerve pierces the fascia medial to the brachioradialis to lie dorsal to the extensor tendons. It divides into a medial branch and a lateral branch to innervate the radial wrist (with some variable overlap from the lateral antebrachial cutaneous nerve), dorsal radial hand, and dorsum of the radial 3½ digits to approximately the middle phalanx level.

The deep branch or posterior interosseous nerve (PIN), winds to the dorsum of the forearm, around the lateral side of the radius, and through the muscle fibres of the supinator. It then divides into medial and lateral branches, each of which supplies different extensor muscles. The PIN supplies ECRB and supinator before entering arcade of Frohse. This arcade is a fibrotendinous structure at the proximal origin of supinator and the most common site for entrapment of the radial nerve. In 25% of individuals, the PIN actually touches the dorsal aspect of radius opposite the bicipital tuberosity; thus fracture fixation (plates) placed high on the dorsal surface of radius may trap the nerve underneath. The most common compression site is at the supinator muscle. However, proximal lesions should be suspected with humeral fractures. Radial nerve palsy associated with fracture is more common after fracture of the middle third of the humerus (Holstein-Lewis fracture) or at the junction of the middle and distal thirds. The nerve also can be compressed by the lateral inter-muscular septum. Less common compression sites include the fibrous arch of the lateral head of the triceps muscle and the accessory subscapularis-teres-latissimus muscle.

The aetiology of PIN syndrome is similar to that of radial tunnel syndrome. PIN compression is most commonly associated with tendinous hypertrophy of the arcade of Frohse and fibrous thickening of the radiocapitellar joint capsule. Lesions, such as lipoma, synovial cyst, rheumatoid synovitis, or vascular aneurysm, may be causative and should be considered where symptoms do not respond to mechanical forces predictably. Hobbies or occupations associated with repetitive and forceful supination predispose the individual to PIN neuropathy. Chronic trauma to the flexion surface of the forearm can also create problems. Crutches that include forearm rings, inappropriately placed forearm braces (e.g. tennis elbow) or tight clothing can provide such external compression.

Compression affects branches innervating the radial wrist extensors and the radial sensory nerve (RSN). After emerging from the supinator, the nerve may be compressed before it bifurcates into medial and lateral branches, causing a complete paralysis of the digital extensors and dorso-radial deviation of the wrist secondary to paralysis of the *extensor carpi ulnaris (ECU)*. If compression occurs after the nerve bifurcates, selective paralysis of muscles occurs, depending on which branch is involved. Compression of the medial branch causes paralysis of the ECU, *extensor digitorum minimi*, and *extensor digitorum communis*. Compression of the lateral branch causes paralysis of the *abductor pollicis longus, extensor pollicis longus*, and *extensor indices*. Other possible aetiologies for posterior interosseous nerve dysfunction include trauma (Monteggia fractures), synovitis (rheumatoid), tumours, and iatrogenic injuries.

Wartenberg syndrome, or RSN entrapment, is unique in that it has isolated sensory symptoms. Insidious onset may occur in association with de Quervain tenosynovitis. Acute onset can occur following post-surgical injury, external compression or trauma on the radial aspect of the wrist. The anatomic site of compression corresponds to the transit of the nerve from its submuscular position beneath the brachioradialis to its subcutaneous position on the ECRL. With pronation, these two muscles can create a scissor-like effect compressing the RSN.

Median nerve

The median nerve arises from both the lateral and medial cords of the brachial plexus and travels with the brachial artery on the medial side of arm between biceps brachii and brachialis. In the upper arm it is lateral to the artery, but then crosses anteriorly to run medial to the artery inside the cubital fossa, in front of the point of insertion of the brachialis muscle and deep to the biceps. The median nerve gives off an articular branch in the upper arm as it passes the elbow joint and then passes between the two heads of pronator teres. It innervates *pronator teres (PT), flexor carpi radialis (FCR)* and *flexor digitorum superficialis (FDS)*; travels between FDS and flexor digitorum profundus before emerging between FDS and FCR. The median nerve gives off two branches as it courses through the forearm: the anterior interosseous branch courses with the anterior interosseous artery and innervates flexor pollicis longus (FPL), FDP to 2nd and 3rd fingers and pronator quadratus. It ends with its innervation of pronator quadratus. The palmar cutaneous branch of the median nerve arises at the distal part of the forearm and supplies sensory innervation to the lateral aspect of the skin of the palm (but not the digits).

Compression of the median nerve in the forearm can arise as a result of anatomic variations (supracondylar process, Struthers ligament, lacertus fibrosus) at the biceps brachii, or overuse/tightness of the pronator teres muscle or flexor superficialis. With less frequency, an anomalous accessory head of the flexor pollicis longus (Ganzer's muscle) or persistent median artery can be found. Rarer causes of extrinsic compression of the median nerve are chronic compartment syndrome or partial rupture of the distal biceps tendon (or bicipital tendon bursitis). The most common site of compression of the median nerve is the tendinous origin of deep head of pronator teres.

PATHOLOGY

Nerve compression can occur directly from anatomic structures as highlighted above. Repetitive or acute trauma to a nerve may result in micro-vascular (ischaemic) changes, oedema, or injury to the myelin sheath and structural alterations in membranes in both the myelin sheath and the nerve axon. Wallerian degeneration of the axons and permanent fibrotic changes in the neuromuscular junction may prevent full reinnervation after compression is relieved. Seddon has classified nerve injuries into three categories:

- Neuropraxia: a transient episode without disruption of the nerve or its sheath – complete recovery is expected
- Axonotmesis: disruption of the axon but maintenance of the Schwann sheath. In this case, motor, sensory and autonomic effects are expected and recovery may be complete or incomplete
- Neurotmesis: nerve and sheath damage and incomplete recovery is usual.

Nerve fibres are not affected uniformly but by their proximity to the source of compression. Superficially located fibres tend to bear the brunt of compression, while central fibres are relatively spared. Since large diameter, heavily myelinated fibres are more sensitive to compression than poorly myelinated fibres, they are more affected. This explains the earlier and more pronounced impairment of light touch (vibration) sensibility in nerve compression disorders. Mild compression produces a transient conduction and disruption of axoplasmic flow which may only be evident with provocative manoeuvres. In chronic compression, segmental demyelination results in slowing of conduction and more persistent symptoms. With progression axolysis occurs in compressed segments, and Wallerian degeneration occurs distally. The critical threshold pressure for initiating changes in nerve has been reported to be 30 mmHg (Mackinnon 2002).

DIAGNOSIS

Nerve compression presents with loss of sensory and motor function where mixed nerves are involved. Radial tunnel and distal sensory nerve compressions are examples of where these symptoms may occur separately. In general progression of motor symptoms may start with a clumsiness or aching and progress to substantial loss of muscular strength and endurance. By the time patients have identified weakness; substantial loss in grip strength is usually measurable. Muscle atrophy is typically a late finding. Sensory abnormalities tend to progress from positional or activity-based paraesthesia that may be associated with pain to persistent symptoms. In later stages, numbness may be so profound that neither pain nor paraesthesias are as pronounced. Sensory abnormalities are first detected in vibration or touch thresholds and later appear in discriminative touch such as two-point discrimination. Tables 29.1–29.3 show the clinical signs, the special tests and common differential diagnosis depending on the site of nerve entrapment.

Ulnar nerve

The presenting symptoms with ulnar nerve are numbness and/or tingling most noted by the patient in the little finger but a loss of sensory function throughout the nerve distribution. Aching pain and loss of hand function are usually reported. Symptoms are aggravated in positions of flexion (and at night). Sensory and motor impairments can be variable, and electrodiagnosis is recommended before proceeding to surgery (Nakazumi & Hamasaki 2001). Patients with an ulnar neuropathy with a gradual non-traumatic onset may report a history of repetitive elbow flexion or prolonged resting of the elbow on a hard surface. Elbow flexion creates narrowing of the cubital tunnel as a result of traction on the arcuate ligament and bulging of the medial collateral ligament. Elbow flexion may also contribute to the injury by increasing the intra-neural pressure. With scarring and adhesion of the epineurium, elongation accentuates the tethering effect on the axons. These effects may be accentuated at night when the patient sleeps with the elbow in flexion.

Sensory and motor examinations of the hand reveal weakness of grip, atrophy of the thenar muscles and weakness of pinch (adductor pollicis muscle). Atrophy of affected muscles is most easily observable in the first dorsal interosseous. Inability to cross fingers may indicate interosseous weakness; although manual muscle testing may also be used. The FCU and FDP to the ring and little finger are usually not affected. Special tests include Froment's sign where pronounced thumb interphalangeal (IP) flexion is observed when grasping a piece of paper between thumb and index finger, as the FPL is used to

Table 29.1 Symptoms and signs depending on the site of nerve entrapment

	Ulnar nerve		Median nerve		Radial nerve	
	Cubital tunnel syndrome	**Guyon's tunnel syndrome**	**Anterior interosseus nerve syndrome**	**Radial tunnel syndrome**	**Posterior interosseus nerve syndrome**	**Distal sensory radial nerve syndrome (Wartenberg's syndrome)**
Area of symptoms	Medial elbow All of 5th and ulnar half of 4th digits	Palmar aspect of 4th and 5th digits only – sensation should be spared over dorsal aspect	Poorly localized to the volar proximal forearm	Approximately 5 cm (2 inches) distal to the lateral epicondyle	Over Arcade of Frohse	Dorsal aspect of the radial 3½ digits, as far distally as the proximal interphalangeal joints. The subungual region[a] should be spared
Nature of symptoms	Pain, numbness or tingling, weakness	Could be any or all of pain, numbness or tingling, weakness	Pain and/or weakness	Pain and fatigue, weakness	Weakness	Pain, numbness or tingling
Motor signs	Grip and/or pinch weakness. Possible Froment's sign.[b] Possible Wartenberg's sign.[c] May have difficulty crossing 2nd and 3rd digits. Specific weakness of 1st dorsal interosseous, abductor digiti minimi and flexor digitorum profundus of the 4th and 5th digits	Froment's sign[b] Wartenberg's sign[c] Weakness of the dorsal and palmar interossei and hypothenar muscles[d]	Weakness of flexor pollicis longus and flexor digitorum profundus of the 2nd digit. Affected individuals will be unable to form a circle by pinching the tips of the thumb and 2nd digit together.	No obvious muscle weakness in early stages[e]	With complete palsy, patients will be unable to extend the thumb or fingers at the MCP joints. Will also have difficulty or be unable to extend the wrist in neutral or ulnar positions[f]	No obvious muscle weakness should be present

[a]The region directly under the nail.
[b]Usually tested by asking the patient to pinch a piece of paper between the thumb and index finger, then the examiner pulls it away. Inability to hold the paper, or excessive flexion of the median innervated flexor pollicis longus (flexion of the 1st IP joint) is considered positive for ulnar nerve palsy.
[c]Abduction and extension of the 5th digit.
[d]Opponens digiti minimi, Abductor digiti minimi, Flexor digiti minimi brevis.
[e]Prolonged compression of the radial nerve may lead to weakness of the radially-innervated muscles of the forearm including extensor digitorum, extensor pollicis longus and brevis, and extensor carpi ulnaris. If weakness is present the condition is usually referred to as posterior interosseous nerve syndrome.
[f]Branches supplying ECRB and ECRL usually come off the radial nerve prior to entering the Arcade of Frohse and therefore are spared.

Table 29.2 Special tests depending on the site of nerve entrapment

Ulnar nerve		Median nerve		Radial nerve	
Cubital tunnel syndrome	**Guyon's tunnel syndrome**	**Anterior interosseus nerve syndrome**	**Radial tunnel syndrome**	**Posterior interosseus nerve syndrome**	**Distal sensory radial nerve syndrome (Wartenberg's syndrome)**
Positive upper limb neurodynamic testing with ulnar nerve bias Positive Tinel's sign at the cubital tunnel[a] Positive elbow flexion test[b] Tenderness or hyperalgesia over the cubital tunnel[c]	Positive upper limb neurodynamic testing with ulnar nerve bias Positive Tinel's sign over Guyon's tunnel	Positive upper limb neurodynamic testing with median nerve bias May reproduce symptoms with deep palpation of the two heads of pronator teres	Positive upper limb neurodynamic testing with radial nerve bias Tenderness over the radial tunnel[d] Pain with resisted extension of the 3rd digit Pain may be reproduced with active or resisted forearm supination with wrist flexion	Positive upper limb neurodynamic testing with radial nerve bias Pain with extreme pronation Tenderness over the radial tunnel Pain with resisted extension of the 3rd digit Pain may be reproduced with active or resisted forearm supination with wrist flexion	Positive upper limb neurodynamic testing with radial nerve bias Positive Tinel's sign over the site of exit of the SRN[e] Symptoms increase when tightly pinching the thumb and 2nd digit together Pain may be reproduced with extreme pronation

[a]Positive Tinel's sign at the cubital tunnel is not an uncommon finding in asymptomatic people.
[b]Flex elbow past 90°, supinate forearm and extend wrists. Positive test is reproduction of pain or discomfort within 60 seconds. Shoulder abduction can be added to increase the symptoms.
[c]Between the medial epicondyle and olecranon.
[d]Approximately 5 cm (2 inches) distal to the lateral epicondyle.
[e]Between the brachioradialis and extensor carpi radialis tendons, approximately two-thirds of the way down the forearm.

Table 29.3 Common differential diagnosis depending on the site of nerve entrapment

Ulnar nerve		Median nerve		Radial nerve	
Cubital tunnel syndrome	**Guyon's tunnel syndrome**	**Anterior interosseus nerve syndrome**	**Radial tunnel syndrome**	**Posterior interosseus nerve syndrome**	**Distal sensory radial nerve syndrome (Wartenberg's syndrome)**
C8/T1 root lesions Guyon's tunnel syndrome Thoracic outlet syndrome Valgus ligament instability Systemic – diabetes, alcoholism Pancoast tumour Medial epicondyle fracture	C8/T1 root lesions Carpal tunnel syndrome Thoracic outlet syndrome Systemic – diabetes, alcoholism Pancoast tumour	Flexor digitorum profundus avulsion Lateral cord lesion C8 radiculopathy (rare) Parsonage-Turner syndrome[a]	Lateral epicondylitis Brachial plexus injury C5–C6 radiculopathy	C5–C8 radiculopathy Lateral epicondylitis Extensor digitorum rupture	De Quervain's tenosynovitis Brachial plexus injury C5–C8 radiculopathy

stabilize the paper substituting for the absent adductor force. If the ulnar nerve is affected below mid-forearm, an ulnar claw (hand of benediction) deformity may be produced as the metacarpophalangeal joints of the fourth and fifth fingers are hyper-extended by the long extensors (owing to a lack of balance because of weak lumbricals to these fingers) with a length residual FDP tension producing flexion of the IP joints. If the ulnar nerve is compromised above the mid-forearm, clawing does not occur, because the FDP is also affected. Deformity usually indicates more profound compression.

Sensory evaluation should include touch threshold or vibration examination to detect milder compression. A Tinel's (percussion) test can also be used, but given the superficial nature of the nerve, a positive test in isolation should not be considered definitive proof of ulnar neuropathy and has been reported in 24% of the asymptomatic people (Rayan et al 1992). A compression test (fingertip pressure over the ulnar nerve) may be more accurate, although evidence is limited. In a small study, it was reported that the most sensitive provocative test in the diagnosis of cubital tunnel syndrome was elbow flexion when combined with pressure on the ulnar nerve. Provocative tests include sustained elbow flexion which is positive if it reproduces symptoms within 1 minute. A study of the elbow flexion test in 216 elbows using Rayan's four positions indicated that the false positive rate was 3.6% at 1 minute and 16.2% at 3 minutes (Rosati et al 1998).

If the ulnar nerve is compromised at the wrist a Tinel's response (electrical, shooting or tingling into the nerve distribution) may be obtained by percussing at Guyon's canal. A wrist flexion test (usually used for carpal tunnel syndrome), that produces paraesthesias in the ring and small fingers is also a positive finding. Both palpation and observation should be used to look for abnormalities at the hamate hook or for swelling that indicates ganglia or masses. A history of 'hammering' or repeated trauma to the palm is not uncommon. The classic presentation is a young man with painless atrophy of the hypothenar muscles and interossei with sparing of the thenar group. Sensory loss and pain involving the ulnar 1½ digits may be present. Distal ulnar compression can be differentiated as the dorsum of the hand is spared, whereas in cubital tunnel compression sensation is affected over both the dorsum of the ulnar half of the ring finger and the little finger. This is because the dorsal cutaneous branch, which leaves the ulnar nerve prior to entering Guyon canal, would be spared if the compression was in Guyon's canal only.

Radial nerve

Radial tunnel syndrome is characterized by pain over the antero-lateral proximal forearm in the region of the radial head and can be aggravated by repetitive elbow extension or forearm rotation. Radial tunnel syndrome can appear similar to symptoms of lateral epicondylitis (Henry & Stutz 2006), although the maximum tenderness is usually located 4 fingerbreadths distal to the lateral epicondyle as opposed to directly over the top of it. Based on a cadaveric study, a clinical test for radial tunnel was proposed that involves constructing nine equal squares on anterior aspect of the forearm, the PIN was confined to the lateral column (crossing two or three of the lateral squares) (Loh et al 2004). Symptoms can be reproduced by extending the elbow and pronating the forearm. In addition, resisted active supination and extension of the long finger cause pain (middle finger test). A compression test where the thumb is used to compress over the radial tunnel (similar to that used for carpal compression) is positive if it reproduces symptoms or aching muscle pain. This has been reported as the most consistent finding radial tunnel syndrome (Rinker et al 2004).

Posterior interosseous nerve syndrome presents with weakness or paralysis of the wrist and digital extensors. Pain may be present, but usually is not a primary symptom. Attempts at active wrist extension often result in weak dorso-radial deviation due to preservation of the radial wrist extensors but involvement of the ECU muscle and extensor digitorum communis. These patients do not have a sensory deficit. Muscle testing should include extension of the metacarpophalangeal joints which will be weak whereas IP extension remains intact because innervation to the lumbricals will be spared (ulnar nerve). Since the EIP and EDM are independent from the EDC and separately innervated, the index and small fingers are less affected than the extension of the third and fourth digits. An extension lag in the middle two fingers, while the index and little fingers extend ('sign of horns') is suggestive of PIN compression.

Patients with compression of the RSN complain of pain over the distal radial forearm associated with paraesthesias over the dorsal radial hand. They frequently report symptom magnification with wrist movement or when tightly pinching the thumb and index digit. These individuals demonstrate a positive Tinel sign over the RSN and local tenderness. Hyperpronation of the forearm can cause a positive Tinel sign. A high percentage of these patients reveal examination findings consistent with de Quervain tenosynovitis, and the synovitis may be a contributing factor in the compression of the nerve. Thus careful examination is required to distinguish isolated diagnosis of either condition versus coexistent pathology. Finkelstein's test may be positive in both cases, but quantitative sensory testing will reveal deficit when the RSN has been compromised.

Median nerve

Patients with pronator syndrome usually complain of pain in the anterior forearm aggravated by forearm rotation. Unlike carpal tunnel patients symptoms are not worse at night. Compression of the median nerve is indicated by sensory motor disturbances affecting the thumb, index and long fingers, and occasionally 'ring-splitting' phenomena, where the lateral side of the ring finger is noted as different from the medial side. If the palm is also affected than confidence is increased that compression is proximal to carpal tunnel. Muscle testing should attempt to differentiate potential compressive structures including lacertus fibrosus (resisted supination and flexion), FDS (independent flexion of the middle finger localizes the level of entrapment to the fibrous arcade of the FDS) or pronator teres (pronation and wrist flexion). A compression test where the thumb is used to create pressure over the pronator muscle that reproduces paraesthesia within 30 seconds is diagnostic. A differential diagnosis for C6/C7 radiculopathy can be determined by examining the function of the muscles innervated by the C6/C7 portions of the radial nerve (wrist extensors and the triceps).

Involvement of the anterior interosseous nerve (AIN) can be distinguished from the median nerve proper because it is primarily a motor nerve except for some sensory branches to the distal radio-ulnar and carpal joints. The latter may contribute to pain in the wrist with this syndrome; however paraesthesia is absent. AIN supplies FPL, the lateral half of FDP, and pronator quadratus. A more common misdiagnosis is an FDP avulsion since loss of terminal joint flexion may be interpreted as a loss of tendon integrity. Patients with AIN syndrome primarily complain of weakness, whereas those with pronator syndrome may present with pain and paraesthesia that can be confused with carpal tunnel syndrome.

PROGNOSIS

The extent of nerve damage affects symptoms and prognosis as discussed above. In general, severe compression detected by electrodiagnosis, atrophy, changes in two-point discrimination and persistent numbness indicate more severe nerve damage and thus poorer prognosis. Dellon et al (1993) followed a cohort of 128 patients treated non-operatively for cubital tunnel syndrome. At 5 years, 89% of patients with symptoms only, 67% of patients with abnormal sensorimotor thresholds, and 38% of patients with abnormal sensorimotor innervations density had not progressed to surgery. A history of elbow injury significantly worsened outcome (P < 0.02), but the results of the pretreatment electrodiagnosis did not. For patients who proceed to cubital tunnel release, outcomes are better if physical therapy is initiated within 3 days rather than if it is delayed for 14 days (Warwick & Seradge 1995).

CONSERVATIVE TREATMENT

General treatment principles

Since the majority of nerve compression syndromes discussed in this chapter are rare, specific high quality evidence on best management approaches is almost lacking. Extrapolation of efficacy of specific techniques studied in more common compression neuropathy (e.g. carpal tunnel syndrome) must be used resulting in lower confidence in the recommendations. A treatment programme generally selects a variety of techniques that address specific objectives such as: alter factors that are contributing to compression or compromise of the nerve, promote nerve recovery, enhance nerve gliding and facilitate normalized cortical reorganization.

Techniques are routinely used to reduce static (compressive) postures, repetitive trauma, or external forces. The specific positions/activities to avoid are discussed by each syndrome below. Careful examination of contractile versus insert structures may delineate the source of compression. Where musculotendinous hypertrophy is a contributing factor, strengthening of these muscles may worsen symptoms. However, strengthening of muscles for postural realignment is needed to reduce positional nerve compression. Muscle endurance may be important to prevent oedema with activity or abnormal movement patterns that contribute to compression. Rest may be required to reduce compression related to inflammation but lack of muscle extensibility is likely to worsen symptoms. Therefore, careful examination of potential sites/aetiologies is required to customize the rest/mobilization/realignment strategy for each patient. A generalized progression of activity would move from rest and gentle nerve gliding exercises to reduce symptoms, to a focus on restoring muscle and nerve length extensibility, and through to functional/postural re-strengthening/rebalancing. An important goal throughout treatment is to ensure that proper body mechanics and muscle recruitment are used during functional and occupational tasks.

Nerve recovery is primarily promoted by removal of compromising/compressive forces and allowing the body to heal nerve fibres that remain viable. Facilitation of this recovery with adjunctive physical agents may promote this process or be used to facilitate mobilization of the nerve. Low dose ultrasound (1.0 w/cm^2), long duration (15-minute session – 5×/wk for 2 weeks, then 2×/wk for 5 weeks) resulted in better nerve conduction velocity in carpal tunnel syndrome patients both at the end of treatment and 6 months later (Ebenbichler et al 1998). Higher doses at shorter intervals have not shown effectiveness. Iontophoresis with dexamethosone and lidocaine was used in one small trial of patients who failed splinting for patients with carpal tunnel syndrome, and 11/19 recovered (Banta 1994). Another trial suggested that in mild to moderate cases, 10 treatments of iontophoresis and ultrasound was effective in reducing symptoms (Dakowicz & Latosiewicz 2005).

The ability of the nerve to glide between different structures in the forearm has been highlighted in the anatomy. More recently there have been suggestions that 'nerve sliding' techniques may enhance mobility of the nerve, while producing less strain (Coppieters & Alshami 2007). An approach that encourages nerve mobility has been suggested as beneficial, but current clinical trials are limited to those using such exercises as an adjunct to splinting and tend to be underpowered (Svernlov et al 2009, Baysal et al 2006, Pinar et al 2005, Coppieters et al 2004). Readers are referred to Chapter 38 of this textbook for nerve neurodynamic. There is rationale (level 5 evidence) to suggest that a detailed examination of muscle mobility, activation and positional effects on symptoms that are characteristic of physical therapy expertise may identify structures that require specific mobilization, although this will remain inherently difficult to study in clinical trials.

Ulnar nerve

The mainstay of treating cubital tunnel syndrome has been night positioning, activity modification (Padua et al 2002), splinting the elbow in extension and nerve gliding exercise. Although custom hard thermoplastic splints are common, compliance can be a problem and soft versions that restrict full flexion may be more acceptable to patients. These can range from inexpensive off-the shelf (neoprene and other materials) or home-made approaches (a pair of socks used to create a sleeve and flexion block) to custom-made individual padded orthoses.

Behavioural changes should include avoiding compression (resting on elbows, elbow flexion, external pressure on elbows) and repetitive flexion or any activity in extremes of position. Office workers may need work station evaluation, postural and ergonomic training.

Nerve mobilization slowly progressed may be useful, but care should be taken to avoid over aggressive mobilization that contributes to the problem through tractioning the ulnar nerve. There is empirical evidence that 'sliding techniques' result in a substantially larger excursion of the ulnar nerve at the elbow than 'tensioning techniques' (8.3 mm versus 3.8 mm), and that this larger excursion is associated with a much smaller change in strain (Coppieters & Butler 2008). Differential stretching of specific muscles (FDS) may also increase mobility. While strength may be compromised, and functional goals may suggest the need for improved strength, therapists should exercise caution as strengthening has the potential to increase compressive factors.

The evidence on conservative management is sparse and inconclusive. A recent small trial suggested that 75% of patients with mild to moderate ulnar neuropathy improve within 6 months but that splinting and nerve gliding provide no additional benefit over activity modification (Svernlov et al 2009). The potential for lack of power in a trial of 70 patients is substantial but indicates the need for more evidence. The potential for natural history of recovery with minor changes (Szabo & Kwak 2007) suggests that activity modification and evaluation of a recovery pathway should be implemented as a first approach. Failure to respond to a more comprehensive physical therapy programme indicates a need for surgical release (Lund & Amadio 2006, Robertson & Saratsiotis 2005).

Radial nerve

Evidence for the effectiveness of conservative management and radial tunnel is lacking (Huisstede et al 2008). Mobilization of the potential compressive structures and differential movement of both muscle and tendon may be useful. Ergonomic changes to workstations may include tilting/split or modified keyboards to reduce excessive rotation or extreme wrist positioning. Tissue pressures suggest that positions of elbow flexion, supination, and wrist extension place the least stress and strain on the radial tunnel. This is not functional, but patients may benefit from a wrist support that places the wrist in moderate wrist extension and advice on avoiding forearm rotation and elbow extended positions during activity. Given that radial nerve symptoms can be confused with lateral epicondylitis patients whose symptoms are improved or worsened by a tennis elbow counterforce bracing should be re-evaluated for potential radial tunnel syndrome and switched to a wrist extension splint.

Median nerve

Changes in activity to reduce median nerve irritation include preventing repetitive forearm rotation and excessive forceful grip. A rest splint that maintains mid-rotation is sometimes used for a short period; although the necessity of this has not been proven (Lee & LaStayo 2004). The natural history of compressive disorders would suggest that activity modification is more important. Stretching of pronator teres and nerve gliding may be useful.

CONCLUSION

Nerves can be compromised in the forearm as a result of anatomic, biomechanical or external forces. Muscle testing and sensory examination should reveal the nerve affected and the most likely site of compression. Quantitative measures of muscle strength and sensory detection threshold are imperative for accurate diagnosis and monitoring progress in treatment. A treatment programme that mitigates the compressive forces, facilitates nerve healing, restores normal gliding, uses postural and cortical retraining to normalize anatomic balance and interpretation of nerve responses, and teaches patients to be proactive in identifying potential sources of compression in their work and behaviour (and how to modify these appropriately) should be successful for mild to moderate cases of nerve compression. Advanced compression may require surgical release, with early physical therapy being indicated. Both the quality and quantity of evidence on physical therapy techniques or programmes is insufficient and studies that look at the immediate impact of specific interventions on nerve function and the more global functional impacts of physical therapy programmes over the longer term are needed.

REFERENCES

Banta, C.A., 1994. A prospective, nonrandomized study of iontophoresis, wrist splinting, and anti-inflammatory medication in the treatment of early-mild carpal tunnel syndrome. J. Occup. Med. 36, 166–168.

Baysal, O., Altay, Z., Ozcan, C., Ertem, K., Yologlu, S., Kayhan, A., 2006. Comparison of three conservative treatment protocols in carpal tunnel syndrome. Journal of Clinical Practice 60, 820–828.

Coppieters, M.W., Alshami, A.M., 2007. Longitudinal excursion and strain in the median nerve during novel nerve gliding exercises for carpal tunnel syndrome. J. Orthop. Res. 25, 972–980.

Coppieters, M.W., Butler, D.S., 2008. Do 'sliders' slide and 'tensioners' tension? An analysis of neurodynamic techniques and considerations regarding their application. Man. Ther. 13, 213–221.

Coppieters, M.W., Bartholomeeusen, K.E., Stappaerts, K.H., 2004. Incorporating nerve-gliding techniques in the conservative treatment of cubital tunnel syndrome. J. Manipulative Physiol. Ther. 27, 560–568.

Dakowicz, A., Latosiewicz, R., 2005. The value of iontophoresis combined with ultrasound in patients with the carpal tunnel syndrome. Rocz. Akad. Med. Bialymst. 50, 196–198.

Dellon, A.L., Hament, W., Gittelshon, A., 1993. Nonoperative management of cubital tunnel syndrome: an 8-year prospective study. Neurology 43, 1673–1677.

Descatha, A., Leclerc, A., Chastang, J.F., Roquelaure, Y., 2004. Incidence of ulnar nerve entrapment at the elbow in repetitive work. Scand. J. Work Environ. Health 30, 234–240.

Ebenbichler, G.R., Resch, K.L., Nicolakis, P., et al., 1998. Ultrasound treatment for treating the carpal tunnel syndrome: randomised 'sham' controlled trial. Br. Med. J. 316, 731–735.

Henry, M., Stutz, C., 2006. A unified approach to radial tunnel syndrome and lateral tendinosis. Tech. Hand Up Extrem. Surg. 10, 200–205.

Huisstede, B., Miedema, H.S., van, O.T., de Ronde, M.T., Verhaar, J.A., Koes, B.W., 2008. Interventions for treating the radial tunnel syndrome: a systematic review of observational studies. J. Hand Surg. [Am.] 33, 72–78.

Lee, M.J., LaStayo, P.C., 2004. Pronator syndrome and other nerve compressions that mimic carpal tunnel syndrome. J. Orthop. Sports Phys. Ther. 34, 601–609.

Loh, Y.C., Lam, W.L., Stanley, J.K., Soames, R.W., 2004. A new clinical test for radial tunnel syndrome, the Rule-of-Nine test: a cadaveric study. J. Orthop. Surg. 12, 83–86.

Lund, A.T., Amadio, P.C., 2006. Treatment of cubital tunnel syndrome: perspectives for the therapist. J. Hand Ther. 19, 170–178.

Mackinnon, E., 2002. Pathophysiology of nerve compression. Hand Clin. 18, 231–241.

Mondelli, M., Giannini, F., Ballerini, M., et al., 2005. Incidence of ulnar neuropathy at the elbow in the province of Siena (Italy). J. Neurol. Sci. 234, 5–10.

Nakazumi, Y., Hamasaki, M., 2001. Electrophysiological studies and physical examinations in entrapment neuropathy: sensory and motor functions compensation for the central nervous system in cases with peripheral nerve damage.

Electromyogr. Clin. Neurophysiol. 41, 345–348.

Okamoto, M., Abe, M., Shirai, H., Ueda, N., 2000. Morphology and dynamics of the ulnar nerve in the cubital tunnel. Observation by ultrasonography. J. Hand Surg. [Br.] 25, 85–89.

Padua, L., Aprile, I., Caliandro, P., Foschini, M., Mazza, S., Tonali, P., 2002. Natural history of ulnar entrapment at elbow. Clin. Neurophysiol. 113, 1980–1984.

Pascarelli, E.F., Hsu, Y.P., 2001. Understanding work-related upper extremity disorders: clinical findings in 485 computer users, musicians, and others. J. Occup. Rehabil. 11, 1–21.

Pinar, L., Enhos, A., Ada, S., Gungor, N., 2005. Can we use nerve gliding exercises in women with carpal tunnel syndrome? Adv. Ther. 22, 467–475.

Rayan, G.M., Jensen, C., Duke, J., 1992. Elbow flexion test in the normal population. J. Hand Surg. [Am.] 17, 86–89.

Richardson, J.K., Green, D.F., Jamieson, S.C., Valentin, F.C., 2001. Gender, body mass and age as risk factors for ulnar mononeuropathy at the elbow. Muscle Nerve 24, 551–554.

Rinker, B., Effron, C.R., Beasley, R.W., 2004. Proximal radial compression neuropathy. Ann. Plast. Surg. 52, 174–180.

Robertson, C., Saratsiotis, J., 2005. A review of compressive ulnar neuropathy at the elbow. J. Manipulative Physiol. Ther. 28, 345.

Roquelaure, Y., Raimbeau, G., Dano, C., et al., 2000. Occupational risk factors for radial tunnel syndrome in industrial workers. Scand. J. Work Environ. Health 26, 507–513.

Rosati, M., Martignoni, R., Spagnolli, G., Nesti, C., Lisanti, M., 1998. Clinical validity of the elbow flexion test for the diagnosis of ulnar nerve compression at the cubital tunnel. Acta Orthop. Belg. 64, 366–370.

Seror, P., Nathan, P.A., 1993. Relative frequency of nerve conduction abnormalities at carpal tunnel and cubital tunnel in France and the United States: importance of silent neuropathies and role of ulnar neuropathy after unsuccessful carpal tunnel syndrome release. Ann. Chir. Main Memb. Super. 12, 281–285.

Svernlov, B., Larsson, M., Rehn, K., Adolfsson, L., 2009. Conservative treatment of the cubital tunnel syndrome. Journal of Hand Surgery European 34, 201–207.

Szabo, R.M., Kwak, C., 2007. Natural history and conservative management of cubital tunnel syndrome. Hand Clin. 23, 311–313.

Warwick, L., Seradge, H., 1995. Early versus late range of motion following cubital tunnel surgery. J. Hand Ther. 8, 245–248.

Wright, T.W., Glowczewskie, F., Cowin, D., Wheeler, D.L., 2001. Ulnar nerve excursion and strain at the elbow and wrist associated with upper extremity motion. J. Hand Surg. [Am.] 26, 655–662.

Chapter | 30 |

Joint mobilization and manipulation

Peter A Huijbregts, Freddy M Kaltenborn, Traudi Baldauf Kaltenborn

INTRODUCTION

Therapists use mobilization and manipulation techniques to reduce pain and increase range of motion (ROM) (Kaltenborn et al 2007). Kaltenborn et al (2007) classify joint restrictions as peri-articular, extra-articular, intra-articular, or combined in aetiology. Peri-articular restrictions due to adaptive shortening of neuromuscular and inert structures (including skin, retinacula, and scar tissue) and extra-articular structures (capsule and ligaments) are best treated with sustained mobilization techniques, whereas peri-articular restriction due to muscle hypertonicity responds best to neurophysiological inhibitory techniques. Intra-articular restrictions are best treated with (traction) manipulation initiated from the actual resting position (Kaltenborn et al 2008).

Guiding both diagnosis and management, Kaltenborn et al (2007) have described grades of movement (Fig 30.1):

- Grade I is a very small traction force that eliminates the normal compressive forces across the joint
- Grade II takes up the slack with initially very little resistance to passive movement (slack zone), then more resistance as tissues are tightened (transition zone), and finally a marked resistance called the first stop
- Grade III occurs after the first stop: as tissues become taut, resistance to movement rapidly increases within this range

© 2011 Elsevier Ltd.
DOI: 10.1016/B978-0-7020-3528-9.00030-3

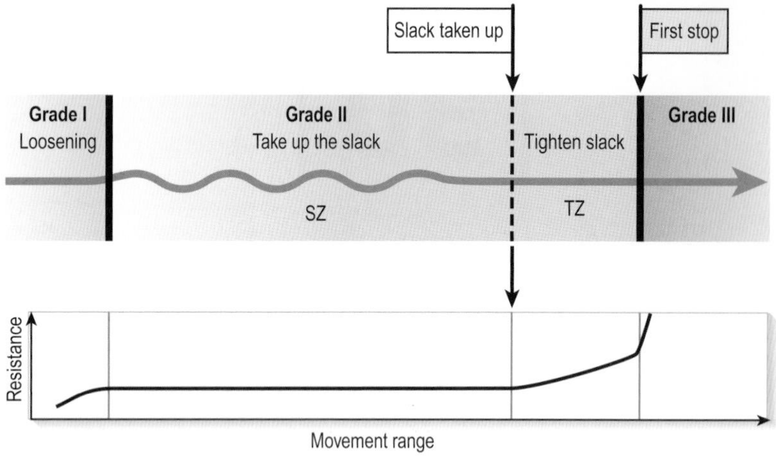

Fig 30.1 Kaltenborn grades of movement

(redrawn from Kaltenborn et al 2007, with permission).

In joint dysfunction both the expected normal excursion and resistance to movement for the various grades will be altered. Grade I traction movements facilitate gliding movements used during examination, mobilization, and manipulation and are applied during all techniques described later. Treatment to relieve pain occurs in the grade I and grade II slack zone ranges. Limited movement in the absence of shortened tissues can be treated by joint mobilization techniques throughout grade II (Kaltenborn et al 2007). Extra-articular restrictions due to capsulo-ligamentous connective tissue shortening are best treated with non-thrust grade III mobilization techniques. Thrust manipulation techniques are used both for diagnosis and management of intra-articular restrictions (Kaltenborn et al 2008). To date, the specific nature of these intra-articular restrictions remains unknown but clinically they may present with restricted ROM; an earlier first stop, abnormal end-feel, and altered through-range resistance (perhaps due to small positional faults or synovial fluid changes with resultant alterations in cohesion and adhesion) with traction and gliding joint play motions; and pain on compression due to possible intra-articular entrapment of sensitive structures.

Without proposing the location of the tissue at fault, Mulligan (2004) has suggested 'minor positional faults' as an alternate aetiology for joint dysfunction that will respond to mobilizations with movement (MWM). With an MWM the therapist applies a sustained accessory glide, long axis rotation, or combination while the patient actively performs a previously painful movement (see Chapter 20 of this textbook for further discussion of MWM in the shoulder). Central to both the Kaltenborn and the Mulligan approach is the emphasis on restoration of the gliding component of the normal joint roll-gliding movement (Exelby 1996). Central to both is also the treatment plane defined as the plane across the concave joint surface. With translatoric techniques encompassing

traction, compression, and gliding techniques, traction and compression are done perpendicular to this treatment plane, whereas gliding techniques induce movement parallel to this plane (Kaltenborn et al 2007).

Whereas Kaltenborn emphasizes gliding techniques in the direction normally associated with the restricted physiological motion, Mulligan often starts with a sustained glide at a right angle to this physiological glide. An iterative process then tests glides in different directions or long axis rotation before settling on the most effective direction allowing for pain-free active range of motion or isometric muscle contraction constituting the MWM (Exelby 1996, Hsieh et al 2002). Two to three sets of 6–10 repetitions are performed supported by a home programme of self-mobilization and corrective taping (Mulligan 2004). An additional difference between Kaltenborn and Mulligan techniques is that the Kaltenborn concept uses only straight-lined (linear) gliding techniques parallel to treatment plane for joint mobilization, whereas Mulligan adapts continuously to the contour of the joint surface with curvilinear gliding techniques. It should be noted that within the Kaltenborn concept curvilinear gliding techniques have traditionally also been used, albeit for assisted active movements and solely according to the convex-concave rule.

SCIENTIFIC EVIDENCE FOR MOBILIZATION OF THE WRIST AND HAND

Research evidence for the use of mobilization and manipulation techniques in the wrist and hand region is limited but emerging. Using animal research, Olson (1987) showed increased passive ROM and ROM during gait in dogs with immobilization-induced radio-carpal hypomobility receiving end range oscillatory traction and gliding mobilization compared to controls not receiving this intervention.

Sucher (1994) provided preliminary clinical evidence for manual therapy for patients with carpal tunnel syndrome (CTS) in the form of an uncontrolled case series showing decreased severity of symptoms and normalization of electrodiagnostic findings. Sucher et al (2005) also provided basic science evidence in cadavers for the use of sustained manual techniques including variations of the opponens roll and transverse carpal extension manoeuvres intended to stretch the flexor retinaculum. Noting significant within-group improvement for self-reported physical and mental distress, nerve conduction studies and finger sensation for both study groups, Davis et al (1998) however found no significant between-group differences in their randomized controlled trial (RCT) of 91 subjects with CTS treated with 16 sessions over 9 weeks of chiropractic cervico-thoracic spine and upper extremity joint and soft tissue manipulation, ultrasound, and night splinting or with medical management consisting of ibuprofen and splinting. In 21 patients with CTS scheduled for surgery, Tal-Akabi & Rushton (2000) compared 3 weeks of treatment with neurodynamic mobilization or with palmar and dorsal carpal gliding mobilization and flexor retinaculum stretching to a control group. They reported significant within-group improvements with regard to pain and active wrist extension ROM for both mobilization groups and significant between-group differences favouring both experimental groups over the control group with regard to pain. Six of seven subjects in the control group proceeded with surgery, whereas 11 of 14 in the mobilization groups cancelled surgery. Two systematic reviews (O'Connor et al 2003, Muller et al 2004) have recommended carpal bone mobilization for the management of patients with CTS.

In an RCT with 30 patients, Taylor & Bennell (1994) compared management of patients with Colles fracture consisting of advice, heat, and a home programme to the same programme combined with manual mobilization and reported no between-group difference in wrist extension ROM. In an RCT with 32 patients, McPhate & Robertson (1998) looked at effects of a home programme with or without manual mobilization and found no between-group difference for wrist extension ROM or grip strength, but significantly lower pain scores in the mobilization group. Kay et al (2000) randomly assigned 39 patients with cast and/or internal fixation post-Colles fracture to a home programme with or without Maitland grade 1–2 accessory mobilization of the distal radio-ulnar and carpal joints progressing to grade 3–4 physiological techniques. They reported significant within-group differences on pain, ROM, grip strength, and function for both groups but only one statistically (but not clinically) significant difference in wrist flexion ROM favouring the mobilization group. Using a single-subject design for eight subjects with stable (type I or III) Colles fractures, Coyle & Robertson (2002) compared six sessions of various combinations of two

60-second end-range oscillatory and sustained palmar gliding radio-carpal mobilization in maximum pain-free extension and noted improvement in wrist extension ROM in both groups. They also noted that oscillation was most effective in increasing ROM if used first in treatment session and in the presence of pain, whereas the sustained technique was more effective in later treatment sessions and when used as a second technique for increasing ROM. A systematic review reflected these equivocal findings in stating that manual mobilization for Colles fracture was not supported by an RCT but did show positive outcomes in a case series design (Michlovitz et al 2004).

Randall et al (1992) randomly assigned 18 subjects after at least 2 weeks of immobilization for a metacarpal fracture to an active ROM home programme or a home programme combined with three sessions of end range oscillatory metacarpophalangeal (MCP) traction and gliding mobilization. Over the course of one week, the mobilization group improved significantly with regard to joint stiffness and ROM as compared to the control group. Two case reports have also lent support to the use of long axis rotation MWM in post-fall MCP I dysfunction, although one report using MRI did not support Mulligan's hypothesis of resolution of a 'minor positional fault' (Folk 2001, Hsieh et al 2002).

One case report indicated the possible benefit of a multimodal management approach in a patient with De Quervain syndrome consisting of neural mobilization and joint mobilization of the cervico-thoracic spine, shoulder, and wrist including palmar and dorsal gliding mobilization of the capitate and lunate bone (Anderson & Tichenor 1994). Backstrom (2002) reported positive outcomes in a patient with De Quervain syndrome using a multi-modal programme including palmar manipulation of the capitate, 'conventional' joint mobilization, and MWM techniques including radial glide of the proximal carpal row during thumb and wrist motion and ulnar glide of the trapezium and trapezoid bones during active thumb motion.

Reflecting the role of the wrist in the upper extremity kinetic chain, Struijs et al (2003) compared (a maximum of) nine treatments over 6 weeks of 15–20 minutes of repeated palmar scaphoid gliding manipulation and passive wrist ROM with a control treatment of friction massage, ultrasound, and strengthening in an RCT on 28 patients with lateral epicondylalgia. They reported a significant between-group difference on a global measure of improvement at 3 weeks and on pain at 6 weeks both favouring the manipulation group.

MOBILIZATION/MANIPULATION OF THE WRIST AND HAND

In the Kaltenborn concept, traction mobilization and manipulation are specific translatoric techniques always performed perpendicular to the treatment plane. When choosing a translatoric gliding mobilization technique, clinicians need to consider the Kaltenborn convex-concave rule describing the arthrokinematic roll-gliding combinations (Kaltenborn et al 2007). When the moving joint partner has a convex joint surface, gliding mobilization occurs in the direction opposite to the direction of restricted bone movement. When the moving joint partner has the concave joint surface, gliding mobilization (in both cases with concurrent grade I traction) occurs in the same direction as the restricted bone movement. Knowledge of joint surface geometry (Mink et al 1990) is, therefore, a necessary prerequisite for appropriate gliding mobilization technique choice. It should be noted that Mulligan MWM techniques generally apply glides perpendicular or even opposite to the directions proposed by the convex-concave rule assuming the presence of undefined 'minor positional faults' interfering with normal arthrokinematic movement behaviour. Unless otherwise indicated all techniques described in this section are taken from Kaltenborn et al (2007).

In the distal radio-ulnar joint the radius is the concave joint partner and the ulna has the convex joint surface. Supination requires a dorsal glide of the distal radius and pronation a palmar glide in relation to the distal ulna.

The proximal row of carpal bones offers a convex articular surface to the concave radius-triangular fibrocartilage complex. This means that roll and glide occur in opposite directions during radio-carpal movements.

The situation is more complex in the articulation between the proximal and distal carpal row. The concave surface on trapezium and trapezoid articulates with a convex surface on the (biconvex) scaphoid. This means that during wrist extension the trapezium and trapezoid roll dorsally and also glide in a dorsal direction and that during wrist flexion roll and glide of the trapezium and trapezoid are both in a palmar direction. In addition, with the trapezium/trapezoid complex able to assume a more dorsal position, radial deviation is made possible. In the central (lunate/capitate) and ulnar (triquetrum and hamate) carpal bones, the proximal row has the concave joint surfaces, whereas the distal carpals have convex joint surfaces. That means that during wrist extension the roll of the capitate and hamate is dorsal, but glides are in a palmar direction. During wrist flexion, the hamate and capitate roll palmar, but glide dorsally. During wrist extension, the radial carpal bones lock early, but an additional 30° occurs lunate and capitate. This requires the presence of a large amount of mobility between the scaphoid and the adjacent lunate.

The CMC II–IV joints are almost flat joints but the CMC V joint is a sellar joint. The concave surface on the fifth metacarpal runs medial–lateral and the convex surface runs dorsal–palmar. The CMC I joint is also a sellar joint. The concave distal surface is involved in flexion and extension of the thumb; the convex distal surface is involved in abduction and adduction of the thumb, i.e. roll and glide are in the same direction for flexion and extension, whereas for abduction and adduction the roll is in the same and the glide is in the opposite direction of the bone movement.

The distal end of the metacarpals I–V is biconvex; the proximal end of the proximal phalanx is biconcave. Therefore, in the MCP II–V joints roll and glide of the proximal phalanx are in the same direction with both flexion-extension and radial-ulnar deviation. The IP joints I–V are hinge joints with the convexity proximal and the concavity distal resulting in roll and glide in the same direction during flexion and extension.

Distal radio-ulnar joint dorsal glide radius (Fig 30.2)

This technique is indicated in patients with restricted supination. The patient is sitting with arm by the side, the forearm supported on table and supinated. The therapist stands facing the palmar side of the patient's forearm. The stabilizing hand of the therapist fixates the distal ulna on its palmar aspect with the thenar and on its dorsal aspect with the fingertips. The thenar portion of therapist's mobilizing hand provides dorsal gliding mobilization to the distal radius. This technique can be performed in various positions of supination up to pathological end range.

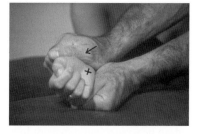

Fig 30.2 Distal radio-ulnar joint dorsal glide radius.

Distal radio-ulnar joint ventral glide radius

This technique is indicated in patients with restricted pronation. The patient is sitting with arm abducted at shoulder, forearm supported on the table and pronated. The therapist stands facing the dorsal side of the patient's forearm. The stabilizing hand of the therapist fixates the distal ulna on its palmar aspect with the fingertips and on its dorsal aspect with thenar or thumb. The thenar portion of therapist's mobilizing hand provides ventral gliding mobilization to distal radius. This mobilization can be performed in various positions of pronation up to pathological end range.

Distal radio-ulnar joint MWM (Mulligan 2004)

This technique is indicated in patients with restricted supination due to minor positional fault (note that the direction of glide is opposite to normal arthrokinematic gliding). The patient is sitting, shoulder flexed, elbow bent, and forearm supinated. The therapist is standing dorsal to the hand. The therapist places the fingers of the ipsilateral hand on the palmar aspect of the distal radius and then covers these with the fingers of the contralateral hand. The ipsilateral thumb is placed over the contralateral thumb on the distal dorsal aspect of the radius. The fingers apply dorsal gliding to ulna and maintaining this, the patient actively supinates (with therapist-applied overpressure).

Radio-carpal traction

This technique serves as an non-specific joint mobilization. The patient is sitting, arm pronated and resting on wedge or table. The therapist stands distal to patient's wrist. The distal forearm is fixated against a wedge by the therapist's stabilizing hand; the thenar portion stabilizes just proximal to the wrist. The mobilizing hand grasps the carpal bones just distal to the wrist joint and performs traction (Fig 30.3).

This technique can be made more effective by various degrees of wrist flexion (Fig 30.4), extension (Fig 30.5), radial deviation, or ulnar deviation; shifting stabilizing and mobilizing hands distally allows for traction between the distal and proximal carpal row. This mobilization can be made more specific when the mobilizing hand grasps one carpal bone with the thumb dorsal and index fingertip ventral.

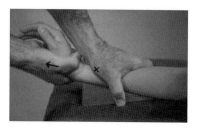

Fig 30.5 Radio-carpal traction in extension.

Radio-carpal palmar glide

This technique is indicated in patients with restricted wrist extension. The patient is sitting, arm pronated and resting on wedge or table. The therapist is standing at the ulnar side of the wrist. The distal forearm is fixated against a wedge by the therapist's stabilizing hand; the thenar portion stabilizes just proximal to the wrist. The mobilizing hand grasps the carpal bones just distal to the wrist joint and performs the palmar glide (Fig 30.6).

This mobilization can be also done in various degrees of wrist extension (Fig 30.7); shifting stabilizing and mobilizing hands distally allows for glide between distal and proximal carpal row. It can be made more specific when the head of metacarpal II of the mobilizing hand is placed on one carpal bone.

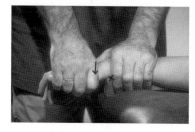

Fig 30.6 Radio-carpal palmar glide.

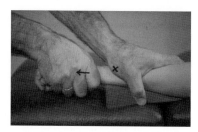

Fig 30.3 Radio-carpal traction.

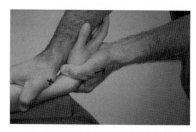

Fig 30.4 Radio-carpal traction in flexion.

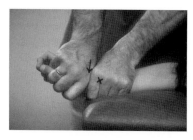

Fig 30.7 Radio-carpal palmar glide in extension.

Radio-carpal dorsal glide

This technique is indicated in patients with restricted wrist flexion. The patient is sitting, arm supinated and resting on a wedge. The therapist is standing at the radial side of the wrist. The distal forearm is fixated against the wedge by the therapist's stabilizing hand; the thenar portion stabilizes just proximal to the wrist. The mobilizing hand grasps the carpal bones just distal to wrist joint and performs the dorsal glide (Fig 30.8).

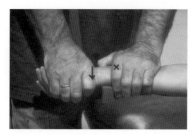

Fig 30.8 Radio-carpal dorsal glide.

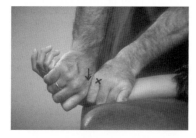

Fig 30.9 Radio-carpal dorsal glide in flexion.

This technique can be also done in various degrees of wrist flexion (Fig 30.9); shifting stabilizing and mobilizing hands distally allows for glide between the distal and proximal carpal row.

Radio-carpal radial glide (Fig 30.10)

This technique is indicated in patients with restricted ulnar deviation. The patient is sitting, shoulder abducted, forearm pronated and resting on a wedge. Patient can be also

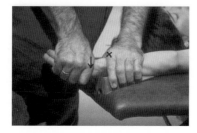

Fig 30.10 Radio-carpal radial glide.

supine, shoulder elevated and externally rotated. The therapist is standing at the palmar side of the wrist. The distal forearm is fixated against a wedge by the therapist's stabilizing hand just proximal to wrist. The mobilizing hand grasps the carpal bones from the ulnar side just distal to the wrist joint and performs the radial glide. This mobilization can be done in various degrees of wrist ulnar deviation.

Radio-carpal ulnar glide (Fig 30.11)

This technique is indicated in patients with restricted radial deviation. The patient is sitting, arm supinated and resting with the ulnar aspect on a wedge. The therapist is standing at the dorsal side of the wrist. The distal forearm is fixated against the wedge by the therapist's stabilizing hand just proximal to the wrist. The mobilizing hand grasps the carpal bones from the radial side just distal to the wrist joint and performs the ulnar glide. The mobilization can be also done in various degrees of wrist radial deviation.

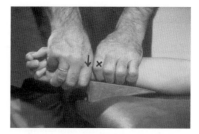

Fig 30.11 Radio-carpal ulnar glide.

Radio-carpal MWM (Mulligan 2004)

This technique is indicated in patients with restricted wrist extension or flexion due to a minor positional fault (note the direction of glide is perpendicular to normal arthrokinematic gliding). The patient is sitting. The therapist is standing proximal to the wrist. The therapist grasps the distal forearm with one hand so that the web between index finger and thumb lies over the distal radius. The other hand grasps the proximal carpal row from the ulnar aspect so that the web space is now over the triquetrum. Radial translation is applied to the proximal carpal row until a direction is found that allows the patient to perform previously painful active wrist flexion or extension.

Opponens roll (Sucher 1994)

This technique is indicated in patients with decreased length of the flexor retinaculum implicated in the aetiology of CTS. The patient is sitting, arm supinated and resting on the table. The therapist is standing distal to patient's hand. The thumb and thenar portion of the ipsilateral hand stabilize the ulnar palmar aspect of hand. The thumb is then brought into abduction with slight extension and supination along the axis of the first metacarpal bone by the contralateral hand of the therapist.

Transverse carpal extension (Sucher et al 2005)

This technique is indicated in patients with decreased length of the flexor retinaculum implicated in the aetiology of CTS. The patient is sitting, arm supinated and resting on the table. The therapist is standing distal to the patient's hand. The mobilization consists of a three-point bending technique whereby the therapist hooks his/her thumbs on the inner palmar edge of the carpal bones (trapezium and hamate distally, scaphoid and pisiform proximally) while his/her fingers wrap around dorsally to converge on the centre of the wrist providing a counterforce. The technique can be done combined with passive thumb and little finger abduction and extension or with the opponens roll technique. Similar three-point techniques over the metacarpal bones causing concave and convex movements of the metacarpal arch can be done as a general mobilization for the inter-metacarpal connections.

Radial carpal palmar glides

This technique is indicated in patients with restricted wrist extension and radial deviation. The patient is sitting, arm pronated and resting on a wedge. The therapist is standing at the ulnar side of the wrist. The distal radius is fixated against the wedge by the therapist's stabilizing hand; the thenar portion stabilizes dorsal just proximal to wrist with the fingers palmar. The mobilizing hand grasps the patient's hand from the radial side; with thenar eminence dorsal against the scaphoid the therapist glides the scaphoid palmar. Moving the fixation distally to include the scaphoid and mobilizing the trapezium and trapezoid in a palmar direction increases restricted flexion and ulnar deviation.

Central carpal palmar glides
(Fig 30.12)

This technique is indicated in patients with restricted wrist extension. The patient is sitting, arm pronated and resting

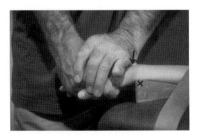

Fig 30.12 Central carpal palmar glides.

on a wedge. The therapist is standing distal to the wrist. The distal radius is fixated against the wedge by a fixation belt. The therapist with one hand grasps the patient's hand from the radial side with the thumb dorsal and index finger palmar over the lunate; the hypothenar of the other hand placed over own thumb glides the lunate palmar. Moving the fixation distally to include the lunate and mobilizing the capitate in a palmar direction increases restricted extension.

Ulnar carpal palmar glides

This technique is indicated in patients with restricted wrist extension. The patient is sitting, arm pronated and resting on a wedge. The therapist is standing distal to the wrist. The distal ulna is fixated against the wedge by a fixation belt. The therapist grasps the patient's hand from ulnar side with the thumb dorsal and index finger palmar over the triquetrum; the hypothenar of the other hand placed over own thumb glides the triquetrum palmar. Moving the fixation distally to include the triquetrum and mobilizing the hamate in a palmar direction increases restricted extension.

Radial carpal dorsal glides

This technique is indicated in patients with restricted wrist flexion and ulnar deviation. The patient is sitting, arm supinated and resting on a wedge. The therapist stands distal to wrist. The distal radius is fixated dorsal against the wedge by a fixation belt. With one hand the therapist grasps the patient's hand from the radial side with the thumb palmar on the scaphoid and fingers dorsal; the hypothenar of the other hand is placed on own thumb and produces the dorsal glide. Moving the fixation distally to include the scaphoid and then mobilizing the trapezium and trapezoid in a dorsal direction will increase restricted extension and radial deviation. With all carpal dorsal glides, the therapist may need to 'soften' contact on the often painful palmar aspect of the carpal bones, for example by using the head of the second metacarpal rather than the thumb as a palmar contact.

Central carpal dorsal glides

This mobilization is indicated in patients with restricted wrist flexion. The patient is sitting, arm supinated and resting on a wedge. The therapist stands distal to the wrist. The distal radius is fixated dorsal against the wedge by fixation belt. The therapist's one hand grasps the hand from the radial side with the thumb (or 'softer' contact) palmar on lunate and index finger dorsal; the other hand places hypothenar on own thumb and produces a dorsal glide. Moving the fixation distally to include the lunate and mobilizing the capitate in a dorsal direction increases restricted flexion.

Ulnar carpal dorsal glides

This mobilization is indicated in patients with restricted wrist flexion. The patient is sitting, arm supinated and resting on a wedge. The therapist is standing distal to the wrist. The distal ulna is fixated dorsal against the wedge by fixation belt. The therapist's hand grasps the hand from the ulnar side with thumb (or 'softer' contact) palmar on triquetrum and index finger dorsal; the other hand places the hypothenar on own thumb and produces a dorsal glide. Moving the fixation distally to include the triquetrum and mobilizing the hamate in a dorsal direction increases restricted flexion.

Carpal glide manipulation with proximal fixation (Fig 30.13)

This manipulation is indicated in patients with restricted wrist extension (in the presence of normal radial and ulnar deviation). The patient stands with the arm flexed forward at the shoulder. The therapist stands in front of the patient and grips the patient's hand from both sides. The index fingers on top of each other stabilize the lunate on its palmar aspect. The capitate bone is contacted with the pads of thumbs on top of each other on its dorsal aspect. Slack is taken up and tightened between the index fingers and thumbs. The impulse consists of a quick downward movement of the patient's arm and wrist from a slightly flexed position. The movement stops suddenly, when the wrist is in the zero position (not in extension). A traction component is maintained throughout the whole procedure. This technique can be applied for wrist extension restrictions resulting from joint restrictions between radius and lunate, lunate and capitate (described above), and radius and scaphoid. The site of restriction in case of restricted extension and radial deviation is mostly between the radius and scaphoid, and/or scaphoid and trapezoid/trapezium complex. A manipulation to restore movement between the scaphoid and trapezoid-trapezium complex in case of restricted extension and radial deviation is described not here but under the next technique. Note that proximal fixation on the palmar aspect of the scaphoid with a thrust applied to the dorsal aspect of the trapezoid/trapezium complex serves to increase wrist flexion.

Carpal glide manipulation with distal fixation (Fig 30.14)

This manipulation is indicated in patients with restricted wrist flexion. The patient stands with the arm flexed forward at the shoulder. The therapist stands in front of the patient and grips the patient's hand from both sides. The index fingers on top of each other stabilize the capitate on its palmar aspect. The lunate is contacted with the pads of the thumbs on top of each other on its dorsal aspect. Slack is taken up and tightened between the index fingers and thumbs. The impulse consists of a quick downward movement of the patient's arm and wrist from a slightly flexed position. The movement stops suddenly, when the wrist is in the zero position (not in extension). A traction component is maintained throughout the whole procedure. Often the palmar aspects of the carpal bones are too sensitive to have a thrust applied to them. Therefore, with distal fixation, the distal bone is stabilized and the proximal bone is moved in a palmar direction resulting in relative dorsal movement of the distal bone. This technique can be used for all bones in the proximal and distal row. Note that carpal glide manipulation of the scaphoid with distal fixation of the trapezoid/trapezium complex is used for restricted wrist extension and radial deviation.

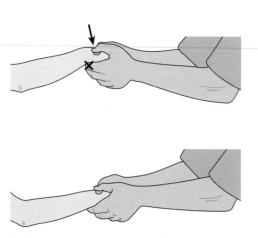

Fig 30.13 Carpal glide manipulation with proximal fixation.

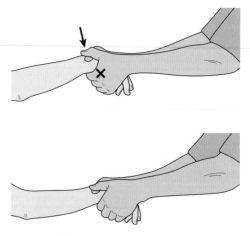

Fig 30.14 Carpal glide manipulation with distal fixation.

Carpometacarpal (CMC) I traction

The patient is sitting, arm stabilized with its ulnar aspect against the table. The therapist is standing proximal to the hand. The stabilizing hand of the therapist fixates the trapezium with the thumb palmar and fingers dorsal. The therapist's mobilizing hand grasps the first metacarpal with the thenar dorsal (radial) and finger palmar and applies traction (Fig 30.15). Similar techniques with the hand pronated on the table, the proximal joint partner stabilized, and the metacarpal bone tractioned can be used for the CMC II–V joints (Fig 30.16).

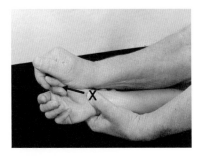

Fig 30.15 Carpometacarpal (CMC) I traction.

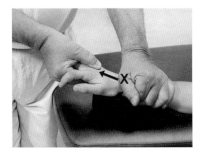

Fig 30.16 Carpometacarpal (CMC) II–V joints traction.

Carpometacarpal (CMC) I glides
(Fig 30.17)

These techniques are indicated in patients with restricted thumb movements. The stabilizing hand grasps the trapezium with the thumb dorsal and index finger palmar and fixates it in a position maximally rotated towards the palm. The mobilizing hand grasps the first metacarpal just distal to the CMC I joint space and applies the glides:

1. For restricted abduction and adduction, the patient sits with the ulnar side of the hand against the therapist's body (Fig 30.17). For restricted abduction, the glide is in a dorsal direction. For restricted adduction, the glide is in a palmar direction (convex rule).
2. For restricted extension and flexion, the patient's hand is turned, so that the dorsal side is against the therapist's body (not pictured). For restricted

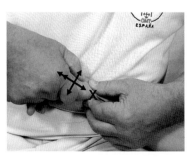

Fig 30.17 Carpometacarpal (CMC) I glides.

extension, the glide is in a radial direction. For restricted flexion, the glide direction is ulnar (concave rule).

Metacarpophalangeal (MCP) I MWM (Folk 2001, Hsieh et al 2002)

This mobilization in indicated in patients with restricted MCP I motion due to a minor positional fault (medial or lateral glide is perpendicular to normal arthrokinematic gliding). The patient is sitting, elbow bent, forearm supinated. The therapist is standing or sitting at the radial aspect of the patient's wrist. The therapist stabilizes the first metacarpal bone between index finger and thumb and applies lateral or medial glide or long-axis rotation that allows the patient to perform a previously painful motion.

Finger joint traction (Fig 30.18)

The patient is sitting, arm supinated, with the dorsum of the hand resting on a wedge or table. The therapist is sitting or standing at the distal aspect of the hand. The thenar eminence of the therapist's stabilizing hand fixates the proximal joint partner. The mobilizing hand grips the distal joint partner and applies traction. The technique can be done in various finger joint positions; shifting fixation distally allows for traction to first MCP, then PIP, then DIP joints.

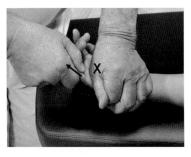

Fig 30.18 Finger joint traction.

Finger joint glides

This technique in indicated in patients with restricted MCP, PIP, or DIP extension. The patient is sitting, arm supinated, the dorsum of the hand resting on the wedge or table. The therapist is sitting or standing at ulnar aspect of the hand. The thenar eminence of the therapist's stabilizing hand fixates the proximal joint partner. The mobilizing hand grips distal joint partner and applies a dorsal glide. With the hand pronated a palmar glide can be applied to mobilize flexion. Radial and ulnar glides can be used at the MCP joints to restore radial and ulnar deviation, respectively.

Finger joint MWM (Mulligan 2004)

This technique is indicated in patients with restricted PIP or DIP flexion due to minor positional fault (the direction of glide is perpendicular to normal arthrokinematic gliding). The patient is sitting. The therapist is standing to the side of the patient. The therapist fixates the proximal partner between thumb and index finger. A medial or lateral glide is applied to the distal joint partner until a direction is found that allows the patient to perform previously painful active PIP or DIP finger flexion.

ACKNOWLEDGEMENT

The authors would like to gratefully acknowledge the librarian of the Physical Therapy Association of British Columbia, Ms. Deb Monkman, MLS, BSc, for her help in retrieving the references used in this chapter.

REFERENCES

Anderson, M., Tichenor, C.J., 1994. A patient with De Quervain's tenosynovitis: A case report using an Australian approach to manual therapy. Phys. Ther. 74, 314–326.

Backstrom, K.M., 2002. Mobilization with movement as an adjunct intervention in a patient with complicated De Quervain's tenosynovitis: A case report. J. Orthop. Sports Phys. Ther. 32, 86–97.

Coyle, J.A., Robertson, V.J., 2002. Comparison of two passive mobilizing techniques following Colles' fracture: A multi-element design. Man. Ther. 3, 34–41.

Davis, P.T., Hulbert, J.R., Kassak, K.M., Meyer, J.J., 1998. Comparative efficacy of conservative medical and chiropractic treatments for carpal tunnel syndrome: A randomized clinical trial. J. Manipulative Physiol. Ther. 21, 317–326.

Exelby, L., 1996. Peripheral mobilisations with movement. Man. Ther. 1, 118–126.

Folk, B., 2001. Traumatic thumb injury management using mobilization with movement. Man. Ther. 6, 178–182.

Hsieh, C.Y., Vicenzino, B., Yang, C.H., Hu, M.H., Yang, C., 2002. Mulligan's mobilization with movement for the thumb: A single case report using magnetic resonance imaging to evaluate the positional fault hypothesis. Man. Ther. 7, 44–49.

Kaltenborn, F.M., Baldauf Kaltenborn, T., Vollowitz, E., 2008. Manual mobilization of the joints: joint examination and basic treatment. vol. III: Traction-manipulation of the extremities and spine, basic thrust techniques. Norli, Oslo.

Kaltenborn, F.M., Evjenth, O., Baldauf Kaltenborn, T., Morgan, D., Vollowitz, E., 2007. Manual mobilization of the extremity joints: joint examination and basic treatment. vol. I: The extremities, sixth revised ed. Norli, Oslo.

Kay, S., Haensel, N., Stiller, K., 2000. The effect of passive mobilization following fractures involving the distal radius: A randomised study. Aust. J. Physiother. 46, 93–101.

McPhate, M., Robertson, V.J., 1998. Physiotherapy treatment of Colles fractures: Hands off or hands on? In: Proceedings of the fifth international Australian physiotherapy association congress. APA, Hobart, p. 235.

Michlovitz, S.L., Harris, B.A., Watkins, M.P., 2004. Therapy interventions for improving joint range of motion: A systematic review. J. Hand Ther. 17, 118–131.

Mink, A.J.F., Ter Veer, H.J., Vorselaars, J.A.C.T., 1990. Extremiteiten: Functie-onderzoek en manuele therapie. Bohn Stafleu Van Loghum, Houten.

Muller, M., Tsui, D., Schnurr, R., Biddulph-Deisroth, L., Hard, J.,

MacDermid, J., 2004. Effectiveness of hand therapy interventions in the primary management of carpal tunnel syndrome: A systematic review. J. Hand Ther. 17, 210–228.

Mulligan, B.R., 2004. Manual therapy: 'NAGS', 'SNAGS', 'MWMS' etc., fifth ed. Plane View Services Ltd, Wellington.

O'Connor, D., Marshall, S.C., Massy-Westropp, N., 2003. Non-surgical treatment (other than steroid injection) for carpal tunnel syndrome. Cochrane Database Syst. Rev. (1). Art. No.: CD003219.

Olson, V.L., 1987. Evaluation of joint mobilization treatment. Phys. Ther. 67, 351–356.

Randall, T., Portney, L., Harris, B.A., 1992. Effects of joint mobilization on joint stiffness and active motion of the metacarpal-phalangeal joint. J. Orthop. Sports Phys. Ther. 16, 30–36.

Struijs, P.A.A., Damen, P.J., Baller, E.W.P., Blankevoort, L., Assendelft, W.J.J., Van Dijk, C.N., 2003. Manipulation of the wrist for management of lateral epicondylitis: A randomized pilot study. Phys. Ther. 83, 608–616.

Sucher, B.M., 1994. Palpatory diagnosis and manipulative management of carpal tunnel syndrome. J. Am. Osteopath. Assoc. 94, 647–663.

Sucher, B.M., Hinrichs, R.N., Welcher, R.L., et al., 2005. Manipulative treatment of carpal tunnel syndrome:

biomechanical and osteopathic intervention to increase the length of the transverse carpal ligament: Part 2. Effect of sex differences and manipulative 'priming. J. Am. Osteopath. Assoc. 105, 135–143.

Tal-Akabi, A., Rushton, A., 2000. An investigation to compare the effectiveness of carpal bone mobilization and neurodynamic mobilization as methods of treatment for carpal tunnel syndrome. Man. Ther. 5, 214–222.

Taylor, N.F., Bennell, K.L., 1994. The effectiveness of passive joint mobilisation on the return of active wrist extension following Colles' fracture: A clinical trial. New Zealand Journal of Physiotherapy 22, 24–28.

Chapter 31

Finger and thumb pathology

Joy C MacDermid, Ruby Grewal, B Jane Freure

INTRODUCTION

Physical therapy for the hand must embrace an understanding of the hand as an 'organ' that interfaces the person with their world by bringing in sensory information, and allowing the person to engage in activity that determines function and quality of life. The hand has intricate anatomical structures in close proximity that contract, glide, and heal following injury. Maintaining joint mobility and stability while the structures in the proximity remain free to glide and resist contractile forces are critical to hand motor performance. Issues of motor control and sensory motor integration are critical to the functionality of the hand. Exquisitely innervated, the hand can serve as a sensory organ or contribute painful stimuli that alter the cortex and produce chronic pain. Manual therapy techniques can contribute to normalizing the neurosensorimotor function of the hand, in combination with other techniques. In the current chapter we highlight the most prevalent conditions affecting the digits.

DIGITAL FRACTURES

Epidemiology: incidence, prevalence, economic impact

Hand fractures are a common traumatic injury usually arising during work place, sporting or recreational activities. Fractures of the metacarpals and phalanges are most

© 2011 Elsevier Ltd.
DOI: 10.1016/B978-0-7020-3528-9.00031-5

common (Hove 1993, Van Onselen et al 2003, Aitken & Court-Brown 2008, Feehan & Sheps 2008a). Border digits are the most commonly affected (thumb/small finger). The majorities are treated conservatively (Feehan & Sheps 2008b). Metacarpal fractures represent 35% of hand fractures.

Anatomy

To better understand hand fractures one must first understand the relationship between both soft tissue and bony factors that contribute to both soft tissue and skeletal stability. We suggest that readers consult a standard anatomy text or The Electronic Textbook of Hand Surgery (http://www.eatonhand.com/hom/hom033.htm) website for details of hand/wrist anatomy as we only will highlight key elements. The latter website has primal pictures used with permission, some radiographic images of anatomy and pathology and information on various bony and soft tissues providing accessible and clearly visualize aspects of key anatomical features. More detailed descriptions of anatomical features are available in classic anatomic textbooks.

Pathology

Bone fractures result from excessive force, in comparison to bone strength. Fracture angulation is determined by the forces exerted by the soft tissues on both the proximal and distal fragment. Movement recovery following fracture can be affected by the nature and severity of the original fracture, associated soft tissue injuries and the extent of malalignment in bony structure that occurs following bony healing.

The mechanism of injury plays a role in the type of fractures that should be anticipated. A direct blow will result in a transverse fracture, a twisting injury will cause a spiral fracture and combination of torque and axial force will result in a short oblique fracture. Fractures are further classified based on the location (head, neck, shaft or base of a specific hand bone) and any associated soft tissue injury.

All fractures are associated with soft tissue injury. The nature of these injuries can be difficult to determine even with imaging and clinical examination. Muscle and ligament injuries can be important aspects of the fracture and may become more evident as the fracture heals and swelling subsides, or when movement is initiated. Scar healing of injured soft tissue can be a substantial component of active movement limitation.

Metacarpal fractures

The metacarpal bones have intrinsic stability provided by strong interosseus ligaments binding them to the carpal bones and proximally by the transverse metacarpal ligament which links all metacarpal heads. Ligaments tend to prevent excessive displacement with injury. The fifth metacarpal is commonly fractured during a 'punch' mechanism (the majority of these injuries occur in males) and are treated conservatively since full motion/function is often obtained despite malrotation. There is generally a good blood supply which supports high rates of healing, usually within 4–6 weeks. The most important soft tissue concerns are preserving MP joint flexion and maintaining EDC glide.

Fractures of the base of metacarpals are intra-articular fractures that result usually from high forces that disrupt the rigid carpal ligaments of the index and middle finger or overwhelm the normal flexibility of the ulnar metacarpals. Shaft fractures are extra-articular fractures that usually arise during a fall or blow and usually angulating dorsally (with components of shortening or rotation). They are described as transverse, oblique or spiral. Intrinsic muscle tension will cause both ends of the metacarpal bone to flex into an apex dorsal presentation. This causes a shortening which compromises the extensor mechanism by altering the muscle length relationship. Metacarpal neck fractures are the most common metacarpal fracture ('boxers fracture'). The impact of a closed fist causes a break at the extra-articular neck. If associated with a bite, infection is a potential complication which can substantially increase tissue damage. Metacarpal head fractures are intra-articular fractures caused by high axial loading that may involve collateral ligaments and substantial comminution. These fractures can lead to chronic pain and joint instability.

Phalangeal fractures

Phalangeal fractures have greater tendency towards instability as the phalanges lack intrinsic muscle support and are adversely affected by the mechanical forces of the extrinsic flexors and extensors. However these fractures are also more likely to become stiff with immobilization (Shehadi 1991) (predicted motion return of 84%). If immobilization is longer than 4 weeks, predicted motion is 66%.

Intra-articular fractures of the base of the proximal phalanx (PP) usually occur following an abduction force most commonly seen in sports injuries or a fall. Displaced fractures may not be reducible conservatively because of collateral ligament avulsion which worsens the fracture displacement with MP flexion. This can lead to higher rates of non-union with conservative management (Shewring & Thomas 2006). PP shaft fractures have the poorest prognosis for regaining full ability as they occur in the flexor zone two. Since 90% of the proximal phalanx surface is covered by gliding structures these can easily become adherent to the fracture callus. PP condyle fractures usually occur with the lateral deviation force and may be associated with collateral ligament injury. This is a common sports injury, and a common missed diagnosis.

The interossei and lumbricals muscles are the prime MCP flexors. The lumbricals originate from the tendons of the flexor digitorum profundus tendon and the three palmar and four dorsal interossei muscles originate from the volar and dorsal surface of the metacarpal respectively (Smith 1975). The interossei insert onto the antero-lateral base of the proximal phalanx and on the extensor mechanism forming part of the lateral band with the lumbricals, which also inserts dorsally into the extensor apparatus. These intrinsic muscles, along with the extrinsic flexor tendons create deforming forces on the fractured metacarpal shaft resulting in apex dorsal angulation (Flatt 1996). A proximal phalanx fracture will typically angulate with an apex volar deformity because the interossei will flex the proximal fragment due to their insertion at the proximal phalangeal base while the distal fragment is pulled into hyperextension by the central slip which inserts at the base of the middle phalanx and acts to extend the distal fragment.

Fractures of the shaft of the MP occur less commonly, and may displace dorsally or volarly. Intra-articular fractures at the base of the middle phalanx (MP) occur commonly from a fall or direct force. These may be associated with PIP joint dislocation and damage to the volar plate and/or central slip. If the compression trauma is severe, a comminuted fracture of the articular surface, with depression of the fragments into the bone shaft or 'pilon' fracture occurs. MP fractures of the distal third tend to angulate with an apex volar deformity as the flexor digitorum superficialis (FDS) acts to flex the proximal fragment. A proximal third fracture usually angulates with an apex dorsal deformity as the FDS will flex the distal fragment while the central slip extends the proximal fragment.

DP fractures are common during crush injuries and may not displace significantly because the presence of a rigid nail plate dorsally helps to preserve alignment. However, due to the space restrictions inherent in the fingertip anatomic structures and their dense innervations, these injuries can be particularly painful. The distal phalanx (DP) accounts first 50% of hand fractures, which may be attributed to its vulnerability as the fingertip. Tendons avulsion alone or with a variable amount of the articular surface 'chip fracture' can occur. This commonly occurs in sports and hence there are sport-related names for these injuries ('jersey' = FDP avulsed from the volar base of the DP or 'baseball' = avulsion of the terminal extensor tendon from the DP). PP shaft fractures are proximal to the nail bed and usually result from direct trauma. PP tuft fractures are the most distal fracture and can be quite painful and difficult to manage since union may be slow.

Thumb fractures

The first CMC joint is a double saddle-joint, which allows movement in both the flexion/extension plane and in abduction/adduction. Because of the wide range of motion present at the thumb CMC joint, angulation of up to 30° is well tolerated allowing rehabilitation to achieve full function even when re-morbid joint mobility is not attained. In extra-articular fractures dorsal angulation occurs because the abductor pollicus brevis, adductor pollicis and flexor pollicis brevis muscles attaching at the base of the proximal phalanx and act to flex the distal fragment while the abductor pollicus longus muscle (which attaches to the metacarpal base) extends the proximal fragment. A Bennett fracture is an intra-articular fracture involving the metacarpal base. The fracture fragment involves the volar ulnar portion of the metacarpal base. This fragment is held undisplaced by the anterior oblique ligament. The remainder of the thumb metacarpal usually subluxes radially, proximally and dorsally by the forces exerted by the abductor pollicus longus.

Diagnosis of digital fractures

The focus of assessment depends on the stage of healing. Clinical and radiographic assessment of fracture union should be performed until union is established. Clinical signs of non-union include exquisite local pain at the fracture site and movement of the fractured components. Computerized tomography can be a useful adjunct to radiographs as they help to accurately delineate the degree of articular displacement and can identify other associated injuries. Radiographs are routinely used to identify fractures and to determine the degree of displacement; however X-ray cannot be used to rule out a rotational deformity. Patients can be asked to actively flex their digits to determine if there is any scissoring of the digits (i.e. overlap). If pain from the acute injury precludes an active flexion effort, passive wrist flexion and extension will place a flexion moment across the fingers with the tenodesis effect allowing an assessment of rotation to be made. A thorough clinical assessment should determine whether there is any associated soft tissue or neurovascular injury and identify any rotational deformity. Assessment should include evaluation of impairments and disabilities arising from fracture complications or treatment sequelae. A summary of these and potential treatment approaches are described in Table 31.1.

Prognosis for digital fractures

Prognosis varies according to the outcome of interest. Successful union of the fracture, restoration of normal anatomy, pre-injury movement/grip strength and function are typical goals and outcomes evaluated. Union is dependent on the person's individual capacity for bone healing and thus affected by prognostic factors that affect bone healing in a generic sense, including individual physical factors (nutrition, comorbidity, age, bone

Table 31.1 Summary of treatment problems and associated treatment techniques for hand fractures*

Problem	Physiotherapeutic treatment strategies
Fracture protection (Fess et al 2004)	• Custom-made or off-the-shelf orthoses
Pain	• Frequent, low intensity active exercise of unaffected joints and affected joints when stable • Adequate fracture protection and oedema management • Desensitization programme • Electro-thermal agents • Co-ordinate pharmacological management and therapy
Nerve irritation/ neuroma	• Desensitization programme (Robinson & McPhee 1986, Waylett-Rendall 1988) • Iontophoresis with lidocaine – evidence in other conditions (Fedorczyk 1997, Baskurt et al 2003, Bolin 2003, Yarrobino et al 2006, Polomano et al 2008) • Mirror box therapy (Altschuler & Hu 2008, Ezendam et al 2009) – limited evidence • Visualization exercises – limited evidence • Nerve gliding/neurodynamic techniques focused on at-risk or symptomatic nerve bias
Oedema	• Exercise in elevation • Compression (compressive gloves, retrograde massage, Coban wrap, string wrapping (Flowers 1988) (especially for digits) • Thermal agents (cold in acute stages for those who can tolerate; heat should be used only in elevation with monitoring of volume) • Physical agents (high voltage stimulation) (Stralka et al 1998)
Loss of joint motion (Michlovitz et al 2004)	• Active exercise of affected joints (stable fixation or healed) • Physiological and accessory joint mobilization • Static progressive splinting • Dynamic splinting • Continuous passive motion (Soffer & Yahiro 1990) (low evidence in other upper extremity joints) • Constrained movement therapy (blocking or casting of adjacent mobile digits to enforce movement of stiff joints)
Loss of power	• Progressive resisted exercise (Hostler et al 2001, Bautmans et al 2009)
Loss of endurance	• Progressive resisted exercise • Progressive functional activity
Scissoring	• Buddy tape to adjacent digit • May require osteotomy
Joint Instability	• Buddy taping, taping, custom or premade orthoses • Activity modification to avoid lateral stress
Non-union	• Low dose ultrasound (Busse et al 2002, Griffin et al 2008)
Abnormal sensorimotor integration or motor control	• Sensorimotor retraining (focused, progressive retraining of normal sensory responses) • Motor control exercises • Dexterity training/functional activity
Prevention of future fractures	• Assess risk for future fracture (based on age mechanism of injury and comorbid status) • Manage modifiable risk factors (safety training, activity modification, protective devices, fall prevention, balance training as needed)

Continued

Table 31.1 Summary of treatment problems and associated treatment techniques for hand fractures*—cont'd

Problem	Physiotherapeutic treatment strategies
General	• In simple, closed metacarpal fractures, early motion has the potential to result in earlier recovery of mobility and strength, facilitate an earlier return to work, and not affect fracture alignment (Feehan & Bassett 2004)
Dorsal skin scar contracture	• Silicone gel/topical agents to superficial scars • Scar massage/ mobilization for adherence • Simultaneous heat, stretch and tendon gliding exercises (Wehbe 1987) • Scar mobilization with hand-held suction device • Ultrasound • Laser
MP joint contracted an extension	• Early positioning MP joint at 70° • Later dynamic or static progressive splinting of MPs
Intrinsic muscle contracture	• Early active intrinsic minus exercises; blocking exercise • Later – dynamic splinting; muscle stimulation
Absence of MP head	• Educate patient about shortening of metacarpal; assess whether any functional implications (may not affect functional outcome) • Assess functionality of extensors; if redundancy is apparent splinting extension at night and strengthen intrinsic • Assess alignment – volar prominence = volar angulation and may require adaptive padding/gloves/positioning or osteotomy • Communicate with health care team
Loss of IP extension	• Blocking exercises • MP block extension splint during the day • PIP extension splint thing at night • Neuromuscular stimulation to EDC and interrosei • Joint mobilizations
Loss of IP flexion	• FDP/FDS tendon glide exercises • Daytime MP flexion blocks blunting • Dynamic or static progressive night's splinting • Heat and composite stretching • Joint mobilizations • Stretch of oblique retinacular ligament
Boutonniere deformity	• Early DIP active flexion to maintain length of lateral bands • Later splinting
Swan neck deformity	• Orthotic to hold MP joint in flexion

*From: Freeland et al 2003, Hardy 2004.

quality), the bone affected (composition, blood supply, biomechanics), behavioural (compliance with fixation, immobilization, re-mobilization, rehabilitation; activity levels), injury (type of fracture, size of defect, soft tissue components, associated injuries) and complications (nerve compression, infection, loss of reduction).

Optimal anatomic outcomes and functional outcomes are moderately related, in that malunion can lead to decreased pain, grip strength, scissoring, or loss of joint motion (Synn et al 2009). However, poor functional outcomes can occur in the presence of good anatomic restoration, particularly where pronounced joint stiffness, chronic pain, or chronic regional pain syndrome exist (Field et al 1992, Field & Atkins 1997). Conversely, adequate functional outcomes are attained in older sedentary individuals despite lack of restoration of normal anatomy (Grewal & MacDermid 2007). When fracture malunion results in scissoring, a corrective rotational osteotomy may be required.

Evidence on prognosis and fractures is generally sparse and poor quality (level IV studies). Functional (DASH), aesthetic and fracture union outcomes in metacarpal shaft and neck fractures were not affected by palmar angular deformity, but functional and aesthetic outcomes were better in non-operatively managed patients (Westbrook et al 2008). Spiral/long oblique fractures of the shaft of the metacarpal are at risk of shortening and resultant extension lag and reduced grip strength. However, there may be progressive recovery of the extension lag by 1 year and a mean of 94% of the contralateral hand motion by 1 year after injury (Al-Qattan 2008). In 51 unstable metaphyseal MP and PP fractures where fixation was maintained with miniature titanium plates union, the final range of total active motion (% TAM) was excellent (> 85%) for 26, good (70–84%) for 17, fair (50–69%) for 5, and poor (< 49%) for 3 (Omokawa et al 2008). Postoperative complications included loss of reduction (2 cases), condylar head collapses (2 cases), and one superficial infection. Plates were removed in 30 cases, and additional surgery was required in 20 cases. Postoperative grip strength averaged 87% of the contralateral side. Older age, intra-articular fracture, phalangeal bone involvement, and soft tissue injury were associated with poorer range of finger motion following fracture (Omokawa et al 2008). A level IIb study of 120 MC and PP emergency room fractures indicated that infection, increased bony defect and associated soft tissue injury increased the risk of nonunion (Ali et al 2007). In another study, 36% of MC or PP fractures showed different complications, PP and open fractures were at higher risk for stiffness, non-union, plate prominence, infection, and tendon rupture (Page & Stern 1998).

Conservative treatment of digital fractures

The general principles of fracture management is to reduce the fracture (open or closed) in a manner that will restore normal anatomy and maintain the reduced position through an immobilization/fixation technique that is sufficient to withstand the potential for loss of reduction through deforming or external forces. Since immobilization leads to comorbid stiffness/weakness, early mobilization is preferable where it does not compromise reduction. In keeping with these goals (Fig 31.1), the general principles of rehabilitation of fractures are divided into two stages (MacDermid 2004):

- *Stage 1 – Early rehabilitation*, which includes protect the healing fracture, minimize pain and oedema, restore normal motion and tissue extensibility, monitor patients for associated injuries or complications, prevent therapy-induced complications, to assist patients in dealing with their injury using appropriate coping mechanisms and

avoidance of patterns that increase the risk of developing chronic pain/disability syndromes and to help patients to understand their injury, the role of healthcare providers, and how to take an active role in their rehabilitation.
- *Stage 2 – Later rehabilitation*, which includes amelioration of joint contracture, restoration of hand and arm strength, adaptation to residual physical impairments, transitioning into normal work or activity and to teach the prevention strategies to reduce risk of a second fracture.

There is a lack of clinical trials comparing different treatment approaches for digital fractures. A single small low-quality trial suggested the use of a compression glove avoided the loss of function imposed by splintage and was associated with a greater range of movement during the second and third weeks following a metacarpal fracture (McMahon et al 1994). Management is based on the stage of bone healing and presenting fracture sequelae (see treatments based on presenting problems in Table 31.1). Poor quality studies support the use of metacarpal bracing for early mobilization.

ULNAR COLLATERAL LIGAMENT (UCL) INJURY OF THE THUMB

Epidemiology

UCL injuries can be acute or chronic. Acute injuries are much more common and are the result of an acute valgus stress rupturing the ligament. Chronic injuries are referred to as gamekeeper's thumb. This is also an injury of the UCL; however, it is the result of attenuation of the ligament due to a chronic, repetitive radially directed force on the ulnar side of the thumb. This was traditionally noticed in Scottish gamekeepers who fractured the necks of the rabbits between their thumbs and index fingers.

Anatomy

The thumb MP joint has both static and dynamic stabilizers. The static restraints include the volar plate, proper and accessory collateral ligaments. The proper collateral ligament acts as the primary stabilizer of the MP joint in flexion, and in extension, the accessory collateral ligament and the volar plate are the primary joint stabilizers (Minami et al 1984, Heyman et al 1993). The dynamic stabilizers include both the thumb extrinsic (EPL, EPB and FPL) and intrinsic (APB, FPB, and adductor pollicis muscles) structures. The adductor pollicis is the most important dynamic stabilizer of the thumb MP joint. It inserts into the extensor hood (through its aponeurosis) and lies superficial to the joint and the UCL.

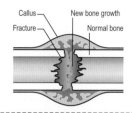

Callus — New bone growth
Fracture — Normal bone

Week 1
- Immobilization
- Early (safe) mobilization

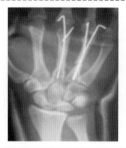

Weeks 2–6
- Manage pain and edema
- ROM unaffected joints
- Safe active motion if fracture stable (closed undisplaced or rigid fixation)

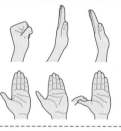

Weeks 4–6+ (graduated mobilization – with clinical union)
- Progressive active, gentle passive techniques
- Assess and treat specific emerging impairments within safety margins (table 1)

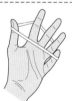

Weeks 8–12+ (remodeling and functional restoration)
- Passive techniques and joint mobilization
- Progressive strength and function program
- Dynamic or progressive static orthotics
- Manage residual disability and future fracture risk

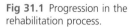

Fig 31.1 Progression in the rehabilitation process.

Pathology

When a valgus stress is applied to the thumb (i.e. a fall onto the abducted thumb) the dynamic and static stabilizers fail sequentially depending on the magnitude of the force. When the injury is limited to the dynamic stabilizers, the thumb will be stable on valgus stress testing. When the proper collateral ligament ruptures valgus instability will be present in MP flexion. When the accessory collateral is also torn, there will be valgus instability in both flexion and extension, indicating a complete tear (Heyman et al 1993). At times, the ruptured distal end of the ligament can become displaced such that it lies superficial and proximal to the adductor aponeurosis. This entity was first described by Stener in 1962 and the lesion bears his name (Stener 1962). Due to interposition of the adductor aponeurosis this injury will not heal without operative intervention.

Diagnosis

Patients will report a history of a valgus injury and complain of pain and swelling over the ulnar aspect of the MP joint. Pain will be exacerbated by forceful pinch and activities such as unscrewing jar tops and holding large objects because of a lack of power from the thumb's inability to generate counter-pressure on the object. Occasionally a Stener lesion may be evident as a palpable mass on the ulnar aspect of the joint; however, lack of such a mass does not rule out a Stener lesion. Radiographs should be obtained and viewed prior to stress testing of the ligament to rule out an avulsion fracture thereby avoiding potential displacement of the fracture fragment. Stress testing of the UCL is performed by placing a valgus stress across the MP joint 30° of flexion and then extension. If there is more than 30° of laxity (or 15° more than the contralateral side) in flexion (30° of MP flexion) rupture of the proper collateral ligament is likely. The valgus stress is then applied in extension. If there is less than 30° of valgus laxity in extension, the accessory collateral is intact, precluding a Stener lesion. If there is greater than 30° of laxity in both flexion and extension, the accessory collateral ligament is also ruptured and the probability of an underlying Stener lesion is approximately 80% (Stener 1962). Radiographs demonstrate radial deviation at the MP joint and possible volar subluxation.

Prognosis

There are no specific prognostic studies on this topic. Inadequate mobilization or failure to detect a Stener lesion can lead to chronic instability and pain.

Conservative treatment of UCL injury

Management consists primarily of immobilization sufficient to permit ligament reattachment/healing. Although biomechanical evidence suggests early control of mobilization might be feasible (Harley et al 2004), it has not been tested in clinical trials. Casting or customized splinting can be used for mobilization but removable splints are best reserved for compliant patients. A Stener lesion or failures to achieve a stable thumb with minimal pain during pinch are indications for surgery (Dinowitz et al 1997): early repair or late ligament reconstruction. Progressive strengthening and protection from lateral stress (functional splinting/taping) will allow remodeling of collagen fibres to ligament orientations that provide tensile strength. Stretching the UCL prematurely can lead to chronic instability.

OTHER DIGITAL TENDON INJURIES

Other tendon injuries that affect the digits can occur through lacerations, avulsion injuries (e.g. mallet/jersey finger), acute boutonniere, pulley ruptures. Lacerations of the flexor tendons that rupture in zones one or two require surgical repair and specific tendon rehabilitation protocols (Groth 2005, Newport & Tucker 2005, Libberecht et al 2006, Koul et al 2008, Soni et al 2009). These may involve active (protected) early mobilization in specially selected cases where repair strength is sufficient. Early passive mobilization protocols remain more common. Consultation with the referring surgeon and awareness of hand therapy rehabilitation protocols are required (Klein 2003, Chai & Wong 2005, Sueoka & LaStayo 2008, Yen et al 2008). Extensor tendon rupture or lacerations in the digits require extension splinting (4–6 weeks), and in some cases surgical repair. Gradually progressed protected active range of motion protocols instituted within the safety margins allowable by the specific

repair are required to ensure tendons glide is restored without compromising repair (tendon rupture or gapping). Active motion with differential gliding is emphasized during rehabilitation. When tendons scarring limits differential gliding, tenolysis may be required.

OSTEOARTHRITIS OF THE DIGITS

Epidemiology

Digital osteoarthritis (OA) is the most prevalent form of degenerative arthritis, although functional consequences vary (Doherty et al 2000, Hunter et al 2004). The DIP is the most affected, although functional consequences tend to be more severe in the carpometacarpal (CMC) joint of the thumb, which affects 1 in 4 women and 1 in 12 men. In patients older than 75 the prevalence of radiographic CMC degeneration increases to 40% in women and 25% in men (Armstrong et al 1994, Doherty et al 2000, Caspi et al 2001).

Anatomy

The CMC joint acts as a universal joint, allowing motion in extension, flexion, adduction and abduction. Together, these movements allow the complex movements of the thumb such as opposition, retro-pulsion, palmar and radial abduction, and adduction. The CMC joint has little intrinsic stability and relies on static ligamentous restraints to limit translation of the metacarpal base during these movements. There are three ligaments that help to stabilize this joint. The primary stabilizer of the CMC joint is the anterior oblique ligament, or volar beak ligament. It is an intra-capsular structure which originates from the palmar tubercle of the trapezium and inserts on the ulnar side of the metacarpal base, along the articular margin. It resists abduction, extension and pronation forces. The secondary stabilizers include the dorso-radial and inter-metacarpal ligaments. The dorso-radial ligament resists dorsal and radial translation of the CMC joint and is the most robust of the CMC joint ligaments. The inter-metacarpal ligament lies between the base of the first and second metacarpals and prevents radial translation of the base of the first metacarpal (Bettinger et al 1999). The thenar muscles also play a role as dynamic stabilizers of the CMC joint. These muscles work in concert, stabilizing the thumb in position to allow activities such as pinching.

Pathology

OA is a degenerative condition characterized by pain, intermittent inflammation and cartilage degeneration. The pathological processes that underlie this degeneration are multifactorial and not fully defined but include genetic and biomechanical factors. Loss of joint space, sub-chondral sclerosis, loss of cartilage, osteophytes and joint deformities occur. The DIP joint can also be affected with mucous cysts which occur during the early stages of degenerative joint disease.

Doerschuk et al (1999) conducted a cadaveric study and demonstrated that the degree of degeneration in the anterior oblique ligament was correlated with the stage of the OA. Eaton & Littler (1973) also demonstrated a strong association between excessive laxity at the thumb CMC joint and premature degenerative changes. Laxity combined with repetitive loading may predispose certain individuals to synovitis, and with continued loading, the articular surfaces gradually wear resulting in joint space narrowing and osteoarthritis. orso-radial subluxation occurs at the base of the thumb metacarpal while distally the adductor pollicis pulls the thumb into an adducted position (Blank & Feldon 1997). This adducted posturing of the thumb leads to difficulty spreading the hand around objects for grasping and leads to compensatory, progressive hyperextension of the MP joint. The aetiology of CMC joint laxity has been attributed to hormonal influences (i.e. prolactin, relaxin and oestrogen), thus potentially explaining the increased incidence of CMC OA seen in women.

Diagnosis

Hand OA is diagnosed using clinical features with radiographic substantiation (Zhang et al 2009). Heberden and Bouchard nodes are clinically defined postero-lateral firm/hard swellings of the IP in PIP joints respectively. Nodal OA exists in the presence of these nodes plus underlying IP joint arthritis defined clinically and/or radiological. Non-nodal OA is defined by IP joint OA in the absence of nodes. Erosive OA is defined radiographically by sub-cortical erosion, cortical destruction and subsequent reparative change and may include bony ankylosis. Generalized OA is when hand arthritis exists in combination with OA at other sites. Thumb base OA is when the first CMC joint is involved in the scaphotrapezial joint.

Typical hand OA symptoms are pain on usage, mild morning pain, inactivity stiffness particularly when affecting only single or a few consistent joints. Lateral deviation of IPs, subluxation or adduction of the thumb base are the common deformities.

The diagnosis of CMC OA is based on history and clinical exam. The typical presentation is a woman in her 50s to 70s with radial sided hand or thumb pain. Clinical examination will reveal tenderness localized to the CMC joint, with a positive grind test (axial compression of the thumb) reproducing pain and crepitus. Radiographs are used to confirm the diagnosis. Various stages of joint involvement can be seen, ranging from a widened joint space (joint effusion or synovitis) to joint space narrowing, subluxation, sclerosis and osteophyte formation. Differential diagnosis includes psoriatic arthritis, rheumatoid arthritis, gout and haemochromatosis, each tends to have different target sites of involvement that can be used to assist with differential (Zhang et al 2009).

Prognosis

Genetic factors, female sex, age over 40, menopausal status, obesity, higher bone density, greater for muscle strength, joint laxity, prior hand injury, higher occupational recreational use are all associated with increased risk of hand OA and its severity and progression (Zhang et al 2009).

Conservative treatment of digital arthritis

Hand OA is a multi-joint problem and treatment approach. EULAR evidence-based recommendations for management suggest a combination of pharmacological and non-pharmacological treatment be individualized to the patient (Klein 2003, Chai & Wong 2005, Sueoka & LaStayo 2008, Yen et al 2008). Education about joint protection and exercise are recommended for all patients. Local application of heat, especially prior to exercise, splints for thumb OA and orthotics to prevent or correct lateral angulation flexion deformities are recommended. Local treatments are preferred over systemic for mild to moderate pain and when only a few joints are affected. Topical NSAIDs and capsaicin are effective and safe treatments. Pharmacological and surgical interventions should be considered in patients with marked pain or disability or when conservative treatments have failed. There is insufficient evidence to choose between different orthotics options (off-the-shelf/custom fit, long/short opponens, dorsal/volar, thermoplastic/neoprene/other materials). Orthotics should be customized according to the joint deformity/damage, functional requirements and patient preferences. It is common for patients with hand arthritis to have multiple orthoses that suit different activities or levels of disease activity. Exercise and education have been shown to be more efficacious than OA information alone (Moe et al 2009).

RHEUMATOID ARTHRITIS AFFECTING THE DIGITS

Rheumatoid arthritis is an inflammatory arthritis that has diffuse digital and other involvement. In the past severe hand deformities were common, but are now uncommon because of pharmacological advances in management of the disease. Older patients may continue to present with severe deformity and for surgical reconstruction.

Rheumatoid arthritis hand deformity can include boutonniere, swan neck, ulnar drift, caput ulna, tendon rupture and sagittal band/tendon subluxation.

CONCLUSION

Injuries to the joints, tendons, ligaments and nerves in the digits are common and require attention to detail during rehabilitation to restore fine precision movement is necessary that essential that function. Principles suggest that protected motion during healing/joint irritability, progressive active movement and strengthening that incorporates functional activities and selected use of joint mobilization techniques to enhance joint kinematics is required. Oedema management and integration of sensory and motor assessment/retraining are particularly important. Reliance on principles is essential given the dearth of physical therapy evidence for digital disorders and the specific lack of attention to this area within manual therapy literature.

REFERENCES

Aitken, S., Court-Brown, C.M., 2008. The epidemiology of sports-related fractures of the hand. Injury 39, 1377–1383.

Al-Qattan, M.M., 2008. Outcome of conservative management of spiral/long oblique fractures of the metacarpal shaft of the fingers using a palmar wrist splint and immediate mobilisation of the fingers. J. Hand Surg. 33, 723–727.

Ali, H., Rafique, A., Bhatti, M., Ghani, S., Sadiq, M., Beg, S.A., 2007. Management of fractures of metacarpals and phalanges and associated risk factors for delayed healing. J. Pak. Med. Assoc. 57, 64–67.

Altschuler, E.L., Hu, J., 2008. Mirror therapy in a patient with a fractured wrist and no active wrist extension. Scand. J. Plast. Reconstr. Surg. Hand Surg. 42, 110–111.

Armstrong, A.L., Hunter, J.B., Davis, T.R., 1994. The prevalence of degenerative arthritis of the base of the thumb in post-menopausal women. J. Hand Surg. [Br.] 19, 340–341.

Baskurt, F., Ozcan, A., Algun, C., 2003. Comparison of effects of phonophoresis and iontophoresis of naproxen in the treatment of lateral epicondylitis. Clin. Rehabil. 17, 96–100.

Bautmans, I., Van, P.K., Mets, T., 2009. Sarcopenia and functional decline: pathophysiology, prevention and therapy. Acta Clin. Belg. 64, 303–316.

Bettinger, P.C., Linscheid, R.L., Berger, R.A., Cooney, W.P., An, K.N., 1999. An anatomic study of the stabilizing ligaments of the trapezium and trapeziometacarpal joint. J. Hand Surg. [Am.] 24, 786–798.

Blank, J., Feldon, P., 1997. Thumb metacarpophalangeal joint stabilization during carpometacarpal joint surgery. Atlas Hand Clinics 2, 217–225.

Bolin, D.J., 2003. Transdermal approaches to pain in sports injury management. Curr. Sports Med. Rep. 2, 303–309.

Busse, J.W., Bhandari, M., Kulkarni, A.V., Tunks, E., 2002. The effect of low-intensity pulsed ultrasound therapy on time to fracture healing: a meta-analysis. Can. Med. Assoc. J. 166, 437–441.

Caspi, D., Flusser, G., Farber, I., Ribak, J., Leibovitz, A., Habot, B., et al., 2001. Clinical, radiologic, demographic, and occupational aspects of hand osteoarthritis in the elderly. Semin. Arthritis Rheum. 30, 321–331.

Chai, S.C., Wong, C.W., 2005. Dynamic traction and passive mobilization for the rehabilitation of zone II flexor tendon injuries: a modified regime. Med. J. Malaysia 60, 59–65.

Dinowitz, M., Trumble, T., Hanel, D., Vedder, N.B., Gilbert, M., 1997. Failure of cast immobilization for thumb ulnar collateral ligament avulsion fractures. J. Hand Surg. [Am.] 22, 1057–1063.

Doerschuk, S.H., Hicks, D.G., Chinchilli, V.M., Pellegrini, V.D., 1999. Histopathology of the palmar beak ligament in trapeziometacarpal osteoarthritis. J. Hand Surg. [Am.] 24, 496–504.

Doherty, M., Spector, T.D., Serni, U., 2000. Epidemiology and genetics of hand osteoarthritis. Osteoarthritis Cartilage 8, 14–S15.

Eaton, R.G., Littler, J.W., 1973. Ligament reconstruction for the painful thumb carpometacarpal joint. J. Bone Joint Surg. [Am.] 55, 1655–1666.

Ezendam, D., Bongers, R.M., Jannink, M.J., 2009. Systematic review of the effectiveness of mirror therapy in upper extremity function. Disabil. Rehabil. 31, 2135–2149.

Fedorczyk, J., 1997. The role of physical agents in modulating pain. J. Hand Ther. 10, 110–121.

Feehan, L.M., Bassett, K., 2004. Is there evidence for early mobilization following an extraarticular hand fracture? J. Hand Ther. 17, 300–308.

Feehan, L.M., Sheps, S.S., 2008a. Treating hand fractures: population-based study of acute health care use in British Columbia. Can. Fam. Physician 54, 1001–1007.

Feehan, L.M., Sheps, S.S., 2008b. Treating hand fractures: population-based study of acute health care use in British Columbia. Can. Fam. Physician 54, 1001–1007.

Fess, E.E., Philips, C.A., Gettle, K., Janson, J.R., 2004. Hand and Upper Extremity Splinting: Principles and Methods. Elsevier Health Sciences, Philadelphia PA.

Field, J., Atkins, R.M., 1997. Algodystrophy is an early complication of Colles' fracture. What are the implications? J. Hand Surg. [Br.] 22, 178–182.

Field, J., Warwick, D., Bannister, G.C., 1992. Features of algodystrophy ten years after Collees' fracture. J. Hand Surg. [Br.] 17B, 318–320.

Flatt, A.E., 1996. Closed and open fractures of the hand: Fundamentals of management. Postgrad. Med. 39, 17–26.

Flowers, K.R., 1988. String wrapping versus massage for reducing digital volume. Phys. Ther. 68, 57–59.

Freeland, A.E., Hardy, M.A., Singletary, S., 2003. Rehabilitation for proximal phalangeal fractures. J. Hand Ther. 16, 129–142.

Grewal, R., MacDermid, J.C., 2007. The risk of adverse outcomes in extra-articular distal radius fractures is increased with malalignment in patients of all ages but mitigated in older patients. J. Hand Surg. [Am.] 32, 962–970.

Griffin, X.L., Costello, I., Costa, M.L., 2008. The role of low intensity pulsed ultrasound therapy in the management of acute fractures: a systematic review. J. Trauma 65, 1446–1452.

Groth, G.N., 2005. Current practice patterns of flexor tendon rehabilitation. J. Hand Ther. 18, 169–174.

Hardy, M.A., 2004. Principles of metacarpal and phalangeal fracture management: a review of rehabilitation concepts. J. Orthop. Sports Phys. Ther. 34, 781–799.

Harley, B.J., Werner, F.W., Green, J.K., 2004. A biomechanical modeling of injury, repair, and rehabilitation of ulnar collateral ligament injuries of the thumb. J. Hand Surg. [Am.] 29, 915–920.

Heyman, P., Gelberman, R.H., Duncan, K., Hipp, J.A., 1993. Injuries of the ulnar collateral ligament of the thumb metacarpophalangeal joint – Biomechanical and prospective clinical-studies on the usefulness of valgus stress-testing. Clin. Orthop. Relat. Res. 165–171.

Hostler, D., Crill, M.T., Hagerman, F.C., Staron, R.S., 2001. The effectiveness of 0.5-lb increments in progressive resistance exercise. J. Strength Cond. Res. 15, 86–91.

Hove, L.M., 1993. Fractures of the hand. Distribution and relative incidence. Scand. J. Plastic Reconstr. Surg. Hand Surg. 27, 317–319.

Hunter, D.J., Demissie, S., Cupples, L.A., Aliabadi, P., Felson, D.T., 2004. A genome scan for joint-specific hand osteoarthritis susceptibility: The Framingham Study. Arthritis Rheum. 50, 2489–2496.

Klein, L., 2003. Early active motion flexor tendon protocol using one splint. J. Hand Ther. 16, 199–206.

Koul, A.R., Patil, R.K., Philip, V., 2008. Complex extensor tendon injuries: early active motion following single-stage reconstruction. Journal Hand Surgery European 33, 753–759.

Libberecht, K., Lafaire, C., Van, H.R., 2006. Evaluation and functional assessment of flexor tendon repair in the hand. Acta Chir. Belg. 106, 560–565.

MacDermid, J.C., 2004. Hand therapy management of intra-articular fractures with open reduction and pi plate fixation: a therapist's perspective. Tech. Hand Up. Extrem. Surg. 8, 219–223.

McMahon, P.J., Woods, D.A., Burge, P.D., 1994. Initial treatment of closed metacarpal fractures. A controlled comparison of compression glove and splintage. J. Hand Surg. [Br.] 19, 597–600.

Michlovitz, S.L., Harris, B.A., Watkins, M.P., 2004. Therapy interventions for improving joint range of motion: A systematic review. J. Hand Ther. 17, 118–131.

Minami, A., An, K., Cooney, W.I., Linscheid, R.L., Chao, E.Y.S., 1984. Ligamentous structures of the metacarpophalangeal joint: A quantitative anatomic study. J. Orthop. Res. 1, 361–368.

Moe, R.H., Kjeken, I., Uhlig, T., Hagen, K.B., 2009. There is inadequate evidence to determine the effectiveness of nonpharmacological and nonsurgical interventions for hand osteoarthritis: An overview of high-quality systematic reviews. Phys. Ther. 89, 1363–1370.

Newport, M.L., Tucker, R.L., 2005. New perspectives on extensor tendon repair and implications for rehabilitation. J. Hand Ther. 18, 175–181.

Omokawa, S., Fujitani, R., Dohi, Y., Okawa, T., Yajima, H., 2008. Prospective outcomes of comminuted periarticular metacarpal and phalangeal fractures treated using a titanium plate system. J. Hand Surg. [Am.] 33, 857–863.

Page, S.M., Stern, P.J., 1998. Complications and range of motion following plate fixation of metacarpal and phalangeal fractures. J. Hand Surg. [Am.] 23, 827–832.

Polomano, R.C., Rathmell, J.P., Krenzischek, D.A., Dunwoody, C.J., 2008. Emerging trends and new approaches to acute pain management. Pain Manag. Nurs. 9, S33–S41.

Robinson, S.M., McPhee, S.D., 1986. Treating the patient with digital hypersensitivity. Am. J. Occup. Ther. 40, 285–287.

Shehadi, S.I., 1991. External fixation of metacarpal and phalangeal fractures. J. Hand Surg. [Am.] 16, 544–550.

Shewring, D.J., Thomas, R.H., 2006. Collateral ligament avulsion fractures from the heads of the metacarpals of the fingers. J. Hand Surg. [Br.] 31, 537–541.

Smith, R., 1975. Intrinsic muscles of the fingers: Function, dysfunction, and surgical reconstruction. Instr. Course Lect. 24, 200–220.

Soffer, S.R., Yahiro, M.A., 1990. Continuous passive motion after internal fixation of distal humerus fractures. Orthopedic Reviews 19, 88–93.

Soni, P., Stern, C.A., Foreman, K.B., Rockwell, W.B., 2009. Advances in extensor tendon diagnosis and therapy. Plastic Reconstructive Surgery 123, 727–728.

Stener, B., 1962. Displacement of the ruptured ulnar collateral ligament of the metacarpo-phalangeal joint of the thumb: A clinical and anatomical study. J. Bone Joint Surg. [Br.] 44, 869–879.

Stralka, S.W., Jackson, J.A., Lewis, A.R., 1998. Treatment of hand and wrist pain. A randomized clinical trial of high voltage pulsed, direct current built into a wrist splint. AAOHN J. 46, 233–236.

Sueoka, S.S., LaStayo, P.C., 2008. Zone II flexor tendon rehabilitation: a proposed algorithm. J. Hand Ther. 21, 410–413.

Synn, A.J., Makhni, E.C., Makhni, M.C., Rozental, T.D., Day, C.S., 2009. Distal radius fractures in older patients: Is anatomic reduction necessary? Clin. Orthop. Relat. Res. 467, 1612–1620.

van Onselen, E.B., Karim, R.B., Hage, J.J., Ritt, M.J., 2003. Prevalence and distribution of hand fractures. J. Hand Surg. [Br.] 28, 491–495.

Waylett-Rendall, J., 1988. Sensibility evaluation and rehabilitation. Orthop. Clin. North Am. 19, 43–56.

Wehbe, M.A., 1987. Tendon gliding exercises. Am. J. Occup. Ther. 41, 164–167.

Westbrook, A.P., Davis, T.R., Armstrong, D., Burke, F.D., 2008. The clinical significance of malunion of fractures of the neck and shaft of the little finger metacarpal. J. Hand Surg. [Eur.] 33, 732–739.

Yarrobino, T.E., Kalbfleisch, J.H., Ferslew, K.E., Panus, P.C., 2006. Lidocaine iontophoresis mediates analgesia in lateral epicondylalgia treatment. Physiother. Res. Int. 11, 152–160.

Yen, C.H., Chan, W.L., Wong, J.W., Mak, K.H., 2008. Clinical results of early active mobilisation after flexor tendon repair. Hand and Surgery 13, 45–50.

Zhang, W., Doherty, M., Leeb, B.F., Alekseeva, L., Arden, N.K., Bijlsma, J. W., et al., 2009. EULAR evidence-based recommendations for the diagnosis of hand osteoarthritis: report of a task force of ESCISIT. Ann. Rheum. Dis. 68, 8–17.

Chapter | **32** |

Referred pain from muscle/myofascial trigger points

César Fernández de las Peñas, Hong-You Ge, Lars Arendt-Nielsen, Jan Dommerholt, David G Simons

INTRODUCTION

Referred pain (pain felt in a different region away from the source of pain) has been known and described for more than a century and has been used extensively as a diagnostic tool in the clinic. In clinical practice, it is very common to see neck or shoulder pain that spreads to the upper arm, the forearm or hand in some patients, whereas in others it spreads to the contralateral side (Carli et al 2002). Pain from deep tissues, e.g. muscle, joints, ligaments, tendons and viscera, is described as deep and diffuse and difficult to locate precisely (Mense 1994). Further, the term 'referred pain' also includes other referred sensations or paraesthesia, since muscle referred pain is not necessarily limited to pain. Therefore, referred pain symptoms can be involved in some arm pain syndromes in which there is no clear diagnosis (Gerwin 1997). For instance, patients with deep pain in the shoulder and posterior deltoid region spreading to the upper arm may be diagnosed as a non-specific arm pain syndrome, since they complain of diffuse arm pain and tenderness with loss of function but lack objective physical signs (Macfarlane et al 2000). Simons et al (1999) described common referred pain patterns from the infraspinatus trigger points (TrPs) which may resemble the clinical picture of these patients. What was considered to be a non-specific arm pain syndrome may in fact originate from infraspinatus TrPs. An additional challenge to this clinical reasoning is

© 2011 Elsevier Ltd.
DOI: 10.1016/B978-0-7020-3528-9.00032-7

that in patients with musculoskeletal pain, the symptoms may be the summation of referred pain from multiple muscle TrPs and even from other structures including joints and viscera, making it more difficult to establish the proper diagnosis. This chapter will describe the clinical and the neurophysiological basis of muscle/myofascial TrPs with referred pain pattern spreading to the shoulder region and the upper extremity.

MUSCLE/MYOFASCIAL TRIGGER POINTS

Definition of muscle/myofascial trigger point

Although there are different definitions of TrPs, the most commonly accepted definition states that 'a TrP is a hyper-irritable spot within a taut band of a skeletal muscle that is painful on compression, stretch, overload or contraction which responds with a referred pain that is perceived distant from the spot' (Simons et al 1999). From a clinical viewpoint, we can distinguish active and latent TrPs. Active TrPs are those in which local and referred pain reproduce the symptoms reported by the patient, and the pain is recognized by the patient as a usual pain (Simons et al 1999). Latent muscle TrPs are those in which local and referred pain did not reproduce any pain symptom familiar or usual for the subject (Simons et al 1999). For instance, a patient with lateral epicondylalgia can have active TrPs, which reproduce the symptoms within the affected arm (Fernández-Carnero et al 2007), but this patient may also have latent TrPs on the non-affected side since the local and referred pain are not usually perceived in this arm (Fernández-Carnero et al 2008). Both active and latent TrPs provoke motor dysfunctions, e.g. muscle weakness, inhibition, increased motor irritability (spasm), muscle imbalance, and altered motor recruitment (Lucas et al 2004), in either the affected muscle or in functionally related muscles (Simons et al 1999).

Characteristics of the referred pain elicited by muscle trigger points

- The duration of referred pain could last for as short as a few seconds or as long as a few hours or days (sometimes indefinitely), depending on the TrP activity.
- The referred pain is described as deep, diffuse, burning, tightening, or pressing pain, which is completely different from neuropathic or superficial (skin) pain.
- The referred pain can spread cranial/caudal or ventral/dorsal, depending on the TrP.

- The referred pain intensity and spreading area is positively correlated to the degree of TrP activity (irritability of the nervous system).
- The referred pain can be accompanied by other symptoms, such as numbness, coldness, stiffness, weakness, fatigue, motor dysfunction (Lucas et al 2004).
- Inactivation of active TrPs should effectively relieve the referred pain.
- TrP referred pain patterns may be similar to joint referred patterns (Bogduk 2004).

Manual identification of muscle/myofascial trigger points

Competent TrPs diagnosis requires adequate manual ability, training, and clinical practice to develop a high degree of reliability in the examination (Gerwin et al 1997, Simons et al 1999, Sciotti et al 2001). There are several signs and symptoms that may be used for TrP diagnosis: (a) presence of a palpable taut band in a skeletal muscle when accessible to palpation; (b) presence of a hyperirritable spot in the taut band; (c) palpable local twitch response on snapping palpation (or needling) of the TrP; and (d) presence of referred pain elicited by stimulation or palpation of the hyperirritable spot (Simons et al 1999). Additional helpful signs for diagnosis are muscle weakness, pain on contraction in the shortened position, or jump sign. However, different systematic reviews investigating the reliability of TrP diagnosis have concluded that it needs to be further investigated with studies of high quality that use current clinical diagnostic criteria in different populations (Tough et al 2007, Myburgh et al 2008, Lucas et al 2009). Factors that may have contributed to the varying reliability of the results from previous studies are lack of identification of taut bands, inexperience of the examiners in assessing muscle TrPs, incorrect positioning of the patient or the assessor, incorrect palpation techniques, variation in the amount of manual force exerted on the palpated point and the duration of force applied. Nevertheless, it has been reported that some muscles may be consistently more reliably examined than others (Gerwin et al 1997, Sciotti et al 2001). Readers are referred to other texts for a more in-depth discussion on TrP diagnosis reliability (Tough et al 2007, Myburgh et al 2008, Fernández-de-las-Peñas et al 2009a, Lucas et al 2009).

Therefore, for clinical purposes Simons et al (1999) and Gerwin et al (1997) recommend that the *minimum* acceptable criteria for TrP diagnosis are the presence of a hyper-irritable spot within a palpable taut band of a skeletal muscle combined with the patient's recognition of the referred pain elicited by the TrP. These criteria, when applied by an experience assessor, have obtained a good inter-examiner reliability (kappa) ranging from 0.84 to

0.88 (Gerwin et al 1997). Recent studies found that taut bands and possibly TrPs can be visualized using magnetic resonance elastography and sonographic elastography (Chen et al 2007, 2008, Sikdar et al 2008, 2009), although future studies are needed to optimize these procedures.

Neurophysiological basis of muscle/myofascial trigger points

TrP referred pain is a process of central sensitization which is mediated by peripheral nociceptive activity and can be facilitated by sympathetic activity or dysfunctional descending inhibition.

TrP: is it a focus of peripheral sensitization?

Muscle pain is associated with activation of muscle nociceptors by a variety of endogenous substances, e.g. neuropeptides or inflammatory mediators, among others. Different algogenic substances are commonly used in experimental pain models for eliciting both local and referred pain from muscle tissues, including hypertonic saline (Arendt-Nielsen & Svensson 2001, Graven-Nielsen 2006), bradykinin and serotonin (Babenko et al 1999a), capsaicin (Witting et al 2000), substance P (Babenko et al 1999b), glutamate (Svensson et al 2003a), nerve growth factor (Svensson et al 2003b), or acidic saline (Sluka et al 2001). It is interesting to note that the referred pain patterns reported with injection of these substances are very similar to the referred pain patterns described in the Trigger Point Manual (Simons et al 1999).

In addition, recent microdialysis studies showed that the concentrations of bradykinin, calcitonin gene-related peptide, substance P, tumour necrosis factor-α, interleukin-1β, serotonin or norepinephrine were significantly higher in active muscle TrPs when compared to latent TrP or control non-TrP points (Shah et al 2005, 2008). These studies suggest that experimental human pain models largely mimic the sensory manifestations of muscle TrPs, which supports that nociceptor hypersensitivity is common at muscle TrPs. A recent study has confirmed the existence of nociceptive hypersensitivity (hyperalgesia) at muscle latent TrPs and also provided evidence of non-nociceptive hypersensitivity (allodynia) at TrPs (Li et al 2009). These studies support that muscle TrPs constitute a focus of sensitization of both nociceptive and non-nociceptive nerve endings.

TrPs and central sensitization mechanisms

When muscles are in a state of sensitization, muscle nociceptors are more easily activated and may respond to normal innocuous or weak stimuli such as light pressure and muscle movement. The presence of multiple TrPs (spatial summation) or the presence of TrPs during prolonged periods of time (temporal summation) would sensitize the spinal cord and supra-spinal structures by continued nociceptive afferent barrage into the central nervous system (Fernández-de-las-Peñas et al 2009c). In these sensitization mechanisms, new receptive fields would appear causing the referred pain (Mense 1994).

Several studies confirmed that the area of the referred pain correlated with the intensity and duration of the muscle pain (Graven-Nielsen et al 1997, Laursen et al 1997). These studies suggest that muscle referred pain is maintained by peripheral sensitization mechanisms. Some clinical studies have demonstrated that sensitization mechanisms related to TrPs may be reversible with proper management (Mellick & Mellick 2003, Hsieh et al 2007). For instance, dry-needling inactivation of primary TrPs inhibits the activity in satellite TrPs situated in their zone of referred pain (Hsieh et al 2007). TrP injection into neck muscles produces rapid relief of palpable scalp or facial tenderness and also alleviates associated symptoms of nausea, photophobia, and phonophobia in migraine (Carlson et al 1993, Mellick & Mellick 2003). However, Sluka et al (2001) determined, in an animal model, that central sensitization is an irreversible process. Kuan et al (2007) demonstrated that spinal cord connections of myofascial TrPs are basically similar to that for a normal tissue region. Nevertheless, TrPs were effective in inducing neuroplastic changes in the dorsal horn neurons (Kuan et al 2007). Further, Niddam et al (2007) demonstrated that pain from TrPs is at least partially processed at supra-spinal levels, particularly the periaqueductal grey substance. Multiple factors can hence influence the degree of sensitization, including dysfunctional descending inhibitory systems, sympathetic activity, or neuropathic activation, and therefore increase the likelihood that myofascial pain syndromes may be reversible.

TrPs and the sympathetic nervous system

There is an emerging interest in the association between muscle TrPs and the sympathetic nervous system. Rabbit (Chen et al 1998b) and human studies (McNulty et al 1994, Chung et al 2004) have shown evidence of a sympathetic contribution to the modulation of spontaneous electrical activity at TrPs. In these studies, increased sympathetic efferent discharge increased both the frequency and the amplitude of spontaneous electrical activity of muscle TrPs, while sympathetic blockers decreased the frequency and amplitude of spontaneous electrical activity. Ge et al (2006) found increased referred pain intensity and tenderness with sympathetic hyperactivity at TrPs, suggesting a sympathetic contribution to the mechanisms responsible for the generation of referred pain. A recent study found an attenuated skin blood flow response after painful stimulation of latent muscle TrPs compared with control non-TrPs, suggesting increased sympathetic vasoconstriction activity at latent TrPs (Zhang et al 2009).

Since both peripheral and central sensitization mechanisms participate in the development of muscle referred pain (for a more complete review see Arendt-Nielsen et al 2000), sympathetic facilitation can involve peripheral, spinal or supra-spinal sympathetic structures. The interaction between the sympathetic and central nervous system, and the sympathetic-sensory and sympathetic-motor coupling at TrPs are still unknown (for a review, see Arendt-Nielsen & Ge 2009). Gerwin et al (2004) have suggested that the presence of alpha and beta adrenergic receptors at the endplate provides a possible mechanism for autonomic interaction (Maekawa et al 2002). Stimulation of the alpha and beta adrenergic receptors stimulated the release of ACh in the phrenic nerve of rodents (Bowman et al 1988).

TrPs: the integrated hypothesis

To expose the hypothesis explaining the pathogenesis of TrPs is beyond the scope of this chapter, but a summary of current data will be reviewed.

The activation of a TrP may result from a variety of factors, e.g. repetitive muscle overuse, acute or sustained overload, psychological stress, or other key myofascial TrPs. Particular attention has been paid to injured or overloaded muscle fibres in the pathogenesis of TrPs (Chen et al 2000, Gerwin et al 2004, Itoh et al 2004, Treaster et al 2006). Some authors have hypothesized that muscle trauma, repetitive low-intensity muscle overload or intense eccentric contractions may create a vicious cycle of events, wherein damage to the sarcoplasmic reticulum or the cell membrane may lead to an increase of the calcium concentration, an activation of actin and myosin filaments, a relative shortage of adenosine triphosphate (ATP), and an impaired calcium pump (Simons et al 1999, Gerwin et al 2004). Based on these events, Simons & Travell proposed the so-called 'energy crisis hypothesis' introduced in 1981 and enhanced by subsequent research leading to the *integrated hypothesis* (Simons 2004).

The *integrated hypothesis* proposes that abnormal depolarization of the post-junctional membrane of motor endplates enhanced by sustained muscular contraction gives rise to a localized hypoxic energy crisis associated with sensory and autonomic reflex arcs that are sustained by sensitization mechanisms (McPartland & Simons 2006). Qerama et al (2004) found higher pain intensity and pain characteristics similar to muscle TrPs when noxious stimuli were applied to motor endplate regions as compared to silent muscle sites. Further, endplate noise and endplate spikes (EMG signals from dysfunctional motor endplate regions) have been significantly associated with muscle TrPs in human and animal studies (Chen et al 1998a, Hong & Yu 1998, Couppé et al 2001, Simons 2001, Kuan et al 2002, Macgregor et al 2006, Chang et al 2008). Findings from these studies support the theory that TrPs are subsequently associated with dysfunctional motor endplates (Simons et al 2002). Although there is evidence to support the integrated hypothesis as an aetiological pathogenesis of TrPs, the hypothesis has some weak links that still need to be addressed in future studies in order to confirm this etiological hypothesis as the genesis of TrPs is becoming increasingly complex (Gerwin 2005, Dommerholt et al 2006, McPartland & Simons 2006).

EXPLORATION OF TRIGGER POINTS RELATED TO ARM PAIN SYNDROMES

Clinical history, examination of active and passive movement patterns, quality and area of pain symptoms, and consideration of referred pain patterns assist clinicians in determining which muscles may be clinically relevant for different neck/arm pain syndromes. Although there is no laboratory or imaging test available that can confirm the presence of TrPs new emerging sonography techniques are promising (Sikdar et al 2009).

TrP palpation starts with the identification of the taut band within the skeletal muscle by palpating perpendicular to the fibre direction. Once the taut band is located, a hypersensitive spot should be identified along the taut band. The presence of a local twitch response (sudden involuntary contraction of the taut band) and referred pain increase the certainty of TrP diagnosis. Sometimes, patients may be asked to contract the muscle to locate the fibres. Muscles may be placed in a relaxed or pre-stretched position for palpation, depending on the clinical presentation of the patient. Clinicians should avoid preconceived expectations of the location and referred pain patterns of TrPs as most textbooks used standard marks for teaching purposes.

TrP can be identified through (a) flat palpation, in which the therapist applies finger or thumb pressure to the muscle against underlying bone tissue (Fig 32.1);

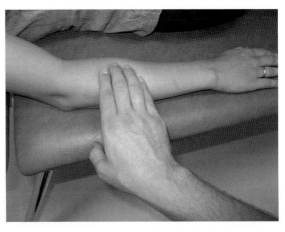

Fig 32.1 Flat palpation of a taut band within the extensor wrist muscles.

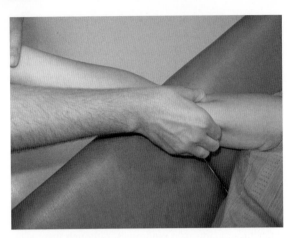

Fig 32.2 Pincer palpation of a taut band within the biceps brachii muscle.

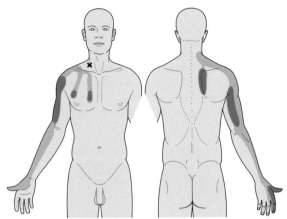

Fig 32.3 Referred pain elicited by myofascial trigger points in the scalene muscle.

(b) pincer palpation where the muscle is rolled between the tips of the digits (Fig 32.2); or (c) snapping palpation, where the clinician moves the fingers back and forth to roll the underlying muscle fibres under the finger.

In this chapter, we will describe the TrPs most commonly involved in the genesis of arm pain syndromes.

Neck-shoulder muscles

There are several neck-shoulder muscles (upper trapezius, sternocleidomastoid, levator scapulae, rhomboid, serratus posterior superior, splenius capitis, or splenius cervicis) from which TrPs referred pain can contribute to arm pain syndromes (Skubick et al 1993, Simons et al 1999). For instance, Fernández-de-las-Peñas et al (2007a) demonstrated, in a blinded controlled study, that the referred pain elicited by the upper trapezius, sternocleidomastoid, sub-occipital and levator scapulae TrPs reproduced the pain pattern in patients with idiopathic neck pain. The referred pain from most of these muscles particularly spreads to the head but not to the neck region, e.g. upper trapezius (Fernández-de-las-Peñas et al 2007b) or sterno-cleidomastoid (Fernández-de-las-Peñas et al 2006) in patients with chronic tension type headache. The levator scapulae and rhomboid TrPs refer pain to the angle of the neck, along the vertebral border of the scapula bone and the posterior part of the shoulder (Simons et al 1999). Readers are referred to other texts for the exploration of neck-shoulder muscles from which TrPs refer pain to the head/neck (Simons et al 1999, Gerwin 2005, Fernández-de-las-Peñas et al 2009b).

Scalene muscles

TrPs may be located in either anterior, medial, or posterior scalene muscle. The referred pain spreads anteriorly to the chest (over the pectoral region), to the anterior shoulder area, to the lateral (radial) border of the upper extremity reaching the thumb and/or index finger, and posteriorly to the medial scapular border and inter-scapular region (Fig 32.3). Spanos (2005) suggested that scalene muscle TrPs are one of the most ignored causes of inter-scapular dorsal pain. Further, since the brachial plexus runs anatomically between the anterior and the medial scalene muscles, TrPs in either scalene muscle may be related to entrapment of peripheral nerves (Chen et al 1998a), contributing to different arm pain syndromes, e.g. carpal tunnel syndrome (Simons et al 1999) and thoracic outlet syndrome (Ferguson & Gerwin 2005). In addition, shortening of these muscles induced by TrPs taut bands may be related to upward dysfunctions of the first rib (Ferguson & Gerwin 2005). It seems that scalene muscle TrPs can have repercussions in both neural and joint tissues in arm pain syndromes.

Pectoralis minor muscle

The pectoralis minor muscle pulls the coracoid process anterior and downward, producing a protracted shoulder position (Ferguson & Gerwin 2005). TrPs within the pectoralis minor muscle refer pain to the anterior part of the chest, the anterior part of the shoulder (coracoid process) and usually to the ulnar aspect of the arm and forearm (Fig 32.4). Since the brachial plexus runs anatomically under the pectoralis minor muscle, an increased tension of this muscle can entrap the lower trunk (C7–C8 nerve trunks) of the brachial plexus, simulating an ulnar radiculopathy (Simons 1991). Langley (1997) suggested that patients with symptoms of brachial plexus irritation and other compression neuropathies should be examined for the presence of TrPs within the pectoralis minor muscle. Hong & Simons (1993) demonstrated that patients with chronic whiplash showed active TrPs in the pectoralis minor muscle reproducing their arm pain symptomatology.

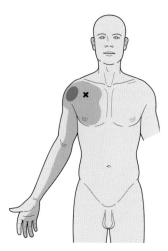

Fig 32.4 Referred pain elicited by myofascial trigger points in the pectoralis minor muscle.

Supraspinatus muscle

The supraspinatus muscle assists abduction of the arm and stabilization of the humerus head during arm movements. TrPs within the supraspinatus muscle elicit a referred pain felt as deep pain around the shoulder, particularly over the mid-deltoid region. Deep pain over the mid-deltoid area may be mistaken with sub-deltoid bursitis (Simons et al 1999). Further, the referred pain may also spread down to the arm and the forearm, and sometimes over the lateral epicondyle of the elbow region (Fig 32.5). Jacobson et al (1989) reported that repetition strain injury over the shoulder joint may be a precipitating factor for supraspinatus TrPs. Chaitow & Delany (2008) suggested that supraspinatus TrPs may lead to imbalance or dysfunction of this muscle inducing non-proper functioning of the

humeral head stabilization during arm elevations. This situation could lead to a compression of supraspinatus tendon against the acromion (Chaitow & Delany 2008). It is clinical experience that TrPs in the supraspinatus muscle can contribute to muscle imbalance or pain symptoms in subjects with sub-acromial impingement.

Srbely et al (2008) reported that treatment of the infraspinatus TrPs reduced the sensitivity of the supraspinatus TrP, since both muscles receive their innervation from the suprascapular nerve (C5 nerve root). Therefore, the Srbely et al (2008) study supports examining all muscles which may contribute to symptoms of shoulder/arm pain.

Infraspinatus muscle

The infraspinatus muscle assists external rotation of the arm and stabilization of the humerus head during arm movements. Simons et al (1999) suggested that TrPs in the infraspinatus muscle may be one of the most ignored causes of shoulder and/or arm pain. Lucas et al (2004) reported that the presence of latent TrPs within the infraspinatus muscle delayed its electromyography activation during arm elevation. The referred pain from this muscle is perceived as deep joint pain in the anterior part of the shoulder area. In addition, the pain also spreads downwards to the antero-lateral (radial) aspect of the arm, forearm and fingers (Fig 32.6). Infraspinatus muscle TrPs usually induce restriction of shoulder internal rotation (Simons et al 1999). Bron et al (2007) found that infraspinatus muscle TrPs showed the best inter-rater reliability (pair-wise agreement 69–80%) when compared to the biceps and deltoid muscles.

Qerama et al (2009) demonstrated that 49% of subjects with normal electrophysiological findings within the median nerve, but pain symptoms mimicking carpal tunnel syndrome, presented with active TrP in the

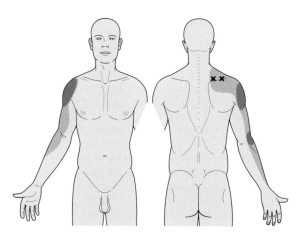

Fig 32.5 Referred pain elicited by myofascial trigger points in the supraspinatus muscle.

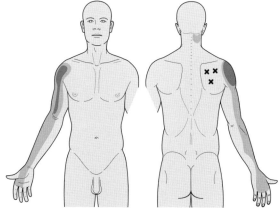

Fig 32.6 Referred pain elicited by myofascial trigger points in the infraspinatus muscle.

infraspinatus muscle associated with paraesthesia and referred pain to the arm and fingers. In the same study, patients with mild electrophysiological signs of carpal tunnel syndrome had a significantly higher occurrence of infraspinatus muscle TrP within the symptomatic arm as compared with patients with moderate to severe electro-physiological signs (33% vs 20%).

Ge et al (2008) found multiple, rather than single, active TrPs in the infraspinatus muscle within the painful side in patients with shoulder arm pain. In addition, this study also reported that most TrPs were located in the mid-fibre region of the muscle belly. Finally, Hong (1994) suggested that infraspinatus muscle TrPs may be considered as primary (key) TrPs of deltoid muscle TrPs. Hsieh et al (2007) confirmed that treating infraspinatus TrPs can inactivate TrPs in the anterior deltoid muscle, whereas others have demonstrated electromyographically that infraspinatus TrPs can inhibit use of the anterior del-toid muscle with full functional recovery with inactivation of the infraspinatus TrP. Infraspinatus muscle TrPs are among the most important to consider in patients with arm pain syndromes.

Teres minor and major muscles

TrPs in the teres minor muscle elicit referred pain in the posterior part of the deltoid region, mimicking a 'painful bursitis' in the posterior part of the shoulder joint (Escobar et al 1988) (Fig 32.7A). TrPs within the teres major refer pain to the posterior deltoid area and shoulder joint, which occasionally can spread to the dorsal forearm (Fig 32.7B).

Subscapularis muscle

Subscapularis TrPs cause severe pain at rest and pain on motion. The referred pain spreads to the posterior aspect

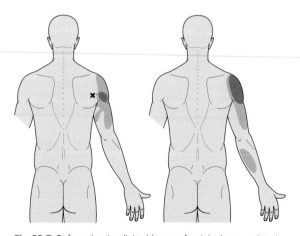

Fig 32.7 Referred pain elicited by myofascial trigger points in the teres minor (A) and major (B) muscles.

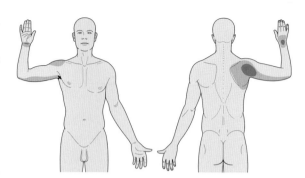

Fig 32.8 Referred pain elicited by myofascial trigger points in the subscapularis muscle.

of the shoulder joint and the scapula, extending down to the posterior aspect of the arm and the volar surface of the wrist (Fig 32.8). The insertion of the subscapularis tendon is usually described on the lesser tuberosity of the humerus; but it seems that this muscle also expands its insertion to the anterior part of the shoulder joint (Cash et al 2009). In addition, the subscapularis muscle has a destabilizing inferior shear potential over the shoulder joint (Ackland & Pandy 2009). Therefore, shortening of this muscle may be implicated in shoulder retraction pathologies, such as the 'frozen shoulder' (Simons et al 1999, Ferguson & Gerwin 2005). Jankovic & Van Zundert (2006) reported that five patients with frozen shoulder syndrome experienced pain relief after TrP injections in the subscapularis muscle. This muscle is one of the most com-monly involved muscles in shoulder dysfunction and pain syndromes and since it serves as antagonist to most of the other shoulder joint stabilizers, its dysfunction encourages development of TrPs in other musculature. Therefore, the subscapularis muscle should not be overlooked in a TrP examination, which takes considerable skill.

Pectoralis major muscle

The shortening of the pectoralis major muscle has been linked clinically to the upper crosses syndrome (Janda 1996). TrPs within the pectoralis major muscle refer pain particularly to the anterior part of the chest, which some-times also spreads to the ulnar aspect of the arm (Fig 32.9). The referred pain from the left pectoralis major muscle may simulate angina pectoris (Simons et al 1999). Further, it is conceivable that angina pectoris may be a precipitating factor for activation of pectoralis major TrPs (viscero-somatic activation). In fact subjects with known or suspected angina pectoris usually present with pain and tenderness in this muscle (Kumarathurai et al 2008). Rinzler & Travell (1948) reported that patients with pain complaint of coronary insufficiency with no history or evidence of cardiac disease are afflicted with active pectoralis major TrPs.

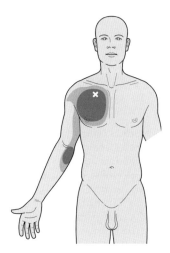

Fig 32.9 Referred pain elicited by myofascial trigger points in the pectoralis major muscle.

Deltoid muscle

The deltoid is one muscle that commonly develops TrPs in any belly (anterior, middle, or posterior). The middle and anterior parts of this muscle are significant potential contributors to a superior shear of the humeral head (Ackland & Pandy 2009); therefore, deltoid muscle TrPs may contribute to shoulder muscle imbalance (Simons et al 1999). Deltoid TrPs refer a burning and deep pain to the region where the muscle is located: (a) TrPs in the anterior part of the deltoid refer pain to the anterior and middle deltoid regions (Fig 32.10A); (b) TrPs in the middle part of the muscle refer pain over the middle and posterior regions (Fig 32.10B); (c) TrPs in the posterior part refer pain to the posterior region of the shoulder (Fig 32.10C). Hsueh et al (1998) reported that C5–C6 disc lesions were associated with active TrPs in the deltoid muscle, suggesting

Fig 32.10 Referred pain elicited by myofascial trigger points in the anterior (A), middle (B) and posterior (C) deltoid muscle.

the clinical relevance of assessing cervical segments related to the innervation of the affected muscle.

Biceps brachii muscle

The referred pain elicited by TrPs in the biceps brachii muscle spreads up the muscle into the anterior region of the shoulder. Referred pain in the region of the biceps tendon can be misdiagnosed as long head bicipital tendonitis (Simons et al 1999). The referred pain can also spread down the muscle to the anterior area of the elbow region (Fig 32.11). It is important to note that the median nerve runs anatomically medial to the muscle belly of the biceps brachii (Maeda et al 2009). Therefore, tension induced by TrP taut bands or abnormal muscle bands (Paraskevas et al 2008) located over the biceps brachii muscle may lead to median nerve tension.

Triceps brachii muscle

Since the radial nerve runs deep to the lateral head of the triceps muscle (Rezzouk et al 2002) TrPs in this muscle may contribute to radial nerve entrapment (Simons et al 1999). TrPs can be located in any of the heads of this muscle: (a) TrPs within the long head of the muscle refer pain upward to the posterior area of the shoulder joint, spreading occasionally to the upper trapezius region, and sometimes down the dorsum of the forearm, skipping the elbow (Fig 32.12A, right arm); (b) TrPs over the lateral head of the muscle refer pain to the posterior part of the arm, sometimes spreading to the dorsum of the forearm or the fourth and fifth digits (Fig 32.12B, right arm); (c) the referred pain elicited by TrPs within the medial head of the muscle are projected to the lateral epicondyle and to the olecranon process (Fig 32.12B, left arm).

Janssens (1991) found, in a study with dogs, that treatment of TrPs in the triceps brachii muscle was critical for their recovery of normal walking and running.

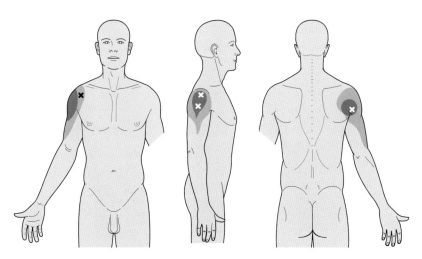

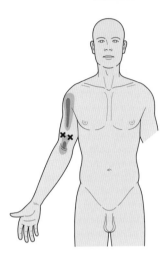

Fig 32.11 Referred pain elicited by myofascial trigger points in the biceps brachii muscle.

Brachioradialis muscle

The brachioradialis is an elbow flexor muscle with the forearm in neutral position inducing symptoms in the forearm or wrist (Simons et al 1999). Brachioradialis TrPs project their referred pain to the lateral epicondyle, the radial aspect of the forearm, the wrist and the base of the thumb, in the space between the thumb and index fingers (Fig 32.13). Referred pain from TrPs in this muscle can mimic a DeQuervain syndrome.

Kao et al (2007) showed that the brachioradialis muscle was significantly more irritable than others, because of the presence of latent TrPs. Fernández-Carnero et al (2007) found that 50% of patients with unilateral lateral

epicondylalgia showed active TrPs within the brachioradialis muscle, supporting its role in this pain condition. Finally, the radial nerve may also be entrapped by shortening of the brachioradialis muscle (Mekhail et al 1999).

Supinator muscle

The supinator muscle is extremely important for a proper functioning of the elbow joint. It is known that the radial nerve crosses the fibrous arch of the supinator muscle, called the arcade of Frohse, the main region of entrapment of this nerve (Tatar et al 2009). Therefore, muscle tension induced by TrP taut bands in this muscle can entrap the radial nerve, particularly the motor branch (posterior interosseus) of the nerve (Simons et al 1999, Schneider 2005). TrPs in the supinator muscle refer pain to the lateral epicondyle, the lateral area of the elbow, and sometimes can project spillover pain to the dorsal aspect of the web of the thumb (Fig 32.14).

Simons et al (1999) suggested that supinator muscle TrPs simulate symptoms in lateral epicondylalgia. This assumption was confirmed by Slater et al (2003) who showed that hypertonic saline injection into the supinator muscle, among others, simulated sensory and motor manifestations of lateral epicondylalgia patients. In a more recent study, Slater et al (2005) found that the injection of hypertonic saline into the supinator muscle in lateral epicondylalgia patients increased the referred pain areas and motor disturbances.

Wrist/hand extensor muscles

The wrist extensor musculature is located over the radial aspect of the forearm and has a complex agonist–antagonist function which makes them vulnerable for

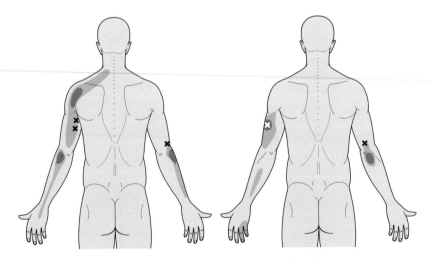

Fig 32.12 Referred pain elicited by myofascial trigger points in the triceps brachii muscle.

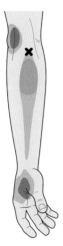

Fig 32.13 Referred pain elicited by myofascial trigger points in the brachioradialis muscle.

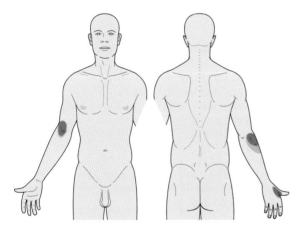

Fig 32.14 Referred pain elicited by myofascial trigger points in the supinator muscle.

Fig 32.15 Referred pain elicited by myofascial trigger points in the extensor carpi radialis longus (A), extensor carpi radialis brevis (B), the extensor digitorum communis (C), and extensor carpi ulnaris (D) muscles.

repetitive strain and overload situations. For instance, the extensor carpi radialis longus muscle induces extension and also radial deviation, whereas the extensor carpi ulnaris muscle also exerts extension of the wrist but ulnar deviation (Livingston et al 2001). Chen et al (2000) found that piano students exhibited significantly decreased pressure thresholds over latent TrPs in these muscles after only 20 minutes of piano playing, which moved them forward – becoming active TrPs and compromising their motor function. The wrist extensor musculature is innervated by the deep branch of the radial nerve (posterior interosseous nerve). The radial nerve may get entrapped in the supero-lateral aspect of the extensor carpi radialis brevis muscle (Clavert et al 2009).

In general, referred pain patterns elicited by wrist extensor muscle TrPs spread upwards to the lateral epicondyle and downwards along the muscle belly toward their insertion in the wrist/hand: (a) TrPs in the *extensor carpi radialis longus* muscle refer pain to the lateral epicondyle and to the dorsum of the hand next to the thumb (Fig 32.15A); (b) TrPs in the *extensor carpi radialis brevis* muscle project pain to the radial and posterior aspects of the hand and the wrist (Fig 32.15B); (c) *extensor digitorum communis* TrPs refer pain downward to the forearm, reaching the same digit that the fibres activate (Fig 32.15C); and, (d) referred pain from the *extensor carpi ulnaris muscle* TrPs is perceived in the ulnar side of the back of the wrist (Fig 32.15D).

Fernández-Carnero et al (2007) found that active TrPs within these muscles (65% extensor carpi radialis brevis, 55% extensor carpi radialis longus and 25% extensor digitorum communis) reproduced the pain pattern symptoms in subjects with lateral epicondylalgia. Therefore, clinicians should examine the wrist extensor muscles in patients with lateral epicondylalgia.

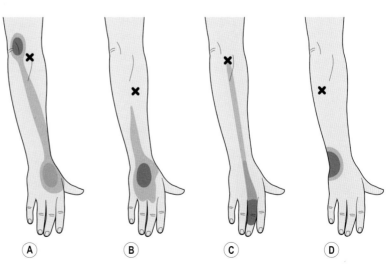

A B C D

Pronator teres muscle

The pronator teres muscle is the main pronator of the forearm. The median nerve passes between the two heads of the pronator teres muscle, making this muscle a common entrapment region of the nerve (Bilecenoglu et al 2005). In fact, an entrapment of the median nerve in the pronator teres muscle is known as the pronator syndrome (Lee & LaStayo 2004). Therefore, tension induced by TrP taut bands in this muscle may be relevant for symptoms associated with median nerve compression (Simons et al 1999). Pronator teres TrPs refer pain downward to the forearm and the volar radial region of the wrist (Fig 32.16).

Wrist/hand flexor muscles

The wrist flexor musculature has a similar complex agonist–antagonist function as the wrist extensor. For instance, the flexor carpi radialis induces wrist flexion and also radial deviation, whereas the flexor carpi ulnaris muscle exerts also wrist flexion but ulnar deviation. The palmaris longus muscle is not present in all subjects. Wrist flexor muscles are innervated by the median and ulnar nerves. Due to anatomical relationships, the median nerve can be entrapped by the flexor digitorum profundus and superficialis muscles, whereas the ulnar nerve can be entrapped by the flexor carpi ulnaris and flexor digitorum profundus muscles (Chaitow & Delany 2008).

In general, referred pain patterns elicited from wrist flexor muscle TrPs usually spread downwards along the muscle belly toward their insertion in the wrist: (a) TrPs in the *flexor carpi radialis* refer pain to the volar aspect of the wrist (Fig 32.17A); (b) *palmaris longus muscle* TrPs

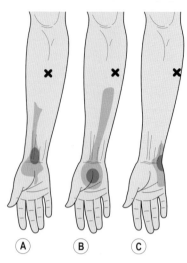

Fig 32.17 Referred pain elicited by myofascial trigger points in the flexor carpi radialis (A), palmaris longus (B), and flexor carpi ulnaris (C), muscles.

project superficial, needle-like pain over the volar area of the palm (Fig 32.17B); (c) referred pain from the *flexor carpi ulnaris muscle* TrPs is perceived in the ulnar side of the volar aspect of the wrist (Fig 32.17C).

Finally, no distinction can be made easily between referred pain patterns of the *flexors digitorum superficialis and profundus* muscles (Simons et al 1999). In these muscles, TrPs will refer pain to the same digit that the fibres activate (Fig 32.18). For instance, TrPs in the fibres of the middle finger flexor muscle refer pain through the length of the middle finger, similarly to the extensor digitorum communis muscle.

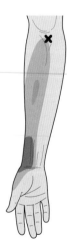

Fig 32.16 Referred pain elicited by myofascial trigger points in the pronator teres muscle.

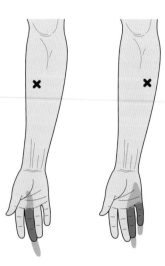

Fig 32.18 Referred pain elicited by myofascial trigger points in the flexors digitorum superficialis and profundus muscles.

Since the median and ulnar nerves may be entrapped between the wrist/hand flexor muscles, clinicians should examine and treat TrPs in this musculature in patients with pain symptoms in either ulnar or median nerve territories, e.g. carpal tunnel syndrome or ulnar neuropathy (Ferguson & Gerwin 2005).

Other muscles

Finally, clinicians should be aware that there is a greater number of muscle TrPs with their own specific referred pain patterns contributing to arm pain syndromes. For example, the brachialis, coracobrachialis, latissimus dorsi, serratus anterior and sub-clavius muscles also refer pain to the arm or the forearm (Simons et al 1999). Several studies have described referred pain from other muscles, such as the pronator quadratus (Hwang et al 2005a) or the abductor pollicis longus (Hwang et al 2005b), which have not been included in the comprehensive book by Simons et al (1999). Furthermore, in the current chapter we did not include any hand musculature (flexor pollicis longus, adductor pollicis, abductor pollicis, opponens pollicis, thumb flexor, or interosseous muscles), which can be also involved in hand pain syndromes (Simons et al 1999).

CONCLUSIONS

In summary, there are numerous neck, shoulder, arm and forearm and hand muscles which can harbour TrPs with referred pain pattern, that can contribute to the origin and maintenance of symptoms in arm pain syndromes such as thoracic outlet syndrome, carpal tunnel syndrome, or lateral epicondylalgia. Clinicians should examine these muscle TrPs to better identify and manage various arm pain syndromes. Although much progress has been made, further studies are required in order to further elucidate the role of muscle TrPs in the evolution of arm pain syndromes.

REFERENCES

Ackland, D.C., Pandy, M.G., 2009. Lines of action and stabilizing potential of the shoulder musculature. J. Anat. 215, 184–197.

Arendt-Nielsen, L., Ge, H.Y., 2009. Pathophysiology of referred muscle pain. In: Fernández-de-las-Peñas, C., Arendt-Nielsen, L., Gerwin, R.D. (Eds.), Tension type and cervicogenic headache: pathophysiology, diagnosis and treatment. Jones & Bartlett Publishers, Boston, pp. 51–59.

Arendt-Nielsen, L., Svensson, P., 2001. Referred muscle pain: Basic and clinical findings. Clin. J. Pain 17, 11–19.

Arendt-Nielsen, L., Laursen, R.J., Drewes, A.M., 2000. Referred pain as an indicator for neural plasticity. Prog. Brain Res. 129, 343–356.

Babenko, V., Graven-Nielsen, T., Svensson, P., et al., 1999a. Experimental human muscle pain and muscular hyperalgesia induced by combinations of serotonin and bradykinin. Pain 82, 1–8.

Babenko, V., Graven-Nielsen, T., Svensson, P., et al., 1999b. Experimental human muscle pain induced by intra-muscular injections of bradykinin, serotonin, and substance P. Eur. J. Pain 3, 93–102.

Bilecenoglu, B., Uz, A., Karalezli, N., 2005. Possible anatomic structures causing entrapment neuropathies of the median nerve: an anatomic study. Acta Orthop. Belg. 71, 169–176.

Bogduk, N., 2004. The neck and headaches. Neurologic Clinics of North America 22, 151–171.

Bowman, W.C., Marshall, I.G., Gibb, A.J., Harborne, A.J., 1988. Feedback control of transmitter release at the neuromuscular junction. Trends Pharmacol. Sci. 9, 16–20.

Bron, C., Franssen, J., Wensing, M., Oostendorp, R.A., 2007. Inter-rater reliability of palpation of myofascial trigger points in three shoulder muscles. J. Man. Manip. Ther. 15, 203–215.

Cash, C.J., MacDonald, K.J., Dixon, A.K., et al., 2009. Variations in the MRI appearance of the insertion of the tendon of subscapularis. Clin. Anat. 22, 489–494.

Carli, G., Suman, A.L., Biasi, G., Marcolongo, R., 2002. Reactivity to superficial and deep stimuli in patients with chronic musculoskeletal pain. Pain 100, 259–269.

Carlson, C.R., Okeson, J.P., Falace, D.A., et al., 1993. Reduction of pain and EMG activity in the masseter region by trapezius trigger point injection. Pain 55, 397–400.

Chaitow, L., Delany, J. (Eds.), 2008. Clinical application of neuromuscular techniques: The upper body, second ed. Shoulder, arm and hand, London: Elsevier, p. 445.

Chang, C.W., Chen, Y.R., Chang, K.F., 2008. Evidence of neuroaxonal degeneration in myofascial pain syndrome: a study of neuromuscular jitter by axonal micro stimulation. Eur. J. Pain 12, 1026–1030.

Chen, D., Fang, Y., Li, J., Gu, Y., 1998a. Anatomical study and clinical observation of thoracic outlet syndrome. Zhonghua Wai Ke Za Zhi 36, 661–663.

Chen, J.T., Chen, S.M., Kuan, T.S., et al., 1998b. Phentolamine effect on the spontaneous electrical activity of active loci in a myofascial trigger spot of rabbit skeletal muscle. Arch. Phys. Med. Rehabil. 7, 790–794.

Chen, S.M., Chen, J.T., Kuan, T.S., et al., 2000. Decrease in pressure pain thresholds of latent myofascial trigger points in the middle finger extensors immediately after continuous piano practice. Journal of Musculoskeletal Pain 8, 83–92.

Chen, Q., Bensamoun, S., Basford, J.R., et al., 2007. Identification and quantification of myofascial taut bands with magnetic resonance elastography. Arch. Phys. Med. Rehabil. 88, 1658–1661.

Chen, Q., Basford, J.R., An, K.N., 2008. Ability of magnetic resonance elastography to assess taut bands. Clin. Biomech. 23, 623–629.

Chung, J.W., Ohrbach, R., McCall Jr., W.D., 2004. Effect of increased sympathetic activity on electrical activity from myofascial painful areas. Am. J. Phys. Med. Rehabil. 83, 842–850.

Clavert, P., Lutz, J.C., Adam, P., et al., 2009. Frohse's arcade is not the exclusive compression site of the radial nerve in its tunnel. Orthop. Traumatol. Surg. Res. 95, 114–118.

Couppé, C., Midttun, A., Hilden, J., et al., 2001. Spontaneous needle electromyographic activity in myofascial trigger points in the infraspinatus muscle: a blinded assessment. Journal of Musculoskeletal Pain 9, 7–16.

Dommerholt, J., Bron, C., Franssen, J.L.M., 2006. Myofascial trigger points: an evidence- informed review. J. Man. Manip. Ther. 14, 203–221.

Escobar, P.L., Ballesteros, J., Teres minor, 1988. Source of symptoms resembling ulnar neuropathy or C8 radiculopathy. Am. J. Phys. Med. Rehabil. 67 (3), p. 120–122.

Ferguson, L., Gerwin, R., 2005. Shoulder dysfunction and frozen shoulder. In: Ferguson, L., Gerwin, R. (Eds.), Clinical mastery in the treatment of myofascial pain. Lippincott Williams & Wilkins, Baltimore, pp. 91–121.

Fernández-Carnero, J., Fernández-de-las-Peñas, C., De-la-Llave-Rincón, A.I., et al., 2007. Prevalence of and referred pain from myofascial trigger points in the forearm muscles in patients with lateral epicondylalgia. Clin. J. Pain 23, 353–360.

Fernández-Carnero, J., Fernández-de-las-Peñas, C., De-la-Llave-Rincón, A.I., et al., 2008. Bilateral myofascial trigger points in the forearm muscles in chronic unilateral lateral epicondylalgia: A blinded controlled study. Clin. J. Pain 24, 802–807.

Fernández-de-las-Peñas, C., Alonso-Blanco, C., Cuadrado, M., et al., 2006. Myofascial trigger points and their relationship with headache clinical parameters in chronic tension type headache. Headache 46, 1264–1272.

Fernández-de-las-Peñas, C., Alonso-Blanco, C., Miangolarra, J., 2007a. Myofascial trigger points in subjects presenting with mechanical neck pain: A blinded, controlled study. Man Ther 12, 29–33.

Fernández-de-las-Peñas, C., Ge, H., Arendt-Nielsen, L., et al., 2007b. Referred pain from trapezius muscle trigger point shares similar characteristics with chronic tension type headache. Eur. J. Pain 11, 475–482.

Fernández-de-las-Peñas, C., Ge, H.Y., Dommerholt, J., 2009a. Manual identification of trigger points in the muscles associated with headache. In: Fernández-de-las-Peñas, C., Arendt-Nielsen, L., Gerwin, R.D. (Eds.), Tension type and cervicogenic headache: pathophysiology, diagnosis and treatment. Jones & Bartlett Publishers, Boston, pp. 183–194.

Fernández-de-las-Peñas, C., Simons, D.G., Gerwin, R.D., 2009b. Muscle trigger points in tension type headache. In: Fernández de las Peñas, C., Arendt-Nielsen, L., Gerwin, R.D. (Eds.), Tension type and cervicogenic headache: pathophysiology, diagnosis and treatment. Jones & Bartlett Publishers, Boston, pp. 61–76.

Fernández-de-las-Peñas, C., Caminero, A.B., Madeleine, P., et al., 2009c. Multiple active myofascial trigger points and pressure pain sensitivity maps in the temporalis muscle are related in chronic tension type headache. Clin. J. Pain 25, 506–512.

Ge, H.Y., Fernández-de-las-Penas, C., Arendt-Nielsen, L., 2006. Sympathetic facilitation of hyperalgesia evoked from myofascial tender and trigger points in patients with unilateral shoulder pain. Clin. Neurophysiol. 117, 1545–1550.

Ge, H.Y., Fernández-de-las-Peñas, C., Madeleine, P., Arendt-Nielsen, L., 2008. Topographical mapping and mechanical pain sensitivity of myofascial trigger points in the infraspinatus muscle. Eur. J. Pain 12, 859–865.

Gerwin, R.D., 1997. Myofascial pain syndromes in the upper extremity. J. Hand Ther. 10, 130–136.

Gerwin, R.D., 2005. Headache. In: Ferguson, L., Gerwin, R.D. (Eds.), Clinical mastery in the treatment of myofascial pain. Lippincott Williams & Wilkins, Baltimore, pp. 1–24.

Gerwin, R.D., Shannon, S., Hong, C.Z., et al., 1997. Inter-rater reliability in myofascial trigger point examination. Pain 69, 65–73.

Gerwin, R.D., Dommerholt, D., Shah, J.P., 2004. An expansion of Simons' integrated hypothesis of trigger point formation. Curr. Pain Headache Rep. 8, 468–475.

Graven-Nielsen, T., 2006. Fundamentals of muscle pain, referred pain, and deep tissue hyperalgesia. Scand. J. Rheumatol. 122, 1–43.

Graven-Nielsen, T., Arendt-Nielsen, L., Svensson, P., Jensen, T.S., 1997. Quantification of local and referred muscle pain in humans after sequential intra-muscular injections of hypertonic saline. Pain 69, 111–117.

Hong, C.Z., 1994. Considerations and recommendations regarding myofascial trigger point injection. Journal of Musculoskeletal Pain 2, 29–59.

Hong, C.Z., Simons, D.G., 1993. Response to treatment for pectoralis minor myofascial pain syndrome after whiplash. J Musculoskeletal Pain 1, 89–131.

Hong, C.Z., Yu, J., 1998. Spontaneous electrical activity of rabbit trigger spot after transection of spinal cord and peripheral nerve. Journal Musculoskeletal Pain 6, 45–58.

Hsieh, Y.L., Kao, M.J., Kuan, T.S., et al., 2007. Dry needling to a key myofascial trigger point may reduce the irritability of satellite MTrPs. Am. J. Phys. Med. Rehabil. 86, 397–403.

Hsueh, T.C., Yu, S., Kuan, T.S., Hong, C.Z., 1998. Associations of active myofascial trigger points and cervical disc lesions. J. Formos. Med. Assoc. 97, 174–180.

Hwang, M., Kang, Y.K., Kim, D.H., 2005a. Referred pain pattern of the pronator quadratus muscle. Pain 116, 238–242.

Hwang, M., Kang, Y.K., Shin, J.Y., Kim, D.H., 2005b. Referred pain pattern of the abductor pollicis longus muscle. Am. J. Phys. Med. Rehabil. 84, 593–597.

Itoh, K., Okada, K., Kawakita, K., 2004. A proposed experimental model of myofascial triggers points in human muscle after slow eccentric exercise. Acupunct. Med. 22, 2–13.

Jacobson, E.C., Lockwood, M.D., Hoefner Jr., V.C., et al., 1989. Shoulder pain and repetition strain injury to the supraspinatus muscle: etiology and manipulative treatment. Journal of American Osteopathy Association 89, 1037–1045.

Janda, V., 1996. Upper cross syndrome. In: Liebenson, C. (Ed.), Rehabilitation of the spine: A practitioner manual. Williams & Wilkins, Baltimore, pp. 97–112.

Jankovic, D., Van Zundert, A., 2006. The frozen shoulder syndrome. Description of a new technique and five case reports using the subscapular nerve block and subscapularis trigger point infiltration. Acta Anaesthesiol. Belg. 57, 137–143.

Janssens, L.A., 1991. Trigger points in 48 dogs with myofascial pain syndromes. Vet. Surg. 20, 274–278.

Kao, M.J., Han, T.I., Kuan, T.S., et al., 2007. Myofascial trigger points in early life. Arch. Phys. Med. Rehabil. 88, 251–254.

Kuan, T.S., Chen, J.T., Chen, S.M., et al., 2002. Effect of botulinum toxin on endplate noise in myofascial trigger spots of rabbit skeletal muscle. Am. J. Phys. Med. Rehabil. 81, 512–520.

Kuan, T.S., Hong, C.Z., Chen, J.T., et al., 2007. The spinal cord connections of the myofascial trigger spots. Eur. J. Pain 11, 624–634.

Kumarathurai, P., Faroog, M.K., Christensen, H.W., et al., 2008. Muscular tenderness in the anterior chest wall in patients with stable angina pectoris is associated with normal myocardial perfusion. J. Manipulative Physiol. Ther. 31, 344–347.

Langley, P., 1997. Scapular instability associated with brachial plexus irritation: a proposed causative relationship with treatment implications. J. Hand Ther. 10, 35–40.

Laursen, R.J., Graven-Nielsen, T., Jensen, T.S., Arendt-Nielsen, L., 1997. Quantification of local and referred pain in humans induced by intramuscular electrical stimulation. Eur. J. Pain 1, 105–113.

Lee, M.J., LaStayo, D.C., 2004. Pronator syndrome and other nerve compressions that mimic carpal tunnel syndrome. J. Orthop. Sports Phys. Ther. 34, 601–609.

Li, L.T., Ge, H.Y., Yue, S.W., Arendt-Nielsen, L., 2009. Nociceptive and non-nociceptive hypersensitivity at latent myofascial trigger points. Clin. J. Pain 25, 132–137.

Livingston, B.P., Segal, R.L., Song, A., et al., 2001. Functional activation of the extensor carpi radialis muscles in humans. Arch. Phys. Med. Rehabil. 82, 1164–1170.

Lucas, K.R., Polus, B.I., Rich, P.A., 2004. Latent myofascial trigger points: their effects on muscle activation and movement efficiency. J. Bodyw. Mov. Ther. 8, 160–166.

Lucas, N., Macaskill, P., Irwig, L., et al., 2009. Reliability of physical examination for diagnosis of myofascial trigger points: a systematic review of the literature. Clin. J. Pain 25, 80–89.

Macfarlane, G.J., Hunt, I.M., Silman, A.J., 2000. Role of mechanical and psychosocial factors in the onset of forearm pain: prospective population based study. Br. Med. J. 321, 676–679.

Macgregor, J., Graf von Schweinitz, D., 2006. Needle electromyographic activity of myofascial trigger points and control sites in equine cleidobrachialis muscle: an observational study. Acupunct. Med. 24, 61–70.

Maeda, S., Kawai, K., Koizumi, M., et al., 2009. Morphological study of the communication between the musculo-cutaneous and median nerves. Anat. Sci. Int. 84, 34–40.

Maekawa, K., Clark, G.T., Kuboki, T., 2002. Intramuscular hypoperfusion, adrenergic receptors, and chronic muscle pain. J. Pain 3, 251–260.

McNulty, W.H., Gevirtz, R., Hubbard, D., Berkoff, G., 1994. Needle electromyographic evaluation of trigger point response to a psychological stressor. Psychophysiology 31, 313–316.

McPartland, J.M., Simons, D.G., 2006. Myofascial trigger points: translating molecular theory into manual therapy. J. Man. Manip. Ther. 14, 232–239.

Mekhail, A.O., Checroun, A.J., Ebraheim, N.A., et al., 1999. Extensile approach to the anterolateral surface of the humerus and the radial nerve. J. Shoulder Elbow Surg. 8, 112–118.

Mellick, G.A., Mellick, L.B., 2003. Regional head and face pain relief following lower cervical intramuscular anesthetic injection. Headache 43, 1109–1111.

Mense, S., 1994. Referral of muscle pain. American Pain Society J 3, 1–9.

Myburgh, C., Larsen, A.H., Hartvigsen, J., 2008. A systematic, critical review of manual palpation for identifying myofascial triggers points: evidence and clinical significance. Arch. Phys. Med. Rehabil. 89, 1169–1176.

Niddam, D.M., Chan, R.C., Lee, S.H., et al., 2007. Central modulation of pain evoked from myofascial trigger point. Clin. J. Pain 23, 440–448.

Paraskevas, G., Natsis, K., Ioannidis, O., et al., 2008. Accessory muscles in the lower part of the anterior compartment of the arm that may entrap neurovascular elements. Clin. Anat. 21, 246–251.

Qerama, E., Fuglsang-Frederiksen, A., et al., 2004. Evoked pain in motor endplate region of the brachial biceps muscle: an experimental study. Muscle Nerve 29, 393–400.

Qerama, E., Kasch, H., Fuglsang-Frederiksen, A., 2009. Occurrence of myofascial pain in patients with possible carpal tunnel syndrome: A single-blinded study. Eur. J. Pain 13, 588–591.

Rezzouk, J., Durandeau, A., Vital, J.M., Fabre, T., 2002. Long head of the triceps brachii in axillary nerve injury: anatomy and clinical aspects. Rev. Chir. Orthop. Reparatrice Appar. Mot. 88, 561–564.

Rinzler, S.H., Travell, J., 1948. Therapy directed at the somatic component of cardiac pain. Am. Heart J. 35, 248–268.

Schneider, M., 2005. Tennis elbow. In: Ferguson, L., Gerwin, R. (Eds.), Clinical mastery in the treatment of myofascial pain. Lippincott Williams & Wilkins. Pgs, Baltimore, pp. 122–144.

Sciotti, V.M., Mittak, V.L., DiMarco, L., et al., 2001. Clinical precision of myofascial trigger point location in the trapezius muscle. Pain 93, 259–266.

Shah, J.P., Phillips, T.M., Danoff, J.V., Gerber, L.H., 2005. An in vitro microanalytical technique for measuring the local biochemical milieu of human skeletal muscle. J. Appl. Physiol. 99, 1977–1984.

Shah, J.P., Danoff, J.V., Desai, M.J., et al., 2008. Biochemicals associated with pain and inflammation are elevated in sites near to and remote from active myofascial trigger points. Arch. Phy. Med. Rehabil. 89, 16–23.

Sikdar, S., Shah, J.P., Gilliams, E., et al., 2008. Assessment of myofascial trigger points (TrPs): a new application of ultrasound imaging and vibration sonoelastography. Conf. Proc. IEEE Eng. Med. Biol. Soc. 5585–5588.

Sikdar, S., Shah, J.P., Gebreab, T., et al., 2009. Novel applications of ultrasound technology to visualize and characterize myofascial trigger points and surrounding soft tissue. Arch. Phys. Med. Rehabil. 90, 1829–1838.

Simons, D.G., 1991. Symptomatology and clinical pathophysiology of myofascial pain. Brachial. Schmerz 5, S29–S37.

Simons, D.G., 2001. Do endplate noise and spikes arise from normal motor endplates? Am. J. Phys. Med. Rehabil. 80, 134–140.

Simons, D.G., 2004. Review of enigmatic MTrPs as a common cause of enigmatic musculoskeletal pain and dysfunction. J. Electromyog. Kinesiol. 14, 95–107.

Simons, D.G., Travell, J.G., Simons, L.S., 1999. Travell & Simons' Myofascial pain and dysfunction: the trigger point manual, vol. 1. second ed. Lippincott William & Wilkins, Baltimore, pp. 278–307.

Simons, D., Hong, C.Z., Simons, L., 2002. Endplate potentials are common to midfiber myofascial trigger points. Am. J. Phys. Med. Rehabil. 81, 212–222.

Skubick, D.L., Clasby, R., Donaldson, C.C., Marshall, W.M., 1993. Carpal tunnel syndrome as an expression of muscular dysfunction in the neck. J. Occupational Rehab. 3 (1), 31–43.

Slater, H., Arendt-Nielsen, L., Wright, A., Graven-Nielsen, T., 2003. Experimental deep tissue pain in wrist extensors: a model of lateral epicondylalgia. Eur. J. Pain 7, 277–288.

Slater, H., Arendt-Nielsen, L., Wright, A., Graven-Nielsen, T., 2005. Sensory and motor effects of experimental muscle pain in patients with lateral epicondylalgia and controls with delayed onset muscle soreness. Pain 114, 118–130.

Sluka, K.A., Kalra, A., Moore, S.A., 2001. Unilateral intramuscular injections of acidic saline produce a bilateral, long-lasting hyperalgesia. Muscle Nerve 24, 37–46.

Spanos, T., 2005. Inter-scapular pain: A myofascial composite syndrome. In: Ferguson, L., Gerwin, R. (Eds.), Clinical mastery in the treatment of myofascial pain. Lippincott Williams & Wilkins, Baltimore, pp. 213–226.

Srbely, J.Z., Dickey, J.P., Lowerison, M., et al., 2008. Stimulation of myofascial trigger points with ultrasound induces segmental anti-nociceptive effects: a randomized controlled study. Pain 139, 260–266.

Svensson, P., Cairns, B.E., Wang, K., Arendt-Nielsen, L., 2003a. Glutamate-evoked pain and mechanical allodynia in the human masseter muscle. Pain 101, 221–227.

Svensson, P., Cairns, B.E., Wang, K., Arendt-Nielsen, L., 2003b. Injection of nerve growth factor into human masseter muscle evokes long-lasting mechanical allodynia and hyperalgesia. Pain 104, 241–247.

Tatar, I., Kocabiyik, N., Gayretli, O., Ozan, H., 2009. The course and branching pattern of the deep branch of the radial nerve in relation to the supinator muscle in fetus elbow. Surgical and Radiological Anatomy 31, 591–596.

Tough, E.A., Write, A.R., Richards, S.S., Campbell, J., 2007. Variability of criteria used to diagnose myofascial trigger point pain syndrome: evidence from a review of the literature. Clin. J. Pain 23, 278–286.

Treaster, D., Marras, W., Burr, D., et al., 2006. Myofascial trigger point development from visual and postural stressors during computer work. J. Electromyog. Kinesiol. 16, 115–124.

Witting, N., Svensson, P., Gottrup, H., et al., 2000. Intramuscular and intra-dermal injection of capsaicin: a comparison of local and referred pain. Pain 84, 407–412.

Zhang, Y., Ge, H.Y., Yue, S.W., et al., 2009. Attenuated skin blood flow response to nociceptive stimulation of latent myofascial trigger points. Arch. Phys. Med. Rehabil. 90, 325–332.

Chapter | 33 |

Manual treatment of myofascial trigger points

César Fernández de las Peñas, Hong-You Ge, Jan Dommerholt

INTRODUCTION

Treatment interventions for muscle/ myofascial trigger points

In clinical practice, there are several intervention modalities aimed at eliminating myofascial/muscle trigger points (TrPs): dry needling therapies (Cummings & White 2001, Dommerholt et al 2006a, Tough et al 2009), ultrasound (Gam et al 1998, Majlesi & Unalan 2004, Srbely & Dickey 2007, Srbely et al 2008), thermotherapy (Lee et al 1997), laser therapy (Pöntinen & Airaksinen 1995, Altan et al 2005, Dundar et al 2007), electrotherapy (Tanrikut et al 2003), magnetic therapy (Brown et al 2002, Smania et al 2005), and manual therapies (Simons et al 1999, Lewit 1999). Among these interventions, manual therapies are the basic treatment options (Dommerholt et al 2006b).

The current chapter will focus on different manual approaches that can be used for inactivating muscle TrPs. Several manual therapies are suggested in the literature: massage (Simons et al 1999), ischaemic compression or TrP pressure release (Hong et al 1993, Simons et al 1999,

© 2011 Elsevier Ltd.
DOI: 10.1016/B978-0-7020-3528-9.00033-9

Fryer & Hodgson 2005, Fernández-de-las-Peñas et al 2006b, Gemmell et al 2008, Dommerholt & McEvoy 2011), myofascial induction (Pilat 2009), spray and stretch (Jaeger & Reeves 1986, Hong et al 1993, Simons et al 1999), passive stretching (Hanten et al 2000), muscle energy or post-isometric relaxation techniques (Lewit 1999, Rodriguez-Blanco et al 2006), neuromuscular approaches (Ibáñez-García et al 2009), active head retraction-extension (Hanten et al 1997), strain/counter strain (Dardzinski et al 2000) and spinal manipulative therapy (Kuan et al 1997, Ruiz-Sáez et al 2007, Fernández-de-las-Peñas 2009).

Best evidence of manual therapies for muscle/myofascial trigger points

The first systematic review of manual therapies in the management of TrPs found inconclusive evidence since few studies have investigated manual therapy approaches for the management of TrPs (Fernández-de-las-Peñas et al 2005a). Later studies reported that the ischaemic compression technique is effective in reducing pain sensitivity of latent (Fryer & Hogson 2005) and active (Fernández-de-las-Peñas et al 2006b) muscle TrPs. No significant differences in the reduction of self-perceived pain and pressure pain sensitivity over upper trapezius muscle TrPs between ischaemic compression and transverse friction massage were found (Fernández-de-las-Peñas et al 2006b). In a clinical study, Gemmell et al (2008) showed that ischaemic compression was superior to sham ultrasound in the immediate reduction of pain in patients with non-specific neck pain and active upper trapezius TrPs, although differences were not clinically relevant. A later systematic review analysing the effectiveness of non-invasive treatments for active TrPs revealed that there is evidence of the short-term effectiveness of manual therapies, but no conclusions can be made relating to medium- and long-term follow-ups (Rickards 2006).

One study not included in these reviews found that neuromuscular approaches were also effective for reducing pressure pain sensitivity of latent TrPs (Ibáñez-García et al 2009). Other studies reported improvements in range of motion after treatment with ischaemic compression (Fernández-de-las-Peñas et al 2004) or post-isometric relaxation technique (Rodríguez-Blanco et al 2006) of latent TrPs in the masseter muscle.

Further, there is preliminary evidence investigating changes in muscle sensitivity after spinal manipulations. Kuan et al (1997) found that spinal manipulation at the C3–C4 and C4–C5 levels was effective in reducing pain and tightness from trapezius muscle TrPs. Additionally, Ruiz-Sáez et al (2007) showed that a manipulation directed at the C3–C4 segment evoked changes in pressure pain sensitivity of latent TrPs in the upper trapezius muscle. Nevertheless, although a clinical relationship

between muscle TrPs and joint impairments has been suggested by some authors (Lewit 1999, Fernández-de-las-Peñas et al 2005b, 2006a, 2009), the clinical effects of spinal manipulations on TrP sensitivity remain unclear.

Finally, the most recent review summarized moderately strong evidence supporting the use of ischaemic pressure for immediate pain relief of muscle TrPs but only limited evidence for long-term pain relief (Vernon & Schneider 2009). Nevertheless, it is difficult to draw clinical conclusions from current evidence since most studies have investigated single modalities, whereas multimodal approaches are usually practised by clinicians. Future clinical studies investigating multimodal interventions including the treatment of myofascial/muscle TrPs with manual therapies are needed.

MANUAL THERAPIES FOR THE MANAGEMENT OF MYOFASCIAL/MUSCLE TRIGGER POINTS

Compression interventions

There are different compression techniques depending on the amount of pressure applied and the presence or absence of pain. Further, the compression may be applied with the muscle in a shortened or lengthening position and for different periods of time.

Simons (2002) proposed that compressing the sarcomeres by direct pressure in a vertical and perpendicular manner combined with active contraction of the involved muscle may equalize the length of the muscle sarcomeres in the involved TrP and consequently decrease the pain; however, this theory has not been scientifically investigated (Dommerholt & Shah 2010). Others have suggested that pain relief from direct pressure may result from reactive hyperaemia within the TrP or a spinal reflex mechanism for the relief of muscle tension (Hou et al 2002).

One of the compression techniques applied over muscle TrPs is the so-called *ischaemic compression* (Simons et al 1999): with the muscle in a lengthened position, the therapist gradually applies manual pressure to the TrP until the sensation of pressure becomes painful. At that moment, the pressure is maintained until the discomfort or pain is eased by around 50–75%, perceived by the patient under treatment – at which moment the pressure is increased until discomfort/pain appears again. This process is usually repeated for 90 seconds (Simons et al 1999), with 2 or 3 repetitions.

Fryer & Hodgson (2005) recommended compression up to 7/10 on a pain scale; however, we believe that this level of pain is excessive. Hou et al (2002) provided alternative compression approaches using either low pressure below pain threshold for prolonged periods (90 seconds) or high pressure over pain threshold (pain tolerance) for a short period (30 seconds). In our clinical practice, the pressure level depends on sensitization mechanisms of the patient and degree of irritability of the TrP.

The ischaemic compression technique has been replaced by *TrP pressure release technique* which consists of an application of pressure over the TrP until an increase in muscle resistance (tissue barrier) is perceived by the therapist (Lewit 1999). The barrier is maintained until the therapist perceives release of the taut band. At this stage the pressure is increased to return to the previous level of muscle tension and the process is repeated for 90 seconds (usually with 2 to 3 repetitions). In most subjects, the moment of increased muscle tension is usually non-painful, but in some subjects, the increase in tissue resistance may correlate with a moderate discomfort perceived by the patient. Gemmell et al (2008) did not find significant differences between ischaemic compression and trigger point pressure release.

A third compression intervention that can be applied for inactivating TrPs is the *strain/counter-strain technique* (Jones 1981, D'Ambrogio & Roth 1997). In this technique the therapist applies pressure until the pain threshold. At that moment, the patient is passively placed in a position that reduces the tension under the palpating fingers and causes a subjective reduction of pain by around 90–100%. This position is maintained for 90 seconds. The patient is passively placed in a relaxed position (Jones 1981). This technique was designed for the management of tender points (Jones 1981). There is no evidence that the tender points described by Jones (1981) are indeed the same entity as TrPs. The relationship between tender points and TrPs has not been investigated. Dardzinski et al (2000) reported a positive immediate improvement in symptoms of 50–75% in a patient after the application of a protocol including strain/counter-strain interventions and body exercises. Rodriguez-Blanco et al (2006) demonstrated that the application of a single session of strain/counter-strain technique over latent TrPs in the masseter muscle induced a small increase of active mouth opening.

Massage therapies

The application of massage for inactivating TrPs was discussed by Simons (2002). A recent study has shown that traditional Thai massage increased heart rate variability and improved stress-related parameters in patients presenting with back pain associated with TrPs (Buttagat et al 2010). Massage can be done along the taut band (longitudinal strokes) or across the taut band (transverse massage or strokes). Hong et al (1993) reported that deep tissue massage was more effective on decreasing pressure pain sensitivity than spray and stretch and other manual therapies. Ibáñez-García et al (2009) showed that neuromuscular approaches were effective for reducing pressure pain sensitivity in latent muscle TrPs. Fernández-de-las-Peñas et al (2006b) found that

transverse massage was equally effective as ischaemic compression for reducing TrP pressure pain sensitivity.

Simons (2002) and Hong et al (1993) have proposed that massage may exert a lengthening effect similar to compression techniques. For instance, transverse friction massage may offer a transverse mobilization to the taut band, whereas muscle strokes may offer a longitudinal mobilization of the taut band. In some muscles, particularly those where clinicians can use the pincer palpation, the therapist's fingers can grasp the taut band from both sides of the muscle TrP, stroking centrifugally and elongating away from the TrP (Simons 2002).

Stretching interventions

There are several applications of stretching approaches: passive stretching (where the therapist passively stretches the muscle without participation of the patient), active stretching (where the patient actively stretches the muscle without participation of the therapist), spray and stretch (Hong et al 1993, Simons et al 1999), or post-isometric relaxation (Lewit 1999). Fryer (2000) suggested that the therapeutic mechanism of stretching interventions may be the combination of 'creep', i.e. temporary elongation of connective tissue during the stretch, and plastic changes in the connective tissues caused by the stretch. Nevertheless, there is little evidence showing that stretching is beneficial for TrP treatment.

Jaeger & Reeves (1986), in a low quality study, found that spray and stretch was effective for reducing pain sensitivity and symptoms in active TrPs. Hong et al (1993) demonstrated that spray and stretch showed immediate positive effects on pressure pain sensitivity and was more effective when combined with deep pressure massage. Hou et al (2002) found that the application of spray and stretch in combination with other modalities was more effective than hot packs for inactivating TrPs.

Dynamic interventions

Since myofascial TrPs are placed in active tissues, i.e. the muscle, we believe that it is important to include dynamic interventions. In these approaches clinicians apply any manual intervention, e.g. TrPs pressure release or longitudinal strokes, combined with contraction or stretching of the affected muscle. For instance, during TrP manual compression, the patient is asked to actively contract the affected muscle (Gröbli & Dommerholt 1997, Gröbli & Dejung 2003). The contraction is thought to stretch the shortened sarcomeres against the compression (Simons 2002). The mechanisms of these techniques are still unknown, but may be related to activation of the intrafascial Pacinian/Paciniform and the Ruffini mechanoreceptors, which are found in all types of dense proper connective tissues (Schleip 2003). Ruffini endings are especially responsive to tangential forces and lateral stretch (Kruger 1987), and stimulation of Ruffini corpuscles is assumed to result in a lowering of sympathetic nervous system activity (Van den Berg & Cabri 1999).

Another combination may be that during the manual compression, the patient is asked to move the segment through a range of motion (Gröbli & Dejung 2003). Dynamic techniques may also include a longitudinal stroke applied by the clinician to locally stretch the TrP taut band, whereas the patient is asked to move the segment (Gröbli & Dejung 2003).

CLINICAL APPLICATIONS OF MANUAL THERAPIES OVER MYOFASCIAL/ MUSCLE TRIGGER POINTS

In this section we describe different manual therapies applied to myofascial TrPs in those muscles with referred pain patterns into the neck and arm. The techniques described here are not the only possibilities and clinicians are encouraged to develop their own techniques based on the principles discussed below. The selection of technique will depend on the TrP irritability and the sensitization of the central nervous system of the patient.

Stretching compression of levator scapulae muscle taut band

A stretching compression technique combines compression, either TrP pressure release or ischaemic compression, with passive or active stretching of the TrP taut band. In our clinical practice, we apply this technique for inactivating levator scapulae TrPs located at the angle of the neck where the levator scapulae muscle emerges from the anterior border of the upper trapezius. For this technique, the patient is seated with the torso resting against the backrest. The therapist brings the upper trapezius muscle in a relaxed position to achieve good contact with the levator scapulae TrP. In that position, a compression technique is applied. When the therapist perceives a slight relaxation of the TrP, the patient's neck is gently turned, either passively or actively, toward the opposite side to increase the tension within the taut band (Fig 33.1). This procedure is repeated until a relaxation within the taut band is perceived or until the referred pain disappears.

Longitudinal strokes of scalene muscle taut band

TrP taut bands in the anterior or medial scalene muscles can entrap the brachial plexus (Chen et al 1998). In addition, tension induced by TrP taut bands within the scalene muscles may be related to upward dysfunctions of the first rib (Ferguson & Gerwin, 2005). In our clinical practice,

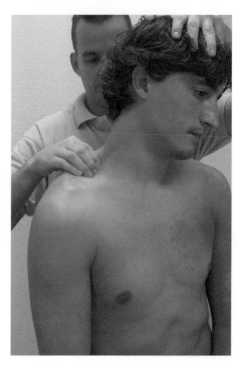

Fig 33.1 Stretching compression of levator scapulae muscle taut band.

the application of longitudinal strokes to both anterior and medial scalene muscles are useful for relaxing TrP taut bands without increasing tension within the brachial plexus.

The anterior scalene is easily palpated below the posterior border of the clavicular division of the sternocleidomastoid muscle. The medial scalene lies deep and lateral to the anterior scalene and anterior to the deep fibres of the levator scapulae muscle.

Longitudinal strokes are usually performed using one thumb in a cranial to caudal direction (Fig 33.2). The degree of pressure applied is determined by the feedback reported by the patient or the tension felt within the patient's tissue.

Compression and contraction of supraspinatus muscle

This technique combines a manual compression with an active contraction of the compressed muscle (Gröbli & Dejung 2003). For the technique, the patient lies prone with the shoulder abducted 90°. The therapist places the upper trapezius muscle in a relaxed position to approximate the supraspinatus fossa of the scapula. In that position, manual compression is applied over supraspinatus TrPs with both thumbs. When the therapist perceives a slight relaxation of the tissue, the patient is asked to

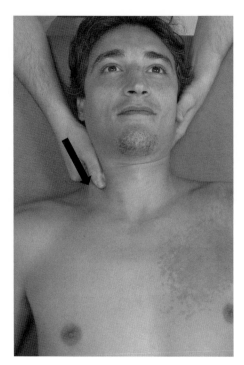

Fig 33.2 Longitudinal stroke of scalene muscle taut band. Black arrow shows the direction of the stroke.

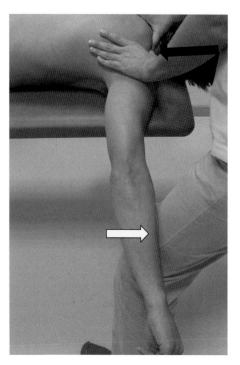

Fig 33.3 Compression and contraction of supraspinatus muscle. The black arrow shows the compression of the therapist and the white arrow shows the direction of the contraction force by the patient (abduction).

contract the muscle abducting the shoulder for 5 seconds. The therapist offers resistance with the leg pushing against the patient's arm in order to achieve an isometric contraction (Fig 33.3). This technique is repeated until the referred pain disappears.

Stretching strokes of infraspinatus muscle taut band

A stretching stroke consists of a longitudinal stroke applied over a muscle placed in a stretched position. With the patient seated, the infraspinatus muscle is stretched by bringing the hand and the arm across the front of the chest to grasp the far armrest of the chair. In this stretched position, longitudinal strokes are performed using one thumb from a medial (thoracic spine) to lateral (spine of the scapula) direction (Fig 33.4).

Stretching longitudinal strokes of infraspinatus muscle taut band

This technique consists of a combination of compression and longitudinal strokes along the TrP taut band. The patient lies prone with the shoulder in 90° of abduction. The fingers of the therapist compress the infraspinatus TrP, grasp the taut band from both sides of the TrP and stroke centrifugally away from the TrP (Fig 33.5).

Stretching compression of teres major muscle taut band

With the patient lying on the opposite side, the teres major muscle can be easily located by pincer palpation. Pincer palpation of the axillary fold a few centimetres below the arm locates the teres major muscle and the lateral border of the scapula. With one hand the therapist pinches the teres major TrP and with the other grasps the forearm of the patient. The therapist passively abducts the patient's shoulder until a tension within the TrP taut band is perceived (Fig 33.6). The tension is usually perceived when the shoulder joint reaches approximately 60° of abduction. The therapist should avoid any compensatory movement of the scapula. The technique is rhythmically repeated until a relaxation in the teres major muscle taut band is perceived.

Stretching compression of subscapularis muscle taut band

The patient is supine with the shoulder abducted between 20–30°. The therapist holds on to the medial border of the scapula and manually brings the scapula laterally. Manual compression is applied cephalad and toward the

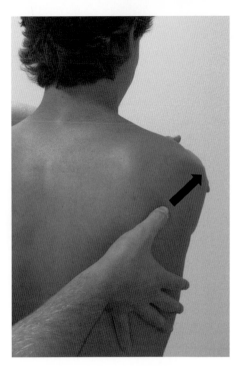

Fig 33.4 Stretching strokes of infraspinatus muscle taut band. Black arrow shows the direction of the stroke.

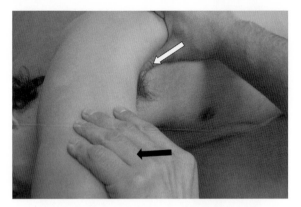

Fig 33.6 Stretching compression of teres major muscle taut band. The black arrow shows the shoulder abduction and the white arrows shows the stabilization force of the therapist.

spine of the scapula. From that position, the therapist dynamically externally rotates and abducts the patient's shoulder until muscle tension is perceived (Fig 33.7).

Dynamic transverse strokes of deltoid muscle trigger points

This technique combines a transverse stroke with passive rotation of the shoulder joint. With the patient supine and the shoulder in 90° of abduction, the therapist grasps the anterior or posterior part of the deltoid muscle.

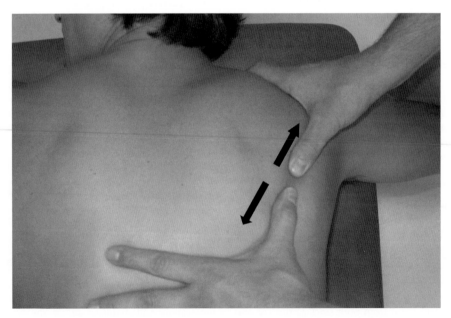

Fig 33.5 Stretching longitudinal strokes of infraspinatus muscle taut band. Both black arrows show the centrifugal direction of the stroke.

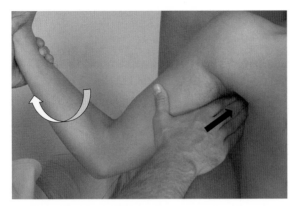

Fig 33.7 Stretching compression of subscapularis muscle taut band. The black arrow shows the compression over the subscapularis whereas the white arrow shows the external rotation and abduction movement.

The thumb of the therapist's hand should be placed over the TrP taut band. The therapist's other hand grasps the forearm. In order to rotate the shoulder joint, the patient's elbow should be extended. For anterior deltoid muscle TrP, the therapist passively internally rotates the shoulder joint and at the same time introduces an anterior to posterior transverse stroke to the anterior part of the deltoid muscle (Fig 33.8). For posterior deltoid muscle TrPs, the

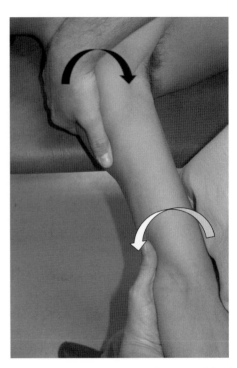

Fig 33.9 Dynamic transverse strokes of posterior deltoid muscle trigger points. Black arrow shows the posterior to anterior stroke of the deltoid and the white arrow shows the external rotation movement.

therapist passively externally rotates the shoulder and at the same time introduces a posterior to anterior transverse stroke to the posterior part of the muscle (Fig 33.9).

Dynamic longitudinal strokes of biceps/triceps brachii muscle taut band

This technique combines longitudinal manual strokes whereas the patient is asked to contract the muscle and move the forearm through its range of motion. For the biceps brachii muscle, the patient lies supine with the shoulder flat on the table, the elbow extended (if possible) and the forearm supinated. The therapist applies longitudinal strokes over the TrP taut band with both thumbs from a cranial (shoulder) to caudal (elbow) direction and at the same time the patient flexes the elbow by contracting the biceps brachii muscle (Fig 33.10). For the triceps brachii muscle, the patient lies prone with the shoulder flat on the table, the elbow flexed (if possible) and hand in neutral position. The therapist applies longitudinal strokes over the taut band with both thumbs from a cranial (shoulder) to caudal (olecranon) direction and at the same time the patient extends the elbow by contracting the triceps brachii (Fig 33.11). It is clinically perceived

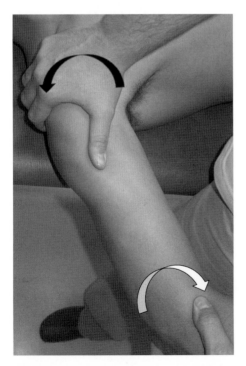

Fig 33.8 Dynamic transverse strokes of anterior deltoid muscle trigger points. Black arrow shows the anterior to posterior stroke of the deltoid and the white arrow shows the internal rotation movement.

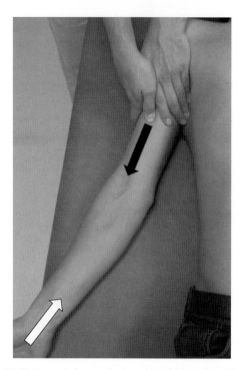

Fig 33.10 Dynamic longitudinal strokes of biceps brachii muscle taut band. The black arrow shows the longitudinal stroke and the white arrow shows the elbow flexion motion.

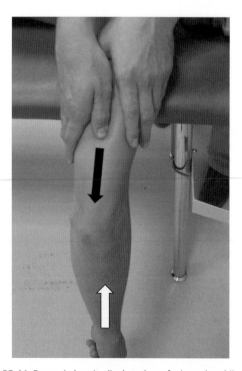

Fig 33.11 Dynamic longitudinal strokes of triceps brachii muscle taut band. The black arrow shows the longitudinal stroke and the white arrow shows the elbow extension motion.

that the strokes should be applied simultaneously to the muscle contraction.

Dynamic longitudinal strokes of hand/wrist extensor muscle taut band

This technique is the same as that described for the biceps/triceps brachii muscle. The patient is seated with the elbow at 90° of flexion, the hand pronated and closed. The therapist applied longitudinal strokes over TrP taut bands with both thumbs from a cranial (elbow) to caudal (wrist) direction and at the same time the patient extends the wrist by contracting the hand/wrist extensor muscles. Since these muscles run longitudinally along the forearm, the therapist can focus the stroke over each hand/wrist extensor muscle (i.e. extensor carpi radialis longus or brevis, extensor digitorum communis or extensor carpi ulnaris muscle).

Transverse massage of hand/wrist flexor muscle trigger points

This technique combines a transverse massage with or without moving the forearm through its range of motion. The patient is asked to actively contract the hand/wrist flexor muscles. The patient is seated with the elbow at 90° of flexion, the hand supinated and opened. The therapist applies a transverse friction massage over TrP taut band of the affected muscle. The patient has two options: (a) to open and close the hand by contracting the hand flexor muscles (Fig 33.12); (b) to close the hand and to flex the wrist by contracting both the hand and wrist flexors (Fig 33.13). Since these muscles also run longitudinal along the forearm, the therapist can focus the transverse massage over the taut band of each hand/wrist flexor muscle (i.e. palmaris longus, flexor carpi radialis or ulnaris, flexor digitorum superficialis or profundus muscle).

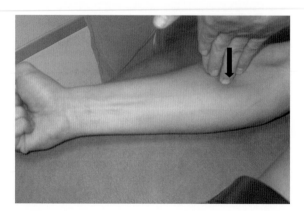

Fig 33.12 Transverse massage of hand flexor muscle trigger points.

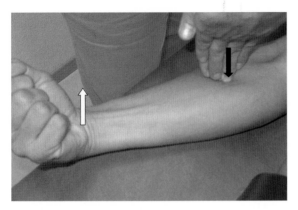

Fig 33.13 Transverse massage of hand/wrist flexor muscle trigger points. The black arrow shows the transverse and the white arrow shows the wrist and finger flexion motion.

Stretching compression of thumb muscles taut bands

Any muscle located in the thenar eminence can develop TrPs. For instance, a TrP within the adductor pollicis muscle refers an aching and deep pain along the thumb and to the radial styloid. TrPs in the opponens pollicis muscle refer pain to the palmar surface of the thumb and to the radial side of the palmar aspect of the wrist.

The stretching compression technique for thenar eminence muscle TrPs consists of compression of the TrP with the thumb of the therapist combined with passive and rhythmical stretching of the muscle. Figure 33.14 shows the technique applied over the opponens pollicis muscle TrPs.

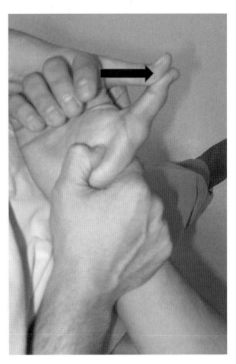

Fig 33.14 Stretching compression of opponens pollicis muscle.

CONCLUSIONS

There are several manual therapies that can be used for inactivating myofascial TrPs within the arm musculature.

Current scientific evidence has investigated single applications of some manual therapies (ischaemic contraction, neuromuscular approach, muscle energy); however, manual therapies are clinically included into a multimodal approach for pain relief. New studies are needed to elucidate the neuro-physiological mechanisms of manual therapies over myofascial TrPs. In addition, the inclusion of manual therapies aimed to inactivating TrPs within multimodal approaches of patients with different arm pain syndromes should be investigated.

REFERENCES

Altan, L., Bingol, U., Aykac, M., Yurtkuran, M., 2005. Investigation of the effect of Ga-As laser therapy on cervical myofascial pain syndrome. Rheumatol. Int. 25, 23–27.

Brown, C.S., Ling, F.W., Wan, J.Y., Pilla, A.A., 2002. Efficacy of static magnetic field therapy in chronic pelvic pain: a double-blind pilot study. Am. J. Obstet. Gynecol. 187, 1581–1587.

Buttagat, V., Eungpinichpong, W., Chatchawan, U., Kharmwan, S.,

2010. The immediate effects of traditional Thai massage on heart rate variability and stress-related parameters in patients with back pain associated with myofascial trigger points. J. Bodyw. Mov. Ther. In Press.

Chen, D., Fang, Y., Li, J, Gu, Y., 1998. Anatomical study and clinical observation of thoracic outlet syndrome. Zhonghua Wai Ke Za Zhi 36, 661–663.

Cummings, T.M., White, A.R., 2001. Needling therapies in the

management of myofascial trigger point pain: a systematic review. Arch. Phys. Med. Rehabil. 82, 986–992.

D'Ambrogio, K.J., Roth, G.B., 1997. Positional Release Therapy. Mosby, St. Louis.

Dardzinski, J.A., Ostrov, B.E., Hamann, L.S., 2000. Myofascial pain unresponsive to standard treatment: successful use of a strain and counter-strain technique with physical therapy. J. Clin. Rheumatol. 6, 169–174.

Dommerholt, J., McEvoy, J., 2011. Myofascial trigger point release approach. In: Wise, C.H. (Ed.), Orthopaedic manual physical therapy: from art to evidence. FA Davis, Philadelphia.

Dommerholt, J., Shah, J., 2010. Myofascial pain syndrome. In: Ballantyne, J.C., Rathmell, J.P., Fishman, S.M. (Eds.), Bonica's management of pain. Lippincott, Williams & Williams, Baltimore, pp. 450–471.

Dommerholt, J., Mayoral-Del-Moral, O., Gröbli, C., 2006a. Trigger point dry needling. J. Man. Manip. Ther. 14, E70–E87.

Dommerholt, J., Bron, C., Franssen, J.L.M., 2006b. Myofascial trigger points: an evidence informed review. J. Man. Manip. Ther. 14, 203–221.

Dundar, U., Evcik, D., Samli, F., Pusak, H., Kavuncu, V., 2007. The effect of gallium arsenide aluminum laser therapy in the management of cervical myofascial pain syndrome: a double blind, placebo-controlled study. Clin. Rheumatol. 26, 930–934.

Ferguson, L., Gerwin, R., 2005. Shoulder dysfunction and frozen shoulder. In: Ferguson, L., Gerwin, R. (Eds.), Clinical mastery in the treatment of myofascial pain. Lippincott Williams & Wilkins, Baltimore, pp. 91–121.

Fernández-de-las-Peñas, C., 2009. Interaction between trigger points and joint hypo-mobility: A clinical perspective. J. Man. Manip. Ther. 17, 74–77.

Fernández-de-las-Peñas, C., Fernández-Carnero, J., Galán-del-Río, F., Miangolarra-Page, J.C., 2004. Are myofascial trigger points responsible of restricted range of motion?: A clinical study (abstract). Journal of Musculoskeletal Pain 12 (Suppl. 9), 19.

Fernández-de-las-Peñas, C., Sohrbeck-Campo, M., Fernández, J., Miangolarra-Page, J.C., 2005a. Manual therapies in the myofascial trigger point treatment: a systematic review. J. Bodyw. Mov. Ther. 9, 27–34.

Fernández-de-las-Peñas, C., Fernández-Carnero, J., Miangolarra-Page, J.C., 2005b. Musculoskeletal disorders in mechanical neck pain: Myofascial trigger points versus cervical joint dysfunctions: A clinical study. Journal of Musculoskeletal Pain 13, 27–35.

Fernández-de-las-Peñas, C., Alonso-Blanco, C., Alguacil-Diego, I.M., Miangolarra, J.C., 2006a. Myofascial trigger points and posterior-anterior joint hypomobility in the mid-cervical spine in subjects presenting with mechanical neck pain: A pilot study. J. Man. Manip. Ther. 14, 88–94.

Fernández-de-las-Peñas, C., Alonso-Blanco, C., Fernández, J., Miangolarra-Page, J.C., 2006b. The immediate effect of ischemic compression technique and transverse friction massage on tenderness of active and latent myofascial triggers points: a pilot study. J. Bodyw. Mov. Ther. 10, 3–9.

Fryer, G., 2000. Muscle energy concepts: a need for change. Journal of Osteopathic Medicine 3, 54–59.

Fryer, G., Hodgson, L., 2005. The effect of manual pressure release on myofascial trigger points in the upper trapezius muscle. J. Bodyw. Mov. Ther. 9, 248–255.

Gam, A.N., Warming, S., Larsen, L.H., et al., 1998. Treatment of myofascial trigger points with ultrasound combined with massage and exercise: a randomised controlled trial. Pain 77, 73–79.

Gemmell, H., Miller, P., Nordstrom, H., 2008. Immediate effect of ischaemic compression and trigger point pressure release on neck pain and upper trapezius trigger points: A randomized controlled trial. Clinical Chiropractics 11, 30–36.

Gröbli, C., Dommerholt, J., 1997. Myofasziale Triggerpunkte; Pathologie und Behandlungsmöglichkeiten. Manuelle Medizin 35, 295–303.

Gröbli, C., Dejung, B., 2003. Nichtmedikamentöse Therapie myofaszialer Schmerze. Schmerz 17, 475–480.

Hanten, W.P., Barrett, M., Gillespie-Plesko, M., et al., 1997. Effects of active head-retraction with retraction/extension and occipital release on the pressure pain threshold of cervical and scapular trigger points. Physiother. Theory Pract. 13, 285–291.

Hanten, W.P., Olson, S.L., Butts, N.L., Nowicki, A.L., 2000. Effectiveness of a home program of ischemic pressure followed by sustained stretch for

treatment of myofascial trigger points. Phys. Ther. 80, 997–1003.

Hong, C.Z., Chen, Y.C., Pon, C.H., Yu, J., 1993. Immediate effects of various physical medicine modalities on pain threshold of an active myofascial trigger point. Journal of Musculoskeletal Pain 1, 37–53.

Hou, C.R., Tsai, L.C., Cheng, K.F., et al., 2002. Immediate effects of various physical therapeutic modalities on cervical myofascial pain and trigger-point sensitivity. Arch. Phys. Med. Rehabil. 83, 1406–1414.

Ibáñez-García, J., Alburquerque-Sendín, F., Rodríguez-Blanco, C., et al., 2009. Changes in masseter muscle trigger points following strain-counter/strain or neuro-muscular technique. J. Bodyw. Mov. Ther. 13, 2–10.

Jaeger, B., Reeves, J.L., 1986. Quantification of changes in myofascial trigger point sensitivity with the pressure algometer following passive stretch. Pain 27, 203–210.

Jones, L.N., 1981. Strain and counter-strain. American Academy of Osteopathy, Newark, OH.

Kruger, L., 1987. Cutaneous sensory system. In: Adelman, G. (Ed.), Encyclopedia of Neuroscience Vol. 1. pp. 293–294.

Kuan, T.S., Wu, C.T., Chen, S., Chen, J.T., Hong, C.Z., 1997. Manipulation of the cervical spine to release pain and tightness caused by myofascial trigger points [abstract]. Arch. Phys. Med. Rehabil. 78, 1042.

Lee, J.C., Lin, D.T., Hong, C.Z., 1997. The effectiveness of simultaneous thermotherapy with ultrasound and electrotherapy with combined AC and DC current on the immediate pain relief of myofascial trigger points. Journal of Musculoskeletal Pain 5, 81–90.

Lewit, K., 1999. Manipulative therapy in rehabilitation of the locomotor system, third ed. Butterworth Heinemann, Oxford.

Majlesi, J., Unalan, H., 2004. High-power pain threshold ultrasound technique in the treatment of active myofascial trigger points: a randomized, double-blind, case-control study. Arch. Phys. Med. Rehabil. 85, 833–836.

Pilat, A., 2009. Myofascial induction approaches for patients with headache. In: Fernández-de-las-Peñas, C., Arendt-Nielsen, L., Gerwin, R. (Eds.), Tension Type and Cervicogenic Headache: pathophysiology, diagnosis and treatment. Jones & Bartlett Publishers, Boston, pp. 339–367.

Pöntinen, P.J., Airaksinen, O., 1995. Evaluation of myofascial pain and dysfunction syndromes and their response to low level laser therapy. Journal of Musculoskeletal Pain 3, 149–154.

Rickards, L.D., 2006. The effectiveness of non-invasive treatments for active myofascial trigger point pain: A systematic review of the literature. International Journal of Osteopathic Medicine 9, 120–136.

Rodríguez-Blanco, C., Fernández-de-las-Peñas, C., Hernández-Xumet, J.E., et al., 2006. Changes in active mouth opening following a single treatment of latent myofascial trigger points in the masseter muscle involving post-isometric relaxation or strain/counter-strain. J. Bodyw. Mov. Ther. 10, 197–205.

Ruiz-Sáez, M., Fernández-de-las-Peñas, C., Rodríguez-Blanco, C., et al., 2007. Changes in pressure pain sensitivity in latent myofascial trigger points in the upper trapezius muscle following a cervical spine manipulation in pain-free subjects. J. Manipulative Physiol. Ther. 30, 578–583.

Schleip, R., 2003. Fascial plasticity: a new neurobiological explanation: Part 1. J. Bodyw. Mov. Ther. 7, 11–19.

Simons, D., Travell, J., Simons, P., 1999. Travell & Simons' Myofascial Pain & Dysfunction: The Trigger Point Manual: The Upper Half of Body. Williams & Wilkins, Baltimore.

Simons, D.G., 2002. Understanding effective treatments of myofascial trigger points. J. Bodyw. Mov. Ther. 6, 81–88.

Smania, N., Corato, E., Fiaschi, A., et al., 2005. Repetitive magnetic stimulation: a novel approach for myofascial pain syndrome. J. Neurol. 252, 307–314.

Srbely, J.Z., Dickey, J.P., 2007. Randomized controlled study of the anti-nociceptive effect of ultrasound on trigger point sensitivity: novel applications in myofascial therapy? Clin. Rehabil. 21, 411–417.

Srbely, J.Z., Dickey, J.P., Lowerison, M., Edwards, A.M., Nolet, P.S., Wong, L.L., 2008. Stimulation of myofascial trigger points with ultrasound induces segmental anti-nociceptive effects: a randomized controlled study. Pain 139, 260–266.

Tanrikut, A., Ozaras, N., Ali-Kaptan, H., et al., 2003. High voltage galvanic stimulation in myofascial pain syndrome. Journal of Musculoskeletal Pain 11, 11–15.

Tough, E.A., White, A.R., Cummings, T.M., et al., 2009. Acupuncture and dry needling in the management of myofascial trigger point pain: A systematic review and meta-analysis of randomised controlled trials. Eur. J. Pain 13, 3–10.

Van den Berg, F., Cabri, J., 1999. Angewandte Physiologie – Das Bindegewebe des Bewegungsapparates verstehen und beeinflussen. Georg Thieme Verlag, Stuttgart, Germany.

Vernon, H., Schneider, M., 2009. Chiropractic management of myofascial trigger points and myofascial pain syndrome: A systematic review of the literature. J. Manipulative Physiol. Ther. 32, 14–24.

Chapter | 34 |

Dry needling of trigger points

Jan Dommerholt

INTRODUCTION

Treating clinically relevant trigger points (TrP) with invasive procedures requires a thorough knowledge of the functional anatomy of muscles and their direct environment. TrPs are identified with manual palpation using either a flat or pincher palpation technique (see Chapter 32). Once a TrP is identified, the clinician must visualize its location in a three-dimensional perspective and appreciate the depth and presence of neighbouring structures, including arteries, veins, nerves, and internal organs. For most muscles, the needle should not be used to locate the TrP, as this would make inactivating TrPs a rather random process (Dommerholt et al 2006). In the neck, shoulder, and arm region, most muscles can be palpated, except parts of the subscapularis and serratus anterior muscles, which are partially in between the scapula and the rib cage. In that case, the clinician can only use the needle to locate and treat TrPs approaching the muscles from the medial border of the scapula. Inactivating TrPs with a needle requires an excellent kinaesthetic sense and awareness, based on training, experience, and anatomical knowledge (Noë 2004). At any time, the clinician must know where in the body the tip of the needle is and which structures will be encountered. Well-developed kinaesthetic perception makes needling procedures safe and accurate as the clinician will be able to appreciate changes in structures and accurately identify when the needle penetrates the skin, the subcutaneous connective tissue and fascial layers, the muscle, and ultimately the taut band and TrP (Mayoral del Moral 2005). When in doubt, stay out!

Invasive TrP therapies can be divided into injection and dry needling. TrP injections are administered with a hypodermic syringe; TrP dry needling is administered with a solid filament needle. Dry needling can be divided into superficial and deep dry needling techniques (Dommerholt et al 2006). Some older studies suggested that dry needling would cause more post-needling soreness (Hong 1994, Kamanli et al 2005), but in these

© 2011 Elsevier Ltd.
DOI: 10.1016/B978-0-7020-3528-9.00034-0

studies, injections were compared to dry needling using a syringe. In a more recent study comparing injections with dry needling using a solid filament needle, there was no significant difference between the two approaches (Ga et al 2007). Dry needling provided longer lasting relief (Ga et al 2007). This chapter covers deep dry needling techniques and does not include specific information about superficial dry needling or TrP injections, but much of the information does apply with minor changes.

Dry needling is within the scope of practice of medicine, acupuncture, and in many jurisdictions of physical therapy and chiropractic. Each practitioner will use discipline-specific philosophy and management approaches to determine when and how dry needling techniques will be applied. Acupuncture practitioners may refer to dry needling as 'TrP acupuncture', but this does not imply that dry needling would be in the exclusive domain of any discipline (Association of Social Work Boards, Federation of State Boards of Physical Therapy et al 2006). Although dry needling is performed with the same needle acupuncturists use, dry needling does not require any knowledge of traditional acupuncture theory or Chinese medicine (Baldry 2005, Amaro 2007, White 2009). Early in the 19th century, physicians used needles, including ladies' hat pins, to treat tender points in the low back region (Churchill 1821, 1828, Elliotson 1827, Osler 1912). Dry needling is an expansion of the TrP injection techniques promoted by Travell, Simons, and others and is based on the observation that the actual mechanical stimulation of a TrP by the needle may be responsible for the therapeutic benefits (Steinbrocker 1944, Travell & Simons 1992, Simons et al 1999).

SCIENTIFIC EVIDENCE OF DRY NEEDLING

One of the first prospective scientific studies of dry needling was published in 1980 and showed its effectiveness in the treatment of injured workers with low back pain (Gunn et al 1980). An authoritative Cochrane review found that dry needling was a potentially useful adjunct in the treatment of individuals with chronic low back pain, but agreed that more high-quality studies are needed (Furlan et al 2005). A study of the effects of latent TrPs on muscle activation patterns in the shoulder region demonstrated that a combination of TrP dry needling and passive stretching restored normal muscle activation patterns (Lucas et al 2004). A prospective, open-label, randomized study on the effect of deep dry needling on shoulder pain in 101 patients following a cerebrovascular accident, showed that after only four dry needling treatments, patients who were treated with dry needling reported significantly less pain during sleep and during physical therapy treatments, had more restful sleep, and

experienced significantly less frequent and less intense pain. They reduced their use of analgesic medications and demonstrated increased compliance with the rehabilitation programme compared to patients who received the regular rehabilitation programme (Dilorenzo et al 2004).

TrP dry needling of the infraspinatus muscle decreased the pain intensity of the shoulder, increased active and passive shoulder internal rotation, and increased the pressure pain threshold of TrPs in the ipsilateral anterior deltoid and extensor carpi radialis longus muscles (Hsieh et al 2007). Dry needling of TrPs in the extensor carpi radialis longus reduced the irritability of TrPs in the ipsilateral trapezius muscle and the overall pain intensity, and improved cervical range of motion (Tsai et al 2010). A similar study of the effect of needling two acupuncture points in the extensor carpi radialis longus and extensor indices muscles reduced the pain intensity and endplate noise associated with a TrP in the trapezius muscle (Chou et al 2009). The authors compared the results to a sham needling procedure, whereby a needle was inserted into a rubber connector with direct contact on the skin. Subjects could feel the sharp needle tip, which makes it questionable whether this was a true sham procedure. Any needling is likely to have a physiological effect, such as a release of endorphins, a change in pain thresholds, or an expectancy of a positive outcome (Pariente et al 2005, Birch 2006, Lund & Lundeberg 2006, Wang et al 2008).

Both actual needling and so-called sham procedures can activate areas involved in sensorimotor processing, and deactivate brain regions more active during rest than during other tasks. Interestingly, in one study areas associated with cognitive functioning were activated by both real and sham needling, but actual needling evoked a stronger response. The authors noted that some of the differences could be due to atypical stimuli from deeper, sub-dermal receptors stimulated by needling, compared to cutaneous receptors stimulated by sham procedures (Napadow et al 2009). Light touch of the skin has been shown to be able to stimulate mechanoreceptors coupled to slow conducting unmyelinated C fibre afferents, which in turn can activate insular regions, but not necessarily the somatosensory cortex (Olausson et al 2002). Kong et al (2006) confirmed that low and moderate pain stimuli were more effective in activating particular areas of the brain than strong pain stimuli.

Dry needling may reduce endplate noise at TrPs (Chen et al 2001) and the chemical concentrations of several nociceptive substances found in the immediate environment of active TrPs (Shah et al 2003, 2005, 2008). Subjects with active TrPs demonstrated abnormal central processing and hyperalgesia in response to electrical stimulation and compression of the TrP (Niddam et al 2007, 2008). Enhanced brain activity was observed in somatosensory and limbic regions, and suppressed activity was noted in the hippocampus (Niddam et al 2008). There is increasing evidence that TrPs contribute to the development of central sensitization (Fernández-de-las-Peñas et al 2007, 2009a,b, Giamberardino et al 2007, Fernández-Carnero et al 2008). There is some evidence from animal studies that needling therapies involve the descending pain inhibitory system (Takeshige et al 1992a,b).

GENERAL GUIDELINES FOR DRY NEEDLING

The following sections provide basic guidance to needling TrPs in the neck, shoulder, and arm muscles. It should be noted that the skills needed to safely and accurately use these techniques can only be learned through attending hands-on courses offered by qualified and experienced tutors. Reading this chapter does not constitute any qualification to use dry needling in clinical practice. There are general guidelines, which should be adhered to. It is recommended that patients are lying down during any needling procedures, because of the risk of vasodepressive syncope. For every muscle, anatomical landmarks should be identified, including the margins of the muscle and any relevant bony structures, i.e. the medial and lateral borders of the scapula and the scapular spine when needling the supraspinatus muscle. Once a TrP is identified, the landmarks are once again verified to assure safe needling.

There is ongoing debate whether disinfection of the skin is necessary and guidelines vary in different countries and regions. For TrP dry needling, using needles in tubes is recommended (White et al 2008). The tube is placed on the skin overlying the TrP and the needle is quickly tapped into the skin. The tube is removed, and the needle is moved in and out into the region of the TrP by drawing the needle back to the subcutaneous tissue and redirecting it. If the needle is not withdrawn sufficiently, the needle will follow the same pathway and the clinician will not be able to alter its direction. The objective of needling is to elicit so-called local twitch responses, which are an indication that the TrP is indeed inactivated (Hong 1994). Following needling procedures, haemostasis must be accomplished to prevent or minimize local bleeding, help restore and maintain range of motion, and facilitate a return to normal function. Only very experienced clinicians should use needling procedures with patients who routinely take warfarin or similar anticoagulants. The use of platelet inhibitors is generally not an absolute contraindication to needling, but requires care to achieve haemostasis.

DRY NEEDLING OF SELECT NECK, SHOULDER, AND ARM MUSCLES

Muscles included in the following sections either cause or contribute to local pain or referred pain in the shoulder or arm. The wrist and finger flexors are not included as the

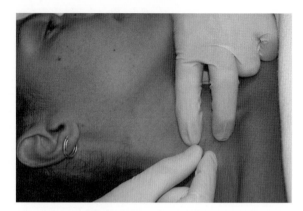

Fig 34.1 Dry needling of the scalene muscles.

treatment is very similar to the treatment of the wrist extensors. The hand muscles are not included as they generally do not cause arm pain.

Scalene muscles (Fig 34.1)

The anterior and middle scalene muscles originate from the first rib, and the posterior scalene muscle comes from the second rib. The muscles insert at the transverse processes of cervical vertebrae C3–C7. For TrP dry needling, the patient is lying either supine or in the lateral position. The medial scalene muscle lies anterior to the transverse processes of the cervical spine. The needle is inserted into the belly of the muscle where the TrP is found. The anterior scalene muscle is identified by asking the patient to sniff sharply (Katagiri et al 2003). The muscle is approached lateral to the clavicular head of the sternocleidomastoid muscle. The posterior scalene muscle is not needled due to its close proximity to the apex of the lungs.

Precautions: The jugular vein should be identified and avoided. The scalene muscles cannot be needled towards the lungs, due to the risk of causing a pneumothorax.

Pectoralis minor muscle (Fig 34.2)

The pectoralis minor muscle originates from the third, fourth and fifth ribs near their costal cartilages and inserts at the coracoid process of the scapula. For TrP dry needling, the patient lies supine. The coracoid process should be identified first. The needle is inserted through the pectoralis muscle and directed either upwards towards the coracoid process, or in a lateral direction tangential to the rib cage.

Precautions: Care must be taken to avoid pneumothorax. Also, the neurovascular bundle of the arm lies under the pectoralis minor muscle close to the coracoid process.

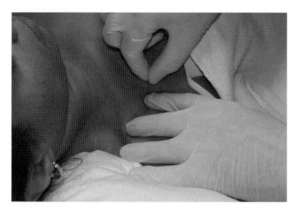

Fig 34.2 Dry needling of the pectoralis minor muscle.

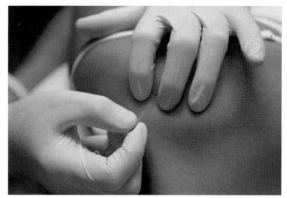

Fig 34.4 Dry needling of the supraspinatus muscle.

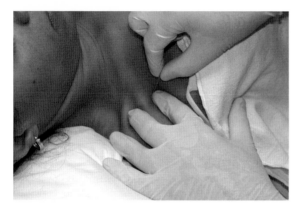

Fig 34.3 Dry needling of the pectoralis major muscle.

Pectoralis major muscle (Fig 34.3)

The pectoralis major muscle has four separate origins; the first arising from the clavicle, the second from the sternum, the third from the ribs, and an abdominal attachment via the aponeuroses of the external abdominal oblique and rectus abdominis muscles. The muscle inserts over the greater tubercle of the humerus along the lateral lip of the bicipital groove. For dry needling, the patient lies supine. When needling over the chest wall, needling is always directed towards a rib with the index and middle fingers placed in the intercostal space to avoid causing pneumothorax. Other portions of the muscle can be needled via a pincer palpation with the needle directed towards the fingers.

Precautions: The ribs must be palpated and used as a guideline to avoid pneumothorax.

Supraspinatus muscle (Fig 34.4)

The muscle arises from the supraspinatus fossa and attaches to the upper part of the greater tubercle of the humeral head. For dry needling, the patient is in side-lying. The needle is directed slightly posteriorly towards the upper border of the scapula and scapular spine.

Precautions: If the needle is directed towards the anterior wall of the supraspinatus fossa, there is a considerable risk of causing a pneumothorax.

Infraspinatus/teres major/teres minor muscles (Fig 34.5)

The three muscles originate from different aspects of the posterior surface of the scapula below the scapular spine. The infraspinatus muscle arises from the infraspinatus fossa and attaches to the middle part of the greater tubercle of the humeral head. The teres major originates at the inferior angle of the scapula and inserts in front of the humerus to its lesser tubercle. The teres minor originates from a higher and more lateral point than the teres major near the axillary border of the scapula. The teres minor inserts behind the humerus to the greater tubercle. For dry needling, the patient lies in the prone position or in

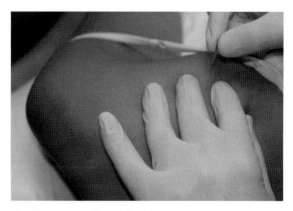

Fig 34.5 Dry needling of the infraspinatus/teres major/teres minor muscles.

side-lying with the arm supported with a pillow. Body landmarks must be palpated before each needle insertion. The medial and lateral border of the scapula should be palpated prior to the needle insertion. For the infraspinatus, the needle is inserted directly into the TrP. When possible, the teres major and minor are grasped between the thumb and the index finger and the needle is inserted towards the finger or the scapula. If the muscles cannot be held in a pincer palpation, careful needling in a lateral direction tangential to the curvature of the rib cage is indicated.

Precautions: Individuals with osteoporosis may present with thin and fenestrated scapulae. By developing a good kinaesthetic awareness of needling, clinicians should notice when the needle leaves the muscle.

Rhomboid major and minor muscles (Fig 34.6)

The rhomboid minor attaches from the spinous processes of C7–T1 and reaches inferior laterally to the medial scapular border at the level of its spine. The rhomboid major muscle originates from the spinous processes of T2–T5 and inserts over the medial border of the scapula to its inferior angle. The muscle is needled in side-lying or prone position. When needling over the chest wall, needling is always directed towards a rib with the index and middle fingers placed in the intercostal space to avoid causing pneumothorax. The needle is inserted in a shallow angle towards the rib in order to avoid penetrating the lung.

Precautions: The rhomboid muscle poses a relatively high risk for pneumothorax. The ribs must be palpated and the needle should always be directed to towards the ribs.

Subscapularis muscle (Fig 34.7)

The subscapularis muscle lies over the anterior surface of the scapula. It originates from the inner surface of the scapula and attaches to the lesser tuberosity of the

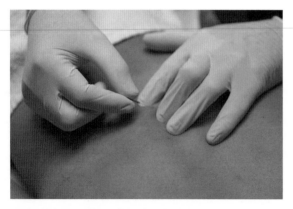

Fig 34.6 Dry needling of the rhomboid major and minor muscles.

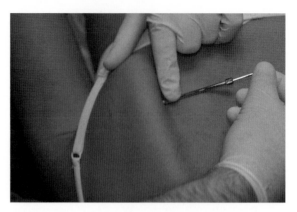

Fig 34.7 Dry needling of the subscapularis muscle.

humerus. For dry needling, the patient lies supine with the arm held in approximately 90 degrees of abduction with the elbow bent. The clinician manually brings the scapula in a protracted and laterally displaced position, which will provide greater access to the lateral aspect of the muscle. The palpating hand is placed against the rib cage and rests on the muscle. The needle is inserted between the palpating fingers towards the undersurface of the scapula. An alternative dry needling may be the following. To treat the more medial TrPs, the patient is placed in the side-lying position on the side that needs to be treated or in prone. The patient's trunk is positioned in such a way that there is winging of the scapula, which makes it possible to needle TrPs in the subscapularis muscle. The needle is directed toward the undersurface of the scapula tangential over the rib cage.

Precautions: With needling the lateral aspect of the muscle, the lungs are protected by keeping the palpating fingers against the chest wall to accurately locate the rib cage. Needling towards the ribs must be avoided for both needle techniques.

Latissimus dorsi muscle (Fig 34.8)

The latissimus dorsi originates from the spinous process of the lower T6 vertebra, the thoracolumbar fascia, iliac crest and inferior three or four ribs. The insertion of the muscle is at the intertubercular groove of the humerus. The muscle can be needled with the patient in supine, prone or side-lying. To needle the latissimus dorsi in the axilla, the patient lies supine with the arm abducted at shoulder level. The muscle is palpated with a pincer palpation and the needle is inserted perpendicularly to the skin. Needling the latissimus dorsi over the trunk requires a similar approach described in the section on the rhomboid muscles.

Precautions: All needle insertions are made in consideration of the chest wall and lungs.

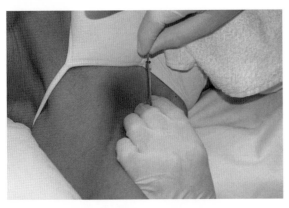

Fig 34.8 Dry needling of the latissimus dorsi muscle.

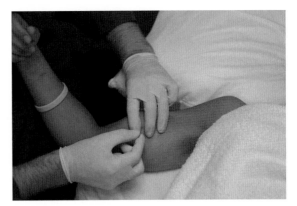

Fig 34.10 Dry needling of the biceps brachii muscle.

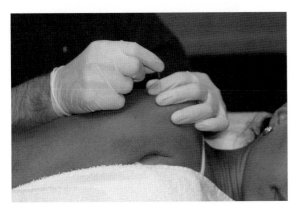

Fig 34.9 Dry needling of the deltoid muscle.

Deltoid muscle (Fig 34.9)

The muscle originates from the anterior border of the lateral third of the clavicle, the lateral border of the acromion bone, lower lip of scapular spine and the fascia over the infraspinatus muscle, and the insertion is over the deltoid tuberosity at the humerus. For dry needling, the patient is either in supine or side-lying position. The needle is inserted perpendicularly through the skin directly into the taut band.

Precautions: None.

Biceps brachii muscle (Fig 34.10)

The long head of the biceps brachii muscle originates from the glenoid fossa with its tendon passing through the glenohumeral joint. The short head originates from the coracoid process without passing through the glenohumeral joint. Both heads attach distally to the lesser tuberosity of the radius. For dry needling, the patient lies in supine. The muscle is palpated and picked up via a

pincer palpation. The needle is inserted perpendicular to the skin and directed towards the practitioner's finger.

Precautions: The neurovascular bundle, which includes the median nerve, the musculocutaneous nerve, the ulnar nerve, and the brachial artery, is located medially to the biceps brachii muscle and must be avoided.

Triceps brachii muscle

The triceps muscle consists of three heads: the long head originates from the scapula inferior to the glenoid fossa, the medial head originates from the medial portion of the humerus and the lateral head originates from the lateral side of the humerus. All three heads insert to the olecranon process on the ulna via a common tendon. For dry needling, the patient can be in supine, prone or side-lying. The muscle is needled via a pincer palpation.

Precautions: The radial nerve passes posteriorly against the humerus and underneath the triceps muscle.

Brachialis muscle (Fig 34.11)

The brachialis muscle originates from the distal two-thirds of the humerus and inserts at the coronoid process of the ulnar tuberosity. The muscle extends into the joint capsule of the elbow. For dry needling, the patient lies supine with the elbow supported and relaxed in a slight flexion. The muscle is palpated with a flat palpation technique. The muscle is needled only from the lateral aspect of the arm to avoid hitting the neurovascular bundle. The needle is directed medially.

Precautions: The neurovascular bundle should be avoided over the medial head of the muscle.

Brachioradialis muscle (Fig 34.12)

The muscle starts from the upper two-thirds of the supracondylar ridge of the humerus and attaches over the distal radius at the styloid process. For dry needling, the patient

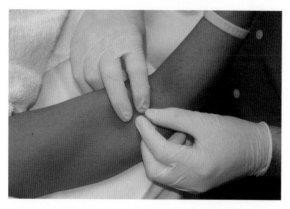

Fig 34.11 Dry needling of the brachialis muscle.

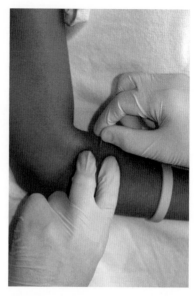

Fig 34.13 Dry needling of the supinator muscle.

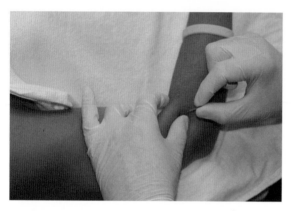

Fig 34.12 Dry needling of the brachioradialis muscle.

lies in supine position. TrPs are identified via pincer palpation. The needle is inserted and directed towards the practitioner's finger.

Precautions: This muscle is the most superficial muscle over the lateral elbow. The radial nerve passes close to it and should be avoided.

Supinator muscle (Fig 34.13)

The supinator muscle originates from the lateral humeral epicondyle, radial collateral ligament, and the annular ligament and the supinator crest of the ulna. The muscle inserts over the radial tuberosity and upper third of the radial shaft. For dry needling, the patient is in supine with the arm supinated. Flat palpation against the radial bone on the volar side of the arm is used to identify the muscle. The needle is inserted pointing proximally towards the humerus. It is possible to needle the supinator muscle at the dorsal aspect of the forearm but there is a risk of hitting the superficial radial nerve, which lies over the muscle, or the posterior interosseus nerve, which lies in between the two heads of the muscle.

Precaution: With the posterior approach, there is a risk of hitting the sensory and motor branches of the radial nerve.

Pronator teres muscle

The pronator teres muscle has a humeral and an ulnar head. They originate from the medial epicondyle and the medial side of the coronoid process of the ulna respectively. Both heads insert over the radius distally from the insertion of the supinator muscle. For dry needling, the patient lies supine with the forearm supinated. The median nerve runs in between the two heads of the pronator teres muscle. The muscle can be needled at the proximal, medial portion approximately 1–2 cm below the elbow joint to avoid the median nerve or at the distal portion close to the insertion over the radius. The muscle is palpated with a flat palpation technique. The needle is inserted perpendicular to the skin and directed towards the ulna or radius respectively.

Precautions: The median nerve runs between the two heads of the muscle and should be avoided.

Wrist and finger extensor muscles (Fig 34.14)

The wrist extensors (extensor carpi radialis longus and brevis muscles) originate from the lateral supracondylar ridge of the humerus, the lateral epicondyle, the radial ligament of the elbow, and the intermuscular septa through a common tendon, which is shared with the extensor carpi ulnaris muscle, and the extensor digitorum muscle.

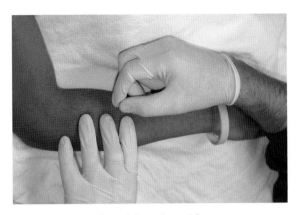

The attachments are at the base of the second and third metacarpal bone, the ulnar side of the base of the fifth metacarpal bone, and the distal phalanx of the fingers respectively. For dry needling, the extensor carpi radialis longus and brevis can be needled with the muscles held in a pincer palpation. The extensor carpi ulnaris and extensor digitorum muscles are treated with a flat palpation.

Precautions: The radial nerve crosses over the extensor digitorum muscle.

Fig 34.14 Dry needling of the wrist and finger extensor muscles.

REFERENCES

Amaro, J.A., 2007. When acupuncture becomes 'dry needling'. Acupuncture Today November 33, 43.

Association of Social Work Boards, Federation of State Boards of Physical Therapy, et al., 2006. Changes in healthcare professions scope of practice: legislative considerations. ASWB, Washington.

Baldry, P.E., 2005. Acupuncture, Trigger Points and Musculoskeletal Pain. Churchill Livingstone, Edinburgh.

Birch, S., 2006. A review and analysis of placebo treatments, placebo effects, and placebo controls in trials of medical procedures when sham is not inert. J. Altern. Complement. Med. 12, 303–310.

Chen, J.T., Chung, K.C., Hou, C.R., et al., 2001. Inhibitory effect of dry needling on the spontaneous electrical activity recorded from myofascial trigger spots of rabbit skeletal muscle. Am. J. Phys. Med. Rehabil. 80, 729–735.

Chou, L.W., Hsieh, Y.L., Kao, M.J., Hong, C.Z., 2009. Remote influences of acupuncture on the pain intensity and the amplitude changes of endplate noise in the myofascial trigger point of the upper trapezius muscle. Arch. Phys. Med. Rehabil. 90, 905–912.

Churchill, J.M., 1821. A treatise on acupuncturation being a description

of a surgical operation originally peculiar to the Japanese and Chinese, and by them denominated zin-king, now introduced into European practice. with directions for its performance and cases illustrating its success. Simpkins & Marshall, London.

Churchill, J.M., 1828. Cases illustrative of the immediate effects of acupuncturation in rheumatism, lumbago, sciatica, anomalous muscular diseases and in dropsy of the cellular tissues, selected from various sources and intended as an appendix to the author's treatise on the subject. Simpkins & Marshall, London.

Dilorenzo, L., Traballesi, M., Morelli, D., et al., 2004. Hemiparetic shoulder pain syndrome treated with deep dry needling during early rehabilitation: a prospective, open-label, randomized investigation. Journal of Musculoskeletal Pain 12 (2), 25–34.

Dommerholt, J., Mayoral-Del-Moral, O., Gröbli, C., 2006. Trigger point dry needling. J. Man. Manip. Ther. 14, E70–E87.

Elliotson, J., 1827. The use of the sulphate of copper in chronic diarrhoea together with an essay on acupuncture. Med. Chir. Trans. 13, 451–467.

Fernández-de-las-Peñas, C., Cuadrado, M.L., Arendt-Nielsen, L., et al., 2007. Myofascial trigger points and sensitization: an updated pain model for tension-type headache. Cephalalgia 27, 383–393.

Fernández-de-las-Peñas, C., Cuadrado, M.L., Barriga, F.J., Pareja, J.A., 2009a. Active muscle trigger points as sign of sensitization in chronic primary headaches. Journal of Musculoskeletal Pain 17 (2), 155–161.

Fernández-de-las-Peñas, C., Galán-del-Rio, F., Fernández-Carnero, J., et al., 2009b. Bilateral widespread mechanical pain sensitivity in women with myofascial temporomandibular disorder: evidence of impairment in central nociceptive processing. J. Pain 10, 1170–1179.

Fernández-Carnero, J., Fernández-de-las-Peñas, C., De-la-Llave-Rincon, A.I., et al., 2008. Bilateral myofascial trigger points in the forearm muscles in patients with chronic unilateral lateral epicondylalgia: a blinded, controlled study. Clin. J. Pain 24, 802–807.

Furlan, A., Tulder, M., Cherkin, D., et al., 2005. Acupuncture and Dry-Needling for low back pain: an updated systematic review within the framework of the cochrane collaboration. Spine 30, 944–963.

Ga, H., Koh, H.J., Choi, J.H., Kim, C.H., 2007. Intramuscular and nerve root stimulation vs lidocaine injection to trigger points in myofascial pain syndrome. J. Rehabil. Med. 39, 374–378.

Giamberardino, M., Tafuri, E., Savini, A., et al., 2007. Contribution of myofascial trigger points to migraine symptoms. J. Pain 8, 869–878.

Gunn, C.C., Milbrandt, W.E., Little, A.S., Mason, K.E., 1980. Dry needling of muscle motor points for chronic low-back pain: a randomized clinical trial with long-term follow-up. Spine 5, 279–291.

Hong, C.Z., 1994. Lidocaine injection versus dry needling to myofascial trigger point. The importance of the local twitch response. Am. J. Phys. Med. Rehabil. 73, 256–263.

Hsieh, Y.L., Kao, M.J., Kuan, T.S., et al., 2007. Dry needling to a key myofascial trigger point may reduce the irritability of satellite MTrPs. Am. J. Phys. Med. Rehabil. 86 (5), 397–403.

Kamanli, A., Kaya, A., Ardicoglu, O., et al., 2005. Comparison of lidocaine injection, botulinum toxin injection, and dry needling to trigger points in myofascial pain syndrome. Rheumatol. Int. 25, 604–611.

Katagiri, M., Abe, T., Yokoba, M., et al., 2003. Neck and abdominal muscle activity during a sniff. Respir. Med. 97, 1027–1035.

Kong, J., White, N.S., Kwong, K.K., et al., 2006. Using fMRI to dissociate sensory encoding from cognitive evaluation of heat pain intensity. Hum. Brain Mapp. 27, 715–721.

Lucas, K.R., Polus, B.I., Rich, P.A., 2004. Latent myofascial trigger points: their effects on muscle activation and movement efficiency. J. Bodyw. Mov. Ther. 8 (2), 160–6.

Lund, I., Lundeberg, T., 2006. Are minimal, superficial or sham acupuncture procedures acceptable as inert placebo controls? Acupunct. Med. 24, 13–15.

Mayoral del Moral, O., 2005. Fisioterapia invasiva del síndrome de dolor miofascial. Fisioterapia 27, 69–75.

Napadow, V., Dhond, R.P., Kim, J., et al., 2009. Brain encoding of acupuncture sensation–coupling on-line rating with fMRI. Neuroimage 47, 1055–1065.

Niddam, D.M., Chan, R.C., Lee, S.H., et al., 2007. Central modulation of pain evoked from myofascial trigger point. Clin. J. Pain 23 (5), 440–448.

Niddam, D.M., Chan, R.C., Lee, S.H., et al., 2008. Central representation of hyperalgesia from myofascial trigger point. Neuroimage 39, 1299–1306.

Noë, A., 2004. Action in perception. MIT Press, Cambridge.

Olausson, H., Lamarre, Y., Backlund, H., et al., 2002. Unmyelinated tactile afferents signal touch and project to insular cortex. Nat. Neurosci. 5, 900–904.

Osler, W., 1912. The principles and practice of medicine. Appleton, New York.

Pariente, J., White, P., Frackowiak, R., Lewith, G., 2005. Expectancy and belief modulate the neuronal substrates of pain treated by acupuncture. Neuroimage 25, 1161–1167.

Shah, J., Phillips, T., Danoff, J.V., et al., 2003. A novel microanalytical technique for assaying soft tissue demonstrates significant quantitative biomechanical differences in 3 clinically distinct groups: normal, latent and active. Arch. Phys. Med. Rehabil. 84, A4.

Shah, J.P., Phillips, T.M., Danoff, J.V., Gerber, L.H., 2005. An in vitro microanalytical technique for measuring the local biochemical milieu of human skeletal muscle. J. Appl. Physiol. 99 (5), 1977–84.

Shah, J.P., Danoff, J.V., Desai, M.J., et al., 2008. Biochemicals associated with pain and inflammation are elevated in sites near to and remote from active myofascial trigger points. Arch. Phys. Med. Rehabil. 89 (1), 16–23.

Simons, D.G., Travell, J.G., Simons, L.S., 1999. Travell and Simons' myofascial pain and dysfunction; the trigger point manual. Williams & Wilkins, Baltimore.

Steinbrocker, O., 1944. Therapeutic injections in painful musculoskeletal disorders. J. Am. Med. Assoc. 125, 397–401.

Takeshige, C., Kobori, M., Hishida, F., et al., 1992a. Analgesia inhibitory system involvement in nonacupuncture point-stimulation-produced analgesia. Brain Res. Bull. 28, 379–391.

Takeshige, C., Sato, T., Mera, T., et al., 1992b. Descending pain inhibitory system involved in acupuncture analgesia. Brain Res. Bull. 29, 617–634.

Travell, J.G., Simons, D.G., 1992. Myofascial pain and dysfunction: the trigger point manual. Williams & Wilkins, Baltimore.

Tsai, C.T., Hsieh, L.F., Kuan, T.S., et al., 2010. Remote effects of dry needling on the irritability of the myofascial trigger point in the upper trapezius muscle. Am. J. Phys. Med. Rehabil. 89, 133–140.

Wang, S.M., Kain, Z.N., White, P.F., 2008. Acupuncture analgesia: II. Clinical considerations. Anesth. Analg. 106, 611–621.

White, A., 2009. Western medical acupuncture: a definition. Acupunct. Med. 27, 33–35.

White, A., Cummings, M., et al., 2008. An introduction to Western medical acupuncture. Churchill Livingstone, Edinburgh.

Chapter | 35 |

Muscle energy approaches

Gary Fryer

INTRODUCTION

Muscle energy technique (MET) is a system of manual procedures that utilizes active muscle contraction effort from the patient, usually against a controlled matching counterforce from the therapist. The MET system was developed by osteopathic physician Fred Mitchell, Sr, in the 1950s although techniques using resisted muscle effort to increase range of motion have been documented in the osteopathic literature as early as 1919 (Swart 1919). The evolution of MET continued with contributions from Fred Mitchell, Jr, who systematized and further developed the methods in published technique manuals (Mitchell et al 1979, Mitchell & Mitchell 1995). The MET approach has since benefited from contributions by many individuals and is now practised by clinicians in different manual therapy disciplines. MET has been used to lengthen shortened muscles, mobilize articulations with restricted

© 2011 Elsevier Ltd.
DOI: 10.1016/B978-0-7020-3528-9.00035-2

mobility, strengthen weakened muscles, and reduce localized oedema and passive congestion (Mitchell et al 1979, Bourdillon et al 1992, Mitchell & Mitchell 1995, Goodridge & Kuchera 1997, Chaitow 2006).

The most commonly described method of MET application is the post-isometric relaxation (or 'contract-relax') technique, especially when the aim is to increase muscle length or joint range of motion. The number of repetitions used is influenced by the response of the involved tissues, but 3–5 repetitions of the procedure have often been recommended (Mitchell et al 1979, Bourdillon et al 1992, Mitchell & Mitchell 1995, Goodridge & Kuchera 1997, Chaitow 2006). The force and duration of isometric effort can be varied depending on the aim of the technique and the tissues involved. A gentle, carefully controlled isometric effort is usually suitable for treatment of specific joint dysfunctions, myofascial trigger points (TrPs), or acute myofascial pain, whereas a stronger contraction can be employed for more fibrotic, shortened muscles. Other variations of this technique exist, like the use of concentric contractions against a yielding resistance to increase strength and recruitment of a muscle, or reciprocal inhibition techniques which facilitate relaxation of a muscle when applied to the antagonist muscle, but these techniques will not be detailed in this chapter.

There are similarities between MET and other forms of post-isometric stretching, such as proprioceptive neuromuscular facilitation techniques, particularly when the techniques are applied to facilitate the lengthening of muscle. However, MET was developed along biomechanical principles for the treatment of spinal and pelvic joint dysfunction, an emphasis which is evident in many MET texts (Mitchell & Mitchell 1995). In this respect, it is very different from other treatment systems which use isometric contraction.

An integrated approach to muscle energy

MET was developed by osteopathic physicians and intended to be applied in a holistic manner consistent with osteopathic philosophy. Osteopathy emphasizes the unity and inter-connectedness of the body, the inter-relationship of structure and function, and the important influence that the musculoskeletal system may exert on other systems and general health. The MET approach was based on a specific diagnostic model that emphasized a global view of body biomechanics and included screening and scanning of global posture, movement patterns, and gross and segmental range of motion (Mitchell et al 1979). For example, in patients presenting with neck and arm pain, the body would be examined from head to toe (posture, static and dynamic symmetry, active and passive range of motion), and treatment would be directed at any or all of the regions believed to be problematic – lower limb, pelvic, lumbar, thoracic,

rib cage, neck, head, upper extremity. Implicit in this approach are the concepts that dysfunction in one region may cause compensation and strain in other regions and that treatment which only addresses the symptomatic site is likely to achieve only short-term relief. In recent years, the remote effects of a manual intervention have received attention from some researchers, resulting in reports of cervical treatment improving shoulder symptoms and hamstring flexibility (Aparicio et al 2009, McClatchie et al 2009), and of thoracic treatment improving neck pain (Cleland et al 2005, González-Iglesias et al 2009) and shoulder pain and disability (Boyles et al 2009).

Assessment and treatment of the thorax – including the spinal joints, the ribs, and the muscles – are extremely important for patients with neck and arm complaints. Treatment of this region should precede treatment of the neck and upper extremity because – in the author's experience – it often produces change and improvement to both symptoms and physical findings in the neck and extremities. Due to limitations of space, techniques for the thorax will not be described here, but the same principles apply to joints in these regions and will be obvious to readers who understand these principles.

MET may be applied in combination with other manual techniques, such as soft tissue manipulation, passive joint articulation, high velocity thrust, and gentle indirect techniques like functional technique and counter-strain (where tissues are held in a position of ease). There is no universal agreement on the criteria for technique selection for a given condition or patient, and probably therapist and patient preferences are significant determinants. Techniques may be selected based on their likely therapeutic mechanisms, despite the speculative nature of those mechanisms. For example, MET may be used where fluid drainage and improved proprioception are desired, high velocity may be used where joint end-feel is particularly hard, end-range articulation may be used where joint motion appears restricted by fibrotic changes in peri-articular tissues, and indirect approaches may be used where significant inflammation and pain is present. The integration of these techniques may involve intuitive cues from palpation and the pragmatic use of alternative techniques when the initial techniques fail to achieve the intended tissue and motion changes.

Evidence of efficacy

As is the case for many manual therapy approaches, there is a lack of high-quality research investigating the clinical effectiveness of MET. This is not surprising given that MET is typically used in conjunction with other techniques, rather than as a single treatment. There is a growing body of evidence demonstrating that MET (and similar post-isometric stretching techniques) increases the extensibility of muscles (Sady et al 1982, Wallin et al 1985, Osternig et al 1990, Magnusson S. et al 1996, Feland et al 2001, Ferber et al 2002, Ballantyne et al 2003) and the range of neck and trunk motion (Schenk et al 1994, 1997, Lenehan et al 2003, Fryer & Ruszkowski 2004, Burns & Wells 2006). However, many of these studies have examined only the immediate or short-term effect of treatment, often in healthy subjects, and there is little evidence that links improvements in flexibility and mobility to positive patient outcomes.

Only one randomized controlled trial of MET as the sole treatment for spinal pain was found during a literature search. This trial reported that acute low back pain patients treated with MET and a home exercise programme had greater improvement in pain and disability than a sham treatment and home exercise programme (Wilson et al 2003). Several clinical trials investigating osteopathic management of spinal pain have included MET as a treatment component, providing additional support for MET as an effective treatment (Licciardone et al 2003, Fryer et al 2005, Chown et al 2008, Schwerla et al 2008). However, these few studies indicate the need for further investigation, particularly for lasting improvement in flexibility and motion and clinical improvement in pain and disability.

Physiological mechanisms

Although the mechanisms by which MET may produce therapeutic benefit are still largely speculative, MET may produce neurological and biomechanical effects, although perhaps through mechanisms that are not typically described in MET texts (Fryer & Fossum 2009b). Traditionally MET has been proposed to produce muscle relaxation via Golgi tendon organ and muscle spindle reflexes (Kuchera & Kuchera 1992, Mitchell & Mitchell 1995), but this explanation seems unlikely since some studies have generally reported increases in electromyographic activity following post-isometric stretching techniques (Osternig et al 1987, 1990). MET has also been proposed to reset the neurological resting length of muscles, but it appears that motor activity does not play a significant role in limiting passive stretch of a muscle, at least in healthy, uninjured subjects (Magnusson et al 1996a,b).

Increased flexibility of muscle groups following isometric contraction is most attributable to an increase in the subject's tolerance to stretch, rather than to lasting biomechanical change in the tissue (Magnusson et al 1996b, Fryer & Fossum 2009b). Increased stretch tolerance may be a result of a decrease in pain perception (hypoalgesia) through the activation of muscle and joint mechanoreceptors which involve centrally mediated pathways, such as the peri-aqueductal grey in the midbrain region and non-opioid serotonergic and noradrenergic descending inhibitory pathways (Souvalis et al 2004, Fryer & Fossum 2009b). Additionally, MET may produce hypoalgesia via peripheral mechanisms associated with increased fluid drainage. Rhythmic muscle contractions increase muscle blood and lymph flow rates (Coates et al 1993, Havas et al 1997). Mechanical forces (such as loading and stretching) acting on fibroblasts in connective tissues may affect fibroblast mechanical signal transduction processes (Langevin et al 2004), changing the interstitial pressure and increasing transcapillary blood flow (Langevin et al 2005). These factors may play an important role in the tissue response to injury and inflammation. MET may support these processes by reducing the concentrations of pro-inflammatory cytokines, resulting in decreased sensitization of peripheral nociceptors.

In addition to hypoalgesia, MET may work in the neurological sphere to enhance proprioception and motor control in patients with pain. Patients with spinal pain have decreased awareness of direction of spinal motion and position (Leinonen et al 2002, Grip et al 2007, Lee et al 2007) and exhibit changes in paraspinal muscle motor strategies (Fryer et al 2004). There is evidence that high velocity manipulation improves head re-positioning in chronic neck pain patients (Rogers 1997, Palmgren et al 2006) and motor recruitment strategies in low back pain patients (Ferreira et al 2007). Although speculative, MET may enhance proprioception, motor control, and motor learning because it involves active and precise recruitment of muscle activity. This area deserves further investigation.

PRINCIPLES OF MUSCLE ENERGY APPLICATION

General principles

The elements comprising the application of MET – restrictive barrier engagement, force of contraction, duration of contraction and post-isometric stretch, number of repetitions – can be varied according to the aim of the technique, the tissue or joint, and the response of tissues to treatment. In general, the precise localization of leverages in one or more planes to a restrictive joint barrier with a gentle contraction effort is important for the application of MET to a single joint dysfunction. These principles may also be applied to irritable or painful myofascial tissues, and the force of stretch and contraction intensity may be progressively increased for muscles that are short and fibrotic without substantial tenderness. In all cases, the therapist should have a well balanced posture to provide control and resistance to the isometric effort in an economical manner; it should not be a struggle. The patient should always be comfortable; the procedures should not be painful even when using a moderate stretching force for large muscles. This chapter describes techniques for a number of commonly encountered joint and muscle dysfunctions; however, the therapist who has a clear understanding of muscle anatomy and joint biomechanics along with the principles of MET should be able to create and modify techniques to affect almost any joint restriction or shortened muscle.

Cautions and contraindications

MET is a safe technique, and no reports of serious adverse reactions have been found in the literature. The cautions and contraindications for MET are similar to those of other soft tissue techniques and involve caution with the use of force and leverage when dealing with acute pain conditions and individuals with weakened bone. In MET, very gentle to moderate application of stretch or isometric contraction is normally performed, so MET is perceived as a safe technique with little risk of serious injury. When applied to previously injured, healing tissues, forces of contraction or stretch should be matched to the stage of healing and repair of the injury to avoid further tissue damage and to promote optimal healing (Lederman 2005).

Cerebrovascular accidents following high velocity manipulation to the cervical spine have been reported as unpredictable rare complications (Di Fabio 1999, Haldeman et al 2001), and, although no such incidents have been reported for MET, care and caution should be taken when treating the cervical spine. Fortunately the leverages advocated for MET applied to the cervical spine are generally subtle and minimal, and the avoidance of end-range rotation and extension leverages may further reduce risks posed by MET.

Caution: All techniques should be applied slowly and carefully with a request for patient feedback. If the patient experiences discomfort or anything other than a pleasant stretching sensation, stop the procedure immediately and reassess the patient. The technique should be stopped and the patient reassessed at any signs of vertebro-basilar insufficiency (Gibbons & Tehan 2006) such as vertigo, visual disturbances, dysphagia, dysarthria, hoarseness, facial numbness, paraesthesias, confusion, or syncope (drop attacks).

Muscle energy application principles for myofascial tissues

Muscle energy technique can be applied to muscles and soft tissues to stretch and lengthen these tissues, to deactivate muscle myofascial TrPs, and to improve lymphatic drainage. The main principles for application of MET are described below:

1. *Stretch the involved muscle.* The muscle should be stretched to its barrier (sense of palpated resistance or end range):
   - Light stretching force to the initial or 'first barrier' if the muscle is acutely painful.

- Moderate stretching force to a comfortable sensation of stretch experienced by the patient if the muscle is only mildly painful or not painful.

2. *Isometric contraction.* Request the patient to contract the targeted muscle (push away from the barrier) against your controlled, unyielding resistance for 5–7 seconds.
   - A light contraction force should be used if the muscle is painful or contains active TrPs.
   - A moderate contraction force may be used for pain-free, fibrotic muscles.

3. *Muscle relaxation.* The patient should fully relax for several seconds, with the stretch maintained. A deep inhalation or exhalation may assist relaxation. Chaitow (2006) recommends maintaining this stretch for up to 60 seconds in the case of chronically shortened muscles (removing the muscle from stretch for a rest period), but this long period of stretch is probably only appropriate for larger muscle groups. A stretch maintained for approximately 10 seconds is generally recommended for neck, shoulder, and upper limb muscles that are judged to be shortened and fibrotic and are not provoked by stretching. A stretch maintained for a few seconds is appropriate for tender and irritable muscles.

4. *Re-engage barrier.* The slack that has developed in the tissues following the contraction and relaxation phases is taken up, and usually the muscle can be stretched to a new barrier without using increased force.

5. *Repetition.* This process is repeated 2–4 times or until a change in length and tissue texture is noted.

6. *Re-examine* to determine if the tissues have changed.

For optimal localization and effectiveness, many of the muscle stretches require subtle fine-tuning for each individual patient. Therapists are encouraged to experiment with small amounts of additional leverage – flexion, rotation, side bending, and traction – using palpation of tissue stretch and patient feedback to maximize the localization of the techniques.

Principles of muscle energy application to the joints of the spine

The application of MET to the intervertebral joints of the spine differs from its application to large muscles in terms of the need for localization, control, and force (Mitchell & Mitchell 1995, Greenman 2003, Fryer & Fossum 2009a). The basic principles of application to intervertebral segments include:

1. *Localization.* Careful attention is required to accurately engage the restricted barrier at the involved level to the initial sense of increasing resistance to motion ('first' or 'feather edge' of barrier) (Mitchell & Mitchell 1995). The primary plane of motion restriction

should be engaged first, and then 'fine-tuning can be performed using secondary planes of motion restriction (if detected) and/or translation'. It is essential that the patient is relaxed, so that active muscle contraction is not helping or hindering the engagement of the restrictive barrier.

2. *Contraction and control.* The patient is instructed to actively push using a very gentle force away from the restrictive barrier against the therapist's controlled, unyielding counterforce for 3–5 seconds. Too strong a contraction recruits larger, multi-segmental muscles and creates difficulty in maintaining accurate localization. The therapist should give clear instructions to the patient, and be relaxed to facilitate patient relaxation.

3. *Relaxation.* The patient should be allowed to relax fully for several seconds.

4. *Re-engage the barrier.* Usually the restrictive barrier is perceived to change or recede, and the therapist should take up the slack to re-engage this barrier.

5. *Repetition.* The procedure is typically performed 3–5 times.

6. *Re-examine.* This will determine if the range or quality of motion has improved.

Box 35.1 shows common errors in MET application.

Spinal coupled motion

Some texts emphasize the importance of the type of coupled motion present and the necessity of determining all planes of restricted motion to perform MET. The traditional MET approach was based on the biomechanical principles of spinal coupled motion proposed by Fryette (1954). Coupled motion, Type 1 or Type 2, was described by Fryette as the involuntary segmental coupling of one plane of motion with another and has been attributed to a combination of anatomical joint plane, ligamentous tension, and intervertebral disc mechanics. Type 1 coupled motion was described as contralateral coupling of

rotation and side bending and was claimed to normally occur when the spine is in a neutral posture; Type 2 coupled motion involved ipsilateral coupling of rotation and side bending and was said to occur when a plane of motion was introduced while the spine was in a non-neutral (flexed or extended) posture. Some authors advocate assessing the spine for asymmetry of the transverse processes while the spine is in different postures (neutral, flexed, and extended) and make inferences concerning motion restrictions from the relative position of these landmarks (Mitchell & Mitchell 1995, Greenman 2003).

The use of this model has been criticized for its prescriptive diagnostic labelling (allowing only three possible combinations of triplanar motion restriction, one Type 1 and two Type 2 combinations) and questionable inferences from static positional assessment (Gibbons & Tehan 1998, Fryer 2000, 2009). Spinal coupled motion in the lumbar region appears to be unpredictable, with variability between spinal levels and between individuals (Gibbons & Tehan 1998, Legaspi & Edmond 2007), and there is little evidence of consistent patterns of thoracic motion coupling although more rigorous studies are required (Sizer et al 2007). The Fryette model described the cervical spine (C2–C7) as having only Type 2 coupled motion. This notion is consistent with some recent studies (Cook et al 2006, Ishii et al 2006), but others suggest there may be variability in the amount and direction of these movements that is influenced by gender, age, and cervical posture (Edmondston et al 2005, Malmstrom et al 2006).

Due to the unpredictability of coupled motions in the lumbar and thoracic region and the possibility of variability in the cervical spine, clinicians are advised to address motion restrictions that present on motion testing, rather than on assumptions based on static palpatory findings and the Fryette model. If a corrective plane of motion is introduced in the primary plane of restricted motion, spinal coupling will occur automatically and without the intervention of the therapist. Therefore, the author recommends a pragmatic approach for addressing the primary motion restriction (in one or more planes) and suggests that associated coupled motions will occur without the need to be intentionally addressed.

> ### Box 35.1 **Common errors in muscle energy application**
>
> - Joint barrier is over-locked
> - Patient pushes too hard
> - Patient's contraction duration is too short
> - The use of too few repetitions (wait for tissue change)
> - Patient does not relax
> - Practitioner does not offer stable support of limb, region, or patient
> - Practitioner allows movement during contraction phase
> - Practitioner is uncomfortable, awkward, poorly positioned, unbalanced, or tense

---

SPECIFIC TECHNIQUES FOR THE CERVICO-THORACIC REGION

Middle and lower cervical spine

Lateral translation, which is most analogous to the primary motion of lateral flexion, is commonly advocated as the initial diagnostic procedure to identify motion restriction in the cervical spine. Side bending activation force can easily be controlled by the therapist. The author recommends introducing either cervical flexion or extension first (where restricted flexion or extension exists). The lateral flexion to the segment can then be localized and, if necessary, fine-tuned with subtle rotation. This order of motion introduction is easily controlled and localized. Although MET texts traditionally describe only Type 2 multiplanar restrictions (flexion and extension dysfunctions), procedures may be adapted and applied for restrictions in a single plane (side bending, rotation, flexion, or extension) or multiple planes, depending on clinical findings. There are two basic variations of this technique, depending on whether the primary restrictions are flexion or extension.

Procedure for primary restriction of flexion, side bending, and rotation
(Fig 35.1, main photo)

1. Patient is supine. The therapist stands or sits at the head of table.
2. Place the fingertips (1st–3rd) of both hands on right and left articular pillars of the upper segment (e.g. C3 pillars for a C3/4 dysfunction).
3. Flex the neck to the level of dysfunction. Introduce side bending / lateral translation until the first barrier at that segment is engaged. Fine-tune with very subtle additional leverage (rotation, more/less flexion or extension) as required.
4. Request the patient to gently push the head towards the midline (side bending away from the restrictive barrier) *or* extend against your resistance for 3–5 seconds.
5. Allow the patient to relax for a few seconds.

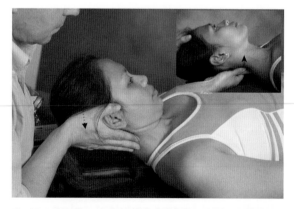

Fig 35.1 Muscle energy technique for the middle and lower cervical spine. The restricted motion barriers are engaged in one or more planes and the patient is instructed to gently push the head back towards the midline against the unyielding counterforce of the therapist. Main photo: for restriction of flexion, side bending, and rotation. Inset: for restriction of extension, side bending, and rotation; note pincer hold on articular pillars producing segmental extension (arrow).

6. Re-engage the new barrier by taking up any slack in side bending or extension.
7. Repeat 2–4 times.
8. Reassess after treatment.

Procedure for primary restriction of extension, side bending, and rotation
(Fig 35.1, inset photo)

1. Patient is supine. The therapist stands or sits at the head of table.
2. Two hand positions are suitable for introducing segmental extension:
   a. Place the fingertips (1st–3rd) of both hands on right and left articular pillars of the upper segment (e.g. C3 pillars for a C3/4 dysfunction).
   b. Place the index and middle finger of one hand on one articular pillar with the thumb on the other pillar of the lower segment. The other hand contacts the patient's head. This pincer hold is useful for introducing highly localized extension (without the need to extend the neck) and lateral translation and for creating a local fulcrum for lateral flexion.
3. Extend the segment by lifting the fingertips on the pillars until the extension barrier is palpated. Introduce side bending (using the cephalic hand to introduce motion and either the fingers or thumb of the pincer hand to act as a fulcrum) and/or lateral translation (using the pincer contact) of the segment until the barrier is engaged. Fine-tune with very subtle additional leverage (rotation, more/less flexion or extension) as required.
4. Request the patient to gently push the head towards the midline (side bending away from the restrictive barrier) *or* flex against your resistance for 3–5 seconds.
5. Allow the patient to relax for a few seconds.
6. Re-engage the new barrier by taking up any slack in side bending (or extension).
7. Repeat 2–4 times.
8. Reassess after treatment.

First rib

Techniques have been described for an elevated first rib, where the rib appears to be held in an elevated position, has a restriction of exhalation motion, and is associated with marked tissue hypertonicity and tenderness (Mitchell & Mitchell 1998, Greenman 2003). This dysfunction has been postulated to involve a superior subluxation of the joint with shortening of the attaching scalene muscles, but this subluxation aetiology is purely speculative. The following technique is proposed to produce reciprocal inhibition of the scalene muscles, but the guiding

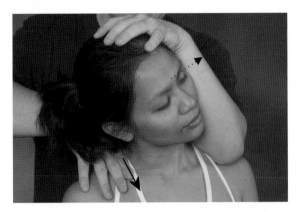

Fig 35.2 Muscle energy technique for an elevated first rib. Note the caudal and anterior pressure applied to the posterior shaft of the first rib (arrow) and the side bending of the patient's neck to relax the tissues around the rib. The patient uses a gentle side bending contraction away from the side of the rib (dotted arrow) against the unyielding counterforce of the therapist.

downward pressure on the rib during patient relaxation may be the crucial element to the success of the technique. It is often helpful to alternate the isometric contraction with the patient taking a deep breath, an exhale, and then relaxation (Fig 35.2):

1. Patient is seated, and the therapist stands behind. Alternatively, this technique may be performed with the patient supine and the therapist sitting at the head of the table.
2. Contact the posterior shaft of the first rib through the trapezius muscle with the thumb and contacting the superior aspect of the shaft with the first phalange or fingers. Exert a caudal and anterior force on the posterior rib shaft to guide it downwards.
3. Side bend and rotate the patient's neck to the side of the rib just before motion of the rib is first sensed.
4. Request the patient to gently push the head towards the midline (side bending away from the side of the rib) for 3–5 seconds.
5. Allow the patient to relax for a few seconds.
6. Re-engage the new barrier by taking up any slack in rib depression or side bending while maintaining the caudal and anterior force on the posterior rib shaft.
7. Repeat 2–4 times.
8. Reassess after treatment.

SPECIFIC TECHNIQUES FOR MUSCLES OF THE CHEST AND NECK

Many of the muscles originating from the chest and neck are susceptible to shortening and may adversely affect posture, causing abnormal stress and strain on other structures that aggravate neck and upper extremity symptoms. Additionally, two muscles – scalene and pectoralis minor – may compress, entrap, and compromise neurovascular structures, which pass by these muscles and aggravate upper extremity symptoms (Simons et al 1999).

Pectoralis major muscle

TrPs in the pectoralis major typically refer pain to the chest and arm (Simons et al 1999), and shortened muscles can produce a round-shouldered, head-forward posture that may lead to ongoing strain to the shoulder and neck regions. Treatment of this muscle should be reinforced by exercises and regular stretching at home to correct the head-forward posture. This technique is not suitable for any patient with an unstable shoulder joint, a previous shoulder injury, or limited shoulder movement due to pain. Do not use external rotation as the primary leverage because this will cause pain and discomfort even in the healthy shoulder joint. Procedure for lengthening the pectoralis major muscle (Fig 35.3):

1. Patient is supine and the therapist stands on the involved side.
2. Abduct the patient's shoulder to 90° and place in comfortable external rotation. The amount of arm abduction can be varied to select particular fibres, with decreasing abduction (below 90°) to localize the clavicular fibres and increasing abduction (above 90°) to localize the sternal fibres.
3. Anchor the tissues by placing your hand or forearm over the patient's sternum (close to the border with the rib cage), using a light compressive and lateral force away from the treated side. Pretension on the

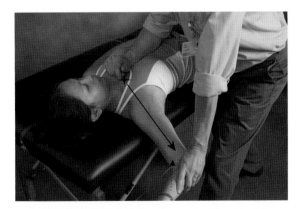

Fig 35.3 Muscle energy technique to lengthen the pectoralis major muscle. Note that the chest is firmly stabilized (star) and the leverages applied to the arm are chiefly horizontal extension and traction (arrow). The patient lifts the arm (dotted arrow) against the unyielding counterforce of the therapist. Note that the applicator arm is straight and the isometric force is easily resisted by the therapist's body weight.

fascia will help minimize the amount of leverage necessary on the shoulder.

4. Grasp the patient's arm close to the elbow.
5. Gently apply horizontal extension and traction (down the length of the humerus) to the shoulder, while maintaining the anchoring pressure near the sternum. The patient should experience a pleasant stretching sensation through the pectoral region. *Note*: The addition of traction frequently produces a much more effective stretch and minimizes the amount of leverage required on the shoulder.
6. Request the patient to gently push the arm towards the ceiling for 5–7 seconds against unyielding resistance. Be positioned so the applicator arm is straight and the isometric force is easily resisted by your body weight.
7. Allow the patient to relax for a few seconds.
8. Re-engage the new barrier by taking up any slack which has developed (the muscle is further lengthened) by gently increasing the horizontal extension.
9. Repeat the procedure 2–4 times.
10. Reassess after treatment.

Pectoralis minor muscle

The pectoralis minor muscle may refer pain to the anterior deltoid region or to the ulnar side of the arm, hand, and fingers and may entrap the axillary artery and brachial plexus to mimic cervical radiculopathy (Simons et al 1999). Like the pectoralis major, shortened pectoralis minor muscles may affect posture, producing round shoulders and a head-forward posture. Procedure for lengthening the pectoralis minor muscle (Fig 35.4):

1. Patient is supine, close to the edge of the bench so that the involved shoulder slightly overhangs the bench. The therapist stands on the involved side.
2. Rest your hand or forearm on the sternum or upper chest and apply a compressive and lateral force to take up tissue slack away from the involved muscle.
3. Cup your hand over the patient's anterior shoulder and slowly apply a force in a posterior and lateral direction with a straight arm (the bench should be low), while maintaining a firm anchor on the pectoral tissues. A small towel can be folded and placed on the patient's anterior shoulder to cushion the therapist's hand if the patient experiences discomfort from the pressure. The patient should feel a pleasant stretching sensation in the pectoral region.
4. Request the patient to gently push the shoulder in an anterior direction towards the ceiling for 5–7 seconds.
5. Allow the patient to relax for a few seconds.
6. Re-engage the new barrier by taking up any slack which has developed (the muscle is further

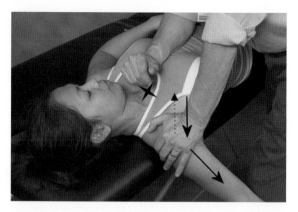

Fig 35.4 Muscle energy technique to lengthen the pectoralis minor muscle. Note that the chest is firmly stabilized (star) and a posterior and lateral force is applied to the anterior shoulder (arrows). The patient attempts to lift the shoulder (dotted arrow) against the unyielding counterforce of the therapist. Note that the applicator arm is straight and the isometric force is easily resisted by the therapist's body weight.

lengthened) by gently increasing the posterior and lateral pressure on the shoulder.
7. Repeat the procedure 2–4 times.
8. Reassess after treatment.

Upper trapezius and levator scapulae muscles

The upper trapezius muscle is reported to be beset by TrPs and is a commonly overlooked source of neck pain and temporal headaches (Simons et al 1999). The levator scapulae muscle, which is reported to produce local pain in the ipsilateral neck, will also be stretched during the treatment of trapezius. Procedure for lengthening the upper trapezius and levator scapulae muscles (Fig 35.5):

1. Patient is supine, with arms resting by side. The therapist stands at the head of the table.
2. Stabilize the shoulder of the treated side with one hand and contact the occiput, mastoid region and upper neck with the other hand. If the patient's head is heavy, support and stabilize your hand using the abdomen or chest. Alternatively, use a crossed arm position, where your hands contact and stabilize both of the patient's shoulders and the crossed arms support the upper neck and head.
3. Fully flex and side bend the neck away from the involved side until a sense of tissue resistance is palpated and the patient reports a pleasant stretching sensation.
4. The addition of cervical rotation may selectively stretch particular fibres. There are different views as to the amount and direction of rotation needed to select specific parts of the muscle (Chaitow 2006, Liebenson

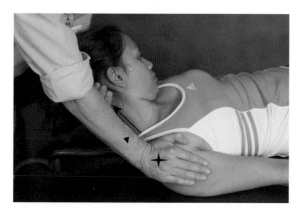

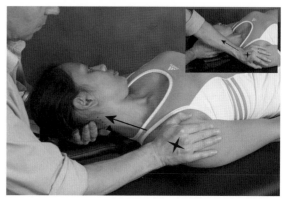

Fig 35.5 Muscle energy technique to lengthen the upper trapezius and levator scapulae muscles. Note that the shoulder is firmly depressed and stabilized (star), with side bending and rotation of the neck according to the fibre direction and sense of stretch (arrow). The patient's isometric effort is side bending towards the involved side or extension (dotted line).

Fig 35.6 Muscle energy technique to lengthen the scalene muscles. Note that the shoulder and upper ribs are stabilized by downward pressure on the shoulder and clavicle (star). Alternatively, the hand and thenar eminence can be placed below the medial clavicle to stabilize the first and second ribs. The neck is slightly extended, laterally flexed and rotated away from the involved side (arrow), and the isometric effort is lateral flexion towards the involved side (dotted arrow). Inset photo: alternative hold where the arms are crossed.

2007). Subtle fine-tuning of rotation using palpatory and patient feedback to determine the most effective position for each individual is recommended.

5. Request the patient to gently push the head and neck back against your controlled, unyielding resistance for 5–7 seconds. The direction of patient force can either be extension or side bending; rotation is not recommended because it is more difficult to control and stabilize. Alternatively, shoulder elevation can be requested and resisted.
6. Allow the patient to relax for a few seconds (or more), maintaining the stretch.
7. Re-engage the new barrier by taking up any slack (the muscle is further lengthened) using shoulder depression.
8. Repeat the procedure 2–4 times.
9. Reassess after treatment.

Scalene muscles

The scalene muscles (anterior, middle, and posterior) are reported as a commonly overlooked source of back, shoulder, and arm pain (Simons et al 1999). Opinions differ on the degree and direction of rotation required for the stretch of the scalene muscles (Gerwin 2005, Chaitow 2006, Liebenson 2007), so experimentation using palpatory and patient feedback is recommended. Procedure for lengthening the scalene muscles (Fig 35.6):

1. Patient is supine, with arms resting by side. The therapist stands at the head of the table.
2. Contact the mastoid, lateral occiput, and upper cervical pillars to stabilize the neck and prevent excessive upper cervical lateral flexion. The other hand is placed over the shoulder to depress and stabilize the

shoulder. The hand and thenar eminence may be placed below the medial clavicle to stabilize the first and second ribs. An alternative hold where the arms are crossed is possible (inset photo).

3. Place the patient's neck in slight extension (remove pillow), laterally flex the neck away from the treated side, and introduce slight rotation. Experiment with varying degrees of rotation for the most effective stretch.
4. Request the patient to gently, laterally flex the head against your resistance for 5–7 seconds.
5. Allow the patient to relax for a few seconds. A deep inhalation and exhalation may assist relaxation of the scalene muscles.
6. Re-engage the new barrier by taking up any slack (the muscle is further lengthened).
7. Repeat the procedure 2–4 times.
8. Reassess after treatment.

SPECIFIC TECHNIQUES FOR JOINTS OF THE UPPER EXTREMITY

Treatment of dysfunctions of joints of the extremities follows the same principles as treatment of spinal joints outlined above. In brief, care should be taken to localize leverage to the restricted barrier in the primary plane of restricted motion with the addition of secondary planes as palpated. Isometric contraction effort should be gentle in order to recruit muscles associated with the joint. In the author's experience, it is useful to combine or alternate MET with other manual techniques, such as end-range passive joint articulation, and to address any associated muscle shortness or TrPs.

Acromio-clavicular joint

Motion of the acromio-clavicular (AC) joint may be assessed by palpation of the joint line during passive motion of the shoulder, specifically when the arm is horizontally flexed and adducted (to gap the joint), during abduction of the shoulder (upward rotation of the scapular) while the shoulder is flexed approximately 30°, and during external and internal rotation while the shoulder is rotated at the abduction barrier (see Chapter 14). MET can be used to address altered range and quality of motion of the AC joint in abduction or in external or internal rotation. Procedure for the AC joint (Fig 35.7):

1. Patient is seated and the therapist stands behind the patient.
2. Palpate the AC joint line with one hand and slightly flex the shoulder (approximately 30° to align leverage with joint line) using the other hand.
3. Abduct shoulder until subtle leverage is palpated at the joint. Additionally, the shoulder may be externally or internally rotated, and the technique directed at any one of these planes. Position the shoulder at the point where the motion of the AC stops.

4. Request the patient to gently adduct or externally rotate or internally rotate the shoulder as appropriate against your unyielding counterforce for 5–7 seconds.
5. Allow the patient to relax for a few seconds.
6. Re-engage and fine-tune the new barrier by taking up any slack which has developed.
7. Repeat the procedure 2–4 times.
8. Reassess after treatment.

Sterno-clavicular joint

The sterno-clavicular (SC) joint connects the upper extremity to the axial skeleton and accommodates motion of the clavicle and scapula by combinations of translation and rotation (Levangie & Norkin 2005). The medial clavicle is typically assessed for inferior glide on the manubrium and costal cartilage at the SC joint during clavicle elevation (bilateral assessment during active elevation of both shoulders) and is assessed for posterior glide during clavicle protraction (when the patient reaches forward with both outstretched arms) (Greenman 2003). For further information about the SC readers are referred to Chapter 15 of this textbook. A decrease in either inferior or posterior glide at one SC may be indicative of dysfunction, and direct manual springing (inferior/posterior) of the joint may confirm the motion restriction.

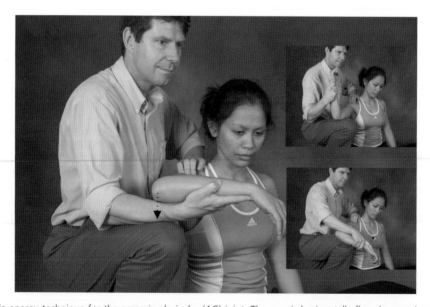

Fig 35.7 Muscle energy technique for the acromio-clavicular (AC) joint. The arm is horizontally flexed approximately 30 degrees and abducted until the motion of the AC is palpated. The technique may be used to address restrictions of abduction, internal or external rotation. The abduction barrier is localized and an isometric adduction effort performed (dotted arrow). Inset (top): application for restriction of external rotation using an isometric internal rotation effort (dotted arrow). Inset (bottom): application for restriction of internal rotation using an isometric external rotation effort (dotted arrow).

Procedure for restricted inferior glide of the medial clavicle at the SC joint (Fig 35.8):

1. Patient is supine and the therapist stands on the involved side. Alternatively, patient may be seated with the therapist standing behind.
2. Palpate the SC joint, and move the humerus and lateral clavicle superiorly by pressure on the elbow to the point where motion of the clavicle at the SC ceases. This leverage is useful where shoulder abduction is uncomfortable or contraindicated. Alternatively, abduction and elevation of the shoulder may be used to elevate the lateral clavicle. Request the patient to gently depress or adduct the shoulder against your unyielding counterforce for 5–7 seconds.
3. Allow the patient to relax for a few seconds.
4. Re-engage and fine-tune the new barrier.
5. Repeat the procedure 2–4 times. Alternating this technique with low velocity springing (mobilization) on the superior medial clavicle at the SC may be helpful for gaining increased motion (Fig 35.8, inset).
6. Reassess after treatment.

Procedure for restricted posterior glide of the medial clavicle at the SC joint (Fig 35.9):

1. Patient is supine and the therapist stands on the involved side.
2. Palpate the SC joint, lifting the shoulder from the table (protract) until motion of the clavicle at the SC ceases. The patient's hand may rest around your neck to lessen the weight of the arm.

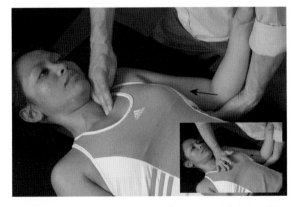

Fig 35.8 Muscle energy technique for restricted inferior glide of the medial clavicle at the sterno-clavicular joint. Note that the lateral clavicle may be elevated by superior pressure through the elbow (arrow) or alternatively by abduction of the arm. The sterno-clavicular joint may be simply monitored (main photo) or an inferior springing force (inset) may assist inferior glide (arrow).

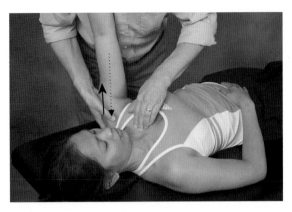

Fig 35.9 Muscle energy technique for restricted posterior glide of the medial clavicle at the sterno-clavicular joint. The lateral clavicle is protracted by lifting the shoulder (arrow) until motion is localized at the sterno-clavicular joint. The patient actively retracts the shoulder and clavicle by drawing the arm back (dotted arrow) against the resistance of the therapist.

3. Request the patient to gently retract the shoulder (draw the arm and shoulder back to the table) against your unyielding counterforce for 5–7 seconds.
4. Allow the patient to relax for a few seconds.
5. Re-engage and fine-tune the new barrier.
6. Repeat the procedure 2–4 times. Alternating this technique with low velocity springing (mobilization) on the anterior medial clavicle at the SC may be helpful for gaining increased motion.
7. Reassess after treatment.

Elbow joint

The three joints of the elbow – humero-ulnar, humero-radial and radio-ulnar – function together as a modified hinge joint (Levangie & Norkin 2005). Restrictions of flexion and extension may be identified by examination, and MET may be performed to increase the range of these motions. These techniques follow the same principles as for increasing motion in other joints and will not be elaborated here. The proximal radio-ulnar joint may be assessed by palpation of the radial head during passive pronation and supination, as well as by assessment of accessory antero-posterior glide. The procedure for restricted pronation (or supination) of the radial head is as follows (Fig 35.10):

1. Patient is supine and the therapist stands on the involved side.
2. Palpate the radial head with your thumb or finger.
3. Flex the elbow and pronate (supinate) the forearm until the end of radial head motion.
4. Request the patient to gently supinate (or pronate) the forearm against your unyielding counterforce for 5–7 seconds.
5. Allow the patient to relax for a few seconds.

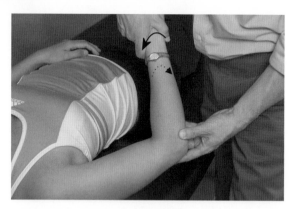

Fig 35.10 Muscle energy technique for restricted pronation of the radial head. The radial head is monitored while the wrist is pronated to a palpated barrier (arrow). The patient performs an isometric effort of wrist supination (dotted arrow) against the unyielding counterforce of the therapist. The opposite directions are employed for restrictions of supination.

6. Re-engage and fine-tune the new barrier.
7. Repeat the procedure 2–4 times.
8. Reassess after treatment.

Wrist and hand

Procedure for restricted carpal joints (Fig 35.11):

1. Patient is supine and the therapist stands on the involved side.
2. Contact a carpal bone using thumb contact on the dorsal surface and the first two fingers on the plantar

surface of the bone. Alternatively, contact two adjacent bones using this hold.
3. Apply slight traction through the carpal bone and wrist.
4. Engage the restrictive barrier in one or multiple planes (flexion, extension, adduction, abduction, or translation).
5. Request the patient to gently oppose the leverage applied against your unyielding counterforce for 5–7 seconds.
6. Allow the patient to relax for a few seconds.
7. Re-engage and fine-tune the new barrier.
8. Repeat the procedure 2–4 times.
9. Reassess after treatment.

SPECIFIC TECHNIQUES FOR MUSCLES OF THE UPPER EXTREMITY

Subscapularis muscle

TrPs in this muscle have been reported to present as deep anterior shoulder pain and may produce substantial limitation of external rotation, thus mimicking adhesive capsulitis (Simons et al 1999). Effective stretch of this muscle requires firm stabilization of the scapula and may be performed with the patient supine or lying on their side. This technique is contraindicated if the patient has an unstable shoulder. The procedure for lengthening the subscapularis muscle is the following (Fig 35.12):

1. Patient is supine and the therapist stands on the involved side.

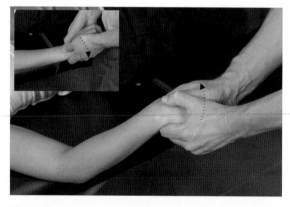

Fig 35.11 Muscle energy technique for restricted carpal joints. The dysfunctional carpal bone is fixed between fingers and thumb, gentle traction applied and one or more restrictive barriers engaged. Main photo: the restrictive barriers of flexion, side bending and translation are engaged and the patient applies a light isometric extension effort (dotted arrow). Inset: the restrictive barriers of extension, side bending and translation are engaged and the patient applies a light isometric flexion effort (dotted arrow).

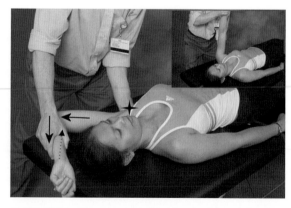

Fig 35.12 Muscle energy technique for the subscapularis muscle. Inset: the arm is lifted to allow the therapist's hand to contact and stabilize the lateral border of the scapular. Main photo: the scapular is firmly stabilized (star) to prevent upward rotation while the shoulder is abducted and externally rotated with slight traction through the arm (arrows). The patient provides isometric effort by lifting the arm (dotted arrow).

2. Lift the patient's arm and place your hand under the scapula, fixing the lateral border with the heel of your hand. Apply firm medial compression to prevent upward rotation of the scapula when moving the arm.

3. Abduct and externally rotate the scapula until a sense of barrier is palpated, and the patient feels a stretching sensation. Firm stabilization of the scapula is important for producing an effective stretch.

4. Request the patient to gently lift the arm towards the ceiling against your unyielding counterforce for 5–7 seconds.

5. Allow the patient to relax for a few seconds.

6. Re-engage the new barrier by taking up any slack (the muscle is further lengthened).

7. Repeat the procedure 2–4 times.

8. Reassess after treatment.

Supraspinatus muscle (Fig 35.13):

1. Patient lies prone and the therapist stands on the side opposite to the muscle to be treated.

2. Internally rotate the patient's shoulder so that the hand rests near the thoracic spine. In order to minimize discomfort on anterior shoulder, place a small folded towel under the patient's shoulder to support and slightly retract the shoulder.

3. Stabilize the scapula by firm posterior-lateral pressure on the medial border.

4. Gently pull the wrist to adduct the shoulder while maintaining the stabilizing pressure on the scapula.

A pleasant stretching sensation in the supraspinatus region should be felt by the patient.

5. Request the patient to gently abduct the arm against your unyielding counterforce for 5–7 seconds.

6. Allow the patient to relax for a few seconds.

7. Re-engage the new barrier by taking up any slack (the muscle is further lengthened).

8. Repeat the procedure 2–4 times.

9. Reassess after treatment.

Supinator muscle

Because it is not possible to isolate the supinator muscle for a strong effective stretch, this technique combines elements from both myofascial release and MET. Procedure for lengthening the supinator muscle (Fig 35.14):

1. Patient is supine and the therapist stands on the involved side.

2. On the supinated forearm, palpate the supinator muscle near the radial head and apply firm – but comfortable – pressure.

3. Slowly pronate the forearm while maintaining a firm pressure on the supinator muscle until resistance or barrier is first sensed.

4. Request the patient to gently supinate the forearm against unyielding counterforce for 5–7 seconds.

5. Allow the patient to relax for a few seconds.

6. Re-engage the new barrier by taking up any slack (the muscle is further lengthened).

7. Repeat the procedure 2–4 times.

8. Reassess after treatment.

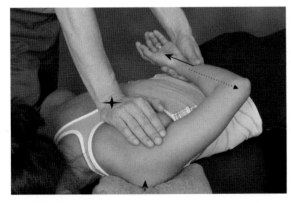

Fig 35.13 Muscle energy technique for the supraspinatus muscle. The anterior shoulder is supported and slightly retracted by a towel (small arrow) and the scapula is firmly stabilized (star) to prevent downward rotation. The therapist draws the wrist (arrow) to adduct the shoulder while preventing movement of the scapula until a barrier or stretching sensation is felt. The patient gently abducts the shoulder against resistance (dotted arrow).

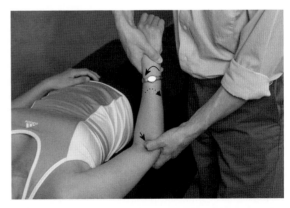

Fig 35.14 Muscle energy technique for the supinator muscle. Firm but comfortable pressure is applied to the supinator muscle overlying the radial head (arrow). The supinated forearm is then slowly pronated (arrow) until a barrier is sensed while maintaining the pressure. The patient performs an isometric effort to supinate the forearm (dotted arrow).

Brachioradialis and forearm muscles
(Fig 35.15):

1. Patient is supine and the therapist stands on the involved side.
2. Fully extend the patient's elbow but support it with one hand (be careful not to overextend elbow). Forearm should be pronated.
3. Apply flexion to the wrist and then gentle traction through the wrist and forearm until a pleasant stretch is felt in the brachioradialis muscle.
4. Request the patient to gently extend the wrist against your unyielding resistance.
5. Allow the patient to relax for a few seconds.
6. Re-engage the new barrier by taking up any slack (the muscle is further lengthened).
7. Repeat the procedure 2–4 times.
8. Reassess after treatment.

This technique can be performed for the wrist flexor muscles when the forearm is supinated and the wrist extended (Fig 35.15, inset photo).

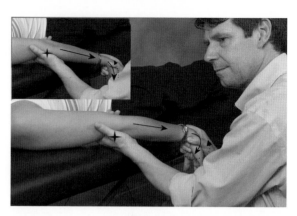

Fig 35.15 Muscle energy technique for brachioradialis and forearm extensor muscles. The extended elbow is stabilized (star), the forearm is pronated, and the wrist is flexed (arrow). Apply gentle traction through the wrist and forearm (arrow) until a pleasant stretch is felt. The patient performs an isometric effort to extend the wrist (dotted arrow). Inset: this technique can be performed for the wrist flexors when the forearm is supinated and the wrist extended.

ACKNOWLEDGEMENTS

The author gratefully acknowledges the assistance of Rolena Stephenson as subject of the photos, and Christian Fossum D.O. for Figure 35.2.

REFERENCES

Aparicio, É.Q., Quirante, L.B., Blanco, C. R., et al., 2009. Immediate effects of the suboccipital muscle inhibition technique in subjects with short hamstring syndrome. J. Manipulative Physiol. Ther. 32, 262–269.

Ballantyne, F., Fryer, G., McLaughlin, P., 2003. The effect of muscle energy technique on hamstring extensibility: The mechanism of altered flexibility. J. Osteopath. Med. 6, 59–63.

Bourdillon, J.F., Day, E.A., Bookhout, M.R., 1992. Spinal Manipulation, fifth ed. Butterworth-Heinemann, Oxford.

Boyles, R.E., Ritland, B.M., Miracle, B.M., et al., 2009. The short-term effects of thoracic spine thrust manipulation on patients with shoulder impingement syndrome. Man. Ther. 14, 375–380.

Burns, D.K., Wells, M.R., 2006. Gross range of motion in the cervical spine: The effects of osteopathic muscle energy technique in asymptomatic subjects. J. Am. Osteopath. Assoc. 106, 137–142.

Chaitow, L., 2006. Muscle Energy Techniques, third ed. Churchill Livingstone, Edinburgh.

Chown, M., Whittamore, L., Rush, M., et al., 2008. A prospective study of patients with chronic back pain randomised to group exercise, physiotherapy or osteopathy. Physiotherapy 94, 21–28.

Cleland, J.A., Childs, J.D., McRae, M., et al., 2005. Immediate effects of thoracic manipulation in patients with neck pain: A randomized clinical trial. Man. Ther. 10, 127–135.

Coates, G., O'Brodovich, H., Goeree, G., 1993. Hindlimb and lung lymph flows during prolonged exercise. J. Appl. Physiol. 75, 633–638.

Cook, C., Hegedus, E., Showalter, C., et al., 2006. Coupling behavior of the cervical spine: A systematic review of the literature. J. Manipulative Physiol. Ther. 29, 570–575.

Di Fabio, R.P., 1999. Manipulation of the cervical spine: Risks and benefits. Phys. Ther. 79, 50–65.

Edmondston, S.J., Henne, S.E., Loh, W., et al., 2005. Influence of cranio-cervical posture on three-dimensional motion of the cervical spine. Man. Ther. 10, 44–51.

Feland, J.B., Myrer, J.W., Schulthies, S.S., et al., 2001. The effect of duration of stretching of the hamstring muscle group for increasing range of motion in people aged 65 years or older. Phys. Ther. 81, 1100–1117.

Ferber, R., Osternig, L.R., Gravelle, D.C., 2002. Effect of pnf stretch techniques on knee flexor muscle emg activity in older adults. J. Electromyogr. Kinesiol. 12, 391–397.

Ferreira, M.L., Ferreira, P.H., Hodges, P.W., 2007. Changes in postural activity of the trunk muscles following spinal manipulative therapy. Man. Ther. 12, 240–248.

Fryer, G., 2000. Muscle energy concepts – a need for change. J. Osteopath. Med. 3, 54–59.

Fryer, G., 2009. Research-informed muscle energy concepts and practice. In: Franke, H. (Ed.), Muscle Energy Technique: History – Model – Research (monograph). Jolandos, Ammersestr, pp. 57–62.

Fryer, G., Fossum, C., 2009a. Muscle energy techniques. In: Fernández-de-las-Peñas, C., Arendt-Nielsen, L., Gerwin, R.D. (Eds.), Tension-Type And Cervicogenic Headache: Pathophysiology, Diagnosis, And Management. Jones and Bartlett Publishers, Sudbury, pp. 309–326.

Fryer, G., Fossum, C., 2009b. Therapeutic mechanisms underlying muscle energy approaches. In: Fernández-de-las-Peñas, C., Arendt-Nielsen, L., Gerwin, R.D. (Eds.), Tension-Type And Cervicogenic Headache: Pathophysiology, Diagnosis, And Management. Jones and Bartlett Publishers, Sudbury, pp. 221–229.

Fryer, G., Ruszkowski, W., 2004. The influence of contraction duration in muscle energy technique applied to the atlanto-axial joint. J. Osteopath. Med. 7, 79–84.

Fryer, G., Morris, T., Gibbons, P., 2004. Paraspinal muscles and intervertebral dysfunction. Part 2. J. Manipulative Physiol. Ther. 27, 348–357.

Fryer, G., Alivizatos, J., Lamaro, J., 2005. The effect of osteopathic treatment on people with chronic and sub-chronic neck pain: A pilot study. Int. J. Osteopath. Med. 8, 41–48.

Fryette, H.H., 1954. Principles of Osteopathic Technic. American Academy of Osteopathy, Newark.

Gerwin, R., 2005. Headache. In: Ferguson, L.W., Gerwin, R. (Eds.), Clinical Mastery in the Treatment of Myofascial Pain. Lippincott Williams & Wilkins, Baltimore, pp. 1–29.

Gibbons, P., Tehan, P., 1998. Muscle energy concepts and coupled motion of the spine. Man. Ther. 3, 95–101.

Gibbons, P., Tehan, P., 2006. Manipulation Of The Spine, Thorax And Pelvis. An Osteopathic Perspective, second ed. Churchill Livingstone, London.

González-Iglesias, J., Fernández-de-las-Peñas, C., Cleland, J.A., et al., 2009. Inclusion of thoracic spine thrust manipulation into an electro-therapy/thermal program for the management of patients with acute mechanical neck pain: A randomized clinical trial. Man. Ther. 14, 306–313.

Goodridge, J.P., Kuchera, M.L., 1997. Muscle energy treatment techniques for specific areas. In: Ward, R.C. (Ed.), Foundations for Osteopathic Medicine. William & Wilkins, Baltimore, pp. 697–761.

Greenman, P.E., 2003. Principles of Manual Medicine, third ed. Lippincott William & Wilkins, Philadelphia.

Grip, H., Sundelin, G., Gerdle, B., et al., 2007. Variations in the axis of motion during head repositioning – a comparison of subjects with whiplash-associated disorders or non-specific neck pain and healthy controls. Clin. Biomech. 22, 865–873.

Haldeman, S., Kohlbeck, F.J., McGregor, M., 2001. Unpredictability of cerebrovascular ischemia associated with cervical spine manipulation therapy: A review of sixty-four cases after cervical spine manipulation. Spine 27, 49–55.

Havas, E., Parviainen, T., Vuorela, J., et al., 1997. Lymph flow dynamics in exercising human skeletal muscle as detected by scintography. J. Physiol. 504, 233–239.

Ishii, T., Mukai, Y., Hosono, N., et al., 2006. Kinematics of the cervical spine in lateral bending: In vivo three-dimensional analysis. Spine 31, 155–160.

Kuchera, W.A., Kuchera, M.L., 1992. Osteopathic Principles In Practice. Kirksville College of Osteopathic Medicine Press, Kirksville.

Langevin, H.M., Cornbrooks, C.J., Taatjes, D.J., 2004. Fibroblasts form a body-wide cellular network. Histochem. Cell Biol. 122, 7–15.

Langevin, H.M., Bouffard, N.A., Badger, G.J., et al., 2005. Dynamic fibroblast cytoskeletal response to subcutaneous tissue stretch ex vivo and in vivo. Am. J. Physiol. Cell Physiol. 288, C747–C756.

Lederman, E., 2005. The Science and Practice of Manual Therapy, second ed. Elsevier Churchill Livingstone, Edinburgh.

Lee, H.Y., Wang, J.D., Yao, G., et al., 2007. Association between cervicocephalic kinesthetic sensibility and frequency of subclinical neck pain. Man. Ther. 13, 419–425.

Legaspi, O., Edmond, S.L., 2007. Does the evidence support the existence of lumbar spine coupled motion? A critical review of the literature. J. Orthop. Sports Phys. Ther. 37, 169–178.

Leinonen, V., Maatta, S., Taimela, S., et al., 2002. Impaired lumbar movement perception in association with postural stability and motor- and somatosensory-evoked potentials in lumbar spinal stenosis. Spine 27, 975–983.

Lenehan, K.L., Fryer, G., McLaughlin, P., 2003. The effect of muscle energy technique on gross trunk range of motion. J. Osteopath. Med. 6, 13–18.

Levangie, P.K., Norkin, C.C., 2005. Joint Structure And Function: A Comprehensive Analysis, fourth ed. F.A. Davis Co., Philadelphia.

Licciardone, J.C., Stoll, S.T., Fulda, K.G., et al., 2003. Osteopathic manipulative treatment for chronic low back pain: A randomized controlled trial. Spine 28, 1355–1362.

Liebenson, C., 2007. Rehabilitation of the Spine: A Therapist's Manual, second ed. Lippincott William & Wilkins, Baltimore.

Magnusson, M., Simonsen, E.B., Aagaard, P., et al., 1996a. A mechanism for altered flexibility in human skeletal muscle. J. Physiol. 497, 293–298.

Magnusson, M., Simonsen, E.B., Dyhre-Poulsen, P., et al., 1996b. Viscoelastic stress relaxation during static stretch in human skeletal muscle in the absence of EMG activity. Scand. J. Med. Sci. Sports 6, 323–328.

Magnusson, S.P., Simonsen, E.B., Aagaard, P., et al., 1996. Mechanical and physiological responses to stretching with and without preisometric contraction in human skeletal muscle. Arch. Phys. Med. Rehabil. 77, 373–377.

Malmstrom, E., Karlberg, M., Fransson, P.A., et al., 2006. Primary and coupled cervical movements. The effect of age, gender, and body mass index. A 3-dimensional movement analysis of a population without symptoms of neck disorders. Spine 31, E44–E50.

McClatchie, L., Laprade, J., Martin, S., et al., 2009. Mobilizations of the asymptomatic cervical spine can reduce signs of shoulder dysfunction in adults. Man. Ther. 14, 369–374.

Mitchell, F.L., Mitchell, P.K.G., 1995. The Muscle Energy Manual. MET Press, East Lansing.

Mitchell, F.L., Mitchell, P.K.G., 1998. The Muscle Energy Manual: Evaluation & Treatment Of The Thoracic Spine Lumbar Spine & Rib Cage. MET Press, East Lansing.

Mitchell, F.L., Moran, P.S., Pruzzo, N.A., 1979. An Evaluation And Treatment Manual Of Osteopathic Muscle Energy Procedures. Mitchell, Moran and Pruzzo, Valley Park.

Osternig, L.R., Robertson, R., Troxel, R.K., et al., 1987. Muscle activation during proprioceptive neuromuscular facilitation stretching techniques. Am. J. Phys. Med. 66, 298–307.

Osternig, L.R., Robertson, R.N., Troxel, R.K., et al., 1990. Differential responses to proprioceptive neuromuscular facilitation stretch techniques. Med. Sci. Sports Exerc. 22, 106–111.

Palmgren, P.J., Sandstrom, P.J., Lundqvist, F.J., et al., 2006. Improvement after chiropractic care in cervicocephalic kinesthetic sensibility and subjective pain intensity in patients with nontraumatic chronic neck pain. J. Manipulative Physiol. Ther. 29, 100–106.

Rogers, R.G., 1997. The effects of spinal manipulation on cervical kinesthesia in patients with chronic neck pain: A pilot study. J. Manipulative Physiol. Ther. 20, 80–85.

Sady, S.P., Wortman, M., Blanke, D., 1982. Flexibility training: Ballistic, static or proprioceptive neuromuscular facilitation? Arch. Phys. Med. Rehabil. 63, 261–263.

Schenk, R.J., Adelman, K., Rousselle, J., 1994. The effects of muscle energy technique on cervical range of motion. J. Man. Manip. Ther. 2, 149–155.

Schenk, R.J., MacDiarmid, J., Rousselle, J., 1997. The effects of muscle energy technique on lumbar range of motion. J. Man. Manip. Ther. 5, 179–183.

Schwerla, F., Bischoff, A., Nurnberger, A., et al., 2008. Osteopathic treatment of patients with chronic non-specific neck pain: A randomised controlled trial of efficacy. Forsch. Komplementärmed. 15, 138–145.

Simons, D.G., Travell, J.G., Simons, L.S., 1999. Myofascial Pain And Dysfunction: The Trigger Point Manual, second ed. William & Wilkins, Baltimore.

Sizer Jr., P.S., Brismee, J.M., Cook, C., 2007. Coupling behaviour of the thoracic spine: A systematic review of the literature. J. Manipulative Physiol. Ther. 30, 390–399.

Souvalis, T., Vicenzino, B., Wright, A., 2004. Neurophysiological effects of spinal manual therapy. In: Boyling, J.D., Jull, G.A. (Eds.), Grieve's Modern Manual Therapy: The Vertebral Column. Elsevier Churchill Livingstone, Edinburgh, pp. 367–380.

Swart, J., 1919. Osteopathic Strap Technic. Joseph Swart, Kansas City.

Wallin, D., Ekblam, B., Grahn, R., et al., 1985. Improvement of muscle flexibility. A comparison between two techniques. Am. J. Sports Med. 13, 263–268.

Wilson, E., Payton, O., Donegan-Shoaf, L., et al., 2003. Muscle energy technique in patients with acute low back pain: A pilot clinical trial. J. Orthop. Sports Phys. Ther. 33, 502–512.

Chapter | 36 |

Myofascial induction approaches

Andrzej Pilat

INTRODUCTION

Fascia represents a connective tissue which forms a continuum network between the different components of the body (Pilat 2003, Langevin 2006, Vanacore et al 2009). Its fibrous construction allows it to accommodate the intrinsic and extrinsic tensional body requirements. Fascia is a tissue mostly represented by anatomical links, but also has extensive functional tasks (Pilat 2003). It has been hypothesized that tension in any part of the tissue could reorient body dynamics (Pilat 2009). The different characteristics of the fascial tissue (density, distribution) allow it to act as a synergistic functional unit, absorbing and distributing local stimulus throughout the whole body. This inherent functional synergy of the fascia can play a relevant role in different functional tasks, e.g. maintenance of body posture against gravity (Langevin 2006).

Further, some authors suggested that fascia could also integrate sensory stimuli (i.e. mechanical, thermal or chemical) from the central nervous system (Pilat 2009, Pilat & Testa 2009). In such a way, sensory information integrated into the fascial tissue may interact with the instructions (inputs) originated in the central nervous system at three different levels:

© 2011 Elsevier Ltd.
DOI: 10.1016/B978-0-7020-3528-9.00036-4

1. *Physical (mechanical – anatomical) link* (Pilat 2003, Ingber 2006, Stecco et al 2008): these links are present at macro and microscopic levels and act in a hierarchical manner (Wang et al 2009). Different studies have observed the transmission and coordination of mechanical impulses in the intrinsic cells structures (Maniotis et al 1997, Hu et al 2003). In these structures, the mechanical impulse (force applied to the collagen filaments) was transmitted from the extracellular matrix through the cellular membrane via integrins and subsequently transferred to the cellular nucleus modifying gene activity (Hu et al 2003). The dynamics of the fascial system movement at the cellular level are associated with contraction of myo-fibroblasts (specialized fibroblasts with dynamic and contractile microfilaments of actin that contract in smooth muscle cell manner) (Gabbiani 2007). At the macroscopic level, some observations on fresh cadavers (Vleeming 1992, Vleeming 1997, Meyer 2003, Stecco et al 2008, Pilat 2009) have shown a mechanical continuity of the fascia tissue where muscles that attach to the fascia act synergistically, creating a myofascial kinetic link (Stecco et al 2008, Pilat 2009).

2. *Functional link*: the fascia is considered a mechano-sensitive structure (Langevin 2006, Vaticón 2009). The mechanical modifications are created primarily in the extracellular matrix which is characterized by piezoelectric and semiconducting properties (Langevin 2006). This connection would permit a real communication between all connective structures, particularly loose connective tissue. Fascial tissue would thus constitute a network of mechanoreceptors, mostly interstitial.

3. *Chemical links* (Wang et al 2009). Ingber (2006) identified the mediating structures for the mechano-chemical integration process in the fascial tissue which is based on mechano-transduction activities. Vanacore et al (2009) identified the networks that provide structural integrity to the tissues and serve as ligands for integrin cell-surface receptors related to the collagen IV which is present in the basement membrane. It is suggested that these networks mediate cell adhesion, migration, growth, and differentiation.

Some theories have suggested that the three-dimensional fascial tissue can be involved in pain transmission processes. For instance, pain experienced in the arm is usually a referred pain, i.e. perceived in areas remote from the site of noxious stimulation, which does not usually follow neuropathic patterns (Travell & Bigelow 1946). The central hyperexcitability theory (Mense 1994) explains the mechanisms of pain from deep structures, but does not clarify the presence of non-segmental patterns of the superficial muscles such as the neck, the latissimus dorsi, trapezius and limb muscles (Han 2009).

The *barrier-dam theory* (Farasyn 2007) suggests that referred pain elicited from neck and arm muscles is mainly peripheral in origin and is manifested by irritation of the peripheral nerves. Liptan (2010) has suggested that fascial dysfunction and inflammation may lead to fibromyalgia syndrome. A study of biopsies showed an increased level of collagen fibres and mediators of inflammation in the intramuscular connective tissue of patients with fibromyalgia syndrome (Liptan 2010). Therefore, it is logical to suggest that fascial inflammation can initiate a peripheral nociceptive input producing pain sensitization, although there is no evidence supporting this hypothesis.

Recently, Han (2009) proposed an alternative hypothesis. Considering the anatomic expansions of the fascial tissue and the formation of myofascial kinetic links, he has suggested *the connective tissue theory*. Han (2009) suggests that the signalling present in the loose connective tissue may be capable of transmitting noxious stimuli from the surface to muscles or other deep structures through the cells of the vascular and neural systems. According to this theory, peripheral pain may also have a direct origin in the connective tissue. Nevertheless, theories related to fascial tissue and pain mechanisms should be confirmed by clinical and scientific research.

This chapter will describe the anatomic continuity of the fascia tissue from the head to the hand, explaining the formation of fascial entrapments and concepts related to its approach through different examples of clinical application of myofascial induction.

DYNAMICS OF THE FASCIA

Fascia represents dense (both regular and irregular) connective tissue involved in various structures (e.g. aponeurosis, tendons, ligaments, joint capsules and nerve sheets) and forms a continuous network between the elements of the locomotor system. Fascia also represents a loose connective tissue that fills the intermediate spaces of the body, creating links between all the anatomic components (vascular, nervous, and visceral). These links not only serve as anatomical connections but also as functional bonds (Pilat 2003). Gerlach & Lierse (1990) suggested an integrated model named the 'bone-fascia-tendon system' for describing the fascia tissue as the linking function of muscular biomechanics. The dissection of fresh cadavers (Meyers 2003, Pilat 2003) and some observations during surgical procedures (Guimberteau et al 2005) reveal that fascial tissue not only surrounds the muscle structure (epimysium), but it also infiltrates muscle itself and fat tissue (in an individual manner). This anatomical situation of the fascial tissue creates a three-dimensional network in macro- and micro-structure levels (Swartz et al 2001, Guimberteau 2005). These connections may also reach cellular and intracellular levels (Chiquet 1999).

Simultaneously, the extracellular matrix of the connective tissue is the medium where the complex mechano-transduction process, in which the cells react dynamically, detecting and interpreting mechanical signals, takes place (Ingber 1998, 2005, 2006, Pilat 2003, 2005, Ghosh & Ingber 2007, Parker & Ingber 2007). It is therefore logical to think that such a multifunctional communication network may have an impact on the biomechanical and biochemical processes related to dysfunctions of the neck and the arm.

ANATOMICAL CONSIDERATIONS RELATED TO THE CONTINUITY OF THE FASCIAL SYSTEM OF THE NECK AND UPPER LIMB

In the upper quadrant, there is no clear division between muscle, nerve and vascular structures related to a single region, since it seems that these structures act in a synergistic form. Fascia tissue appears to facilitate anatomical and functional continuity between the head, the trunk and the upper extremity (Pilat 2003, Vanacore et al 2009).

Fascial anatomy of the cervical region

The fascial cervical system forms several spaces with a longitudinal orientation (Bienfait 1987, Upledger 1987, Bochenek & Reicher 1997, Pilat 2003) which divide, envelop, support and connect muscles, bones, viscera, vascular vessels and peripheral nerves. In this region fascia can be compared to a system of tubes concentrically placed inside one another, with interconnections at different levels and of several forms (Pilat 2003, 2009) (Fig 36.1). These interconnections unfold between the muscles

establishing mechanical links which determine the direction and the amplitude of motion (Bochenek & Reicher 1997). The lubrication of these compartments, due to the greater amount of fatty tissue or loose connective tissue present, allows a greater freedom of movement (particularly sliding) of the fascial system (Pilat 2009).

The fascial system is responsible for the transmission of dynamic (active) forces between the cranium, mandible, hyoid, sternum, clavicles, scapula, the first two ribs and the neck. The fascial system deeply communicates the endo-cranium with the endo-thorax, influencing not only the mechanics of the cervical region, the shoulder complex, the arm and the temporomandibular joint, but also the mechanics of the respiratory and vascular systems (Pilat 2009).

The route and the connections between the different fascial layers are individual for each subject. This is why it is difficult to classify the exact anatomy in relation to the trajectory and inter-relations. Most anatomists agree with the following classification and distribution of the fascial system (Pilat 2009):

- Superficial fascia
- Deep fascia

This system forms complex links with the shoulder girdle, and continuity with the arm.

Superficial cervical fascia

The superficial fascia is located under the skin forming a firm link (Pilat 2009). It closely surrounds the entire structure of the cervical spine (Figs 36.1–36.3), and can vary in thickness, elasticity, resistance and fat content. It contains the platysma muscle, cutaneous nerves, capillaries, lymphatic vessels and is an elastic structure. The dynamic activity of the superficial fascia is related to the platysma muscle, which expands superficially over the antero-lateral region of the neck. On the upper side,

Fig 36.1 Scheme showing the continuity of the fascial system of the cervical region and its links with the scapular-thoracic region. (A) Sagittal projection.(B) Horizontal projection. *(C)The superficial sheet of the deep cervical fasciae communicating the craneal structures and the chewing system with the scapular-thoracic region. (D) Prevertebral fascia creating the bond between the sub-occipital region and the shoulder girdle.*

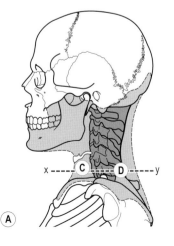

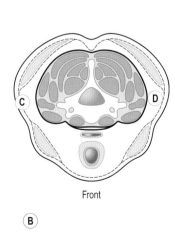

Front

(A)

(B)

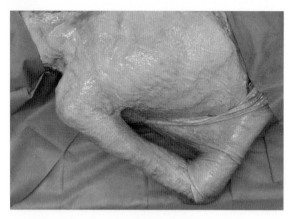

Fig 36.2 Continuity of the superficial fascia in the front part of the body, from the cervical region to the arm. Note the skin withdrawn at the level of the forearm as a glove. There is no independent movement between the superficial fascia and the skin.

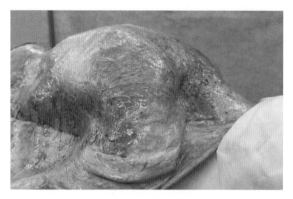

Fig 36.3 Continuity of the superficial fascia of the cervical, scapular and dorsal regions.

the superficial fascia envelops the mandible and it continues to the superficial face muscles (depressor anguli, depressor labii inferioris and orbicularis oris). On its inferior side, the superficial fascia extends beyond the level of the clavicle and inserts into the second and third ribs. Finally, on the lateral side, superficial fascia continues to the platysma insertion (Pilat 2009).

Deep cervical fascia

The deep cervical fascia is located under the skin, the superficial fascia, and the platysma muscle. It is a thin lamina that envelops the neck region like a collar. At the upper side, the fascia inserts on the periostium of the occipital external protuberance, the mastoid process of the temporalis bone, the external acoustic meatus, the inferior border of the zygomatic arch and the masseter fascia. Posteriorly, deep fascia inserts on the spinous

processes of the cervical spine, the nuchal and supraspinous ligaments.

From the posterior insertions, the superficial lamina of the deep cervical fascia is divided bilaterally into two compartments enveloping first the upper trapezius and then the sternocleidomastoid muscle (Fig 36.1A). At the anterior border of the trapezius muscle, the deep fascia expands into a fibrotic lamina that attaches to the fascia of the scalene muscles. The sternocleidomastoid fascial envelop is asymmetric, with a deep layer that is thin and low-load resistant and a superficial layer that is thicker and stronger, particularly at the superior part of the muscle belly. At the superior border, the cervical fascia of the sternocleidomastoid muscle forms fibrotic trabecules crossing the subcutaneous tissue as far as the dermis. The sternocleidomastoid and the upper trapezius muscles surround the borders of the neck region, establishing several free spaces, which allow access to the deepest lamina of the cervical fascia. Furthermore, the cranial and clavicle insertions of upper trapezius and sternocleidomastoid muscles appear as only one muscle. Finally, other structures mechanically related to the superficial lamina of the deep cervical fascia are the sub-mandible glandule and the fibrotic capsule of the parotid glandule. This span forms a complex structure that can participate into the dynamics of the shoulder girdle.

The deepest level of the cervical fascia is represented by the pre-vertebral fascia (Fig 36.1B) that envelops all the cervical muscles except the sternocleidomastoid, the upper trapezius and the infrahyoid muscles. The inferior insertions, at the third thoracic vertebrae, join the thoracolumbar fascia and continue to the lumbar region. In its lateral projection the pre-vertebral fascia runs bilaterally to the axillary fascia. Further, at the antero-inferior border, the pre-vertebral fascia continues toward the vertebral anterior longitudinal ligament and the posterior border of the mediastinum. Finally, laterally the pre-vertebral fascia covers the three scalene muscles and anteriorly the longus collis and longus cervicis muscles. This fascia rests superficially over the transverse processes of the cervical vertebrae (Gallaudet 1931, Bochenek & Reicher 1997, Pilat 2009). Readers are referred to other textbooks for a greater detail of cervical fascial anatomy (Pilat 2009).

Fascial anatomy of the upper extremity

Superficial fascia layer of the upper extremity

The fascial continuity between the neck and the arm on the superficial level is clear on fresh cadaver (Figs 36.4 & 36.5). Along the shoulder and arm region, the fat content is high. In the forearm, the fat content depends on the physical build of each person, although it seems that fat is reduced along the extremity (Fig 36.6). In the hand

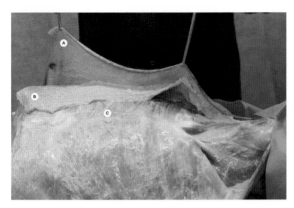

Fig 36.4 Superficial fascia of the cervical and pectoral region. Note the continuity of the fascial structure and its considerable thickness with high fat content. (A) Skin. (B) Superficial fascia. (C) Deep fascia at a pectoral level.

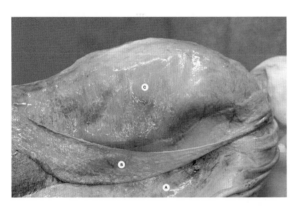

Fig 36.5 Superficial fascia of the scapular-thoracic region. Note the continuity of the fascial structure and its smaller thickness in relation to the pectoral region. (A) Skin. (B) Superficial fascia. (C) Deep fascia at dorsal level.

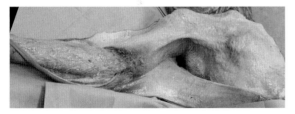

Fig 36.6 Superficial fascia in the forearm. Its thickness is smaller in comparison with the arm.

there is a marked difference between the dorsal and palmar regions, probably resulting from their different functions. In the dorsal region of the hand the fascia is loose and thin, enabling mobility for flexing the fingers (Fig 36.7). The fascia of the palmar region of the hand is

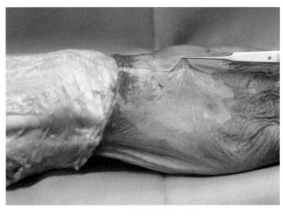

Fig 36.7 Areolar fascia in the dorsum of the hand. Note how easily it separates from the deep fascia.

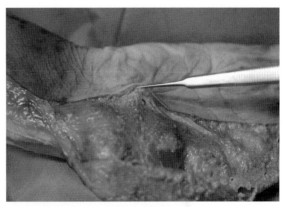

Fig 36.8 Superficial fascia in the palm of the hand. Note how firmly it adheres to the skin.

firmly adhered to the skin (Fig 36.8); however as the fascia runs through the thenar and hypothenar eminence, the superficial fascia is more loose and thin. The superficial fascia has various names: subcutaneous fascia (Rouviere & Delmas 2005), cellular cutaneous tissue (Testut & Latarjet 2007) and subcutaneous adipofascial tissue (Avelar 1989). The characteristics of hand fascia have been studied in relation to plastic surgery and the skin healing process (Congdon et al 1946, Markmann & Barton 1987, Avelar 1989).

Deep fascia layer of the upper extremity

The main anatomical fascial link between the cervical region and the upper extremity is the superficial sheet of the deep cervical fasciae (Fig 36.9). The lower span extends the length of the upper extremity (Pilat 2003) and forms numerous links which continue towards the spine of the scapula, the acromion process and the

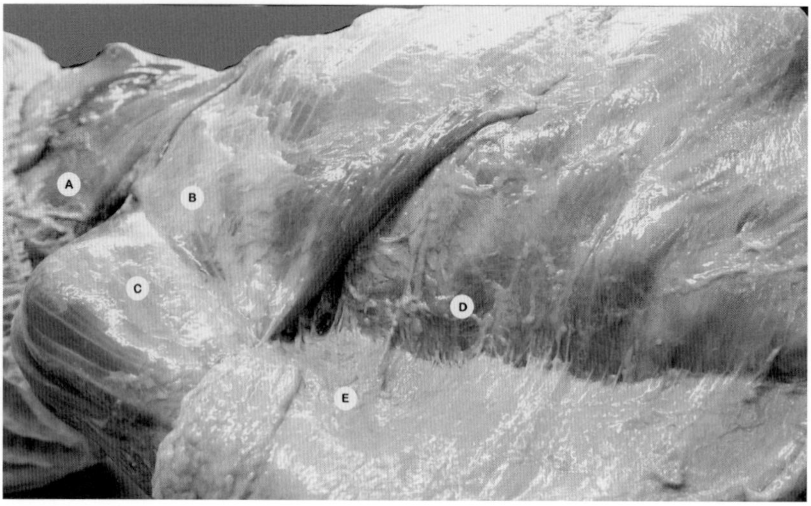

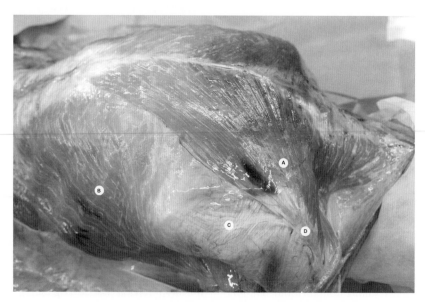

Fig 36.9 The anterior and lateral view of the deep fascia. (A) External lamina of the deep cervical fascia. (B) Pectoral fascia. (C) Deltoid fascia. (D) Serratus anterior muscle fascia. (E) Superficial fascia. The first four (A–D) form a continuous and thin lamina that infiltrates the muscle mass through fine expansions in the form of intra-muscular septa.

clavicle. They then link together projecting towards the pectoralis major, the deltoid, the trapezius, the infraspinatus, teres minor, the teres major and the latissimus dorsi muscles (Fig 36.10). The intermediate and deep fascial layers (Figs 36.11 & 36.12) involve the pectoralis minor, supraspinous, levator scapulae, rhomboid and subscapularis muscles. This span forms a complex structure that can be involved in the function and the

dynamics of the shoulder girdle. These spans can be divided into two groups:

Frontal and antero-lateral span

- The pectoralis fascia (Fig 36.13) forms a thin sheet over the anterior thorax and is firmly inserted in the sternum bone. This fascia continues, covering the front of the pectoralis major muscle to enfold over the

Fig 36.10 (A) Trapezius muscle. (B) Latissimus dorsi muscle. (C) Infraspinatus fascia. Note a large density of the fibres of the insertions of the muscles on the spine of the scapula (D) and also the density, thickness and multidirectional span of the infraspinatus fascia (C).

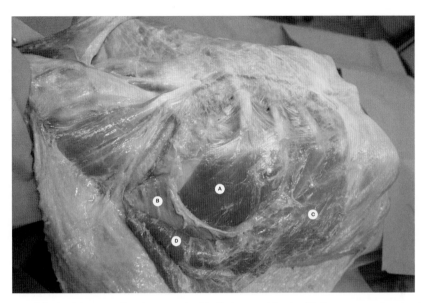

Fig 36.11 Clavi-pectoral fascia. (A) Pectoralis minor muscle. (B) Clavipectoral fascia. (C) Serratus anterior muscle. (D) The pectoralis major muscle is sectioned in its sternal and clavicular insertions, turned and resting on the arm.

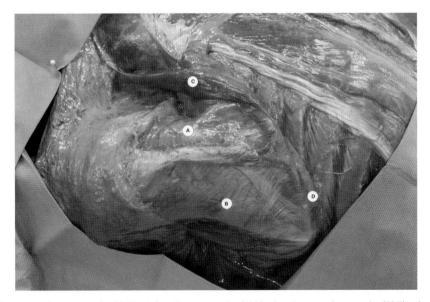

Fig 36.12 (A) The supraspinatus muscle. (B) The infraspinatus muscle. (C) The levator scapulae muscle. (D) The rhomboid muscle is hidden under the scapula.

lower edge, then upholstering the inner face. Under the pectoralis major it is continuous with the fascia of the anterior abdominal wall (Pilat 2003, Testut & Latarjet 2007).

• The deltoid fascia (Fig 36.9) extends as a lateral expansion of the pectoralis fascia. This fascia enfolds the deltoid muscle and, in the posterior span, is linked to the infraspinatus muscle. This lower span continues with the brachial fascia.

• The clavi-pectoral fascia is suspended starting at the front edge of the clavicle, then the coracoid process and the coraco-clavicular ligament. This fascia encases the sub-clavian muscle, continues over the front part of the sternum and laterally joins the deltoid fascia.

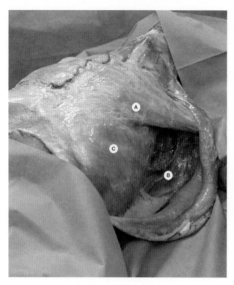

Fig 36.13 Panoramic view of the axillar fossa. (A) The pectoralis major muscle. (B) The latissimus dorsi muscle. (C) The serratus major muscles.

It also expands from its lower edge to encompass the pectoralis minor muscle. Further, its deep span is firmly integrated to the inter-costal muscles and the ribs. Its lower end continues to the axillar fossa, where it joins the pectoralis fascia (Fig 36.11) (Gallaudet 1931, Bochenek & Reicher 1997).

- The serratus anterior fascia is very thin and it covers all the muscle (Fig 36.13).

Posterior and postero-lateral span

- The trapezius fascia (Fig 36.10) is a continuation of the superficial sheet of the deep cervical fasciae which, in its posterior portion from the spina scapulae, continues with the trapezius fascia.
- The supraspinatus fascia (Fig 36.12) encompasses the supraspinatus muscle, enclosing it with the osseous channel of the supraspinatus fossa within an osteo-fascial compartment (Rouviere & Delmas 2005).
- The infraspinatus fascia (Fig 36.12) is a very resistant structure starting on the spine of the scapula. This fascia provides support to the infraspinatus, teres minor and teres major muscles, adjoining them at their insertions (Rouviere & Delmas 2005). It is firmly united to both the medial and lateral borders of the scapula showing strong and multidirectional fibre connections.
- The latissimus dorsi fascia (Figs 36.10 and 36.13) is continuous with the fascia of the teres major muscle. It is strengthened in its lower portion by the deep layer of the axillar fascia.
- The fascia of the levator scapulae muscle (Fig 36.12) represents a thin sheet that accompanies the muscle throughout its length.
- The fascia of the subscapularis muscle covers the area of the subscapularis fossa separating the subscapularis and serratus major muscles.
- The rhomboid muscle fascia (Fig 36.12) is more robust in its span in the lower end, where it is continuous with the trapezium and latissimus dorsi fascia.
- The axillar fascia (Figs 36.13–36.14) forms the axillar base. It spans from the lower border of the pectoralis

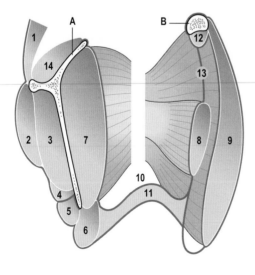

A Scapula
B Cavicle
1 Trapezius muscle
2 Deltoid muscle
3 Infraspinatus muscle
4 Teres minor muscle
5 Teres major muscle
6 Latissimus dorsi muscle
7 Subscapularis muscle
8 Pectoralis minor muscle
9 Pectoralis major muscle
10 Deep lamina of the axillar fascia
11 Superficial lamina of the axillar fascia
12 Subclavian muscle
13 Clavipectoral fascia
14 Supraspinatus muscle

Fig 36.14 Sagittal section of the axillar fossa.

fascia toward the lower end of the teres major and latissimus dorsi muscles. Its deep layer is suspended from the lower border of the pectoralis minor muscle running through the axillar edge of the scapula, entering the insertions of the subscapularis, teres major and teres minor muscles and finally approaching the glenoid cavity. In its medial span, it travels close to the anterior serratus muscle (Bochenek 1997, Rouviere & Delmas 2005, Testut & Latarjet 2007).

This complex distribution of the fascia tissue allows integration of the fascial and muscle structures of the cervical region with the scapular girdle, the brachial fascia, antebrachial fascia and finally to the structures in the hand.

- The brachial fascia encompasses the structure of the arm. In the superior end it is continuous with the pectoralis fascia (Fig 36.15), the deltoid, the axillar and the dorsal fasciae, and continues to the thoraco-lumbar fascia (Rouviere & Delmas 2005, Testut & Latarjet 2007). Stecco et al (2008) analyzed structures of the shoulder in fresh cadavers and clearly identified the connections and continuity in all the specimens

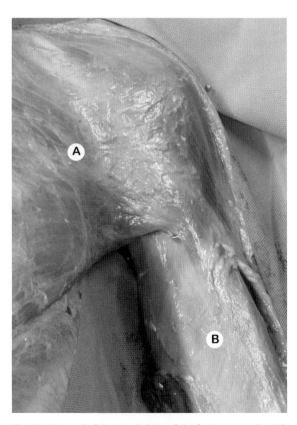

examined. Stecco et al (2008) also noted the presence of muscle fibres of those muscles connected directly to the intramuscular septa of the arm. These septa are continuous with the fascia that envelops the overlying muscular fascia that connects to the brachial fascia. This finding was confirmed in the observation of the transverse sections (Stecco et al 2008). When there is a muscle contraction, some bundles tense the intramuscular septa and indirectly strengthen the brachial fascia. Stecco et al (2008) suggested that these expansions and insertions strengthen the anatomical design of the brachial fascia, placing this fascia in a selective tension according to the contraction of the muscles which may increase the effectiveness of the arm's movement. The brachial fascia expands two fibrous sheets that are transversally oriented forming the flexor and extensor compartments (Rouviere & Delmas 2005), that involve the two main muscles of the arm: triceps and biceps brachii. In the upper third section of the arm, there is the third compartment that contains the coraco-brachial muscle.

- The ante-brachial fascia arises as a direct continuation of the brachial fascia in its inferior section (Fig 36.16). In the ventral aspect there is a connection between the brachial fascia, the ante-brachial fascia, and the lower insertion of the brachial biceps muscle, through a fibrous link described as lacertus fibrosus (Fig 36.17). This aponeurosis extends in the form of a fan (Testut & Latarjet 2007) from the lower tendon of the biceps and continues distally over the proximal end of the ante-brachial fascia. Then it inserts in the cubital region of the common mass of the epitrochlear muscles (Blemker et al 2005, Chew & Giuffrè 2005). The lacertus fibrosus connection is perhaps one of the best examples of the dynamic links in which the strength is transmitted directly from the fascia to the fascia reinforcing the bone-tendon connection. In the posterior part of the upper extremity there is a direct link between the triceps muscle and the ante-brachial fascia. One portion of the triceps' tendon is firmly inserted in the olecranon and the other continues to attach to the ante-brachial fascia.

- The palmar fascia extends in a fan pattern and is continuous with the ante-brachial fascia. It is a thick structure reinforced by the palmaris longus muscle. Laterally it continues to the thenar and hypothenar eminences (Elliot 1988) (Fig 36.18).

- The dorsal fascia of the hand is continuous with the dorsal fascia of the forearm. It covers the tendons of the extensor muscles and becomes thicker forming the extensor retinaculum (Fig 36.19). The main function of the retinaculum is to maintain the extensors' tendons in their functional positioning.

Fig 36.15 Detail of the interlinking of the fascia pectoralis with the brachial fascia. (A) Pectoralis fascia. (B) Brachial fascia

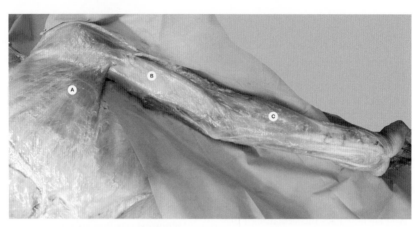

Fig 36.16 Fascial continuity of the anterior face of the upper limb. (A) Pectoralis fascia. (B) Brachial fascia. (C) Ante-brachial fascia.

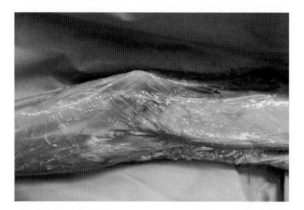

Fig 36.17 Lacertus fibrosus.

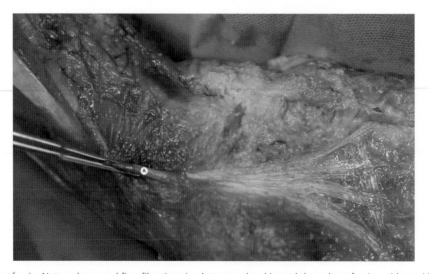

Fig 36.18 Palmar fascia. Note a dense and firm fibrotic union between the skin and the palmar fascia, evidenced by the presence of longitudinal and transverse fibres. (A) The tendon of the palmaris longus muscle

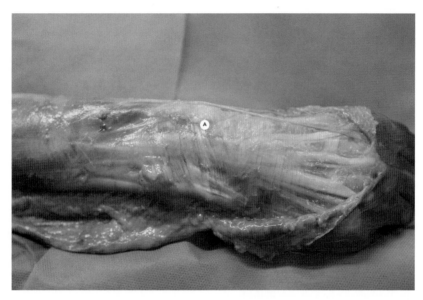

Fig 36.19 Dorsal fascia of the hand. (A) Extensor retinaculum.

THEORETICAL ASPECTS RELATED TO THE TREATMENT OF THE MYOFASCIAL DYSFUNCTION SYNDROME

Myofascial dysfunction syndrome mechanics

Proper fascial dynamics are necessary for the optimal functioning of all the body's systems. A reduction in mobility of the fascial tissue may alter blood circulation, which becomes slow and heavy, leading in extreme cases to ischaemia and deterioration of the muscle fibres. An excessive stimulation of collagen production is created in the myofascial system, causing loss of quality. Further, this stimulation of collagen tissue can facilitate the formation of areas of tissue trapping or restriction, that is, an alteration of physiological movement as regards to amplitude, speed, resistance and coordination (Pilat 2009).

These fascial restrictions (Fig 36.20) promote the formation of compensatory (substitute) movement patterns, although further research is needed to support these hypotheses. Regardless of the cause of the restriction, if this situation persists for long periods of time it can lead to excessive loads and dysfunction (Pilat 2003). These changes impact the loose connective tissue structure, resulting in remodeling of the specialized structures (dense regular and irregular connective tissue) and producing a reorientation of fibres. All these specialized structures include the tendons, ligaments and the articular

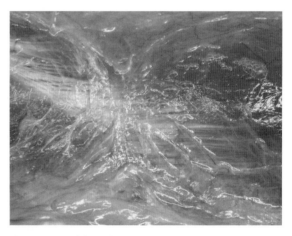

Fig 36.20 Fascial restriction.

capsules. Short-term tissue changes will affect the local function, but long-term changes could create global dysfunction patterns.

Fascial restriction regions

The zones that are most vulnerable to fascial restriction formation generally are:

- Bonding zones between fascial structures in areas of extensive loads. For example, the lacertus fibrosus (Fig 36.17) in which the strength of the muscle contraction is transmitted not only to the tendon but also through the intrinsic/extrinsic connective tissues related to the muscle (Huijing et al 1998, 2001a,b). The lacertus fibrosus not only protects the neurovascular bundle, but it also dynamically stabilizes the biceps' tendon at its lower insertion (Eames at al 2007). It is possible that the traction force in the lower insertion of the biceps is so large – as compared to that received by its two superior insertion tendons – that it requires this reinforcement. A similar anatomical design is noted in numerous structures including the tendon of the quadriceps muscle where it inserts to the patella.

- Zones with excessive friction (tendons with tendinous sheaths reinforced by the retinacula) (Fig 36.19). An increase in compression between tendon and retinacula leads to degenerative changes (Benjamin et al 1995).
- Zones where there are numerous insertions of fascial structures with considerable fibrous density (i.e. scapular spine) (Fig 36.10). When the fascial restriction occurs, this may create a change in the local movement and result in a compensation pattern (Pilat 2009).
- Zones with prolonged and/or repeated hypo-mobility are typically a result of incorrect posture.
- Body segments affected by traumatic or surgical processes.
- Places that tend to bear excessive loads as a result of prolonged and/or repeated emotional stress.

Neurophysiologic mechanisms for releasing the restrictions of the fascial system

The fascia is considered as a mechano-sensitive system. The application of myofascial induction techniques creates a mechanical stimulus in the connective tissue. The effect of this mechanical stimulus may occur at micro- or macroscopic levels and may include the whole organism, the viscera, or a group of cells. It has been shown that this is also recognized in the fascial network where the series of structural molecules form the extracellular conjunctive matrix (Langevin 2006, Vaticón 2009).

Three main mechanisms used for releasing and restructuring the fascial system include piezoelectricity, the attitude of the interstitial mechanoreceptors along with the dynamics of the myofibroblasts, and visco-elasticity.

Piezoelectricity

Piezoelectricity is a phenomenon exhibited by certain crystals. When subjected to mechanical tension they acquire a polarization in their mass with different electrical potentials and loads on their surface (Pilat 2003). The crystals in the human body are liquid (Szent-Gyorgi

1994, Bouligard 1978). When a mechanical drive is applied to these crystals, a minute electrical pulse is generated, particularly in the matrix of the connective tissue which becomes harmonic and oscillating. The information is transmitted electrically through the connective tissue (Oschman 2003). Since collagen is a semi-conductor (Cope 1975) it may be capable of forming an integrated electronic network that enables the interconnection of all the facial system components (O'Connell 2003). Thus, the basic properties of the system (i.e. elasticity, flexibility, elongation, resistance) will depend to a great extent upon the ability to maintain a continuous flow of information (Pilat 2009).

Dynamics of the myofibroblasts

The muscle is a contractile tissue that enables the body to move. The fascia should be considered as an intramuscular connective tissue that forms a functional unit with the muscle fibres. The fascial system is highly innervated by mechanoreceptors included in the somato-sensory system. There are two methods of reception, transmission and interpretation of each mechanical stimulus (Vaticón 2009):

- *Epicritical* sensitivity, that is knowledge, exploration, quantitative information, transmitted through the lemniscal path, from the Paccini and paciniform corpuscles, the Golgi organs and the Ruffini corpuscles.
- *Protopathic* sensitivity, that is qualitative and plastic information, transmitted through extra-lemniscal path. The interstitial receptors that make up a protection and alarm system are located in this process. These are polymodal receptors that may act as mechanoreceptors or nociceptors.

Consequently, the mechanical input (manual pressure or traction) received by the mechanoreceptors creates a broad range of responses in the fascial system that may turn into a movement at both macro- and microscopic levels (Pilat 2003, 2009)

The possibility of the fascial system having its own system of movement is controversial. Some authors (Staubesand & Li 1997, Schleip et al 2006, 2007) believe that this phenomenon is related to the dynamics of the myofibroblasts. These authors suggest that the activation of the actin microfilaments is the origin or motor of movement. Schleip et al (2007) recorded the movement of the lumbar fascia in rats. Further research on the dynamics of myofibroblasts in pathologies such as Dupuytren contracture, plantar fasciitis, frozen shoulder or fibromyalgia support this observation. Some studies focused on skin healing process also strongly support this reasoning (Fidzianska & Jablonska 2000, Gabbiani 2003, 2007, Satish et al 2008). Chaudhry et al (2008) developed a 3-D mathematical model for deformation of human fascia. They suggest that the mechanical forces applied during the manual techniques cannot modify the length of the structures of the dense connective tissue (i.e. plantar fascia), but can create mechanical changes in the loose connective tissue (i.e. superficial nasal fascia). It should also be considered that the handling of the patient may stimulate fascial mechanoreceptors and trigger changes in skeletal muscle tone. This could potentially be sensed manually by the therapist. The movement may be visible or perceived by careful palpation. The manual palpation of the movement without simultaneous visual confirmation of that phenomenon has several possible explanations:

- During surgical procedures Guimberteau et al (2005) found, with 25× microscope enlargement and video camera, the presence of an uninterrupted network of Multi-microvacuolar Collagenous Absorbing Systems (MVCS). These systems have been explained as a 'chaotic matrix' which maintains its form as a result of the action of physical forces that link them into a hierarchical complexity related to time and space factors (Guimberteau et al 2005).
- Different studies (Ingber 1998, 2005, 2006, Ghosh & Ingber 2007, Parker et al 2007, Stamenovic et al 2007, Wang et al 2009) have shown that cellular dynamics and active response of the cytoskeleton, following the action of mechanical forces from the extracellular matrix, induce tissue remodeling at both cell and sub-cell levels.
- Ingber's theory focused on intercommunication systems based on the tensegrity principles (Ingber 1998, Pilat & Testa 2009). The tensegrity theory determines a system of shared tension in the distribution of the mechanical forces at multiple body levels, which can also explain the global reaction of the fascial system when it receives adequate mechanical stimulus during manual treatment.

Visco-elasticity

Visco-elasticity defines the long-term behaviour of the material. The application of a force to a material with visco-elastic properties causes deformation. After some time, the deformation increases without increasing the force.

The visco-elastic properties of the fascia have been observed in numerous studies which have analyzed various fascial structures: thoracolumbar fascia (Yahia et al 1993), fascia lata (Wright & Rennels 1964), and subcutaneous fascia of rats (Latridies et al 2003). Other authors defined the concepts for practical applications: Rolf (1977), Threlkeld (1992), Barnes (1990), Cantu & Grodin (2001), Pilat (2003, 2009), and Schleip et al (2005). Recent theories hypothesized that different chemical mediators may be involved in this process (Vaticón 2009), although further research is needed.

Visco-elasticity is related to the remodelling process of the extracellular matrix, to changes in tissue density and to the proper orientation of the collagen fibres. A study (ex vivo) conducted on the fascia lata, plantar fascia and nasal fascia confirmed the visco-elastic properties of this tissue (Chaudhry et al 2007). Some of the observations found in this study are:

- The visco-elastic response begins 60 seconds after applying a constant traction or compression force.
- To avoid the blocking the release response, it is suggested that the clinician should *not* gradually increase the applied force but that the force should be constant.
- Different fascial structures require different magnitudes of force application; however the time for the response throughout the movement remains the same.

The three different responses of the fascial system are the result of the application of a proper mechanical impulse with adequate force, time and speed. Each of these mechanisms occurs at different levels of the system (micro and/or macro) and also at different time scales (Pilat 2003, 2009, Langevin 2006, Huijing 2009, Vaticón 2009). Any of these mechanisms has the potential to influence the behaviour of the others (Langevin 2006). According to the response of the fascial system during treatment, all the mechanisms may interact (Pilat 2003, Vaticón 2009). As a result of therapy, there is an increase of the blood flow to the restricted areas caused by the release of histamine, a proper orientation in fibroblast mechanics, an increase in blood supply to the nervous tissue and an increase of the flow of metabolites to and from the tissue, thus accelerating the healing process (Evans 1980, Barnes 1990, Barlow & Willoughby 1992, Hamwee 1999, Pilat 2003).

THERAPEUTIC STRATEGIES APPLIED IN THE MYOFASCIAL INDUCTION PROCESS

General observations related to the therapeutic process

There are various concepts related to the treatment of the fascial system (Barnes 1990, Rolf 1977, Manheim 1998, Paoletti 1998, Cantu & Grodin 2001, Chaitow & Delany 2002, Pilat 2003). Evidence provided by the basic sciences regarding the mechanical phenomena related to the therapeutic induction of the fascial system as discussed above provides a proper theoretical frame for therapeutic applications. However, there is need for unification and validation of clinical procedures by clinical research (Remving 2007).

The clinical applications suggested below are based on the clinical experience of the author (Pilat 2003) and are based on the theoretical framework discussed previously. Myofascial induction process may be combined with other manual therapy strategies or as an exclusive treatment procedure.

Definition of the myofascial induction process

Myofascial induction is a simultaneous evaluation and treatment process, which uses tridimensional movements of sustained pressures applied to the entire myofascial system with the aim of releasing the facial restrictions. The term induction is related to the fact that clinicians do not release or stretch the system, since they will apply the correct mechanical stimulus for changing the properties of the tissue. The aim of the process is the recovery of the motion amplitude, force, and coordination.

Basis for clinical applications

General observations (Pilat 2003):

- The evaluation of fascial dysfunction should be included in clinical reasoning processes. We suggest using the same techniques when investigating the movement dysfunctions of every region treated, after taking an exhaustive patient history. In this regard, the patient's retrospective pathology is generally summarized as one of three types of behaviour (Pilat 2007a):
  - **Misuse** – reduced coordination and/or stability
  - **Abuse** – trauma
  - **Overuse** – repetitive movements and/or excess load.

This will lead, in time, to the fourth factor:

  - **Disuse** – atrophy or reduced load capacity (the disuse may become a pathology, in itself).
- At this time there are no objective tests to isolate myofascial dysfunction from other pathologies. During physical examination, the fascia tissue is also being tested by different musculoskeletal tests; however, it is sometimes very difficult to differentiate between muscle, nerve or fascia lesion. Exploration is further complicated by the close anatomic bond between muscle fibres and the fasciae. However, recent studies using high-resolution sonography techniques anticipate a diagnostic procedure for muscle impairments (see Chapter 32).
- Biomechanically, the myofascial system responds to compression and traction forces. These two mechanical strategies can be used when applying myofascial induction techniques.
  - Restrictions may occur in various directions and planes. They may even occur in different directions in a same plane, or in the same direction in various planes, or in different planes in various directions.
  - The direction of the releasing movement is towards facilitation. The therapist should refrain from performing movements in arbitrary directions.
  - There is no need for active muscle contraction performed by the patient. The patient may be asked to maintain a state of active passiveness.

Clinical procedure principles (Pilat 2003, 2009)

- The therapist applies a slow three-dimensional compression or traction causing the tissue to become tense. This is referred to as the first restriction barrier.
- The applied pressure is constant for the first 60–90 seconds. This is the time required for releasing the first restriction barrier according to the visco-elastic response (Chaudhry et al 2007).
- During the first phase of the technique, the therapist barely causes the tissue to move.
- Upon overcoming the first restriction barrier, the therapist accompanies the movement in the direction of the restriction, pausing at each next barrier.
- In each technique, the therapist must overcome at least three to six consecutive barriers and a minimum time of application is usually 3–5 minutes.
- The tension applied to the tissue must be constant, but the pressure applied by the therapist may be modified after overcoming the first barrier. Pressure should be reduced if there is an increase in pain and/or abundant activity.

Examples of practical applications

The following techniques are examples of the therapeutic strategies used to treat myofascial restrictions and are related to the most common clinical neck and arm pain syndromes.

Techniques targeted to the cervical segment (Pilat 2003)

A forward head posture can result in an exaggerated extension of the upper cervical spine, increasing tension in the hyoid muscles (Pilat 2003, 2009). The prolonged and repetitive tension may lead to the depression and posterior transfer of the jaw, forcing the subject's mandible to depress. This action is countered by contraction of the temporal and masseter muscles, tensing the fascial system. This may result in limitations of jaw movement.

The hyoid bone is involved in daily activities such as swallowing, talking, chewing, playing wind instruments. The hyoid bone is fixed to the pre-vertebral and superficial fascia. Therefore a fascial dysfunction may directly affect its proper functioning, which may result in altered dynamics of the muscles inserted to the hyoid bone.

The scalene muscles laterally flex the cervical spine while the sub-occipital muscles extend the head. The scalene muscles also stabilize the first rib. Since these muscles have a vertical anatomy, some authors have hypothesized that they can exert a traction force from the cervical vertebrae downwards.

Sub-occipital induction (Fig 36.21)

With the patient in supine, the therapist is seated on a chair. The therapist places both hands under the patient's head. Then the therapist touches the sub-occipital space with the second to the fifth fingers attempting to place the fingers vertically. Applying a three-dimensional pressure, the principles of induction are followed.

Suprahyoid region induction (Fig 36.22)

With the patient supine, the therapist places their caudal hand above the hyoid bone surrounding it. The endings of the index and medium fingers of the cranial hand should be placed on the mandible. With the caudal hand the therapist applies slight traction in the caudal direction, whereas with the cranial hand applies a traction towards the head. Applying a three-dimensional pressure, the principles of induction are followed.

Induction of scalene muscles (Fig 36.23)

With the patient lying supine, the therapist places both thumbs along the supra-clavicular space. By maintaining this position for approximately 60–90 seconds, there is a rotation of the head to one side (clinical observation). The therapist makes contact with the patient's head on the side in order to turn the head. The other hand's thumb continues the releasing manoeuvre. *Note*: Pressure over the brachial plexus should be avoided. If any sensation of pins and needles is felt towards the upper limb, the fingers must release from the brachial plexus.

Induction of pre-vertebral fascia (Fig 36.24)

With the patient supine, the therapist slightly turns the patient's head to one side and then places their fingers

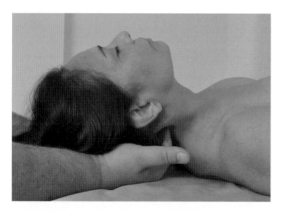

Fig 36.21 Sub-occipital induction approach.

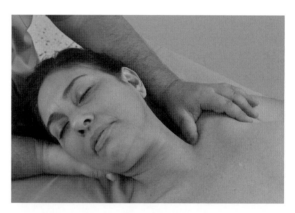

Fig 36.23 Induction of scalene muscles.

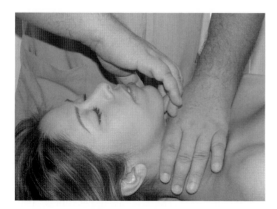

Fig 36.22 Suprahyoid region induction.

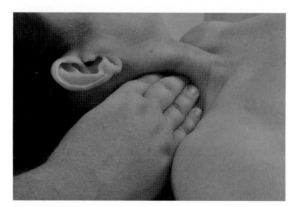

Fig 36.24 Induction of pre-vertebral fascia.

underneath the belly of the sternocleidomastoid muscle (over the scalene and above the transverse processes of the cervical vertebrae). The induction principles are followed as always. *Note*: Do not apply pressure over the trachea or the carotid artery.

Techniques targeted to the shoulder girdle (Pilat 2003)

The shoulder girdle links the trunk with the upper extremity. The link is functionally produced through the sternoclavicular articulation (see Chapter 14). Further, the trapezius, infraspinatus, supraspinatus, and deltoid muscles are connected to the scapula. The fascial insertions of these muscles form a fibrous link (Fig 36.12). The restriction of fascial tissue in this region can modify the distribution of tensional lines of the scapular region, contributing to neck and arm pain.

Induction of the pectoralis and deltoid fascia (Fig 36.25)

With the patient supine, the therapist crosses the hands placing the cranial hand over the front of the shoulder, and the caudal over the homo-lateral edge of the sternum. Applying a three-dimensional force, the principles of induction are followed.

Induction of clavi-pectoral and pectoralis minor muscle fascia (Fig 36.26)

With the patient lying supine, the therapist holds the arm of the patient with the cranial hand. The arm of the patient is abducted approximately at 90°. The caudal hand, in a pronation position, is introduced into the space between

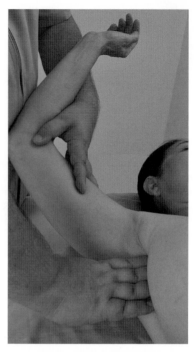

Fig 36.26 Induction of clavi-pectoral and pectoralis minor muscle fascia.

the pectoralis major and the ribs. In that position, the therapist slowly directs the fingers medially and cranially.

Integrated induction of the arm (Fig 36.27)

With the patient supine, the therapist places the caudal hand at the sternum level whereas the cranial hand holds the patient's arm, with an elevation of approximately 120°. The therapist applies a slight traction. Applying a thee-dimensional force the principles of induction are followed.

Induction of the spine of scapula (Fig 36.28)

With the patient seated, the therapist contacts the supraspinous space by pressing the fingers in the direction of the scapula's spine. The other hand of the therapist is gently placed on the patient's head. By applying a three-dimensional force, the therapist follows the principles of induction. In the author's clinical experience, it is normal to observe some head movement – the therapist should follow it.

Induction of the trapezius muscle (Fig 36.29)

This technique follows the same principles as previously. The fingers contact the upper edge of the trapezius muscle while the therapist contacts its upper fibres. Painful reactions should be avoided and treated with special care.

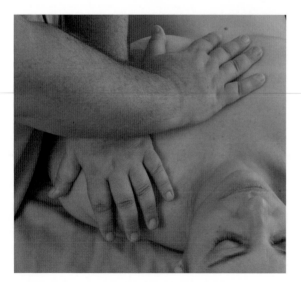

Fig 36.25 Induction of pectoralis and deltoid fascia.

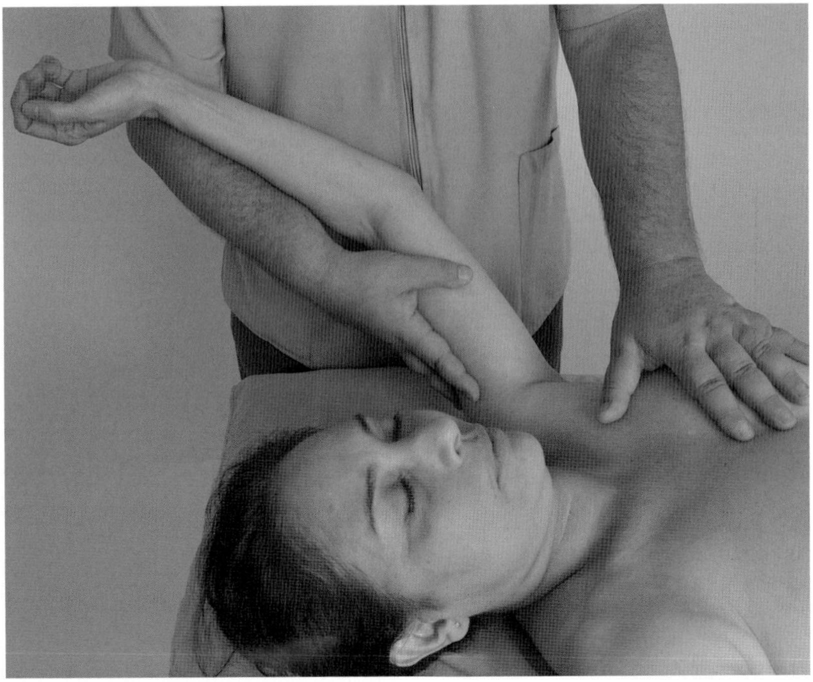

Fig 36.27 Integrated induction of the arm.

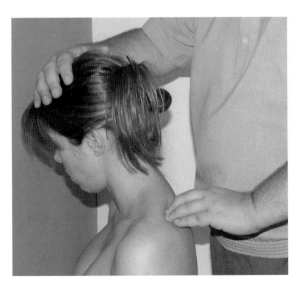

Fig 36.28 Induction of the spine of the scapula.

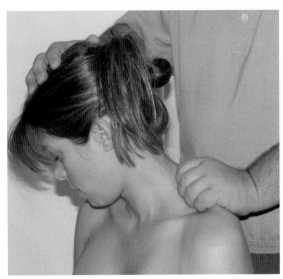

Fig 36.29 Induction of the trapezius muscle.

Techniques targeted to the brachial and ante-brachial fascia

Lateral epicondylalgia is one of the most common pathologies in the elbow region and is associated with an excessive traction generated by the extensor muscles. The muscle most often involved in this pathology is the extensor carpi radialis brevis. It is believed that the pathology is caused by the exaggerated traction of its tendon (see Chapter 26). Briggs & Elliott (1985) found that of 139 dissected upper extremities, only 29 cases showed a direct insertion of the tendon of the extensor muscles into the epicondyle. In the other cases, the tendon was fixed on the fascia of the extensor carpi radialis longus, extensor digitorum communis, supinator and radial collateral ligament. This example reveals the need to analyze and focus the therapy to the broad fascial bonds.

Induction of brachial and ante-brachial fascia connection (Fig 36.30)

The patient is supine with the arm abducted approximately 90° and the forearm in a relaxed supination. The therapist places one hand over the ventral surface of the medium third of the forearm. The inner hand is placed underneath, embracing the elbow and the proximal end of the forearm. Both hands softly compress the forearm – the cranial hand applies traction in the caudal direction and the lower hand in the cranial direction.

Induction of the bicipital fascia (Fig 36.31)

The patient is supine with the forearm supinated. The therapist places the hands (without crossing them) with the fingers contacting both ends of the bicipital fascia. In that position, the therapist applies pressure toward the extremity and towards the cubital fossa of the elbow. The principles of induction are followed.

Induction of the extensor retinacle (Fig 36.32)

With the patient supine and the forearm pronated, the therapist places the hands (crossing them) as follows.

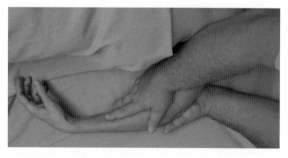

Fig 36.30 Induction of the brachial and ante-brachial fascia connection.

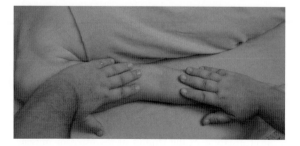

Fig 36.31 Induction of the bicipital fascia.

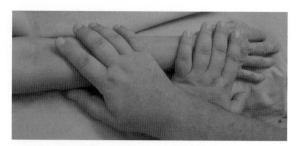

Fig 36.32 Induction of extensor retinacle.

The caudal hand contacts the retinacle region and the cranial hand the posterior third of the forearm. In that position, the therapist applies pressure towards the limb and in cranial and caudal directions. The principles of induction are followed.

Techniques targeted to the fascia of the hand

Kalin & Hirsch (1987) found that only 8 of 69 interosseous muscles showed bone insertions exclusively. In the remaining examples, the insertions were produced through the fascial structures. Additionally, the palmar fascia is linked to the palmaris longus muscle which represents a fascial link that is directly related to the functional integrity.

Induction of the carpal tunnel and palmar fascia (Fig 36.33)

The therapist places the thumbs on the region of the carpal tunnel and flexes the index fingers over the back of the wrist, forming a clamp. Holding the patient's wrist,

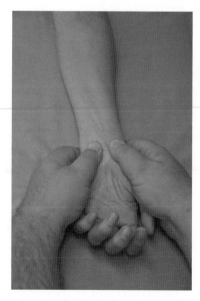

Fig 36.33 Induction of the carpal tunnel and palmar fascia.

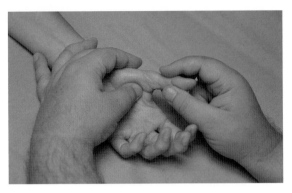

Fig 36.34 Three-dimensional telescopic induction.

the therapist applies a three-dimensional traction while slightly extending the wrist. The principles of induction are followed. *Note*: Considerable pressure should be maintained and the therapist should not allow the fingers to slip over the patient's skin. The same strategy is used to treat the palmar fascia, placing the fingers into the palmar fascia.

Telescopic three-dimensional induction (Fig 36.34)

The therapist, with the non-dominant hand, stabilizes the metacarpal bone or phalanx of the finger to be treated. The level of the stabilization depends on the site of the symptoms. With the other hand the therapist holds the distal phalanx of the patient's finger between the thumb, the index, and the middle fingers. A global treatment may be performed or only at a given level. The facilitated movement is followed.

Inter-osseous induction (Fig 36.35)

The therapist places the thumbs over the palmar surface of the metacarpophalangeal joints, so that it may separate the proximal phalanxes of the patient's fingers. The other

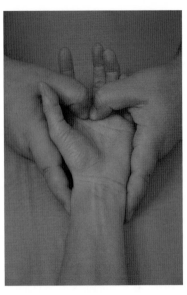

Fig 36.35 Inter-osseous induction.

fingers stabilize the patient's hand. With the thumbs, the therapist exerts a three-dimensional pressure. The same strategy may be applied over the dorsal inter-osseous.

CONCLUSIONS

From an anatomical and functional viewpoint, the fascia represents a structure communicating throughout the body. Research on the dynamics of connective tissue at all levels of its construction is permitting a better understanding of the phenomena that accompanies myofascial induction approaches. However, continuous multidisciplinary research is required to validate the practical applications (Remving 2007).

REFERENCES

Avelar, J., 1989. Regional distribution and behavior of the subcutaneous tissue concerning selection and indication for liposuction. Aesth. Plast. Surg. 13, 155–162.

Barlow, Y., Willoughby, S., 1992. Pathophysiology of soft tissue repair. Br. Med. Bull. 48, 698–711.

Barnes, J., 1990. Myofascial Release. MFR Seminars, Paoli.

Benjamin, M., Qin, S., Ralphs, J.R., 1995. Fibrocartilage associated with human tendons and their pulleys. J. Anat. 187, 625–633.

Bienfait, M., 1987. Estudio e tratamento do esqueleto fibroso: Fascias e pompages. Summus Editorial, Sao Paulo.

Blemker, S.S., Pinsky, P.M., Delp, S.L., 2005. A 3D model of muscle reveals the causes of nonuniform strains in the biceps brachii. J. Biomech. 38, 657–665.

Bochenek, A., Reicher, M., 1997. Anatomia czlowieka. PZWL, Warszawa.

Bouligard, Y., 1978. Liquid crystals and their analogs in biological systems. Solid State Physics 14, 259–294.

Briggs, C.A., Elliott, B.G., 1985. Lateral epicondylitis. A review of structures associated with tennis elbow. Clin. Anat. 7, 149–153.

Cantu, T.I., Grodin, A.J., 2001. Myofascial manipulation: Theory and clinical application. Aspen Publishers, Maryland.

Chaitow, L., Delany, J., 2002. Clinical application of neuromuscular techniques. In: The Lower Body, vol. 2. Churchill Livingstone, London.

Chaudhry, H., Huang, C.h., Schleip, R., et al., 2007. Viscoelastic behavior of human fasciae under extension in manual therapy. J. Bodyw. Mov. Ther. 11, 159–167.

Chaudhry, H., Schleip, R., Zhiming, J.I., et al., 2008. Three-Dimensional Mathematical Model for Deformation of Human Fasciae in Manual Therapy. J. Am. Osteopath. Assoc. 108, 379–390.

Chew, M.L., Giuffrè, B., 2005. Disorders of the distal biceps brachii tendon. Radiographics 25, 1227–1237.

Chiquet, M., 1999. Regulation of extracellular matrix gene expression by mechanical stress. Matrix Biol. 18, 417–426.

Congdon, E.D., Edson, J., Ynitelli, S., 1946. Gross structure of subcutaneous layer of anterior and lateral trunk in the male. Am. J. Anat. 79, 399–429.

Cope, F.W., 1975. A review of the applications of solid state physics concepts to biological systems. J. Biol. Phys. 3, 1–41.

Eames, M.H., Bain, G.I., Fogg, Q.A., van Riet, R.P., 2007. Distal biceps tendon anatomy: a cadaveric study. Am. J. Bone Joint Surg. 89, 1044–1049.

Elliot, D., 1988. The early history of contracture of the palmar fascia. Part 1: the origin of the disease: the curse of the MacCrimmons: the hand of benediction: Cline's contracture. J. Hand Surg. [Br.] 13, 246–253.

Evans, P., 1980. The healing process at cellular level: A review. Physiotherapy 66, 256–259.

Farasyn, A., 2007. Referred muscle pain is primarily peripheral in origin: the 'barrier–dam' theory. Med. Hypotheses 68, 144–150.

Fidzianska, A., Jablonska, S., 2000. Congenital fascial dystrophy: abnormal composition of the fascia. J. Am. Acad. Dermatol. 43, 797–802.

Gabbiani, G., 2003. The myofibroblast in wound healing and fibrocontractive diseases. J. Pathol. 200, 500–503.

Gabbiani, G., 2007. Evolution and clinical implications of the myofibroblast concept. In: Findley, T.W., Schleip, R. (Eds.), Fascia research. Basic science and implications for conventional and complementary health care. Urban and Fischer, Munich, pp. 56–60.

Gallaudet, B.B., 1931. A description of the planes of fascia of the human body. Columbia University Press, New York.

Gerlach, U.J., Lierse, W., 1990. Functional construction of the superficial and deep fascia system of the lower limb in man. Acta Anat. (Basel) 139, 11–25.

Ghosh, K., Ingber, D.E., 2007. Micromechanical control of cell and tissue development: Implications for tissue engineering. Adv. Drug Deliv. Rev. 59, 1306–1308.

Guimberteau, J., Sentucq-Rigall, J., Panconi, B., 2005. Introduction to the knowledge of subcutaneous sliding system in humans. Ann. Chir. Plast. Esthet. 50, 19–34.

Hamwee, J., 1999. Zero balancing: Touching the energy of bone. North Atlantic Books, Berkeley.

Han, D.G., 2009. The other mechanism of muscular referred pain: The 'connective tissue' theory. Med. Hypotheses 73, 292–295.

Hu, S., Chen, J., Fabry, B., et al., 2003. Intracellular stress tomography reveals stress focusing and structural anisotropy in cytoskeleton of living cells. Am. J. Physiol. Cell Physiol. 285, C1082–C1090.

Huijing, P.A., 2009. Epimuscular miofascial force transmission: A historical review and implications for new research. J. Biomech. 42, 9–21.

Huijing, P.A., Baan, G.C., 2001a. Extramuscular myofascial force transmission within the rat anterior tibial compartment: proximo-distal differences in muscle force. Acta Physiol. Scand. 173, 297–311.

Huijing, P.A., Baan, G.C., 2001b. Myofascial force transmission causes interaction between adjacent muscles and connective tissue: effects of blunt dissection and compartmental fasciotomy on length force characteristics of rat extensor digitorum longus muscle. Arch. Physiol. Biochem. 109, 97–109.

Huijing, P.A., Baan, G.C., Rebel, G.T., 1998. Non-myotendinous force transmission in rat extensor digitorum longus muscle. J. Exp. Biol. 201, 683–691.

Ingber, D.E., 1998. The architecture of life. Sci. Am. 278, 48–57.

Ingber, D.E., 2005. Tissue adaptation to mechanical forces in healthy, injured and aging tissues. Scand. J. Med. Sci. Sports 15, 199–204.

Ingber, D.E., 2006. Cellular mechanotransduction: putting all the pieces together again. FASEB J. 20, 811–827.

Kalin, P.J., Hirsch, B.E., 1987. The origins and function of the interosseous muscles of the foot. J. Anat. 152, 83–91.

Langevin, H.M., 2006. Connective tissue: a body-wide signaling network? Med. Hypotheses 66, 1074–1077.

Latridies, J., Wu, J., Yandow, J., Langevin, H., 2003. Subcutaneous tissue mechanical behavior is linear and viscoelastic under uniaxial tension. Connect. Tissue Res. 44, 208–217.

Liptan, L., 2010. Fascia: A missing link in our understanding of the pathology of fibromialgia. J. Bodyw. Mov. Ther. in press.

Manheim, C., 1998. The Miofascial Release Manual. Slack Inc, New York.

Maniotis, A., Chen, C., Ingber, D., 1997. Demonstration of mechanical connections between integrins, cytoskeletal filaments, and nucleoplasm that stabilize nuclear structure. Proc. Natl. Acad. Sci. U.S.A. 94, 849–854.

Markmann, B., Barton, F.E., 1987. Anatomy of the subcutaneous tissue of the trunk and lower extremity. Plastic Reconstructive Surgery 80, 248–254.

Mense, S., 1994. Referral of muscle pain. J. Pain 3, 1–9.

Meyers, T., 2003. Anatomy trains. Elsevier, Amsterdam.

O'Connell, J.A., 2003. Bioelectric responsiveness of fascia. Tech. Orthop. 18, 67–73.

Oschman, J., 2003. Energy medicine in therapeutics and human performance. Nature's Own Research Association, Dover, New Hampshire.

Paoletti, S., 1998. Les fascias: role des tissus dans la mécanique humaine. Sully, Paris.

Parker, K.K., Ingber, D.E., 2007. Extracellular matrix, mechanotransduction and structural hierarchies in heart tissue engineering. Philosophical Transactions of the Royal Society of London 362, 1267–1279.

Pilat, A., 2003. Inducción Miofascial. Madrid, MacGraw-Hill.

Pilat, A., 2005. El peligro de moverse y el peligro de no moverse. Interpretación del dolor desde la práctica fisioterapéutica. Libro de Ponencias XV Jornadas de Fisioterapia de la Escuela de Fisioterapia de la ONCE. Universidad Autónoma de Madrid, Madrid.

Pilat, A., 2007a. El lenguaje del dolor (el proceso de interpretación del dolor en fisioterapia), Libro de Ponencias XV Jornadas de Fisioterapia EUF ONCE. Universidad Autónoma de Madrid, Madrid.

Pilat, A., 2009. Myofascial induction approaches for headache. In: Fernández-de-las-Peñas, C., Arendt-Nielsen, L., Gerwin, R.D. (Eds.), Tension Type and Cervicogenic Headache: pathophysiology, diagnosis and treatment. Jones & Bartlett Publishers, Boston.

Pilat, A., Testa, M., 2009. Tensegridad: El Sistema Craneosacro como la unidad biodinámica, Libro de Ponencias XIX Jornadas de Fisioterapia, 95-111, EUF ONCE. Universidad Autónoma de Madrid, Madrid.

Remving, L., 2007. Fascia Research. Myofascial release: 5.4.5 - 140: An evidence based treatment concept. Elsevier Urban & Fischer, New York.

Rolf, I., 1977. La integración de las estructuras del cuerpo humano. Ediciones Urano, Barcelona.

Rouviere, H., Delmas, A., 2005. Anatomía Humana. Masson, Barcelona.

Satish, L., Laframboise, W.A., O'Gorman, D.B., et al., 2008. Identification of differentially expressed genes in fibroblasts derived from patients with Dupuytren's Contracture. BMC Med. Genomics 1, 1–10.

Schleip, R., Klingler, W., Lehmann-Horn, F., 2005. Active fascial contractility: fascia may be able to contract in a smooth muscle-like manner and thereby influence musculoskeletal dynamics. Med. Hypotheses 65, 273–277.

Schleip, R., Naylor, I.L., Ursu, D., et al., 2006. Passive muscle stiffness may be influenced by active contractility of intramuscular connective tissue. Med. Hypotheses 66, 66–71.

Schleip, R., Kingler, W., Lehmann-Horn, F., 2007. Fascia is able to contract in a smooth muscle-like manner and thereby influence musculoskeletal mechanics. In: Findley, T.W., Schleip, R. (Eds.), Fascia research. Basic science and implications for conventional and complementary health care. Urban and Fischer, Munich, pp. 76–77.

Stamenovic, D., Rosenblatt, N., Montoya-Zavala, M., et al., 2007. Rheological Behavior of Living Cells is Timescale Dependent. J. Biophys. 93, 39–41.

Staubesand, J., Li, Y., 1997. Begriff und Substrat der Fazienslerose bei chronisch-venöser Insuffizienz. Phlebologie 26, 72–77.

Stecco, C., Porzionato, A., Macchi, V., et al., 2008. The expansions of the pectoral girdle muscles onto the brachial fascia: morphological aspects and spatial disposition. Cells Tissues Organs 188, 320–329.

Swartz, M.A., Tschumperlin, D.J., Kamm, R.D., et al., 2001. Mechanical stress is communicated between different cell types to elicit matrix remodeling. Proc. Natl. Acad. Sci. U.S.A. 98, 6180–6185.

Szent-Gyorgyi, A., 1994. The study of energy-levels in biochemistry. Nature 148, 157–159.

Testut, L., Latarjet, A., 2007. Compendio de la anatomía descriptiva. Masson, Madrid.

Threlkeld, A.J., 1992. The effects of manual therapy on connective tissues. Phys. Ther. 72, 893–902.

Travell, J., Bigelow, N.H., 1946. Referred somatic pain does not follow a simple 'segmental' pattern. Federal Proceedings 5, 106.

Upledger, J., 1987. Craniosacral therapy II. Eastland Press, Seattle.

Vanacore, R., Ham, A., Voehler, M., et al., 2009. Sulfilimine Bond Identified in Collagen IV. Science 325, 1230–1234.

Vaticon, D., 2009. Sensibilidad Myofascial: El Sistema Craneosacro como la unidad biodinámica, Libro de Ponencias XIX Jornadas de Fisioterapia, 24-30, EUF ONCE. Universidad Autónoma de Madrid, Madrid.

Vleeming, A., 1992. The posterior layer of the thoracolumbar fascia. Its function in load transfer from spine to legs. In: Vleeming, A. et al., (Eds.), First interdisciplinary world congress on low back pain. ECO, Rotterdam.

Vleeming, A., Stoeckart, R., 1997. The role of the pelvic girdle in couplin the spine and legs: a clinical-anatomical perspective on pelvic stability. In: Vleeming, et al., (Eds.), Movement, Stability & Lumbopelvic Pain Elsevier.

Wang, N., Tytell, J., Ingber, D., 2009. Mechanotransduction at a distance: mechanically coupling the extracellular matrix with the nucleus. Science 10, 75–81.

Wright, D.G., Rennels, D.C., 1964. A study of the elastic properties of plantar fascia. J. Bone Joint Surg. [Am.] 46, 482–492.

Yahia, L.H., Pigeon, P., DesRosiers, E.A., 1993. Viscoelastic properties of the human lumbodorsal fascia. J. Biomed. Eng. 15, 425–429.

Chapter | 37 |

Peripheral mechanisms of chronic upper limb pain: nerve dynamics, inflammation and neurophysiology

Jane Greening, Andrew Dilley

INTRODUCTION

Chronic upper limb pain represents a significant social economic health care problem. The Health and Safety Executive in the UK places upper limb pain second only to low back pain in terms of incidence and lost work days. To the frustration of clinicians and patients, too little is known regarding the causes of chronic upper limb pain. Treatments tend not to be evidence based and are often focussed on diagnostic labels rather than individual patient presentations. Diffuse repetitive strain injury (RSI), also referred to as non-specific arm pain, chronic arm pain following whiplash injury and complex regional pain syndrome type 1 (CRPS1) that affects the upper limb are common conditions seen in the clinic. Despite differences in initial cause of symptoms, many of these patients experience ongoing pain in their upper limbs with little sign of tissue injury. Patients describe spontaneous pain, pain with limb movements, deep muscle aches, paraesthesia, hyperalgesia (i.e. increased sensitivity to noxious stimuli), allodynia (i.e. increased sensitivity to non-noxious stimuli) and difficulties with the coordination of fine movement, all of which suggests a neuropathic contribution to their symptoms. Studies have also shown subtle changes to upper limb peripheral nerve function in both whiplash patients and those with RSI (Chien et al 2008, Greening & Lynn 1998, Greening et al 2003). However, nerve conduction studies show that there is no objective sign of a frank nerve injury (Alpar et al 2002, Harrington et al 1998, Rodriquez et al 2004, Wallis et al 1998). Central nervous system changes account for some of these symptoms, although there is no evidence that such changes are the primary cause.

In these patient groups, previous investigations of cytokine levels suggest that inflammation affecting nerve tissue may contribute to symptoms (Carp et al 2007,

© 2011 Elsevier Ltd.
DOI: 10.1016/B978-0-7020-3528-9.00037-6

Gerdle et al 2008, Uceyler et al 2007a). Animal studies have shown that nerve inflammation can result in significant peripheral and central changes that may account for painful symptoms described by these patients (Bove et al 2003, Carp et al 2007, Dilley et al 2005, Elliott et al 2008). It has also been suggested that increased nerve strain and changes to neural dynamics may contribute to symptoms (Byng 1997, Dilley et al 2005, Greening 2005, Greening et al 2005, Lynn et al 2002, Quintner 1989, Sterling et al 2002). Following an overview of peripheral nerve trunk anatomy, this chapter will review studies in the upper limb that have used ultrasound imaging and magnetic resonance imaging (MRI) to measure nerve movement and identify possible nerve inflammation in these patient populations. We will also review the now compelling evidence for altered nerve function, morphology and neuropathic symptoms following nerve inflammation.

ANATOMY OF A PERIPHERAL NERVE

The peripheral nerve trunk has been described as consisting of an inner 'neural core' and an outer connective tissue tube or sheath (Ushiki & Ide 1990, Walbeehm et al 2004). The inner core consists of the endoneurium and perineurium, whereas the outer connective tissue sheath is formed of the epineurium (Fig 37.1). The axons are located within the endoneurium of a peripheral nerve and are arranged into bundles called fascicles, which are surrounded by the perineurium. Axons are closely associated with Schwann cells, either individually (myelinated axons), or in small groups (unmyelinated axons in Remak bundles). The axons and cells of the endoneurium (i.e. Schwann cells, fibroblasts, macrophages and mast cells), plus the extensive endoneurial capillary network are supported by longitudinally aligned collagen fibrils that form the endoneurial connective tissue. The axons follow an undulating course which is supported by these endoneurial collagen fibrils (Haninec 1986). These undulations appear as a light/dark optical effect under light microscopy and are referred to as Bands of Fontana. This wave-like alignment of the axons may represent a reserve length during nerve elongation that protects the axons from high strain levels.

The perineurium is a highly specialized connective tissue structure formed of a tightly woven network of myofibroblasts. It is up to 15 cells deep in humans (Thomas et al 1993) and contains collagen fibrils that run longitudinally, obliquely and circumferentially to provide strength (Gamble & Eames 1964, Sunderland 1978). Although not as effective as the blood–brain barrier, the perineurium act as a diffusion barrier that helps maintain the endoneurial microenvironment surrounding the axons. A positive fluid pressure within the endoneurium is maintained by the impermeability of the perineurium and its circular arrangement of collagen fibrils (Sunderland 1978, Walbeehm et al 2004). When the nerve is under strain, the increased pressure within the endoneurium will act to resist the reduction in nerve cross-sectional area and will contribute to nerve stiffness. A movement plane exists between the perineurium and the epineurium. Bridging these layers are a series of visco-elastic connections that increase in stiffness as nerve strain is increased (Tillett et al 2004). Also passing obliquely between the perineurium and endoneurium are transperineurial blood vessels that may contribute to this mechanical connection.

The epineurium forms the outer sheath of the nerve and consists of axially arranged undulating, thick, collagen bundles (Ushiki & Ide 1990). It provides some degree of nerve extensibility and will cushion against external

Fig 37.1 Cross-sectional diagram of a peripheral nerve trunk.

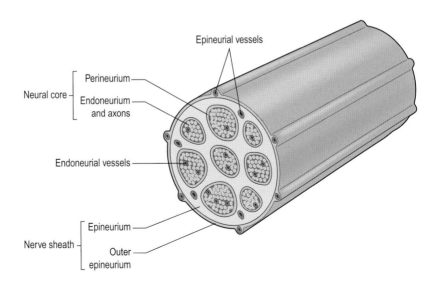

Epineurial vessels

Neural core — Perineurium

Endoneurium and axons

Endoneurial vessels

Nerve sheath — Epineurium

Outer epineurium

trauma. The epineurium is surrounded by a loose thin connective tissue, the adventitia, which, while connecting the peripheral nerve trunk to adjacent tissue, allows considerable nerve movement.

Both axonal conduction and axoplasmic transport are metabolic processes that require an uninterrupted blood supply. This is provided by the extensive interconnected vascular systems within the endoneurium, perineurium and epineurium. Extrinsic longitudinal vessels run along the loose adventitia in a sinuous course that allows the nerve considerable mobility. These connect to the intrinsic vessels within the epineurium, which follow a similar sinuous course. These epineurial vessels in turn communicate with the endoneurial vessels (Lundborg 1988).

The connective tissue of the nerve trunk is itself innervated by the nervi nervorum. There is also a contribution from axons forming the perivascular plexus (Hromada 1963). These unmyelinated axons (Thomas 1963) contain both substance P and calcitonin gene related peptide, which classifies them as C fibre axons (Sauer et al 1999, Zochodne & Ho 1992, 1993). Activation of these axons in response to nerve damage or capsaicin application to the nerve sheath causes nerve hyperaemia (i.e. increased blood flow) (Zochodne & Ho 1992). Electrophysiological studies have also demonstrated the nociceptive function of the nervi nervorum (Bove & Light 1995).

While peripheral nerves have a thick layer of epineurium, nerve roots are bathed in cerebrospinal fluid and have a thin pial covering. Compared to peripheral nerve trunks, nerve roots are relatively vulnerable to mechanical stress and the effects of inflammatory mediators. The distal part of the nerve root is surrounded by a dural sleeve that is continuous with the thin epineurium of the spinal nerve. While dural connections to the intervertebral foramina ensure that during limb movements strain is not transmitted onto the nerve roots, movements of the cervical spine will impose a degree of strain on to these structures.

MECHANICAL PROPERTIES OF A PERIPHERAL NERVE

Since most peripheral nerves pass across joints at some distance from the centre of joint rotation, their path length will change as the joint is rotated. Consequently, peripheral nerves have to move to accommodate changes in their path length. Nerve movements can be longitudinal or transverse and can also occur in response to changes in surrounding soft tissues. When the nerve path is shortened, peripheral nerves will become slack and are said to be unloaded. In this shortened position, nerves tend to run a tortuous course (Sunderland 1978). When the nerve path is lengthened, the nerve will initially straighten. This is referred to as loading the nerve (i.e.

tensioning the nerve). Further lengthening of the nerve path (beyond the length of the nerve) will result in elongation (i.e. stretch) of the nerve. These increases in the nerve length usually occur without any detrimental effect on nerve function. The measure of elongation is strain, which is often expressed as a percentage increase in the nerve length. The greatest increase in nerve strain occurs in the segments closest to the joint that is moving (Dilley et al 2003).

Stress–strain curves have been described for excised nerves undergoing stress (Fig 37.2). Stress is defined as the force/load applied divided by the area over which it acts (e.g. a larger diameter nerve is under less stress compared to a smaller diameter nerve when the same load is applied). Stress can be applied to the nerve trunk as longitudinal, compressive or shear stress or any combination of these forces (Topp & Boyd 2006). In excised nerves, when load is initially applied to a nerve, it is seen to elongate considerably (i.e. increase in strain) with minimal increase in longitudinal stress (toe region on the stress–strain curve) (Kwan et al 1992) (Fig 37.2). With increasing load, the nerve continues to elongate at a steady rate with a linear increase in longitudinal stress in what is termed the linear region of the stress–strain curve, until the nerve mechanically fails. The slope of the curve relates to the inherent stiffness of the nerve (a steeper slope indicating increased stiffness). The 'toe' region has been proposed as a region that protects axons against loading damage and may reflect the initial straightening of the neural connective tissue and axons (Kwan et al 1992, Rydevik et al 1990). However, the stress–strain curve of excised nerves may not completely apply to nerves in situ (Walbeehm et al 2004).

The positive fluid pressure within the endoneurium provides a mechanism to protect excessive loading of the mechanically weaker inner neural core during nerve elongation (Walbeehm et al 2004). This endoneurial fluid pressure (Lundborg 1988), which is maintained by the arrangement of collagen fibrils and impermeability of the perineurium, causes the inner neural core to act as a

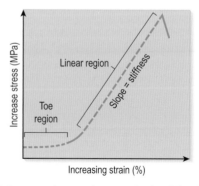

Fig 37.2 Stress–strain curve for an excised peripheral nerve.

relatively incompressible inner chamber. Such a mechanism would resist a decrease in epineurial diameter during elongation and act to increase nerve stiffness.

Should the ability of nerves to elongated and slide freely become compromised by adhesion to surrounding tissues, then limb movements would result in a localized increase in nerve strain that may lead to a loss of function, fibrosis and painful symptoms (Mackinnon 2002, Millesi et al 1990). Studies have investigated the limits to which nerves can be stretched before their function is compromised. Levels of strain exceeding 6% can lead to changes in blood supply and therefore nerve function (Grewel et al 1996). Since nerves have to slide and stretch during limb movements, the inherent mechanical properties of the nerve are of extreme importance.

Physical tests of nerve movement

As well as tests of nerve function and nerve conduction, clinicians use physical tests (both active and passive) to apply strain and pressure (palpation) to nerve plexuses and peripheral nerve trunks. Historically, tests that apply nerve strain have been used to look for mechanical change in the peripheral nervous system. However, more recently, it has become clear that nerve mechanical sensitivity will result in positive responses to these physical tests. In the upper limb, tests of nerve movement and nerve trunk palpation are particularly useful in cases where a neuropathic contribution is suspected and there is no overt sign of nerve injury, for e.g. RSI and chronic arm pain following whiplash injury. Movement tests of the brachial plexus, median, ulnar and radial nerves are considered to give a positive response when upper limb movements that apply strain to these nerve trunks and the brachial plexus result in symptom reproduction and consequent loss of joint rotation due to a protective flexor withdrawal response. Moderate digital pressure applied over nerve trunks is also shown to produce painful symptoms in patients with RSI or arm pain following whiplash injury (Greening et al 2005).

Positive responses to upper limb nerve movement tests are expected in patients where there is an obvious impairment of nerve movement. An impairment of nerve movement could result from frank compression or nerve transection (Lundborg 1988). Such restrictions in nerve movement in the presence of ongoing movements of the upper extremity could lead to local increases in nerve strain sufficient to affect the local nerve blood supply and nerve function. An increase in nerve strain may lead to epineurial bleeding and oedema, perpetuating a vicious circle of scarring and further increases in strain. Severe injury would result in axon degeneration with complete conduction block. In the upper limb there are well documented sites where the peripheral nerve trunk

may be more susceptible to 'irritation' and 'entrapment'. Lundborg (1988) describes these sites as where the nerve passes through a fibrous or fibro osseous tunnel (e.g. thoracic aperture, carpal tunnel, cubital tunnel), under a constricting fibrous band or fascial edge (e.g. ulnar nerve, under flexor carpi ulnaris; median nerve, through pronator teres) or through any repetitively contracting muscle (e.g. with repeated forearm, finger, wrist movements).

The sensitivity and specificity of applying additional strain to individual cords of the brachial plexus and peripheral nerves during these upper limb nerve movement tests has been measured in cadaveric studies (Kleinrensink et al 2000). Interestingly, only the median nerve upper limb tension test (ULTT) was shown to be specific in applying strain to the medial cord of the brachial plexus and the median nerve trunk. Other nerve movement tests apply substantial strain to all the cords of the brachial plexus and to all peripheral nerve trunks.

IN VIVO MEASUREMENTS OF NERVE MOVEMENT

It is important to understand how peripheral nerves cope with limb movements and normal levels of strain before examining neural dynamics in patients. Until fairly recently the pattern of longitudinal nerve movement in vivo was not well understood, most information having been obtained from cadavers.

Cadaveric studies examined longitudinal movement of the median, ulnar and radial nerves in response to shoulder, elbow and wrist movements (Kleinrensink et al 1995, Wilgis & Murphy 1986, Wright et al 1996, 2001, 2005). Early observations of longitudinal movement of the median nerve were also reported in vivo using a microneurography recording electrode inserted into the nerve (McLellan & Swash 1976). These studies indicated that movements of 5–10 mm are readily produced. It was also claimed that strain values for the median nerve of over 10% are obtained for joint movement within the physiological range (Wright et al 1996), values that are likely to cause reduced blood flow and impaired nerve conduction (Grewel et al 1996).

We have examined in detail nerve movement in the upper limb using high frequency ultrasound imaging. In these studies, sequences of ultrasound images were analysed using a frame-by-frame cross correlation algorithm that measured pixel shifts between images (Dilley et al 2001, 2003). With this technique, we have measured median and ulnar nerve movement and strain during neck and upper limb movements (Dilley et al 2003, 2007, Julius et al 2004).

Median nerve

Longitudinal nerve movement

Median nerve movement values that we obtained for wrist, shoulder and elbow movements were consistent with values obtained from cadavers (Wilgis & Murphy 1986, Wright et al 1996). When the upper limb was fully extended (i.e. 90° shoulder abduction, elbow extended, wrist in 40° extension) with contralateral neck side flexion, a position that was similar to the median nerve upper limb tension test + (ULTT +) (Kleinrensink et al 2000), nerve strain in the forearm was estimated to be only 2.5–3%. This is very different from the 10% strain measured in cadavers (Wright et al 1996) and while this may reflect the difference in method, our results indicate that even with the limb extended, median nerve strain is at a level unlikely to produce pathological change.

Nerve compliance

Peripheral nerves are well adapted to cope with large changes in their path length. This means that high strain levels that are detrimental to nerve function are never reached. Importantly, ultrasound studies show that the

median nerve is easily unloaded (Dilley et al 2003, 2007). This unloading is due to localized regions of high compliance that exist at the shoulder and elbow joints (Fig 37.3), i.e. where nerves follow a non-linear course when unloaded and/or exhibit less stiffness.

Evidence for a region of compliance through the shoulder was obtained from nerve movement data during neck and shoulder movements. Firstly, during the first 50° of shoulder abduction, with the elbow extended, there is virtually no median nerve movement in the arm and forearm. Nerve movement only occurs towards the end of abduction, once the nerve is loaded and begins to elongate along its whole length (Fig 37.3A,B). Secondly, during contralateral cervical lateral flexion, with the shoulder adducted (i.e. shortened nerve path length), there is no nerve movement in the arm at the start of cervical movement. In contrast, with the shoulder at 90° abduction (i.e. extended nerve path length), nerve movement occurs throughout contralateral cervical lateral flexion. Thirdly, as the elbow joint is extended from 90° flexion to 45° with the shoulder in 90° abduction, the nerve moves in the arm but not in the forearm. At 45° with the shoulder in 90° abduction of elbow extension, slack is taken up through shoulder region and the nerve becomes loaded.

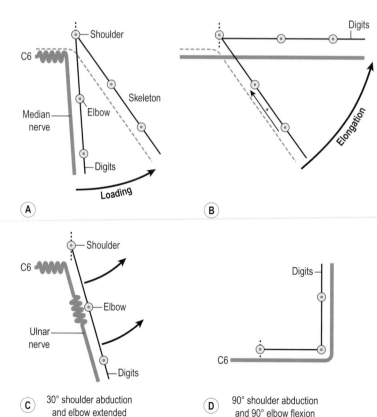

Fig 37.3 (A) & (B) The pattern of median nerve movement during shoulder abduction. (A) 10–50° shoulder abduction. The median nerve at 10° shoulder abduction showing a region of high compliance (i.e. slack) in its proximal segment. As the shoulder is abducted to 50°, the nerve will initially straighten from its proximal segment as it becomes loaded. (B) 50–90° shoulder abduction. At approximately 50°, the nerve will start to elongate (stretch) as the shoulder is abducted to 90°. During stretching, the nerve will elongate towards the moving joint (indicated by the starred arrow). (C) and (D) The pattern of ulnar nerve movement during elbow flexion. (C) 30° shoulder abduction and elbow extended. The ulnar nerve at 30° shoulder abduction and the elbow straight showing regions of high compliance at the shoulder and across the elbow. (D) 90° shoulder abduction and 90° elbow flexion. As the shoulder is abducted to 90° and the elbow flexed to 90°, the nerve straightens at the proximal segment and across the elbow with negligible movement in the arm and forearm

(A and B from Dilley et al 2003, with permission).

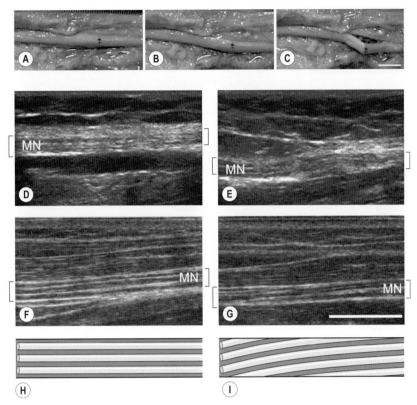

Fig 37.4 (A) to (C) Images showing median nerve folding (just proximal to the bicipital aponeurosis) during elbow flexion with the shoulder in 90° abduction. (A) Elbow extended with the median nerve stretched. (B) Elbow at 45° flexion with slight nerve bowing as it unloads. (C) Elbow at 90° flexion with clear folding of the nerve. A similar pattern can be seen with the shoulder adducted. Note that during dissection of the median nerve, the surrounding adventitia has been cut. (D) & (E) Ultrasound images of the median nerve just proximal to the bicipital aponeurosis. In (D) the elbow is extended and the median nerve appears straight. In (E) the elbow is flexed to 90° and the nerve follows a non-linear course. (F) & (G) Ultrasound images of the median nerve in the forearm showing the clearly defined fascicular structure. In (F), the limb is in an extended position (with the wrist and elbow extended) and the fascicles appear straight. In a flexed position (G), the fascicles appear curved. (H) & (I) represent the fascicular structure in the extended (H) and flexed (I) positions.
(F and G from Dilley et al 2003, with permission).

At this point, the nerve also moves in the forearm. This pattern of nerve movement is also accounted for by extensive folding of the median nerve in the arm with the elbow flexed (Fig 37.4A–E). Examination of median nerve movement during elbow flexion reveals a region of compliance proximal to the elbow that exists even with the shoulder in 90° abduction (Fig 37.4A–C).

As well as folding and bowing of the nerve trunk as a mechanism to prevent excessive loading, the fascicles themselves are also able to bow independent of the outer connective tissue sheath (i.e. the epineurium and adventitia). The fascicles are likely to undergo loading at a later stage during stretch of the connective tissue sheath. This forms a protective mechanism that prevents excessive stretching of the axons. Fascicular folding is readily observed from ultrasound images of the median nerve when the nerve is unloaded (Fig 37.4F–I).

Nerve loading

It is only when the limb is extended that the median nerve will become loaded and behave like a continuous spring (i.e. the linear region of a stress-strain curve; Fig 37.2). During normal physiological joint movements, the maximum strain in the median nerve is unlikely to exceed 4%. Therefore, the median nerve is well designed to cope with changes in its path length caused by limb movements. Any stretching that does occur, is unlikely to threaten the intraneural blood supply or nerve conduction.

Transverse median nerve movement

Transverse nerve movements occur during limb movements in response to deformation of adjacent soft tissues. This is not an active movement but rather the nerve is pushed by movement of the adjacent soft tissue into a

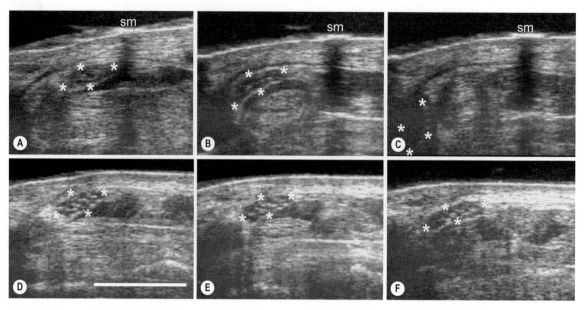

Fig 37.5 Cross sectional (transverse) ultrasound images of the median nerve (outlined *) at the proximal carpal tunnel. (A) to (C) Images of the **non-symptomatic** side in a patient with RSI during wrist flexion ((A) wrist 30° extension, (B) mid position and (C) wrist 30° flexion) showing median nerve excursion in a lateral and posterior direction during wrist flexion. (D) to (E) Images of the **symptomatic** side in a patient with RSI during wrist flexion ((D) wrist 30° extension, (E) mid position and (F) wrist 30° flexion) showing very little transverse movement of the median nerve. In the flexed wrist position (F), the nerve remains compressed between the flexor retinaculum and the flexor tendons. sm = skin marker.

new position. For example, at the wrist the median nerve is observed to slide transversely in a lateral direction during wrist or digit flexion (Greening et al 2001). During this movement, the flexor tendons move anteriorly towards the roof of the carpal tunnel, which causes the median nerve to slide transversely (laterally) and in some cases posteriorly (Fig 37.5A–C). In this instance, transverse sliding ensures that the nerve is not compressed between the tendons and the flexor retinaculum in positions of wrist and finger flexion.

Ulnar nerve

Ultrasound studies of longitudinal ulnar nerve movement (Dilley et al 2007) suggest that, similar to the median nerve, the ulnar nerve is unloaded in most functional upper limb positions. Nerve movement observations indicate a similar region of high compliance at the shoulder and elbow joint (see Fig 37.3C,D). For example, shoulder abduction, with the elbow flexed, produces negligible movement of the ulnar nerve in the arm or forearm. Elbow movements also cause negligible movement of the ulnar nerve in the arm or forearm (Dilley et al 2007). This latter result is surprising as elbow flexion produces an increase of approximately 18 mm in nerve path length, since the nerve lies approximately 12 mm from the centre of rotation of this joint. However, with the

elbow flexed and the shoulder adducted, the ulnar nerve appears folded proximal to elbow joint, which indicates a region of high compliance at this joint. Unfortunately this study did not measure transverse movement of the nerve at the cubital tunnel during elbow flexion, which would likely bring the nerve closer to the centre of rotation. Additionally, transverse movement could also explain the small degree of longitudinal nerve movement observed.

NERVE MOVEMENT STUDIES IN PATIENTS

Using ultrasound imaging we have investigated median nerve movement in the most common nerve entrapment syndrome, namely carpal tunnel syndrome, in patients following repair surgery for median nerve transection as well as in patients with RSI and chronic arm pain following whiplash injury. All patients examined had painful symptoms with the application of the median nerve ULLT, apart from patients with nerve repair following complete transection where this test was not applied.

In RSI, painful symptoms are spread throughout the upper limb and therefore it has been postulated that longitudinal median nerve movement might be restricted at multiple sites. These sites include the shoulder region, at the pronator teres muscle and the carpal tunnel. However, ultrasound studies of longitudinal nerve movement revealed no significant difference through the shoulder, the forearm or carpal tunnel in the RSI patients studied compared to control subjects (Dilley et al 2008). We have also failed to find a reduction in longitudinal median nerve movement through the carpal tunnel in patients with carpal tunnel syndrome (CTS) (Erel et al 2003), despite its clinical labelling as an entrapment neuropathy. Similarly, at surgery longitudinal median nerve movement remained unchanged following carpal tunnel release (Tuzuner et al 2004). Using laser Doppler imaging, a small reduction in median nerve movement in CTS patients was noted when the nerve was loaded (i.e. wrist and elbow extension) but no change when the nerve was unloaded (i.e. elbow flexion) (Hough et al 2007). This small reduction in the loaded position by no means indicates a longitudinal entrapment of the median nerve.

Interestingly, studies of median nerve movement in patients with RSI and those with arm symptoms following whiplash injury do indicate a reduction in proximal longitudinal movement of the median nerve in the forearm during deep inspiration (Greening et al 2005). This decrease is however not sufficient to cause detrimental increases in nerve strain. Instead, this change may be caused by a restriction in motion of the first rib. In the RSI patients, poor and prolonged cervical spine posture might result in shortening of the scalene muscles (Pascarelli & Hsu 2001), causing an elevated first rib. During whiplash injury the first rib may also be elevated (based on clinical observations), possibly due to the excessive stretch applied to the scalene muscles and their subsequent reflex shortening. Elevation of the first rib will compromise the space available to the trunks of the brachial plexus within the scalene triangle, possibly leading to neurogenic thoracic outlet syndrome.

Patients with RSI and CTS have a reduction in lateral transverse median nerve movement at the proximal carpal tunnel and there is a significantly altered pattern of movement in patients with arm pain following whiplash (Allmann et al 1997, Erel et al 2003, Greening et al 1999, 2001, 2005, Lynn et al 2002, Nakamichi & Tachibana 1995) (Fig 37.5D–F). The lack of lateral transverse nerve movement of the median nerve at this osseous fibrous tunnel would, as previously described, subject the nerve to increasing pressure and irritation during wrist and finger movements. This would account for painful symptoms experienced by these patients during functional hand activities.

While it is important to understand that small reductions in longitudinal and transverse nerve movement are unlikely to cause significant increases to longitudinal nerve strain, symptoms may occur as a result of nerve pathology at the first rib and within the carpal tunnel. The only example to date that we have of a reduction in longitudinal nerve sliding of the median nerve was found in patients who had undergone median nerve repair following traumatic nerve transection (Erel et al 2009). In these patients there was a 8% reduction of median nerve movement in the forearm during metacarpal extension on the repaired side compared to the uninjured side. The observed reduction on the repaired side was mainly due to three of the ten patients who showed a substantial change (up to 54% reduction compared to the uninjured side). Of particular interest was a correlation between a reduction in nerve sliding and time until surgery. Since nine of the ten patients had surgery within one week of injury, a delay (in days), may result in excessive scar formation and subsequent impairment in nerve movement.

In vivo measurement of ulnar nerve movement in conditions such as cubital tunnel syndrome and the radial nerve in radial tunnel syndrome for example, remains to be evaluated. In the patients we have examined, namely RSI and arm pain following whiplash injury, despite 'positive' results for the median nerve ULTT and/or digital pressure over the nerve trunk, these patients do not show significant changes to longitudinal nerve movement. Clearly, these patients have a painful response to neural mechanical stimulation and have therefore developed nerve mechanical sensitivity. This poses some important questions: why should elongating a nerve within its normal physiological range or applying digital pressure over the nerve trunk cause painful symptoms i.e. how has the nerve become mechanically sensitive? Secondly, how does this inform our understanding of the aetiology of these conditions and modify treatment and rehabilitation?

INFLAMMATION OF A PERIPHERAL NERVE

Trauma, either repetitive or a defined insult, underlies the onset of symptoms in patients with RSI, arm pain following whiplash and CRPS1. It is interesting to speculate that while there is no indication of frank nerve injury, a more minor neural injury such as inflammation may be a cause of ongoing symptoms.

Despite differences in the mechanism of trauma, symptoms appear similar in these patients. Patients complain of spontaneous pain, pain with limb movements, deep muscle aches, paraesthesia, hyperalgesia, allodynia and difficulties with the coordination of fine movement. Importantly, all of the patients that we have examined have clear signs of nerve mechanical sensitivity (i.e. painful responses to nerve movement tests and to digital pressure over affected nerve trunks). The lack of sufficient evidence for restricted, or altered, longitudinal nerve movement in patients, coupled with the inherent biomechanical compliance of the upper limb peripheral nerves, suggests that strain increases into the pathological range are not an obvious cause of these symptoms. The lack of frank nerve injury on clinical testing also suggests that significant axonal degeneration and demyelination are an unlikely cause of symptoms for many patients. Therefore, what are the mechanisms that lead to pain in these patients?

The physiological mechanisms underlying symptoms in patients with chronic upper limb pain, including those with RSI, arm pain following whiplash and also CRPS1, are undoubtedly complex and will involve central neuropathic changes. Neuropathic symptoms that include clinical signs of nerve mechanical sensitivity suggest a mechanism of symptom production that extends beyond the central nervous system to the periphery. A peripheral mechanism is further supported by evidence of changes to Aβ, Aδ and C fibre sensory and autonomic function in the peripheral nerves of patients with RSI and whiplash injury (Chien et al 2008, Greening & Lynn 1998, Greening et al 2003). Examination of sera from these patient groups reveals raised levels of inflammatory mediators, which is indicative of an inflammatory component (Carp et al 2007, Gerdle et al 2008, Huygen et al 2002, Kivioja et al 2001, Uceyler et al 2007a). Mediators that are up-regulated in RSI, CRPS1 and arm pain following whiplash include cytokines such as tumour necrosis factor (TNF) α, interleukin (IL) 1β, and IL6. Cytokines are a group of signalling molecules secreted by immune cells that help regulate the inflammatory response. Cytokine levels frequently correlate with patient symptoms (Carp et al 2007, Maihofner et al 2005), indicating a role for inflammation in the pathophysiology of these chronic pain conditions. Physiological studies performed in animals have shown that inflammation can affect peripheral nerve function (see below). Together with reports of raised levels of immune mediators, these findings indicate a major role for inflammation in chronic pain.

Causes of inflammation

Inflammation of a peripheral nerve is triggered by a direct insult to the nerve itself, infection or by local inflammation of adjacent tissues. In the latter situation, the nerve is an innocent bystander, where the diffusion of inflammatory mediators released at a neighbouring injury site will cause disruption to, or cross, the blood–nerve barrier to reach the endoneurium. Examples of pathologies where peripheral nerves are vulnerable to indirect insult include muscle injury, disc herniation or tumours growing close to nerve trunks. It is important to remember that clinically many patients with chronic upper limb pain do not show signs of frank nerve injury. Therefore, the trauma associated with such conditions will be subtle, sufficient to cause inflammation without significant axonal degeneration and demyelination. In whiplash injury for example, nerve roots and spinal nerves may be subjected to a direct traction injury as well as to the effects of inflammatory mediators from adjacent injured structures. In CRPS1,

which usually occurs as a complication following injury or surgery (Janig & Baron 2003), peripheral nerves may also be subjected to the effects of inflammatory mediators from adjacent injured tissues.

In RSI, the prolonged repetitive motion of the forearm muscles is considered sufficient to induce inflammation of the median nerve. Evidence for this mechanism has been provided by an animal model of the condition (Clark et al 2003). In this model, animals were trained to perform a high or low repetition, negligible force task over a period of up to 12 weeks. This task involved repeated reaching and grasping of food pellets. Both high (8 reaches/min) and also low (3 reaches/min) repetition tasks were sufficient to cause inflammation of the median nerve and the forearm tendons and muscles (Barbe et al 2003, Clark et al 2003, Elliott et al 2008). Inflammation occurred from four weeks as macrophages that are activated by the immune response invaded the peripheral tissues. Cytokines (IL1α, IL1β, IL6, IL10 and TNFα) were also expressed within the endoneurium by resident cells (Al-Shatti et al 2005).

Inflammation and the microenvironment of the nerve

Subtle changes in the endoneurial microenvironment underlie the development of neuropathic symptoms (Sommer et al 1993). The endothelial wall of the endoneurial capillaries and the perineurium comprise the blood–nerve barrier. The role of this barrier is to maintain the microenvironment of the endoneurium. It helps regulate the entry of molecules into the endoneurium and maintains the ionic milieu that is essential for normal axonal conduction. Although not as effective as the blood–brain barrier, circulating cells and proteins cannot easily cross the blood–nerve barrier (Olsson 1990). Activated T lymphocytes are however an exception and these cells circulate freely between the capillaries and the endoneurium (Watkins & Maier 2002). Many of the resident cells within the endoneurium function as immune cells, and when activated, can secrete inflammatory mediators. These cells include fibroblasts, Schwann cells, macrophages, dendritic cells and mast cells (Moalem & Tracey 2006, Watkins & Maier 2002). Immediately following nerve trauma, the calcium-activated protease calpain causes the release of early proinflammatory cytokines such as TNFα and IL1β (Uceyler et al 2007b). These cytokines are secreted within the endoneurium by resident immune cells. The release of cytokines (e.g. TNFα) and growth factors (e.g. vascular endothelial growth factor) triggers the breakdown of the blood–nerve barrier (Creange et al 1997) to allow immune cells and proteins that could not previously cross this barrier to enter the endoneurium. Chemokines such as CCL2 attract neutrophils and macrophages to the inflammatory site (Toews et al 1998), further enhancing the inflammatory response.

Animal models of nerve inflammation

A number of animal models have been developed that result in sensory behavioural changes similar to those observed in patients. These models include the chronic constriction injury model (CCI) (Bennett & Xie 1988), the spinal nerve ligation model (SNL) (Kim & Chung 1992) and the neuritis model (Bennett 1999). Laboratory studies using these models have shown that inflammation can alter the physiological properties of sensory axons. Many of these studies have focussed on the development of ongoing activity (i.e. spontaneous firing of axons) and axonal mechanical sensitivity (i.e. responses of axons to direct mechanical stimulation), both of which are likely to contribute to a peripheral mechanism leading to painful symptom production. In particular, the development of axonal mechanical sensitivity provides a mechanism for pain in response to nerve movement tests and direct palpation of peripheral nerve trunks.

Both the CCI and SNL model produce marked mechanical allodynia and thermal hyperalgesia (Bennett & Xie 1988, Kim & Chung 1992) as well as ongoing activity (Chen & Devor 1998, Djouhri et al 2006, Kajander & Bennett 1992, Tal & Eliav 1996, Wu et al 2001, 2002) and axonal mechanical sensitivity (Chen & Devor 1998, Dilley & Bove 2008b). In the SNL model, intact axons within the sciatic nerve comingle with injured axons that are undergoing the processes of Wallerian degeneration. Wallerian degeneration is the degeneration of injured axons and involves the recruitment of macrophages for the removal of axonal debris. The presence of activated macrophages implies the release of inflammatory mediators, which would induce a form of intraneural neuritis. A major finding in the SNL model is that uninjured C-fibre axons develop ongoing activity and respond to direct mechanical stimulation (Wu et al 2001, Dilley & Bove 2008b). However, both the CCI and spinal nerve ligation model cause significant neuropathy due to extensive Wallerian degeneration and therefore do not reflect the subtle injury that is possibly associated with RSI, arm pain following whiplash injury or CRPS1.

Neuritis model

The neuritis model is an animal model of localized peripheral nerve inflammation that more closely resembles the clinical presentation in many patients with chronic upper limb pain. It produces a minor nerve injury with inflammation in the absence of gross neuropathology, i.e. degeneration or demyelination (Bove et al 2003, Chacur et al 2001, Dilley et al 2005, Eliav et al 1999) (Fig 37.6A). In this model, an immune-stimulant (either complete Freund's adjuvant (killed bacterial cell wall) or zymosan (killed yeast cell wall)) is applied locally around the sciatic nerve or nerve of interest. Over a period of

days, a robust local inflammatory response occurs that is confined mainly to the epineurium (Bove et al 2009) (Fig 37.6B). Within hours, activated macrophages, neutrophils and T lymphocytes begin to congregate outside of the perineurium, eventually peaking in numbers at four weeks (Bove et al 2003, 2009, Eliav et al 1999, Gazda et al 2001). Surprisingly, the immune cells do not penetrate across the perineurium to enter the endoneurium (Bove et al 2009), which is likely to reflect the diffusion properties of the perineurium. In contrast, very small numbers of T lymphocytes have been reported within the endoneurium that have probably entered from the endoneurial vessels (Eliav et al 1999). Within the first week, the perineurium becomes oedematous but by 4 weeks it has thickened to become consolidated (Bove et al 2009). The early oedematous, less consolidated appearance of the perineurium provides a short window that allows inflammatory factors to diffuse across the barrier into the endoneurium. Following induction of the neuritis, animals develop cutaneous hypersensitivity with signs of mechanical allodynia (Bove et al 2003, Chacur et al 2001, Eliav et al 1999) as well as heat and mechanical hyperalgesia and cold allodynia (Eliav et al 1999). Interestingly, in the zymosan-induced model, mechanical allodynia was reported to be bilateral, which infers a central mechanism initiated by the localized peripheral nerve inflammation (Gazda et al 2001). Therefore, it is possible that a single inflammatory site may cause contralateral symptoms in patients.

These studies of locally induced inflammation in the absence of axonal degeneration result in significant neuropathic signs that are consistent with neuropathic pain in patients. However, the mechanisms underlying these sensory changes are unclear. Much of the current work on the neuritis model has focussed on the physiological effects of inflammation on peripheral axons. These studies have shown that inflammation causes the development of ongoing activity in both unmyelinated (C-) and myelinated (A-) axons (Bove et al 2003, Dilley et al 2005, Eliav et al 2001). Most of the myelinated axons that develop ongoing activity are Aδ-fibres (Eliav et al 2009), which, like C-fibre axons, are largely nociceptive. The observation of ongoing activity in nociceptors corresponds to the painful sensations described by patients, especially the symptoms of apparent un-evoked spontaneous pain. Such increases in ongoing activity may also contribute to centrally driven neuropathic symptoms. While central sensitization is considered to play a significant role in the development of neuropathic symptoms (Campbell & Meyer 2006, Campbell et al 1988), central sensitization is dependent upon the continued firing of peripheral axons into the central nervous system (Gracely et al 1992, LaMotte et al 1991). It has been shown that by blocking the firing of axons from an irritated peripheral nerve, central neuropathic changes can reverse (Gracely et al 1992).

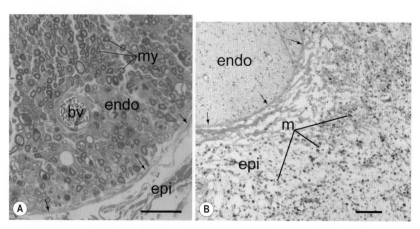

Fig 37.6 Microscopic appearance of the neuritis site. (A) Toluidine blue stained transverse section through the neuritis showing the relatively normal appearance of the myelinated axons (examples labelled 'my') with very few abnormal axons. Note the oedematous, less consolidated appearance of the perineurium (arrows). (B) Haematoxylin and eosin stained transverse section immuno-reacted against activated macrophages (ED1+) at the neuritis. There are considerable numbers of macrophages in the epineurium (dark stain; examples labelled with 'm') with only minimal numbers in the endoneurium. Note the oedematous, less consolidated appearance of the perineurium (arrows). endo = endoneurium; arrows = perineurium. epi = Epineurium. bv = blood vessel. Scale bar in (A) = 50 μm and in (B) = 100 μm.

The neuritis model was the first to show that inflammation causes otherwise normally conducting, C- and A-fibre axons to develop mechanical sensitivity that is localized to the site of inflammation (Bove et al 2003, Dilley & Bove 2008b, Dilley et al 2005, Eliav et al 2001). Axonal mechanical sensitivity was tested with both direct pressure and by applying short stretches to the inflamed nerve (Fig 37.7). Less than 5% stretch is sufficient to cause firing of axons in inflamed nerves (Dilley et al 2005), with the most sensitive axons responding to less than 3% stretch. Importantly, these stretch values are consistent with those obtained from human studies of median nerve stretch when the arm is fully extended in a position similar to the median nerve movement ULTT (Dilley et al 2003). This finding also suggests that, in patients, pathological increases in nerve strain are not a prerequisite for symptoms and that in the presence of nerve mechanical sensitivity, arm pain may be experienced during normal physiological limb movements.

Normally, it is only the terminals of peripheral nerves that respond to mechanical stimulation by transduction through mechanically sensitive ion channels. It is important to state that mechanical sensitivity and ongoing activity originating part way along an axon does not occur in the absence of inflammation. It should be noted that these observations of axonal mechanical sensitivity contrast from the original findings in the CCI model, where it was the tips of degenerated axons that became mechanically sensitive (Chen & Devor 1998, Tal & Eliav 1996). The neuritis model instead provides an inflammatory environment in the absence of axonal degeneration that is likely to be comparable to that in patients.

It is reported that C- and Aδ-fibre axons are more susceptible to the development of axonal mechanical sensitivity (Bove et al 2003). The increased susceptibility of these axons to the effects of inflammation is consistent with the nociceptive properties of these nerve fibres and also the symptoms of pain described by patients. Interestingly, mechanically sensitive axons mainly innervate deep structures such as muscles and joints (Bove et al 2003, Dilley & Bove 2008b) (Fig 37.7B). These findings fit well with the 'deep ache' described by patients and which is frequently complained of when nerve movement tests are applied. Localized peripheral nerve inflammation may also contribute to sympathetic changes in patients with CRPS1. In the neuritis model, the rate of ongoing activity in postganglionic sympathetic axons passing through the inflammatory site is reduced (Bove 2009).

In the neuritis model, axonal mechanical sensitivity is a relatively short lived phenomena and peaks within one week of developing neuritis (Dilley & Bove 2008b). By two months the axonal mechanical sensitivity has resolved. Despite the resolution of abnormal sensory responses, macrophages and T lymphocytes still persist in the epineurium at two months (Bove et al 2009). It is likely that consolidation of the perineurium soon after the peak of the axonal mechanical sensitivity prevents inflammatory components released by these cells from entering the endoneurium.

It is evident from these laboratory studies that localized inflammation can be detrimental to axonal physiology. It has already been suggested that inflammation-induced increases in axonal excitability appear to drive central

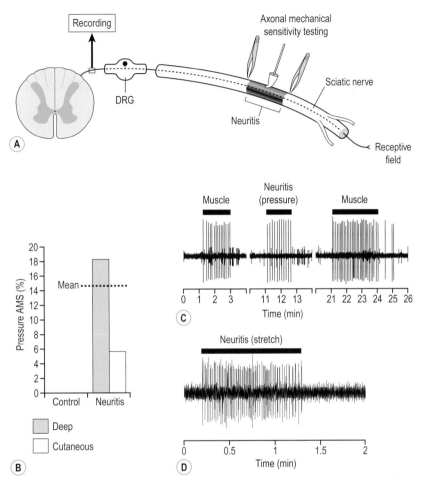

Fig 37.7 Electrophysiological recordings of axonal mechanical sensitivity in C-fibre axons. (A) Diagram of the experimental setup. The sciatic nerve trunk is locally inflamed (neuritis) mid thigh. Recordings are made from isolated C-fibre axons within the L5 dorsal root (recording) that pass through the neuritis. The nerve is mechanically stimulated at the neuritis either by direct pressure using a silicone tipped probe or by stretching with fine forceps. Note the relationship of the L5 dorsal root to the dorsal root ganglia (DRG) and also the spinal cord. (B) The percentage of deep and cutaneous C-fibre axons that responded to pressure at the neuritis at one week. The average number of C-fibre axons that responded to pressure was 14.5% (9 of 62 axons) following neuritis (denoted by heavy horizontal line) compared to 0% (0 of 36 axons) in untreated animals. The majority of axons that developed axonal mechanical sensitivity innervated deep (8 of 44 axons) rather than cutaneous (1 of 18 axons) structures. (C) Typical response to pressure at the neuritis from an axon innervating the gastrocnemius muscle. Short horizontal lines above the responses represent the duration of the mechanical stimuli. The gastrocnemius muscle was mechanically stimulated initially to show that the axon had a functioning peripheral field (denoted by Muscle). This was followed by mechanical stimulation of the nerve at the test site (denoted by Neuritis). Mechanical responses from the periphery after stimulating the nerve demonstrated that the mechanical stimulus did not adversely affect the conduction of the axon. (D) Typical response to stretch across the neuritis site. The short horizontal line above the response represents the duration of the stretch.
(B & C from Dilley & Bove 2008; D from Dilley et al. 2005 with permission).

mechanisms leading to central sensitization. Localized neuritis also triggers physiological changes to peripheral neurons that extend beyond the site of inflammation. Following neuritis, phenotypic changes (i.e. the expression of new proteins) occur in the cell bodies of sensory neurons (Dilley et al 2005). It is not yet clear what these changes represent. It is possible that they correspond to the up-regulation of ion channels that contribute to the ongoing activity and axonal mechanical sensitivity. Accordingly, in other models of nerve injury, there are reports of the up-regulation of sodium channels and mechanically sensitive channels that contribute towards painful symptoms (Black et al 2004, Duan et al 2007, Pertin et al 2005). Following neuritis, physiological changes also occur along the length of the axon. A reduction in the conduction velocity of C-fibre axons proximal to the neuritis has been reported that actually recovers at a similar time to the axonal mechanical sensitivity (Dilley & Bove 2008b). Local neuritis has also been shown to reduce the number of functioning peripheral nerve terminals (Dilley et al 2005). This is consistent with findings in patients with RSI, where peripheral nerve function is altered (Greening & Lynn 1998, Greening et al 2003).

PHYSIOLOGICAL ROLE OF INFLAMMATORY MEDIATORS

It is apparent that local nerve inflammation can alter the properties of peripheral sensory axons, inducing ongoing activity and axonal mechanical sensitivity, both of which may contribute to painful symptoms in patients. However, it is important to understand what inflammatory components are responsible for these physiological changes and the neuronal mechanisms that lead to such changes.

The lack of large numbers of activated macrophages, T cells and neutrophils within the endoneurium following neuritis suggests that the physiological effects are probably due to diffusible inflammatory mediators produced during the inflammatory response. In the neuritis model, raised levels of cytokines IL1, IL6 and TNFα are reported at the inflammatory site within hours of induction (Eliav et al 2009, Gazda et al 2001). These cytokines are secreted by inflammatory cells that congregate outside of the perineurium and by resident cells, e.g. Schwann cells and fibroblasts. As well as orchestrating the immune response, cytokines also play an important physiological role. Nerve growth factor (NGF), which is better known for its role supporting the development of peripheral neurons, is also up-regulated during inflammation (McMahon et al 2005) and has a similar physiological role to that of cytokines. The administration of small doses of cytokines IL1β, IL6 and TNFα causes hyperalgesia and allodynia in animals (Cunha et al 1992, Eliav et al 2009, Schafers et al 2003a,b, Sorkin & Doom 2000, Zelenka et al 2005).

The acute perineural exposure of TNFα to the sciatic nerve also increases ongoing activity in C-fibre axons (Leem & Bove 2002, Sorkin et al 1997). IL1β is similarly reported to induce ongoing activity in myelinated axons following direct exposure (Ozaktay et al 2006) and IL1β and IL6 both sensitize heat-activated (Obreja et al 2002, 2005) and sodium channels (Liu et al 2006). The cytokines IL1β and IL6 have both been implicated in the development of axonal mechanical sensitivity and ongoing activity (Eliav et al 2009). The administration of NGF causes hyperalgesia in animals (Lewin et al 1993). It also induces ongoing activity (Kitamura et al 2005) and sensitizes peripheral terminals (Rueff & Mendell 1996) following its direct exposure to sensory neurons. From this data it can be seen that elevated levels of cytokines and NGF close to a peripheral nerve can lead to changes in the physiological function of sensory axons that may contribute towards painful symptoms in patients.

Chemokines are a group of inflammatory mediators with similar properties to cytokines. Along with cytokines, chemokines are also able to interact with both the immune and nervous systems. Of particular interest is the chemokine CCL2, which is up-regulated following nerve injury (White et al 2005). Administration of CCL2 rapidly induces mechanical allodynia in animals (Tanaka et al 2004). Its acute exposure also directly excites neurons (Oh et al 2001, Sun et al 2006) and sensitizes the transient receptor potential vanilloid 1 channel (TRPV1) (Jung et al 2008). TRPV1 is a channel that is widely expressed on nociceptive axons and is sensitive to capsaicin and mechanical stimulation. It is thought to play a significant role in the development of neuropathic pain.

The mechanisms by which these inflammatory mediators interact with peripheral neurons are unclear. Following nerve injury, cytokine and chemokine receptors located on sensory neurons are up-regulated (Bhangoo et al 2007, Schafers et al 2003a). Therefore, cytokines and chemokines may interact with their receptors on neurons to alter axonal function. Cytokines, chemokines and NGF also act to change the sensitivity and expression of ion channels that are associated with an increase in axonal excitability (e.g. TRPV1 and sodium channels) (Gould et al 2000, Jung et al 2008, Tanaka et al 1998, Zhang et al 2005, Zhu & Oxford 2007).

Disruption of axoplasmic transport

Mechanically sensitive ion channels at the peripheral terminals of axons are constantly being replaced by newly synthesized ion channels. New ion channel components are synthesized within cell bodies in the dorsal root ganglia and transported to the terminals by fast axoplasmic transport (Koschorke et al 1994). Inflammatory mediators can disrupt axoplasmic transport (Amano et al 2001, Armstrong et al 2004). This is consistent with the disruption of axoplasmic transport without Wallerian degeneration of axons following acute nerve trunk compression (Kitao et al 1997). It has been shown that the disruption of axoplasmic transport in the sciatic nerve can cause axonal mechanical sensitivity to develop at the site of disruption (Dilley & Bove 2008a). It is therefore hypothesized that in patients, local nerve inflammation may disrupt axoplasmic transport in sensory axons to cause the accumulation and insertion of mechanosensitive ion channel components at the

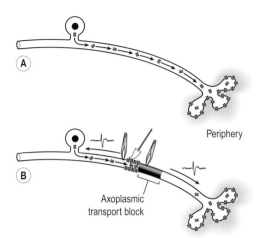

Fig 37.8 Inflammation-induced disruption of axoplasmic transport as a mechanism for the development of axonal mechanical sensitivity. (A) The components required for mechanical sensitivity are transported from the cell body of a sensory axon to the periphery for insertion at the terminal. (B) Inflammation-induced disruption of axoplasmic transport leads to the accumulation and insertion of mechanosensitive components proximal to the site of axoplasmic blockade. Mechanical stimulation of the axon membrane at the inflamed site (by pressure or stretch) will result in the generation of action potentials (denoted by arrows).

inflamed site (Dilley & Bove 2008a) (Fig 37.8). The lack of functioning peripheral terminals in some conducting axons might have also resulted from a disruption of axonal transport at the neuritis (Dilley et al 2005). Therefore, axoplasmic transport disruption may have widespread effects on the health of the neuron. Changes to axoplasmic transport develop over days and therefore represent a chronic pathway that can lead to altered axonal physiology. This chronic mechanism contrasts to the acute effects of inflammatory mediators on peripheral sensory axons. Therefore, in patients, the peripheral mechanisms are likely to involve multiple pathways that ultimately contribute to painful symptoms.

NERVI NERVORUM

The nervi nervorum also provides a potential mechanism that may account for nerve mechanical sensitivity, since axons of the nervi nervorum respond to mechanical stimulation of the nerve trunk (Bove & Light 1995). However, innervation of the nerve sheath by the nervi nervorum is sparse and mechanical stimulation of the sciatic nerve in untreated (control) animals has failed to find these axons (Bove et al 2003, Dilley & Bove 2008a, Dilley et al 2005,

Eliav et al 2001). Sensitization of the nervi nervorum is unlikely to form a major contribution to symptom production.

IMAGING NERVE INFLAMMATION

Magnetic resonance imaging has been used as an indicator of inflammation in peripheral nerves (Filler et al 1993, 1996, 2004, Koltzenburg & Bendszus 2004). As part of the inflammatory process, the water content in neural tissues increases, which causes the nerve to appear hyper-intense on T2-weighted MRI (Filler et al 1996, Koltzenburg & Bendszus 2004). For example, in carpal tunnel syndrome, the median nerve appears abnormally bright at the carpal tunnel on T2-weighted MRI, a change that suggests local nerve inflammation in this region (Cudlip et al 2002). We have demonstrated an increase in median and ulnar nerve signal intensity at the carpal tunnel and distal forearm in two patients with RSI and also ulnar nerve signal intensity at the cubital tunnel in a patients with CRPS1 (Fig 37.9). Prior to imaging, all three patients had painful responses to nerve movement tests, as well as palpation over the nerve trunks, at the hyperintense sites. These findings fit well with inflammation-induced nerve mechanical sensitivity and an underlying peripheral mechanism for the painful symptoms experienced by these patients.

CONCLUSIONS

Peripheral nerves are extremely well adapted to cope with limb movements within the physiological range. The only evidence that we have of altered longitudinal nerve sliding is in a small proportion of patients following median nerve repair. Patients with RSI, whiplash injury and CRPS1 have raised levels of inflammatory mediators, which indicate a role for inflammation. There is also some clinical evidence from MRI of peripheral nerve inflammation in RSI and CRPS1. In these patient groups and perhaps others, such as non-specific back pain and fibromyalgia, axons may become mechanically sensitive following exposure to inflammatory mediators. Animal studies using a model of localized nerve inflammation clearly demonstrate nerve mechanical sensitivity. This would suggest a peripheral neuropathic mechanism contributing to painful symptoms and a painful response to nerve movement tests.

Clinically, tests that demonstrate nerve mechanical sensitivity, i.e. nerve movement tests and digital palpation, provide the clinician with the rationale to focus treatment, at an early date, towards alleviating a neuropathic condition. Treatment strategies should include drugs that can reduce the excitability of neurons, for example, pregabalin,

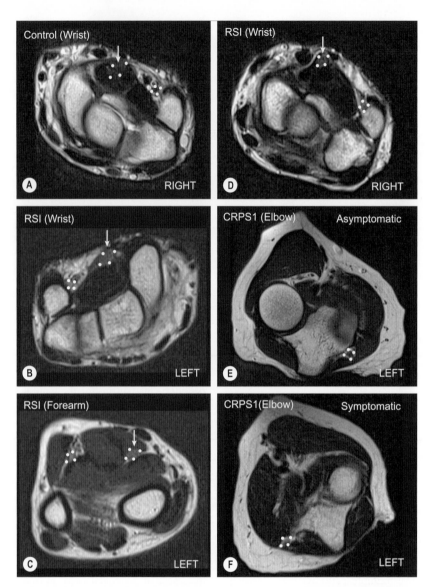

Fig 37.9 MRI scans of the wrist and elbow in patients with diffuse RSI and CRPS1. (A) to (D) T2-weighted images of the median and ulnar nerve (A) at the carpal tunnel in a control subject, (B) at the carpal tunnel and (C) distal forearm on the symptomatic side in a patient with diffuse RSI and (D) at the carpal tunnel on the symptomatic side of a second patient with diffuse RSI. Note the bright appearance of both the median and ulnar nerves in the patient images, which indicates inflammation. (E) to (F) T2-weighted images of the ulnar nerve on the (E) asymptomatic and (F) symptomatic side in a patient with CRPS1. Note the bright appearance of the ulnar nerve on the symptomatic side compared to the asymptomatic side. White dots represent the median and ulnar nerve boundaries. Arrows indicate the median nerve.

amitriptyline, carbamazepine and lidocaine. Symptom production is likely to involve complex mechanisms, which means that simple analgesics and non-steroidal anti-inflammatory drugs may not be effective. Future treatments may include inflammatory mediator receptor antagonists and neutralizing antibodies to reduce the effects of the inflammatory response. It is important that normal pain-free movement patterns are re-established in these chronic pain patients. There are many physical and cognitive treatment strategies available that may be helpful in achieving this. However, techniques that are applied to 'mobilize' the peripheral nervous system are not effective in CTS (O'Connor et al 2009) and are therefore unlikely to be of any benefit in these chronic pain patients. Nerve mobilization exercises may in fact be detrimental if they result in further noxious input. Sliding techniques that claim not to increase nerve strain, have been suggested to reduce intraneural oedema and even affect nerve physiology (Coppieters & Butler 2008).

However, to date, there is no scientific evidence that sliding techniques improve the axonal microenvironment or alter axonal physiology, or that these techniques improve outcomes for patients over and above other treatment strategies.

REFERENCES

Al-Shatti, T., Barr, A.E., Safadi, F.F., et al., 2005. Increase in inflammatory cytokines in median nerves in a rat model of repetitive motion injury. J. Neuroimmunol. 167 (1–2), 13–22.

Allmann, K.H., Horch, R., Uhl, M., et al., 1997. MR imaging of the carpal tunnel. Eur. J. Radiol. 25 (2), 141–145.

Alpar, E.K., Onuoha, G., Killampalli, V.V., et al., 2002. Management of chronic pain in whiplash injury. J. Bone Joint Surg. 84 (6), 807–811.

Amano, R., Hiruma, H., Nishida, S., et al., 2001. Inhibitory effect of histamine on axonal transport in cultured mouse dorsal root ganglion neurons. Neurosci. Res. 41 (2), 201–206.

Armstrong, B.D., Hu, Z., Abad, C., et al., 2004. Induction of neuropeptide gene expression and blockade of retrograde transport in facial motor neurons following local peripheral nerve inflammation in severe combined immunodeficiency and BALB/C mice. Neuroscience 129 (1), 93–99.

Barbe, M.F., Barr, A.E., Gorzelany, I., et al., 2003. Chronic repetitive reaching and grasping results in decreased motor performance and widespread tissue responses in a rat model of MSD. J. Orthop. Res. 21 (1), 167–176.

Bennett, G.J., 1999. Does a neuroimmune interaction contribute to the genesis of painful peripheral neuropathies? Proc. Natl. Acad. Sci. U. S. A. 96 (14), 7737–7738.

Bennett, G.J., Xie, Y.K., 1988. A peripheral mononeuropathy in rat that produces disorders of pain sensation like those seen in man. Pain 33 (1), 87–107.

Bhangoo, S., Ren, D., Miller, R.J., et al., 2007. Delayed functional expression of neuronal chemokine receptors following focal nerve demyelination in the rat: a mechanism for the development of chronic sensitization of peripheral nociceptors. Mol. Pain 3, 38.

Black, J.A., Liu, S., Tanaka, M., et al., 2004. Changes in the expression of tetrodotoxin-sensitive sodium channels within dorsal root ganglia neurons in inflammatory pain. Pain 108 (3), 237–247.

Bove, G.M., 2009. Focal nerve inflammation induces neuronal signs consistent with symptoms of early complex regional pain syndromes. Exp. Neurol. 219 (1), 223–227.

Bove, G.M., Light, A.R., 1995. Unmyelinated nociceptors of rat paraspinal tissues. J. Neurophysiol. 73 (5), 1752–1762.

Bove, G.M., Ransil, B.J., Lin, H.C., et al., 2003. Inflammation induces ectopic mechanical sensitivity in axons of nociceptors innervating deep tissues. J. Neurophysiol. 90 (3), 1949–1955.

Bove, G.M., Weissner, W., Barbe, M.F., 2009. Long lasting recruitment of immune cells and altered epi-perineurial thickness in focal nerve inflammation induced by complete Freund's adjuvant. J. Neuroimmunol. 213 (1–2), 26–30.

Byng, J., 1997. Overuse syndromes of the upper limb and the upper limb tension test: a comparison between patients, asymptomatic keyboard workers and asymptomatic non-keyboard workers. Man. Ther. 2 (3), 157–164.

Campbell, J.N., Meyer, R.A., 2006. Mechanisms of neuropathic pain. Neuron 52 (1), 77–92.

Campbell, J.N., Raja, S.N., Meyer, R.A., et al., 1988. Myelinated afferents signal the hyperalgesia associated with nerve injury. Pain 32, 89–94.

Carp, S.J., Barbe, M.F., Winter, K.A., et al., 2007. Inflammatory biomarkers increase with severity of upper-extremity overuse disorders. Clin. Sci. 112 (5), 305–314.

Chacur, M., Milligan, E.D., Gazda, L.S., et al., 2001. A new model of sciatic inflammatory neuritis (SIN): induction of unilateral and bilateral mechanical allodynia following acute unilateral peri-sciatic immune activation in rats. Pain 94 (3), 231–244.

Chen, Y., Devor, M., 1998. Ectopic mechanosensitivity in injured sensory axons arises from the site of spontaneous electrogenesis. Eur. J. Pain 2 (2), 165–178.

Chien, A., Eliav, E., Sterling, M., 2008. Whiplash (grade II) and cervical radiculopathy share a similar sensory presentation: an investigation using quantitative sensory testing. Clin. J. Pain 24 (7), 595–603.

Clark, B.D., Barr, A.E., Safadi, F.F., et al., 2003. Median nerve trauma in a rat model of work-related musculoskeletal disorder. J. Neurotrauma 20 (7), 681–695.

Coppieters, M.W., Butler, D.S., 2008. Do 'sliders' slide and 'tensioners' tension? An analysis of neurodynamic techniques and considerations regarding their application. Man. Ther. 13 (3), 213–221.

Creange, A., Barlovatz-Meimon, G., Gherardi, R.K., 1997. Cytokines and peripheral nerve disorders. Eur. Cytokine Netw. 8 (2), 145–151.

Cudlip, S.A., Howe, F.A., Griffiths, J.R., et al., 2002. Magnetic resonance neurography of peripheral nerve following experimental crush injury, and correlation with functional deficit. J. Neurosurg. 96 (4), 755–759.

Cunha, F.Q., Poole, S., Lorenzetti, B.B., et al., 1992. The pivotal role of tumour necrosis factor alpha in the development of inflammatory hyperalgesia. Br. J. Pharmacol. 107 (3), 660–664.

Dilley, A., Bove, G.M., 2008a. Disruption of axoplasmic transport induces mechanical sensitivity in intact rat C-fibre nociceptor axons. J. Physiol. 586 (2), 593–604.

Dilley, A., Bove, G.M., 2008b. Resolution of inflammation-induced axonal mechanical sensitivity and conduction slowing in C-fiber nociceptors. J. Pain 9 (2), 185–192.

Dilley, A., Greening, J., Lynn, B., et al., 2001. The use of cross-correlation analysis between high-frequency ultrasound images to measure longitudinal median nerve movement. Ultrasound Med. Biol. 27 (9), 1211–1218.

Dilley, A., Lynn, B., Greening, J., et al., 2003. Quantitative in vivo studies of median nerve sliding in response to wrist, elbow, shoulder and neck movements. Clin. Biomech. 18 (10), 899–907.

Dilley, A., Lynn, B., Pang, S.J., 2005. Pressure and stretch mechanosensitivity of peripheral nerve fibres following local inflammation of the nerve trunk. Pain 117 (3), 462–472.

Dilley, A., Summerhayes, C., Lynn, B., 2007. An in vivo investigation of ulnar nerve sliding during upper limb movements. Clin. Biomech. 22 (7), 774–779.

Dilley, A., Odeyinde, S., Greening, J., et al., 2008. Longitudinal sliding of the median nerve in patients with non-specific arm pain. Man. Ther. 13 (6), 536–543.

Djouhri, L., Koutsikou, S., Fang, X., et al., 2006. Spontaneous pain, both neuropathic and inflammatory, is related to frequency of spontaneous firing in intact C-fiber nociceptors. J. Neurosci. 26 (4), 1281–1292.

Duan, B., Wu, L.J., Yu, Y.Q., et al., 2007. Upregulation of acid-sensing ion channel ASIC1a in spinal dorsal horn neurons contributes to inflammatory pain hypersensitivity. J. Neurosci. 27 (41), 11139–11148.

Eliav, E., Herzberg, U., Ruda, M.A., et al., 1999. Neuropathic pain from an experimental neuritis of the rat sciatic nerve. Pain 83 (2), 169–182.

Eliav, E., Benoliel, R., Tal, M., 2001. Inflammation with no axonal damage of the rat saphenous nerve trunk induces ectopic discharge and mechanosensitivity in myelinated axons. Neurosci. Lett. 311 (1), 49–52.

Eliav, E., Benoliel, R., Herzberg, U., et al., 2009. The Role of IL-6 and IL-1beta in Painful Perineural Inflammatory Neuritis. Brain Behav. Immun. 23 (4), 474–484.

Elliott, M.B., Barr, A.E., Kietrys, D.M., et al., 2008. Peripheral neuritis and increased spinal cord neurochemicals are induced in a model of repetitive motion injury with low force and repetition exposure. Brain Res. 1218 (2), 103–113.

Erel, E., Dilley, A., Greening, J., et al., 2003. Longitudinal sliding of the median nerve in patients with carpal tunnel syndrome. J. Hand Surg. 28 (5), 439–443.

Erel, E., Dilley, A., Turner, S., et al., 2009. Sonographic measurements of longitudinal median nerve sliding in patients following nerve repair. Muscle Nerve 41 (3), 350–354.

Filler, A.G., Howe, F.A., Hayes, C.E., et al., 1993. Magnetic resonance neurography. Lancet 341 (8846), 659–661.

Filler, A.G., Kliot, M., Howe, F.A., et al., 1996. Application of magnetic resonance neurography in the evaluation of patients with peripheral nerve pathology. J. Neurosurg. 85 (2), 299–309.

Filler, A.G., Maravilla, K.R., Tsuruda, J.S., 2004. MR neurography and muscle MR imaging for image diagnosis of disorders affecting the peripheral nerves and musculature. Neurol. Clin. 22 (3), 643–647.

Gamble, H.J., Eames, R.A., 1964. An Electron Microscope Study of the Connective Tissues of Human Peripheral Nerve. J. Anat. 98, 655–663.

Gazda, L.S., Milligan, E.D., Hansen, M.K., et al., 2001. Sciatic inflammatory neuritis (SIN): behavioral allodynia is paralleled by peri-sciatic proinflammatory cytokine and superoxide production. J. Peripher. Nerv. Syst. 6 (3), 111–129.

Gerdle, B., Lemming, D., Kristiansen, J., et al., 2008. Biochemical alterations in the trapezius muscle of patients with chronic whiplash associated disorders (WAD): a microdialysis study. Eur. J. Pain 12 (1), 82–93.

Gould III, H.J., Gould, T.N., England, J.D., et al., 2000. A possible role for nerve growth factor in the augmentation of sodium channels in models of chronic pain. Brain Res. 854 (1–2), 19–29.

Gracely, R.H., Lynch, S.A., Bennett, G.J., 1992. Painful neuropathy: altered central processing maintained dynamically by peripheral input. Pain 51 (2), 175–194.

Greening, J., 2005. How inflammation and minor nerve injury contribute to pain in nerve root and peripheral neuropathies. In: Boyling, J., Jull, G. (Eds.), Grieves Modern Manual: Therapy The Vertebral Column. Churchill Livingstone, London.

Greening, J., Lynn, B., 1998. Vibration sense in the upper limb in patients with repetitive strain injury and a group of at-risk office workers. Int. Arch. Occup. Environ. Health 71 (1), 29–34.

Greening, J., Smart, S., Leary, R., et al., 1999. Reduced movement of median nerve in carpal tunnel during wrist flexion in patients with non-specific arm pain. Lancet 354 (9174), 217–218.

Greening, J., Lynn, B., Leary, R., et al., 2001. The use of ultrasound imaging to demonstrate reduced movement of the median nerve during wrist flexion in patients with non-specific arm pain. J. Hand Surg. 26 (5), 401–406.

Greening, J., Lynn, B., Leary, R., 2003. Sensory and autonomic function in the hands of patients with non-specific arm pain (NSAP) and asymptomatic office workers. Pain 104 (1–2), 275–281.

Greening, J., Dilley, A., Lynn, B., 2005. In vivo study of nerve movement and mechano-sensitivity of the median nerve in whiplash and non-specific arm pain patients. Pain 115 (3), 248–253.

Grewel, R., Jiangming, X., Sotereanos, D.G., et al., 1996. Biomechanical properties of peripheral nerve. Hand Clin. 12 (2), 195–204.

Haninec, P., 1986. Undulating course of nerve fibres and bands of Fontana in peripheral nerves of the rat. Anat. Embryol. (Berl.) 174 (3), 407–411.

Harrington, J.M., Carter, J.T., Birrell, L., et al., 1998. Surveillance case definitions for work related upper limb pain syndromes. J. Occup. Environ. Med. 55 (4), 264–271.

Hough, A.D., Moore, A.P., Jones, M.P., 2007. Reduced longitudinal excursion of the median nerve in carpal tunnel syndrome. Arch. Phys. Med. Rehabil. 88 (5), 569–576.

Hromada, J., 1963. On the nerve supply of the connective tissue of some peripheral nervous tissue system components. Acta Anat. (Basel) 55, 343–351.

Huygen, F.J., De Bruijn, A.G., De Bruin, M.T., et al., 2002. Evidence for local inflammation in complex regional pain syndrome type 1. Mediators Inflamm. 11 (1), 47–51.

Janig, W., Baron, R., 2003. Complex regional pain syndrome: mystery explained? Lancet Neurol. 2 (11), 687–697.

Julius, A., Lees, R., Dilley, A., et al., 2004. Shoulder posture and median nerve sliding. BMC Musculoskelet. Disord. 5, 23.

Jung, H., Toth, P.T., White, F.A., et al., 2008. Monocyte chemoattractant protein-1 functions as a neuromodulator in dorsal root ganglia neurons. J. Neurochem. 104 (1), 254–263.

Kajander, K.C., Bennett, G.J., 1992. Onset of a painful peripheral neuropathy in rat: a partial and differential deafferentation and spontaneous discharge in A beta and A delta primary afferent neurons. J. Neurophysiol. 68 (3), 734–744.

Kim, S.H., Chung, J.M., 1992. An experimental model for peripheral neuropathy produced by segmental spinal nerve ligation in the rat. Pain 50 (3), 355–363.

Kitamura, N., Konno, A., Kuwahara, T., et al., 2005. Nerve growth factor-induced hyperexcitability of rat sensory neuron in culture. Biomed. Res. 26 (3), 123–130.

Kitao, A., Hirata, H., Morita, A., et al., 1997. Transient damage to the axonal transport system without Wallerian degeneration by acute nerve compression. Exp. Neurol. 147 (2), 248–255.

Kivioja, J., Rinaldi, L., Ozenci, V., et al., 2001. Chemokines and their receptors in whiplash injury: elevated RANTES and CCR-5. J. Clin. Immunol. 21 (4), 272–277.

Kleinrensink, G., Stoeckart, R., Vleeming, A., et al., 1995. Peripheral nerve tension due to joint motion. A comparison between embalmed and unembalmed human bodies. Clin. Biomech. 10 (5), 235–239.

Kleinrensink, G.J., Stoeckart, R., Mulder, P.G., et al., 2000. Upper limb tension tests as tools in the diagnosis of nerve and plexus lesions. Anatomical and biomechanical aspects. Clin. Biomech. 15 (1), 9–14.

Koltzenburg, M., Bendszus, M., 2004. Imaging of peripheral nerve lesions. Curr. Opin. Neurol. 17 (5), 621–626.

Koschorke, G.M., Meyer, R.A., Campbell, J.N., 1994. Cellular components necessary for mechanoelectrical transduction are conveyed to primary afferent terminals by fast axonal transport. Brain Res. 641 (1), 99–104.

Kwan, M.K., Wall, E.J., Massie, J., et al., 1992. Strain, stress and stretch of peripheral nerve. Rabbit experiments in vitro and in vivo. Acta Orthop. Scand. 63 (3), 267–272.

LaMotte, R.H., Shain, C.N., Simone, D.A., et al., 1991. Neurogenic hyperalgesia: psychophysical studies of underlying mechanisms. J. Neurophysiol. 66 (1), 190–211.

Leem, J.G., Bove, G.M., 2002. Mid-axonal tumor necrosis factor-alpha induces ectopic activity in a subset of slowly conducting cutaneous and deep afferent neurons. J. Pain 3 (1), 45–49.

Lewin, G.R., Ritter, A.M., Mendell, L.M., 1993. Nerve growth factor-induced hyperalgesia in the neonatal and adult rat. J. Neurosci. 13 (5), 2136–2148.

Liu, L., Yang, T.M., Liedtke, W., et al., 2006. Chronic IL-1β signaling potentiates voltage-dependent sodium currents in trigeminal nociceptive neurons. J. Neurophysiol. 95 (3), 1478–1490.

Lundborg, G., 1988. Nerve Injuries and Repair. Churchill Livingstone, Edinburgh.

Lynn, B., Greening, J., Leary, R., 2002. Sensory and autonomic function and ultrasound nerve imaging in RSI patients and keyboard workers (No. CRR 417/2002). Health and Safety Executive, London.

Mackinnon, S.E., 2002. Pathophysiology of nerve compression. Hand Clin. 18 (2), 231–241.

Maihofner, C., Handwerker, H.O., Neundorfer, B., et al., 2005. Mechanical hyperalgesia in complex regional pain syndrome: a role for TNF-alpha? Neurology 65 (2), 311–313.

McLellan, D.L., Swash, M., 1976. Longitudinal sliding of the median nerve during movements of the upper limb. J. Neurol. Neurosurg. Psychiatry 39, 566–570.

McMahon, S.B., Cafferty, W.B., Marchand, F., 2005. Immune and glial cell factors as pain mediators and modulators. Exp. Neurol. 192 (2), 444–462.

Millesi, H., Zoch, G., Rath, T., 1990. The gliding apparatus of peripheral nerve and its clinical significance. Annals of Hand and Upper Limb Surgery 9 (2), 87–97.

Moalem, G., Tracey, D.J., 2006. Immune and inflammatory mechanisms in neuropathic pain. Brain Res. Rev. 51 (2), 240–264.

Nakamichi, K., Tachibana, S., 1995. Restricted motion of the median nerve in carpal tunnel syndrome. J. Hand Surg. 20 (4), 460–464.

O'Connor, D., Marshall, S.C., Massy-Westropp, N., 2009. Non-surgical treatment (other than steroid injection) for carpal tunnel syndrome (Review). Cochrane Database Syst. Rev. (1):CD003219.

Obreja, O., Rathee, P.K., Lips, K.S., et al., 2002. IL-1 beta potentiates heat-activated currents in rat sensory neurons: involvement of IL-1RI, tyrosine kinase, and protein kinase C. FASEB J. 16 (12), 1497–1503.

Obreja, O., Biasio, W., Andratsch, M., et al., 2005. Fast modulation of heat-activated ionic current by proinflammatory interleukin 6 in rat sensory neurons. Brain 128 (7), 1634–1641.

Oh, S.B., Tran, P.B., Gillard, S.E., et al., 2001. Chemokines and glycoprotein120 produce pain hypersensitivity by directly exciting primary nociceptive neurons. J. Neurosci. 21 (14), 5027–5035.

Olsson, Y., 1990. Microenvironment of the peripheral nervous system under normal and pathological conditions. Crit. Rev. Neurobiol. 5 (3), 265–309.

Ozaktay, A.C., Kallakuri, S., Takebayashi, T., et al., 2006. Effects of interleukin-1 beta, interleukin-6, and tumor necrosis factor on sensitivity of dorsal root ganglion and peripheral receptive fields in rats. Eur. Spine J. 15 (10), 1529–1537.

Pascarelli, E.F., Hsu, Y.P., 2001. Understanding work-related upper extremity disorders: clinical findings in 485 computer users, musicians, and others. J. Occup. Rehabil. 11 (1), 1–21.

Pertin, M., Ji, R.R., Berta, T., et al., 2005. Upregulation of the voltage-gated sodium channel beta2 subunit in neuropathic pain models: characterization of expression in injured and non-injured primary sensory neurons. J. Neurosci. 25 (47), 10970–10980.

Quintner, J.L., 1989. A study of upper limb pain and paraesthesiae following neck injury in motor vehicle accidents: assessment of the brachial plexus tension test of Elvey. Br. J. Rheumatol. 28 (6), 528–533.

Rodriquez, A.A., Barr, K.P., Burns, S.P., 2004. Whiplash: pathophysiology, diagnosis, treatment, and prognosis. Muscle Nerve 29 (6), 768–781.

Rueff, A., Mendell, L.M., 1996. Nerve growth factor NT-5 induce increased thermal sensitivity of cutaneous nociceptors in vitro. J. Neurophysiol. 76 (5), 3593–3596.

Rydevik, B.L., Kwan, M.K., Myers, R.R., et al., 1990. An in vitro mechanical and histological study of acute stretching on rabbit tibial nerve. J. Orthop. Res. 8 (5), 694–701.

Sauer, S.K., Bove, G.M., Averbeck, B., et al., 1999. Rat peripheral nerve components release calcitonin gene-related peptide and prostaglandin E-2 in response to noxious stimuli: Evidence that nervi nervorum are nociceptors. Neuroscience 92 (1), 319–325.

Schafers, M., Sorkin, L.S., Geis, C., et al., 2003a. Spinal nerve ligation induces transient upregulation of tumor necrosis factor receptors 1 and 2 in injured and adjacent uninjured dorsal root ganglia in the rat. Neurosci. Lett. 347 (3), 179–182.

Schafers, M., Sorkin, L.S., Sommer, C., 2003b. Intramuscular injection of tumor necrosis factor-alpha induces muscle hyperalgesia in rats. Pain 104 (3), 579–588.

Sommer, C., Galbraith, J.A., Heckman, H.M., et al., 1993. Pathology of experimental compression neuropathy producing hyperesthesia. J. Neuropathol. Exp. Neurol. 52 (3), 223–233.

Sorkin, L.S., Doom, C.M., 2000. Epineurial application of TNF elicits an acute mechanical hyperalgesia in the awake rat. J. Peripher. Nerv. Syst. 5 (2), 96–100.

Sorkin, L.S., Xiao, W.H., Wagner, R., et al., 1997. Tumour necrosis factor-alpha induces ectopic activity in nociceptive primary afferent fibres. Neuroscience 81 (1), 255–262.

Sterling, M., Treleaven, J., Jull, G., 2002. Responses to a clinical test of mechanical provocation of nerve tissue in whiplash associated disorder. Man. Ther. 7 (2), 89–94.

Sun, J.H., Yang, B., Donnelly, D.F., et al., 2006. MCP-1 enhances excitability of nociceptive neurons in chronically compressed dorsal root ganglia. J. Neurophysiol. 96 (5), 2189–2199.

Sunderland, S., 1978. Nerve and Nerve Injuries. Churchill Livingstone, Edinburgh.

Tal, M., Eliav, E., 1996. Abnormal discharge originates at the site of nerve injury in experimental constriction neuropathy (CCI) in the rat. Pain 64 (3), 511–518.

Tanaka, M., Cummins, T.R., Ishikawa, K., et al., 1998. SNS Na$^+$ channel expression increases in dorsal root ganglion neurons in the carrageenan inflammatory pain model. Neuroreport 9 (6), 967–972.

Tanaka, T., Minami, M., Nakagawa, T., et al., 2004. Enhanced production of monocyte chemoattractant protein-1 in the dorsal root ganglia in a rat model of neuropathic pain: possible involvement in the development of neuropathic pain. Neurosci. Res. 48 (4), 463–469.

Thomas, P.K., 1963. The connective tissue of peripheral nerve: a electron microscope study. J. Anat. 97 (1), 35–44.

Thomas, P.K., Berthold, C.H., Ochoa, J., et al., 1993. Microscopic anatomy of the peripheral nervous system. In: Dyck, P.J., Thomas, P.K. (Eds.), Peripheral Neuropathy. Saunders, Philadelphia.

Tillett, R.L., Afoke, A., Hall, S.M., et al., 2004. Investigating mechanical behaviour at a core-sheath interface in peripheral nerve. J. Peripher. Nerv. Syst. 9 (4), 255–262.

Toews, A.D., Barrett, C., Morell, P., 1998. Monocyte chemoattractant protein 1 is responsible for macrophage recruitment following injury to sciatic nerve. J. Neurosci. Res. 53 (2), 260–267.

Topp, K.S., Boyd, B.S., 2006. Structure and biomechanics of peripheral nerves: nerve responses to physical stresses and implications for physical therapist practice. Phys. Ther. 86 (1), 92–109.

Tuzuner, S., Ozkaynak, S., Acikbas, C., et al., 2004. Median nerve excursion during endoscopic carpal tunnel release. Neurosurgery 54 (5), 1155–1160.

Uceyler, N., Eberle, T., Rolke, R., et al., 2007a. Differential expression patterns of cytokines in complex regional pain syndrome. Pain 132 (1–2), 195–205.

Uceyler, N., Tscharke, A., Sommer, C., 2007b. Early cytokine expression in mouse sciatic nerve after chronic constriction nerve injury depends on calpain. Brain Behav. Immun. 21 (5), 553–560.

Ushiki, T., Ide, C., 1990. Three-dimensional organization of the collagen fibrils in the rat sciatic nerve as revealed by transmission- and scanning electron microscopy. Cell Tissue Res. 260 (1), 175–184.

Walbeehm, E.T., Afoke, A., de Wit, T., et al., 2004. Mechanical functioning of peripheral nerves: linkage with the 'mushrooming' effect. Cell Tissue Res. 316 (1), 115–121.

Wallis, B.J., Lord, S.M., Barnsley, L., et al., 1998. The psychological profiles of patients with whiplash-associated headache. Cephalalgia 18 (2), 101–105.

Watkins, L.R., Maier, S.F., 2002. Beyond neurons: evidence that immune and glial cells contribute to pathological pain states. Physiol. Rev. 82 (4), 981–1011.

White, F.A., Sun, J., Waters, S.M., et al., 2005. Excitatory monocyte chemoattractant protein-1 signaling is up-regulated in sensory neurons after chronic compression of the dorsal root ganglion. Proc. Natl. Acad. Sci. U. S. A. 102 (39), 14092–14097.

Wilgis, E.F., Murphy, R., 1986. The significance of longitudinal excursion in peripheral nerves. Hand Clin. 2, 761–766.

Wright, T.W., Glowczewskie, F., Wheeler, D., et al., 1996. Excursion and strain of the median nerve. J. Bone Joint Surg. 78, 1897–1903.

Wright, T.W., Glowczewskie Jr., F., Cowin, D., et al., 2001. Ulnar nerve excursion and strain at the elbow and wrist associated with upper extremity motion. J. Hand Surg. 26 (4), 655–662.

Wright, T.W., Glowczewskie Jr., F., Cowin, D., et al., 2005. Radial nerve excursion and strain at the elbow and wrist associated with upper-extremity motion. J. Hand Surg. 30 (5), 990–996.

Wu, G., Ringkamp, M., Hartke, T.V., et al., 2001. Early onset of spontaneous activity in uninjured C-fiber nociceptors after injury to neighboring nerve fibers. J. Neurosci. 21 (8), RC140.

Wu, G., Ringkamp, M., Murinson, B.B., et al., 2002. Degeneration of myelinated efferent fibers induces spontaneous activity in uninjured C-fiber afferents. J. Neurosci. 22 (17), 7746–7753.

Zelenka, M., Schafers, M., Sommer, C., 2005. Intraneural injection of interleukin-1beta and tumor necrosis factor-alpha into rat sciatic nerve at physiological doses induces signs of neuropathic pain. Pain 116 (3), 257–263.

Zhang, N., Inan, S., Cowan, A., et al., 2005. A proinflammatory chemokine, CCL3, sensitizes the heat- and capsaicin-gated ion channel TRPV1. Proc. Natl. Acad. Sci. U. S. A. 102 (12), 4536–4541.

Zhu, W., Oxford, G.S., 2007. Phosphoinositide-3-kinase and mitogen activated protein kinase signaling pathways mediate acute NGF sensitization of TRPV1. Mol. Cell. Neurosci. 34 (4), 689–700.

Zochodne, D.W., Ho, L.T., 1992. Hyperemia of injured peripheral nerve: sensitivity to CGRP antagonism. Brain Res. 598 (1–2), 59–66.

Zochodne, D.W., Ho, L.T., 1993. Evidence that capsaicin hyperaemia of rat sciatic vasa nervorum is local, opiate-sensitive and involves mast cells. J. Physiol. 468, 325–333.

Chapter | 38 |

Neurodynamic interventions and physiological effects: Clinical neurodynamics in neck and upper extremity pain

Paul Mintken, Emilio Puentedura, Adriaan Louw

CHAPTER CONTENTS

INTRODUCTION

Manual Therapy involves the selective examination and evaluation of the effects of movement, position and activities on the signs and symptoms of a neuro-musculoskeletal disorder (Maitland 1986). This allows the clinician to formulate a working hypothesis regarding the movement problem which can be confirmed or denied following the careful reassessment during and after specific treatment applications. Manual Therapy is therefore a useful approach to examine, evaluate and treat movement problems affecting the neuromusculoskeletal system. We have found that it is useful to think of the mechanics of the body's moving parts in terms of components comprising a chassis (skeletal framework), articulations (joints and supporting ligaments), motors (muscles and tendons) and electrical wiring (nervous system). Each of the components that make up the neuromusculoskeletal system plays an important and interdependent role in its overall health and function.

One could argue that many of the early Manual Therapy systems of the 1960s and 1970s placed a greater emphasis on the health and function of the joints and hence, 'manual therapy' became synonymous with 'passive joint mobilization' and 'thrust joint manipulation' (Butler 1991). Despite an underlying awareness of the interdependency of the components of the neuromusculoskeletal system, relatively little attention was paid to the physical health

© 2011 Elsevier Ltd.
DOI: 10.1016/B978-0-7020-3528-9.00038-8

and movement of the nervous system. This changed dramatically following the published works of Gregory Grieve, Alf Breig, Geoffrey Maitland, Robert Elvey and David Butler. Their collective works opened a new frontier in Manual Therapy – the hypothesis that the entire nervous system is a mechanical organ that could develop 'adverse tension,' or impaired mobility, which could then be treated with various movement therapies.

When the concept of mobilizing the nervous system took root within the physical therapy community in the late 70s and early 80s it was met with some significant scepticism by the other health professions (Di Fabio 2001). The concept originally focused on the mechanical 'stiffness' within the nervous system, and it was thought at the time that this stiffness required aggressive stretching. Needless to say, neurologists and neurosurgeons did not greet this new branch of physical therapy with much enthusiasm. While a subset of patients benefited from treating this 'adverse neural tension' with 'stretching' and mobilization, many manual therapists soon found that some patients got significantly worse following these interventions, and therefore very quickly abandoned the use of these neural mobilization techniques.

What should we call it then?

'Adverse neural tension' has been defined as the abnormal physiological and mechanical responses produced by nervous system structures when testing its normal range of movement and stretch capabilities (Butler 1991). A 'neural tension test' is therefore designed to examine the physical (mechanical) abilities of the nervous system (Butler 2000). The use of the term 'tension' has significant limitations because it fails to take into account other aspects of nervous system function, such as movement, pressure, viscoelasticity and physiology (Shacklock 1995a,b, 2005a,b). A more appropriate term is 'neurodynamic test' (Shacklock 2005a) and it is one our profession should embrace.

The term 'neurodynamics' refers to the mechanics and physiology of the nervous system within the musculoskeletal system and how these systems relate to each other (Shacklock 1995a). This term allows for the consideration of movement-related neurophysiological changes as well as the neuronal dynamics that is postulated to occur in the central nervous system (CNS) during physical and mental activity. A key tenet of this definition is that the nervous system is capable of movement and stretch, and that there is a 'normal' response (as well as abnormal) of the nervous system to movement and tension. Both Butler and Shacklock have advocated the transition to the term 'neurodynamic' as opposed to 'neural tension', because 'neurodynamics' places less emphasis on 'stretching' and 'tension' and more emphasis on the nervous system, the 'container' in which it lives, and the mechanisms that can alter the function of the nervous system. These

other mechanisms include changes to intraneural blood flow (Ogata & Naito 1986); neural inflammation (Zochodne & Ho 1991); mechanosensitivity (Calvin et al 1982, Nordin et al 1984) and muscle responses (Hall et al 1995, 1998, Van der Heide et al 2001).

Neurodynamic impairments should really be conceptualized as any specific physical dysfunction (whether it be neural, muscular or skeletal) which presumes to physically challenge normal functioning of the nervous system. These impairments can arise from mechanical, chemical or sensitivity changes anywhere in the neuro-musculoskeletal system. Therefore in neurodynamics, neural tissues may have a tension problem (mechanical) or be hypersensitive (a problem of pathophysiology) or a combination of both (Shacklock 2005b). Instead of a length or 'tension' problem, the primary mechanical fault within the nervous system may be one of reduced sliding (neural sliding dysfunction) and/or it could be a compression problem that relates to the tissues that form a mechanical interface to the nervous system. Therefore, the time has come for us to embrace the current nomenclature: 'Neurodynamics'.

OPERATING DEFINITIONS

In order to facilitate understanding the rest of this chapter, some operational definitions are provided.

Clinical neurodynamics

This can be defined as the examination, evaluation and treatment of the mechanics and physiology of the nervous system as they relate to each other and how they are integrated with musculoskeletal function (Shacklock 1995a).

Neurodynamic test

The testing procedures used in clinical neurodynamics. These can be defined as a series of body movements that produces mechanical and physiological events in the nervous system according to the movements of the test (Shacklock 2005b). A neurodynamic test aims to physically challenge or test the mechanics and/or physiology of a part of the nervous system. For example, a mechanical component of a Median Neurodynamic Test (MNT) would be the ability of the median nerve tract to slide and glide in relation to surrounding tissues such as the lower cervical discs, scalenes, biceps and carpal tunnel. The physiological components may relate to blood flow within the median nerve tract, ion channel activity within axons of the median nerve, inflammation within various sections of the median nerve and representation changes in the CNS of the median nerve, arm, forearm and their movements.

Neurogenic pain

Pain that is initiated or caused by a primary lesion, dysfunction, or transitory perturbation in the peripheral or central nervous system (Merskey & Bogduk 1994).

Sensitizing movements

Movements that increase forces in the neural structures in addition to those movements employed in the standard neurodynamic test (Butler 1991, 2000, Shacklock 2005b). Sensitizing movements should not be confused with differentiating movements. Sensitizing movements can be useful in loading or moving the nervous system beyond the effects of the standard neurodynamic test, i.e. strengthening the test. However, they also load and move musculoskeletal structures and are therefore not as helpful in determining the existence of a neurodynamic problem as a differentiating movement.

Differentiating movements

Movements that emphasize or isolate the nervous system by producing movement in the neural structures in the area in question rather than moving the musculoskeletal structures in the same area (Butler 2000, Shacklock 2005b). Differentiating movements place emphasis on the nervous system without affecting the other structures and are therefore used to help establish the existence of a neurodynamic problem. An example of a differentiating movement for a patient with carpal tunnel pain would be the addition of cervical ipsilateral side bending (see later in this chapter for further examples).

Sliders

Neurodynamic manoeuvres performed in order to produce a sliding movement of neural structures in relation to their adjacent tissues (Butler 2000, Shacklock 2005b). Sliders involve application of movement/stress to the nervous system proximally while releasing movement/stress distally, and then reversing the sequence. Sliders allow larger ranges of motion, provide a means of distraction from the painful area, should provide multi-tissue, non-painful, and, it would be hoped, fear-reducing novel inputs into the CNS (Butler 2000). Research has shown that sliders actually result in greater excursion than simply stretching the nerve (Coppieters & Butler 2008).

Tensioners

Neurodynamic manoeuvres performed in order to produce an increase in tension (not stretch) in neural structures which theoretically may improve neural viscoelastic and physiological functions (help neural tissue cope better with increased tension) (Butler 2000,

Shacklock 2005b). Tensioners are the opposite of sliders in that movement/stress is applied proximally and distally to the nervous system at the same time, and then released. Tensioners may better challenge stiffness and more long-lasting physical dysfunction (Butler 2000).

NEUROPHYSIOLOGY IN CERVICO-BRACHIAL PAIN

Initially, manual therapists were more interested in the mechanical aspects of neurodynamics (Brieg 1978, Elvey 1979, 1986, Butler 1991). Unfortunately it has led to a very 'mechanistic' view of the nervous system (Butler 2000). Most textbooks describe normal nerve mechanics related to various positions, postures or movements, subsequent abnormal mechanics (pathomechanics) and finally movement-based treatment aimed at restoring normal nerve movement (Butler 1991, 2000, Shacklock 2005b). None of this is disputed. However, increased knowledge in our understanding of nerve pain related to neurophysiological changes and the processing within the brain of nerve movement (and pain) warrants investigation and discussion.

Pathologies that affect peripheral nerves usually result in dysaesthetic pain and/or nerve trunk pain (Asbury & Fields 1984). Dysaesthetic pain (where light touch causes pain) often manifests as burning and/or tingling pain due to abnormal impulses from hyperexcitable afferent nerve fibres, which, due to injury, may become abnormal impulse generating sites (AIGS) (Devor et al 1979, Asbury & Fields 1984, Woolf & Mannion 1999). AIGS may spontaneously fire as the result of mechanical or chemical stimuli (Butler 2000) such that dysaesthetic pain may present as very bizarre patterns, from bursts of pain in response to a stimulus to pain that presents spontaneously with no apparent stimuli.

In contrast, nerve trunk pain commonly presents as deep, achy pain arising from nociceptors within the nervous tissue that are sensitized to mechanical or chemical stimuli (Asbury & Fields 1984, Kallakuri et al 1998). Nerve trunk pain usually has a fairly straightforward stimulus-response relationship (Asbury & Fields 1984). These two types of pain can be evoked by a variety of chemical or mechanical stimuli, and may lead to allodynia or hyperalgesia. Allodynia is a pain sensation that is evoked from stimuli that are not normally painful while hyperalgesia is an exaggerated pain response to stimuli that would normally be painful (Asbury & Fields 1984, Woolf & Mannion 1999, Nee & Butler 2006).

Nerve sensitivity

In order to understand nerve sensitivity, knowledge of ion channels is required. Although the complexity of ion channel regulation is not yet properly understood and the research is based on animal studies, scientists and clinicians are using the information about ion channels to improve patient care (Barry 1991, Butler 2000). Ion channels are essentially proteins clumped together with an opening – to allow ions to flow in/out of a membrane (Devor 2006). They are synthesized in the dorsal root ganglion (DRG) based on a genetic coding, and are distributed along an axon to allow ions to flow in/out of the nerve to polarize or depolarize the membrane. Ion channels are not uniformly distributed along the axolemma with certain areas known to have higher concentrations of ion channels, such as the DRG, axon hillock, nodes of Ranvier and areas where the axon has lost myelin (Devor et al 1993, Devor 1999, 2006).

Adding to the complexity is the fact that there are countless types of ion channels, including channels that seem to respond to movement, pressure, blood flow, circulating adrenaline levels, etc. (Fig 38.1). From a survival perspective, this seems logical as a means for the nervous system to become 'sensitive' to various stimuli. However, the amount and type of ion channels found in the axolemma is in a constant state of change (Devor et al 1993, Devor 2006). Research has shown that the half-life of some ion channels may be as short as 2 days (Barry 1991), and ion channels that drop out of the membrane are not necessarily replaced by the same type. Ion channel deposition is directly impacted by the environment the organism finds itself in (Barry 1991). For example, changes in temperature around an animal with experimentally removed myelin produce higher concentrations of 'cold-sensing' channels in that area, animals in stressful environments produce higher concentrations of adreno-sensitive channels, and animals that have joints with restricted movement cause upregulation of movement sensitive ion channels (Devor et al 1993, Devor & Seltzer 1999, Devor 2006). With higher concentrations of similar ion channels in an area, the chances for the nerve to depolarize and cause an action potential increase. In essence, the nerve may develop an AIGS. The nervous system can then become sensitive to various types of stimuli, such as temperature, movement, pressure, anxiety, stress, the immune system and more (Devor & Seltzer 1999, Butler 2000, Butler & Moseley 2003) (Fig 38.2). The nervous

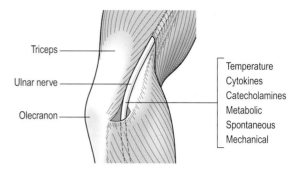

Fig 38.2 Ulna nerve at the elbow – depicting types of ion channels.

system can therefore be viewed as an alarm system beautifully designed to protect the organism and the amount and type of ion channels at any given time may be a fair representation of what the brain computes is needed for survival (Butler & Moseley 2003).

Central nervous system processing in neurodynamic tests

Many clinicians are familiar with the term 'central sensitivity'. Central sensitivity is defined as a condition in which peripheral noxious input into the CNS leads to an increased excitability where the response to normal inputs is greatly enhanced (Woolf 2007). Repeated painful stimuli, such as easily excitable AIGS, may cause low-threshold neurons with large receptive fields to depolarize in response to stimuli that would normally be benign (Woolf 2007). It has been shown that injured neural tissue may alter its chemical makeup and reorganize synaptic contacts in the CNS such that innocuous stimuli are directed to cells that normally receive only noxious inputs (Woolf 2007). Hence, the CNS becomes 'hyperexcitable' due to a combination of decreased inhibition and increased responsiveness (Woolf 2000). This is analogous to turning up the volume on the system such that innocuous stimuli begin to generate painful sensations while noxious stimuli result in an exaggerated pain

Fig 38.1 Ion channels.

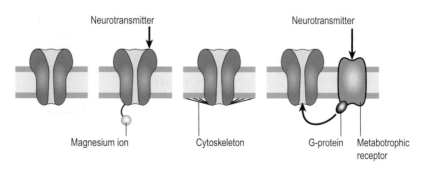

response. Woolf (2000) described this process as a change in both the software and the hardware of the CNS, and we would argue that clinicians have the tools to impact both of these.

CLINICAL NEUROBIOMECHANICS IN THE UPPER EXTREMITY

Neurobiomechanics is the study of the normal and pathological range of motion of the nervous system. Unfortunately, what we know is based upon somewhat limited research, largely animal and cadaver studies. There is no doubt that this is an area in need of further research efforts, and the interest shown by researchers in this area is certainly helping to expand our knowledge. For recent work, see Zoech et al (1991), Szabo et al (1994), Kleinrensink et al (1995, 2000), Wright et al (2001) and Dilley et al (2003).

A key issue in the understanding of neurobiomechanics is the concept of the nervous system being considered as a continuous tissue tract. The system is continuous mechanically via its continuous connective tissue formats, electrically via conducted impulses and, chemically via its common neurotransmitters. The nervous system being a mechanical continuum is probably most relevant to the study of neurodynamics, because it implies transmission of movement (sliding/gliding) and the development of tension (stretching) within and along the system. That is, wrist extension and elbow extension lengthens and moves the median nerve distally within its neural pathway, and contralateral cervical lateral flexion adds a pull in the proximal direction. This has been demonstrated in cadaveric studies in which the nerve roots are marked with paper markers or pins. When the shoulder is depressed and abducted in external rotation, the cervical nerve roots are pulled out of the vertebral foramen (Elvey 1979).

Another key concept in neurodynamics is that of the mechanical interface. The mechanical interface is defined as 'that tissue or material adjacent to the nervous system that can move independently to the system' (Butler 1991). Mechanical interfaces are central to an understanding of neurodynamics, because they represent the most likely sites for the development of movement or force transmission problems. Mechanical interfaces can be hard or bony (e.g. ulnar nerve at the cubital tunnel); ligamentous (e.g. ligament of Struthers in the forearm); joints (e.g. zygapophyseal joints); or muscular (e.g. supinator muscle in the forearm). Mechanical interfaces can be normal, where movement and function is optimal and symptom-free, or they can be pathological, where something happens to restrict movement of the nervous system at the interface, or compress the nervous tissue. Examples would include osteophytes, extensive bruising, or swelling which could occupy space at the mechanical interface

resulting in restricted range of motion and independence of the nervous system and the interface. Numerous studies have shown that if the interface is injured or damaged, it may have repercussions for the adjacent neural tissues. Examples include the cubital tunnel (Coppieters et al 2004), carpal tunnel (Mackinnon 1992, Nakamichi & Tachibana 1995, Coveney et al 1997, Rozmaryn et al 1998, Greening et al 1999), intervertebral foramen (De Peretti et al 1989, Chang et al 2006, Siddqui et al 2006), spinal canal (Fritz et al 1998, Chang et al 2006) and piriformis (Kuncewicz et al 2006). If this happens, range of motion of the nervous system can be impaired, and this would presumably lead to the abnormal mechanical response in our definition of neurodynamics.

As the nervous system winds its way through its anatomical course, it will be forced to stretch, slide (longitudinal or transverse), bend and become compressed. Stretch will be defined here as the elongation of the nerve relative its starting length. However, nerves are not solid structures and stretch causes internal compression due to displacement of nerve tissue/fluid (Fig 38.3). The physiological effects of stretch and compression include changes to intra-neural blood flow, conduction, and axoplasmic transport. Studies have shown that if a peripheral nerve is held on an 8% stretch for 30 minutes, it will cause a 50% decrease in blood flow; 8.8% stretch for 1 hour will cause 70% decrease in blood flow and 15% stretch for 30 minutes will cause 80–100% blockage in blood flow (Ogata & Naito 1986, Driscoll et al 2002). Wall et al (1992) were able to demonstrate that a 6% stretch/strain of a peripheral nerve for 1 hour resulted in a 70% decrease in action potentials, and a 12% stretch/strain for 1 hour caused complete conduction block. Interestingly other studies, Millesi (1986) and Zoech et al (1991) reported that from full wrist and elbow flexion to full wrist and elbow extension, the median nerve has to adapt to nerve bed that becomes 20% longer. Similar data has been provided by Beith et al (1995) with respect to the sciatic/tibial nerve. Research by Breig (1960, 1978), Breig & Marions (1963), Breig & el-Nadi (1966), Breig et al (1966) and Breig & Troup (1979) has demonstrated that flexion of the cervical spine leads to tension in the

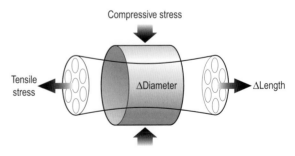

Fig 38.3 Stretching a nerve leads to increased intraneural pressure.

dura and spinal cord resulting in a cephalad movement of the cauda equina. This ultimately limits the available mobility of the sciatic nerve. Obviously, there must be some mechanical and physiological adaptations within peripheral nerves to accommodate such significant changes in length and to cope with prolonged stretching or strain. The effects of compression have also been studied with as little as 20–30 mmHg causing decreased venous blood flow and 80 mmHg causing complete blockage of intraneural blood flow (Rydevik et al 1981, Ogata & Naito 1986). Compression also is shown to alter axonal transport (Dahlin et al 1993) and action potential conduction (Fern & Harrison 1994).

Nerves can be seen to move relative to their adjacent tissues, and this motion has been described as sliding or excursion (McLellan & Swash 1976, Wilgis & Murphy 1986). Excursion is seen to occur both longitudinally and transversely. This sliding or excursion is considered an essential aspect of neural function because it serves to dissipate tension and distribute forces within the nervous system. Instead of stretching (and thereby developing tension) the nervous system can move longitudinally and/or transversely and distribute itself along the shortest course between fixed points, and hence, it can equalize tension throughout the neural tract.

As joints move, there is nerve bed elongation (increase in length of the neural container) on the convex side of the joint, and nerve bed shortening (decrease in length of the neural container) on the concave side of the joint. When there is nerve bed elongation, the nerve glides towards the joint that is moving and this is referred to as convergence. When there is nerve bed shortening, the nerve glides away from the joint that is moving and this is referred to as divergence. Dilley et al (2003) used real-time ultrasound to examine the effects on elbow extension on the median nerve and found the magnitude of excursion for the median nerve in the mid-upper arm to be 10.4 mm distally towards the elbow and in the mid-forearm to be 3.0 mm proximally towards the elbow. With the elbow held in extension while applying wrist extension, they recorded excursion of the median nerve at the mid-upper arm 1.8 mm distally towards the elbow, and in the mid-forearm 4.2 mm distally towards the wrist. It can be argued that some degree of excursion must occur in the hand proximally towards the wrist also.

Studies have shown that the starting position and the sequencing of limb movement during neurodynamic tests affect the degree of excursion along the nerve. In the same study referenced above, Dilley et al (2003) also examined the median nerve at the distal arm and mid-forearm using two different start positions: elbow in full extension and shoulder at 45° or at 90° abduction, then performed wrist extension from neutral to 45°. They found that greater excursion of the median nerve occurred when the shoulder was in a more slackened position (45° abduction). For the shoulder at 45° abduction, excursion was 2.4 mm

distally at the distal arm and 4.7 mm distally at the mid-forearm. For shoulder at 90° abduction, excursion was 1.8 mm distally at distal arm and 4.2 mm distally at mid-forearm. The sequence of movements has also been shown to affect the distribution of symptoms in response to neurodynamic testing (Shacklock 1989, Zorn et al 1995). These authors reported a greater likelihood of producing a response that is localized to the region that is moved first or more strongly. Tsai (1995) conducted a cadaveric study in which strain in the ulnar nerve at the elbow was measured during ulnar neurodynamic testing in three different sequences, proximal-to-distal, distal-to-proximal, and elbow-first sequence. The elbow-first sequence consistently produced 20% greater strain in the ulnar nerve at the elbow than the other two sequences. Therefore, it can be argued that greater strain in the nerves occurs at the site that is moved first, that is, the first component of a neurodynamic test or treatment technique.

THE BASE TESTS FOR THE UPPER EXTREMITY

Butler (1991) proposed a base test system for neurodynamic evaluation. It is a clinically intuitive system evolved for ease of handling and to fulfill a perceived clinical demand. It is based on existing tests and the basic principles of neurodynamics already discussed, and in most clinical situations, the tests are refined or adapted based upon reasoned diagnoses and the clinical presentation of the patient with neck and arm symptoms. Nee & Butler (2006) described a positive neurodynamic test as one that reproduces a familiar symptom, is changed by the movement of a body segment away from the site of symptoms, or there are differences in the test response from side to side or what is known to be normal in asymptomatic individuals. A positive test does not allow the identification of a specific area of injury, it is merely suggestive of increased mechanosensitivity somewhere along the neural tissue tract (Nee & Butler 2006).

The main tests for the upper extremity involve four varieties of the upper limb neurodynamic test (ULNT) and were evolved from Elvey's initial test (Elvey 1979). They include attention to the major neural pathways and major sensitizing movements. The four tests will now be described in detail and are: ULNT1 (median nerve bias), ULNT2 (median nerve bias), ULNT2 (radial nerve bias), ULNT3 (ulnar nerve bias) (Table 38.1).

The numbers refer to the powerful sensitizing movements where 1 is shoulder abduction, 2 is shoulder girdle depression and 3 is elbow flexion (Butler 2000). Two tests for the median nerve have been developed as this nerve is more commonly injured than the other nerves in the upper limb, and it was felt that a test was required to evaluate shoulder girdle depression and gleno-humeral

Table 38.1 Illustrating the major components, movements, sensitizing motions and differentiating motions for the four distinct upper limb neurodynamic tests (ULNT)

	ULNT1 median	ULNT2 median	ULNT2 radial	ULNT ulnar
Nerves Tested	Median, Anterior Interosseous (C5–C7)	Median, Anterior Interosseous (C5–C7)	Radial	Ulnar, C8 and T1 nerve roots
Shoulder	Stabilized from elevating and Abducted (90–110°)	Depressed and Abducted (10°)	Depressed and Abducted (10°)	Depressed and Abducted (10–90°), hand to ear
Elbow	Extended	Extended	Extended	Flexed
Forearm	Supinated	Supinated	Pronated	Pronated
Wrist	Extended	Extended	Flexed and Ulnarly Deviated	Extended and Radially Deviated
Fingers and Thumb	Extended	Extended	Flexed	Extended
Rotation of Shoulder	Lateral	Lateral	Medial	Lateral
Cervical Spine (Sensitizing)	Contralateral side flexed	Contralateral side flexed	Contralateral side flexed	Contralateral side flexed
Cervical Spine (Differentiating)	Ipsi-lateral side flexed	Ipsi-lateral side flexed	Ipsi-lateral side flexed	Ipsi-lateral side flexed

elevation independently (Butler 2000). Additionally, ULNT2 is useful in patients that have limited glenohumeral abduction.

It is recommended that all ULNTs be performed actively before passively. This allows the therapist to gauge the patient's ability and willingness to move and provides an approximate measure of the range of motion likely to be encountered during the passive test. It also may decrease the patient's fears and anxieties about the test and symptoms likely to be elicited during the test. Finally, if the active movement is found to be extremely sensitive, a reasoned decision may be made not to perform the tests passively in order to avoid symptom exacerbation.

Some important handling issues with respect to performance of the ULNTs include:

- Only perform the ULNTs if you have a clinical rationale for doing so. Establish clinical reasoning hypotheses prior to tests regarding pathobiology, likely specific dysfunctions to be found on examination, precautions, and sources of symptoms.
- Explain to the patient exactly what you are going to do and what you want them to do. It is vital to have the patient comfortable about reporting any responses to testing, anywhere in their body.
- Perform the test on the less painful side or non-painful side first. If there is little difference between

sides, perform the test on the left side first for consistency.
- Starting positions should be consistent each time, and any variations from normal practice should be noted/recorded (use of pillows, etc.).
- Note symptom responses including area and nature (type of response) with the addition of each component of the test.
- Watch for antalgic postures and other compensatory movements during the test (e.g. cervical movements or trapezius muscle activity).
- Test for symmetry between sides.
- Explain your findings to your patient.
- Repeat the test gently a number of times before recording an actual measurement.

ULNT1 (median) active test

If the patient has described a symptom provoking position or movement, have them demonstrate it for you and observe the mechanics involved. If possible, perform a quick structural differentiation. For example, the patient may demonstrate a symptomatic position for their elbow pain, and you could have them maintain that elbow position and then ask them to move their neck to see if that alters their elbow symptoms.

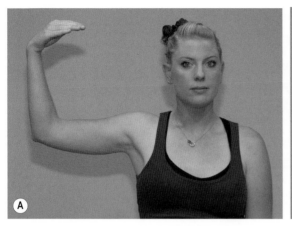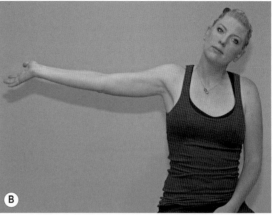

Fig 38.4 Active ULNT1 – Median. Have the patient abduct and externally rotate the shoulder with the elbow flexed to 90 degrees and the wrist flexed (A). Then have the patient extend the elbow, followed by wrist extension and cervical side bending away from the affected side (B).

A simple protocol for the active evaluation of the median neurodynamic test (ULNT1) has been described (Butler 2000). Have the patient abduct and externally rotate the shoulder with the elbow flexed to 90° and the wrist flexed (Fig 38.4A). Then ask the patient to extend the elbow and wrist, and finally tilt the head away from the affected side (Fig 38.4B). Compare to the opposite side, and note symptom responses as well as what happens to the shoulder girdle. Where the nervous system is sensitive, the shoulder girdle will often elevate (Butler 2000).

ULNT1 (median) passive test

A detailed description of the ULNT1 test is available in previous texts (Butler 1991, 2000, Shacklock 2005b). The key points involved are that the patient lies supine, both arms by the side, shoulder close to the edge of the examination table, no pillow if possible, and body straight. The therapist stride stands with the near foot placed forward, near hip approximating the table and is facing the patient's head. The therapist's near hand presses on the table above the patient's shoulder in either a knuckles or fist position (Fig 38.5A) but there should not be any downward or caudad pressure on the superior aspect of the patient's shoulder. The focus is to maintain the shoulder position during the performance of the test and prevent any shoulder elevation rather than to passively depress the shoulder girdle. With the other hand, the therapist holds the patient's hand with the thumb extended to apply tension to the motor branch of the median nerve. The therapist's fingers wrap around the patient's fingers distal to the metacarpophalangeal joints. The patient's elbow is flexed at 90° and supported on the therapist's near (front) thigh (Fig 38.5B).

The movements performed in sequence are glenohumeral abduction up to 90–110°, if available, in the frontal plane. This is followed by wrist and finger extension and forearm supination. Then, gleno-humeral external rotation is added to available range, although it is generally stopped at 90° if the patient is very mobile. The next component of the test is elbow extension and this should be done gently and with care not to cause any shoulder motion, especially adduction, which would thereby ease off the developing neurodynamic test (Fig 38.5C). After the addition of each component the patient is asked to relate any and all symptoms which may be evoked. Attention is paid to differences in the test response between the involved and uninvolved sides, and may include asymmetries resistance perceived by the examiner in the range of motion available or the sensory response. The final component of the test involves structural differentiation with cervical spine movements. The selection of the proper structural differentiation motion will be based on where the symptoms (if any) are located. If distal symptoms have developed (e.g. forearm and wrist pain) and are to be differentiated, the neck is moved into contralateral lateral flexion and any change in the distal symptoms would constitute a positive structural differentiation. If cervical contralateral flexion increases the symptoms and cervical ipsilateral flexion decreases the symptoms, this would constitute a positive structural differentiation and perhaps lead to a positive neurodynamic test. If proximal symptoms have developed (e.g. neck and shoulder pain) and are to be differentiated, the wrist is released from its extended position and again, any change in the proximal symptoms would constitute a positive structural differentiation.

A pattern of frequently reported and observed responses has been noted in young asymptomatic subjects

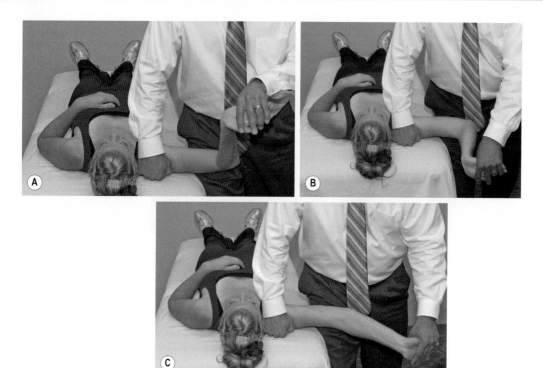

Fig 38.5 Passive ULNT1 – Median. Shoulder abduction is introduced while preventing shoulder girdle elevation (A). Next, wrist and finger extension is introduced with forearm supination, followed by shoulder external rotation (B). Finally, the elbow is extended to tolerance (C). Cervical side bending away (sensitizing movement) or towards (differentiating movement) or can be introduced.

(Kenneally 1985). 'Stretching', 'pulling', 'pain', 'tingling' and 'numbing' are commonly reported sensations even in individuals who are asymptomatic prior to the test. Kenneally et al (1988) summarized the responses of 400 asymptomatic individuals to the ULNT1 as follows:

- A deep stretch or ache in the cubital fossa (99% of volunteers) extending down the anterior and radial aspect of the forearm and into the radial side of the hand.
- A definite tingling sensation in the thumb and first three fingers.
- A small percentage felt stretch in the anterior shoulder.
- Cervical lateral flexion away from the side tested increased evoked responses in 90% of subjects.
- Cervical lateral flexion towards the side tested decreased the test response in 70% of subjects.

Indications for the ULNT1

A therapist would consider using the ULNT1 in their clinic where, after detailed subjective evaluation, objective examination and evaluation, there is a hypothesis of neurogenic pain in the upper limb or there may be a hypothesis that the source of the disorder lies in the median nerve pathways and receptive fields. Alternatively, the patient may have indicated a pain provoking movement or position which is similar to the test (e.g. hanging washing on the line) or a part of the test (e.g. forearm pronation and supination activities).

ULNT2 (median) active test

In some cases, it may not be possible or appropriate to abduct the shoulder and this is where the ULNT2 can be quite useful by using shoulder girdle depression as the sensitizing movement. For the active test, the patient can hang their arm naturally by their side and look at their thumb (Fig 38.6A). Have the patient point their thumb away, extend the wrist and then reach their hand down towards the floor (Fig 38.6B). They can use their other hand to depress their shoulder girdle. If necessary, they can then side-bend the cervical spine away from the test side and compare responses with the other side.

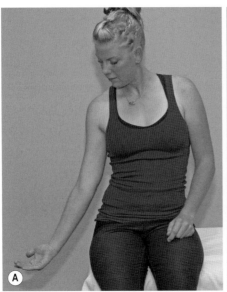 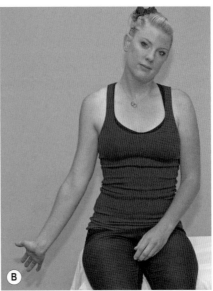

Fig 38.6 Active ULNT2 – Median. With the arm by the side, have the patient point their thumb away (A), then extend the wrist and reach their hand down towards the floor (B). Side bending away from the affected side can be added, as well as shoulder depression and abduction.

ULNT2 (median) passive test

For detailed description of the ULNT2 test see previous texts (Butler 1991, 2000, Shacklock 2005b). Once again, the key points involved are that the patient lies supine on a slight diagonal with their shoulder just over the edge of the treatment table to allow for contact with the therapist's thigh. The therapist stands near the patient's shoulder and uses his thigh to carefully depress the shoulder girdle. The therapist's right hand cradles the patient's left elbow and the left hand controls the patient's wrist and hand. The patient's arm is in approximately 10° of abduction (Fig 38.7A). The second component of the test is elbow extension and then whole arm external rotation (Fig 38.7B). Next, add wrist and finger extension and some specific handholds are suggested by authors (Butler 2000, Shacklock 2005b) (Fig 38.7C). Throughout this test, as each component is added, the patient is asked to relate any and all symptoms which may be evoked. Gleno-humeral abduction is then added if necessary. In most cases, there will be sufficient symptoms evoked without adding abduction, and structural differentiation can be achieved through cervical contralateral lateral flexion. Once again, for positive structural differentiation, the therapist is looking for alteration of evoked symptoms by the addition or subtraction of test components distant to the symptoms. If symptoms are reported distally (e.g. forearm and wrist) then change in the symptoms with cervical movements (increase with contralateral lateral flexion and decrease with ipsilateral lateral flexion) would represent positive structural differentiation.

ULNT2 (radial) active test

There are many ways to have the patient perform an active ULNT2 (Radial) test. The most common method is to have the patient hold their arm to their side, flex their wrist, look at their palm and then internally rotate their arm so that they can look at their palm over their shoulder (Fig 38.8A). The patient can then depress and abduct the shoulder and look away to introduce contralateral cervical side bending if needed (Fig 38.8B). Symptoms evoked during the performance of the test actively may obviate the need for performing the test passively.

ULNT2 (radial) passive test

Further detailed descriptions of this test can be found in texts (Butler 1991, 2000, Shacklock 2005b). The key points involved in this test, much like ULNT2 (median), are that the patient lies supine on a slight diagonal with their shoulder just over the edge of the treatment table to allow for contact with the therapist's thigh. The therapist stands near the patient's shoulder and uses his thigh to carefully depress the shoulder girdle. The therapist's right hand cradles the patient's left elbow and the left hand controls the patient's wrist and hand. The patient's

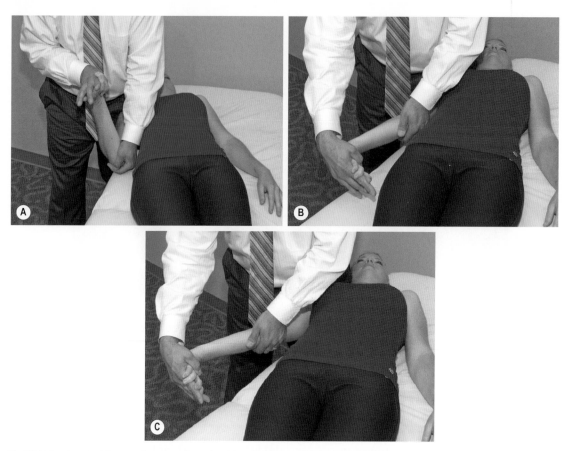

Fig 38.7 Passive ULNT2 – Median. Introduce shoulder girdle depression with the hip while supporting patient's elbow with your inside hand and supporting patient's wrist and hand with your outside hand (A). The elbow is then extended, and the whole arm is externally rotated. Finally, the forearm is fully supinated, the wrist and fingers are extended (B) and the arm is slowly abducted (C) to symptom tolerance. Cervical side bending away (sensitizing movement) or towards (differentiating movement) or can be introduced.

arm is in approximately 10° of abduction (Fig 38.9A). The second component of the test is elbow extension and then whole arm internal rotation (Fig 38.9B). Next, add wrist and finger flexion and it may be appropriate to add in wrist ulnar deviation and thumb flexion (Fig 38.9C). As with all the neurodynamic tests, as each component is added, the patient is asked to relate any and all symptoms which may be evoked. Gleno-humeral abduction can be added if necessary but as with ULNT2 (median) in most cases, there will be sufficient symptoms evoked without adding abduction and structural differentiation can be achieved through cervical contralateral lateral flexion.

Yaxley & Jull (1991) investigated the most common responses to the ULNT2 (radial) test on 50 asymptomatic 18–30-year-old subjects. Their findings were a strong painful stretch over the radial aspect of the proximal forearm (84% of all responses), often accompanied by a stretch pain in the lateral aspect of the upper arm (32%) or biceps brachii (14%) or the dorsal aspect of the hand (12%). Such a symptom response area would make the radial nerve at the elbow a candidate for a source of pain (Butler 2000).

ULNT3 (ulnar) active test

The active ULNT3 (ulnar) can be performed by asking the patient to look at their hand and hold it up as though they were holding a tray of drinks (in wrist extension) (Fig 38.10A). Further loading can then be added by having the patient look away, add more elbow flexion, depress the shoulder girdle and add in forearm pronation (Fig 38.10B). Cervical spine retraction is also thought to be another worthwhile sensitizing movement (Butler 2000). In patients with good range of movement, and especially

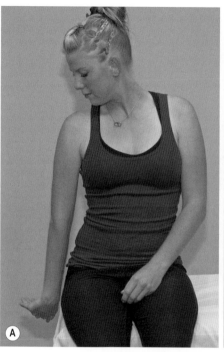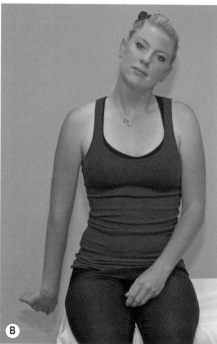

Fig 38.8 Active ULNT2 – Radial. With the arm by the side, have the patient flex their wrist, look at their palm and then internally rotate their arm so that they can look at their palm over their shoulder (A). Shoulder depression and abduction can be added as well as contralateral cervical side bending (B).

in younger flexible patients, have them attempt the 'mask' position

ULNT3 (ulnar) passive test

As with ULNT1 (median), this test has the patient lying supine, arms by the side, shoulder close to the edge of the examination table, no pillow if possible, and body straight. The therapist stride stands with the near foot placed forward, near hip approximating the table and is facing the patient's head. The therapist's near hand presses on the table above the patient's shoulder in either a knuckles or fist position and this time, applies a downward or caudad pressure on the superior aspect of the patient's shoulder to achieve shoulder girdle depression. With the other hand, the therapist holds the patient's hand palm against palm and the elbow starts in flexion (Fig 38.11A). The wrist and fingers are extended (and perhaps some radial deviation) as the elbow is flexed. The forearm is then pronated and the shoulder taken into lateral rotation and abduction (Fig 38.11B). This is achieved by the therapist 'walking' around the point of the patient's elbow within the groin. The final components added can be cervical contralateral lateral flexion or shoulder girdle depression, depending upon symptoms evoked and structural differentiation. Flanagan (1993) reported normal values for this distal to proximal sequencing of the test and found that 82% of subjects reported responses in the hypothenar eminence and medial two fingers, and 64% reported pins and needles in the same area.

The ULNT3 (ulnar) test is often performed from proximal to distal, with shoulder girdle depression and shoulder abduction followed by shoulder external rotation, then elbow flexion and finally wrist and finger extension with forearm pronation. Butler (2000) has suggested that in order to standardize the base test system, clinicians should make all the tests start from the shoulder girdle.

CLINICAL APPLICATION OF NEURODYNAMICS IN NECK AND UPPER EXTREMITY PAIN

An important consideration to always keep in mind is that healthy mechanics of the nervous system within the upper quadrant enables pain-free posture and movement. In the presence of mechanical impairment (pathomechanics) of

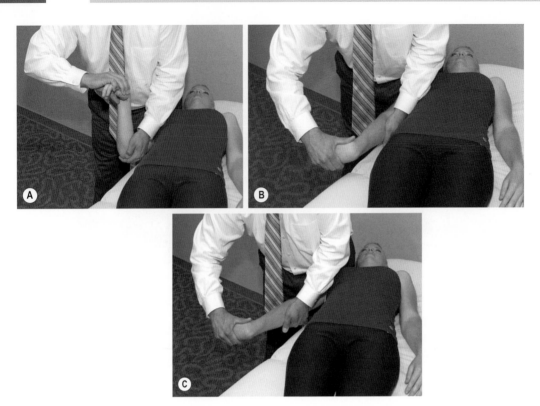

Fig 38.9 Passive ULNT2 – Radial. Introduce shoulder girdle depression with the hip while supporting patient's elbow with your inside hand and supporting patient's wrist and hand with your outside hand (A). The elbow is then extended, the wrist and fingers are flexed, the wrist is ulnarly deviated and the whole arm is internally rotated (B). Finally, the arm is slowly abducted to symptom tolerance (C). Cervical side bending away (sensitizing movement) or towards (differentiating movement) or can be introduced.

neural tissues, e.g. nerve entrapment, symptoms may be provoked during activities of daily living such as combing one's hair or tucking in one's shirt. The aim of using neurodynamic tests in assessment is to stimulate mechanically by moving neural tissues in order to gain an impression of their mobility and sensitivity to mechanical stresses. The purpose of treatment via these tests is to improve their mechanical and physiological function (Shacklock 1995a).

Mechanosensitivity is the chief mechanism that enables nerves to cause pain with movement. If a nerve is not mechanically sensitive, then it won't respond (cause pain) to mechanical forces applied to it. Mechanosensitivity can be defined as the ease with which impulses can be activated from a site in the nervous system when a mechanical force is applied. Normal nerves can be mechanosensitive (given sufficient force) and therefore, respond to applied forces (Rosenbleuth et al 1953, Lindquist et al 1973). This is a key fact to keep in mind when making judgments about whether the neural tissues within the cervical spine and upper limb

are a problem. Responses to neurodynamic tests in the upper limb are either normal or abnormal, and then relevant or irrelevant (Shacklock 2005b). Normal neurodynamic test responses would be considered as those that are in a normal location (relative to normative data), normal quality of symptoms, and normal range of movement for the upper limb. Abnormal neurodynamic test responses would be considered as those that are in a different location than normal, different quality of symptoms and/or range of movement of the limb is less than the uninvolved side. In most cases, there may be reproduction of the patient's symptoms. The next clinical question to consider would be whether the test responses are relevant or irrelevant. Relevance, in this case, would mean that the test responses are causally related to the patient's current problem, and an irrelevant finding would be where the test responses are not causally related to the patient's current problem. Many times this can be elucidated by asking the patient, 'is that a familiar symptom to you?'

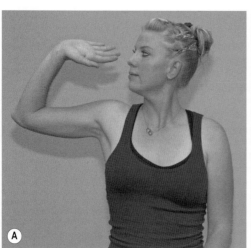
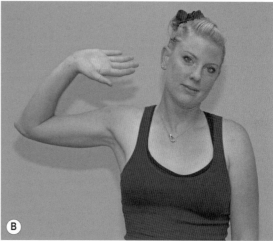

Fig 38.10 Active ULNT3 – Ulnar. The patient is asked to look at their hand and hold it up as though they were holding a tray of drinks (in wrist extension as depicted in A). The nerve can be further challenged by increasing elbow flexion and contra-lateral cervical side bending (B).

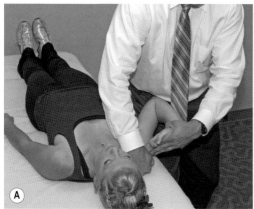
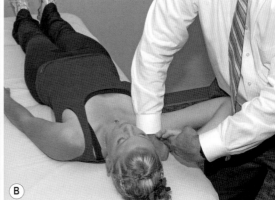

Fig 38.11 Passive ULNT3 – Ulnar. Face the patient and block the shoulder to prevent shoulder girdle elevation. The elbow is then flexed and stabilized by the therapist's hip. Wrist and finger extension is then introduced along with full pronation, radial deviation and shoulder external rotation (A). The shoulder is then abducted through the frontal plane to tolerance (B). Cervical side bending away (sensitizing movement) or towards (differentiating movement) or can be introduced.

The symptoms evoked on a neurodynamic test can be inferred to be neurogenic (positive test in a clinical sense):

- if structural differentiation supports a neurogenic source
- if there are differences left to right and to known normal responses
- if the test reproduces the patient's symptoms or associated symptoms

- if there is support from other data such as history, area of symptoms, imaging tests, etc.

The greater the number of 'ifs' present, the stronger the case for a clinically relevant test. Clinically, the information required from neurodynamic tests is symptom response, resistance encountered, changes to symptom response and resistance encountered as each component of the test is added or subtracted. This information, along with the patient history, subjective and objective examination, etc., should give the clinician the ability to provisionally diagnose the site of neuropathodynamics and then re-assess after whatever treatment might be administered. It is important to realize that the treatment need not be a mobilizing technique for the nervous system, as the clinician may decide to mobilize or treat the mechanical interface, or perhaps he/she may decide the problem is not peripheral neurogenic in nature but rather a 'central processing enhancement' in which patient education/reassurance/discussion may be the treatment of choice. It is also important to remember that sensitivity to a neurodynamic test could be from a combination of primary (tissue-based) or secondary (CNS-based) processes.

Treatment

In a randomized controlled trial, Tal-Akabi & Rushton (2000) compared neural mobilizations, joint mobilizations or no treatment in patients with carpal tunnel syndrome (CTS) and found that both interventions were more effective than no treatment at reducing pain and ultimate need for surgery. In contrast to the above study, Heebner & Roddey (2008) reported that the addition of neural mobilization to standard care did not result in improved outcomes in patients with CTS. Neural mobilizations in the upper quarter have also been utilized with success in patients with cervical radiculopathy (Coppieters et al 2003, Cleland et al 2005, Costello 2008, Young et al 2009); lateral epicondylalgia (Vicenzino et al 1996, 1998, Ekstrom & Holden 2002); and cubital tunnel syndrome (Coppieters et al 2004).

Management of neuropathic pain should focus on reducing mechanosensitivity and restoring normal movement to both the nervous tissue and its mechanical interface. Reassessment should be continual, and include clinical evaluation along with patient feedback. We believe that patient education is paramount and should include a brief discussion of neurodynamics, the neurobiology of pain and the continuity of the nervous system. Additionally, if there is a central sensitization component to the symptoms, this should also be addressed, along with any perceived or real fear of movement the patient may have. This can reduce the threat value associated with their pain experience.

Next, we have found it useful to treat any impairment in the non-neural tissues to reduce any mechanical forces that the 'container' may be placing on the nervous tissue. Interventions utilized may include joint mobilization/manipulation, stretching, soft tissue work and therapeutic exercise. Detailed discussion of these interventions is beyond the scope of this chapter and are detailed in other chapters of this textbook. Any of the above interventions, if utilized, should be followed by a reassessment of the provocative ULNT to determine if change

has occurred. If change occurred, treatment may be discontinued for that day, or specific neurodynamic interventions (either active or passive) may be added to the treatment.

We like to further break neurodynamic interventions down into one of two approaches, 'sliders' or 'tensioners', each of which has its own indications and clinical usefulness (Nee & Butler 2006, Coppieters & Butler 2008). With a sliding or gliding technique, combined movements of at least two joints are alternated in such a way that one movement elongates the nerve bed while the other movement shortens the nerve bed. This results in a situation where the nerve is mobilized through a large degree of longitudinal excursion with a minimum amount of tension. These techniques should be non-provocative, and may be more tolerable to patients than tensioning techniques. For example, abundant literature supports the use of cervical lateral glide mobilizations (Fig 38.12) to effect changes in neck and/or arm symptoms (Vicenzino et al 1998, Vicenzino et al 1999a,b, Cowell & Phillips 2002, Coppieters et al 2003, Cleland et al 2005, Costello 2008, McClatchie et al 2009, Young et al 2009) as this intervention has been shown to produce immediate reductions in mechanosensitivity and pain in patients with lateral epicondylalgia (Vicenzino et al 1996) and cervico-brachial pain (Elvey 1986, Cowell & Phillips 2002, Coppieters et al 2003). This can be done with or without the arm in an ULNT position.

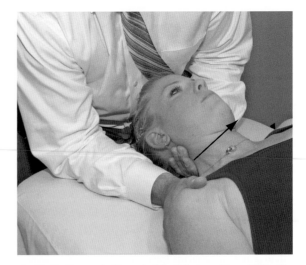

Fig 38.12 The cervical lateral glide technique (Elvey 1986). The hand used to perform the lateral glides is the hand opposite of the patient's affected side. The motion should be purely transverse away from the affected side, and the clinician's other hand is used to stabilize (rather than depress) the scapula on the affected side. The arm can also be placed in an ULNT position (Vicenzino et al 1999).

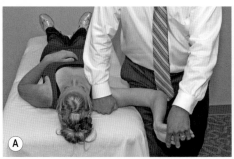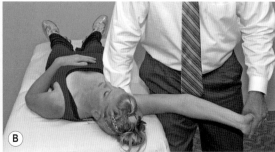

Fig 38.13 Passive 'slider' technique for the median nerve utilizing ULNT1 (Median). The patient is set up just prior to the onset of symptoms as per the passive ULNT1 (Median) passive test (A). To then 'slide' the median nerve, the cervical spine is actively side bent to the ipsilateral side as the clinician extends the elbow (B).

Elvey (1986) reported that gliding techniques were more effective than no intervention at reducing pain and disability in patients with cervico-brachial pain, and was more effective than manual therapy directed at the shoulder and thoracic spine in reducing pain in these patients. Furthermore, Rozmaryn et al (1998) reported in a non-randomized controlled trial that the addition of neural gliding techniques to conservative management of patients with CTS reduced the need for surgery by 29.8%. An example of a passive slider mobilization for the median nerve would include positioning the patient's arm in 90–110° of abduction with 90° of shoulder external rotation with the elbow flexed to 90° with wrist and finger extension and forearm supination (Fig 38.13A). To then passively 'slide' the median nerve, wrist extension could be relaxed as the elbow is extended (distal slider) or the cervical spine could be actively side bent to the ipsilateral side as the elbow is extended (proximal slider) (Fig 38.13B). This could also be given as an active technique performed by the patient at home (Fig 38.14A,B). Another example of an active 'sliding' technique is illustrated in Figure 38.15A,B.

With a tensioning technique, elongation of the nerve bed is obtained by moving one or several joints such that the 'tension' within the nerve is elevated (Coppieters & Butler 2008). These techniques are, by nature, more stressful to the neural tissue and should be used with caution as they may irritate the mechanosensitive patient. They are not static stretches and should always involve gentle oscillations in and out of resistance. These techniques are generally indicated for patients who experience symptoms as a result of impairments in the neural tissue's ability to elongate; hence the goal is to restore the physical capabilities of the neural tissue to tolerate movement. The tension is increased to the point of a mild stretching sensation, or,

in the case of non-irritable patients, may be taken to the onset of mild symptoms at the end of the oscillation. Any of the active or passive ULNT's can be used as 'tensioners.' Sets and repetitions are determined by the irritability of the patients as well as the response (positive/negative) to the interventions. We have found that starting with 1–3 sets of 10 oscillations is useful, followed by a reassessment of the ULNT to determine if the interventions had any effect. Finally, techniques aimed at non-neural structures can be combined with neurodynamic interventions, such as the cervical lateral glide technique while holding the arm in an ULNT position (Vicenzino et al 1998, 1999b, Cowell & Phillips 2002, Coppieters et al 2003, Cleland et al 2005, Young et al 2009).

CONCLUSIONS

Clinicians should keep in mind the underlying principles of neurobiomechanics; that is, the nervous system is a continuous tract that is subject to slide, glide, bend, and stretch as it travels through its mechanical interface. Symptoms can arise as a result of intrinsic or extrinsic impairments anywhere along this tortuous course. Clinicians can render meaningful interventions that have a direct impact on the space, movement and blood supply for the nervous system, in addition to producing beneficial neuro-physiological effects. Neurodynamic interventions (passive or active) should involve smooth, controlled, gentle, large amplitude movements. Sustained stretching is rarely indicated. Finally, we caution readers that neurodynamic interventions are but a small part of an overall patient-centred treatment approach encompassing multiple treatment interventions.

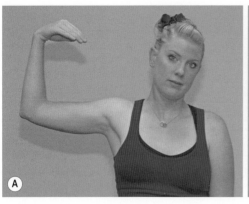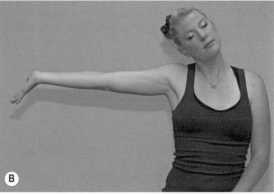

Fig 38.14 Active 'slider' technique for the median nerve utilizing ULNT1 (Median). The patient's arm is positioned in 90–110° of abduction with 90° of shoulder external rotation with the elbow flexed to 90° with the wrist and fingers flexed with forearm supination (A). To then 'slide' the median nerve, the cervical spine is actively side bent to the ipsilateral side as the patient actively extends the elbow and the wrist (B).

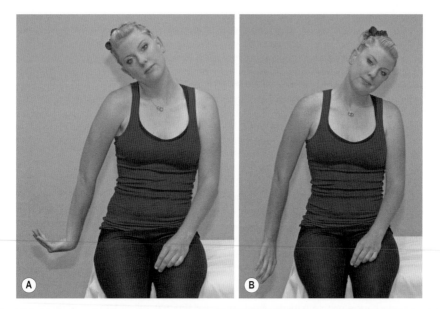

Fig 38.15 Active 'slider' technique for the radial nerve utilizing ULNT2 (Radial). With the cervical spine side bent to the affected side, the patient positions the affected arm in shoulder internal rotation, elbow extension, forearm pronation and wrist and finger flexion (A). The patient then actively side bends away while releasing the wrist and finger flexion (B).

REFERENCES

Asbury, A.K., Fields, H.L., 1984. Pain due to peripheral nerve damage: an hypothesis. Neurology 34, 1587–1590.

Barry, S.R., 1991. Clinical implications of basic neuroscience research. I: Protein kinases, ionic channels, and genes. Arch. Phys. Med. Rehabil. 72, 998–1008.

Beith, I.D., Robins, E.J., et al., 1995. An assessment of the adaptive mechanisms within and surrounding the peripheral nervous system, during changes in nerve bed length resulting from underlying joint movement. In: Shacklock, M.O. (Ed.), Moving in on Pain. Butterworth-Heinemann, Melbourne.

Breig, A., 1960. Biomechanics of the central nervous system. Almqvist and Wiksell, Stockholm.

Breig, A., 1978. Adverse Mechanical Tension in the Central Nervous System. Almqvist and Wiksell, Stockholm.

Breig, A., El-Nadi, A.F., 1966. Biomechanics of the cervical spinal cord. Relief of contact pressure on and overstretching of the spinal cord. Acta Radiol. Diagn. (Stockh.) 4, 602–624.

Breig, A., Marions, O., 1963. Biomechanics of the Lumbosacral Nerve Roots. Acta Radiol. Diagn. (Stockh.) 1, 1141–1160.

Breig, A., Troup, J., 1979. Biomechanical considerations in the straight leg raising test. Spine 4, 242–250.

Breig, A., Turnbull, I., Hassler, O., 1966. Effects of mechanical stresses on the spinal cord in cervical spondylosis: a study on fresh cadaver material. J. Neurosurg. 25, 45–56.

Butler, D.S., 1991. Mobilisation of the Nervous System. Churchill Livingstone, Melbourne.

Butler, D.S., 2000. The Sensitive Nervous System. Noigroup, Adelaide.

Butler, D.S., Moseley, G.L., 2003. Explain Pain. NOI Publications, Adelaide.

Calvin, W.H., Devor, M., Howe, J.F., 1982. Can neuralgias arise from minor demyelination? Spontaneous firing, mechanosensitivity, and afterdischarge from conducting axons. Exp. Neurol. 75, 755–763.

Chang, S.B., Lee, S.H., Ahn, Y., et al., 2006. Risk factor for unsatisfactory outcome after lumbar foraminal and far lateral microdecompression. Spine 31, 1163–1167.

Cleland, J.A., Whitman, J.M., Fritz, J.M., et al., 2005. Manual physical therapy, cervical traction, and strengthening exercises in patients with cervical radiculopathy: a case series. J. Orthop. Sports Phys. Ther. 35, 802–811.

Coppieters, M.W., Butler, D.S., 2008. Do 'sliders' slide and 'tensioners' tension? An analysis of neurodynamic techniques and considerations regarding their application. Man. Ther. 13, 213–221.

Coppieters, M.W., Stappaerts, K.H., Wouters, L.L., et al., 2003. Aberrant protective force generation during neural provocation testing and the effect of treatment in patients with neurogenic cervico-brachial pain. J. Manipulative Physiol. Ther. 26, 99–106.

Coppieters, M.W., Bartholomeeusen, K.E., Stappaerts, K.H., 2004. Incorporating nerve-gliding techniques in the conservative treatment of cubital tunnel syndrome. J. Manipulative Physiol. Ther. 27, 560–568.

Costello, M., 2008. Treatment of a patient with cervical radiculopathy using thoracic spine thrust manipulation, soft tissue mobilization, and exercise. J. Man. Manip. Ther. 16, 129–135.

Cowell, I.M., Phillips, D.R., 2002. Effectiveness of manipulative physiotherapy for the treatment of a neurogenic cervico-brachial pain syndrome: a single case study experimental design. Man. Ther. 7, 31–38.

Coveney, B., Trott, P., Grimmer, K., 1997. The upper limb tension test in a group of subjects with a clinical presentation of carpal tunnel syndrome. Tenth Biennial Conference. Manipulative Physiotherapists Association of Australia, Melbourne.

Dahlin, L.B., Archer, D.R., McLean, W.G., 1993. Axonal transport and morphological changes following

nerve compression. An experimental study in the rabbit vagus nerve. J. Hand Surg. [Br.] 18, 106–110.

de Peretti, F., Micalef, J.P., Bourgeon, A., et al., 1989. Biomechanics of the lumbar spinal nerve roots and the first sacral root within the intervertebral foramina. Surg. Radiol. Anat. 11, 221–225.

Devor, M., 1999. Unexplained peculiarities of the dorsal root ganglion. Pain Suppl. 6, S27–S35.

Devor, M., 2006. Sodium channels and mechanisms of neuropathic pain. J. Pain 7, S3–S12.

Devor, M., Seltzer, Z., 1999. Pathophysiology of damaged nerves in relation to chronic pain. In: Wall, P.D., Melzack, R. (Eds.), Textbook of Pain. Churchill Livingstone, Edinburgh.

Devor, M., Schonfeld, D., Seltzer, Z., et al., 1979. Two modes of cutaneous reinnervation following peripheral nerve injury. Journal of Complementary Neurology 185, 211–220.

Devor, M., Govrin-Lippmann, R., Angelides, K., 1993. Na$^+$ channel immuno-localization in peripheral mammalian axons and changes following nerve injury and neuroma formation. J. Neurosci. 13, 1976–1992.

Di Fabio, R., 2001. Neural Mobilization: The Impossible. J. Orthop. Sports Phys. Ther. 31, 224–225.

Dilley, A., Lynn, B., Greening, J., et al., 2003. Quantitative in vivo studies of median nerve sliding in response to wrist, elbow, shoulder and neck movements. Clin. Biomech. (Bristol, Avon) 18, 899–907.

Driscoll, P.J., Glasby, M.A., Lawson, G.M., 2002. An in vivo study of peripheral nerves in continuity: biomechanical and physiological responses to elongation. J. Orthop. Res. 20, 370–375.

Ekstrom, R.A., Holden, K., 2002. Examination of and intervention for a patient with chronic lateral elbow pain with signs of nerve entrapment. Phys. Ther. 82, 1077–1086.

Elvey, R.L., 1979. Brachial plexus tension tests and the pathoanatomical origin of arm pain. In: Idczak, R. (Ed.), Aspects of manipulative therapy. Manipulative Physiotherapists Association of Australia, Melbourne, pp. 105–110.

Elvey, R.L., 1986. Treatment of arm pain associated with abnormal brachial plexus tension. Aust. J. Physiother. 32, 225–230.

Fern, R., Harrison, P.J., 1994. The contribution of ischaemia and deformation to the conduction block generated by compression of the cat sciatic nerve. Exp. Physiol. 79, 583–592.

Flanagan, M., 1993. Normative responses to the ulnar nerve bias tension test. University of South Australia, Adelaide.

Fritz, J.M., Delitto, A., Welch, W.C., et al., 1998. Lumbar spinal stenosis: a review of current concepts in evaluation, management, and outcome measurements. Arch. Phys Med. Rehabil. 79, 700–708.

Greening, J., Smart, S., Leary, R., et al., 1999. Reduced movement of median nerve in carpal tunnel during wrist flexion in patients with non-specific arm pain. Lancet 354, 217–218.

Hall, T., Zusman, M., Elvey, R., 1995. Manually detected impediments in the straight leg raise test. Clinical Solutions. Ninth Biennial Conference of the Manipulative Physiotherapists' Association of Australia, G. Jull. Gold Coast, Queensland, pp. 48–53.

Hall, T., Zusman, M., Elvey, R., 1998. Adverse mechanical tension in the nervous system? Analysis of straight leg raise. Man. Ther. 3, 140–146.

Heebner, M.L., Roddey, T.S., 2008. The effects of neural mobilization in addition to standard care in persons with carpal tunnel syndrome from a community hospital. J. Hand Ther. 21, 229–240.

Kallakuri, S., Cavanaugh, J.M., Blagoev, D.C., 1998. An immunohistochemical study of innervation of lumbar spinal dura and longitudinal ligaments. Spine 23, 403–411.

Kenneally, M., 1985. The upper limb tension test. In: Proceedings. Fourth Biennial Conference, Manipulative Therapists Association of Australia.

Manipulative Therapists Association of Australia, Brisbane.

Kenneally, M., Rubenach, H., Elvey, R.L., 1988. The upper limb tension test: the SLR of the arm. In: Grant, R. (Ed.), Physical Therapy of the Cervical and Thoracic Spine. Churchill Livingstone, New York.

Kleinrensink, G.J., Stoeckart, R., Vleeming, A., 1995. Mechanical tension in the median nerve. The effects of joint positions. Clin. Biomech. (Bristol, Avon) 10, 240–244.

Kleinrensink, G.J., Stoeckart, R., Mulder, P.G., et al., 2000. Upper limb tension tests as tools in the diagnosis of nerve and plexus lesions. Anatomical and biomechanical aspects. Clin. Biomech. (Bristol, Avon) 15, 9–14.

Kuncewicz, E., Gajewska, E., Sobieska, M., et al., 2006. Piriformis muscle syndrome. Ann. Acad. Med. Stetin. 52, 99–101.

Lindquist, C., Nilsson, B.Y., Skoglund, C.R., 1973. Observations on the mechanical sensitivity of sympathetic and other types of small-diameter nerve fibers. Brain Res. 49, 432–435.

Mackinnon, S.E., 1992. Double and multiple 'crush' syndromes. Double and multiple entrapment neuropathies. Hand Clin. 8, 369–390.

Maitland, G.D., 1986. Vertebral Manipulation, fifth ed. Butterworths, Ontario.

McClatchie, L., Laprade, J., Martin, S., et al., 2009. Mobilizations of the asymptomatic cervical spine can reduce signs of shoulder dysfunction in adults. Man. Ther. 14, 369–374.

McLellan, D.L., Swash, M., 1976. Longitudinal sliding of the median nerve during movements of the upper limb. J. Neurol. Neurosurg. Psychiatry 39, 566–570.

Merskey, H., Bogduk, N., 1994. Classification of Chronic Pain. IASP Press, Seattle.

Millesi, H., 1986. The nerve gap: theory and clinical practice. Hand Clin. 2, 651–663.

Nakamichi, K., Tachibana, S., 1995. Restricted motion of the median nerve in carpal tunnel syndrome. J. Hand Surg. [Br.] 20, 460–464.

Nee, R.J., Butler, D.S., 2006. Management of peripheral neuropathic pain: Integrating neurobiology, neurodynamics, and clinical evidence. Phys. Ther. Sport 7, 36–49.

Nordin, M., Nystrom, B., Wallin, U., et al., 1984. Ectopic sensory discharges and paresthesiae in patients with disorders of peripheral nerves, dorsal roots and dorsal columns. Pain 20, 231–245.

Ogata, K., Naito, M., 1986. Blood flow of peripheral nerve: Effects of dissection, stretching and compression. J. Hand Surg. [Am.] 11B, 10–14.

Rosenbleuth, A., Buylla, A., Ramos, G., 1953. The responses of axons to mechanical stimuli. Acta Physiologica Latinoamericana 3, 204–215.

Rydevik, B., Lundborg, G., Bagge, U., 1981. Effects of graded compression on intraneural blood flow: An in-vivo study on rabbit tibial nerve. J. Hand Surg. 6, 3–12.

Rozmaryn, L.M., Dovelle, S., Rothman, E.R., et al., 1998. Nerve and tendon gliding exercises and the conservative management of carpal tunnel syndrome. J. Hand Ther. 11, 171–179.

Shacklock, M.O., 1989. The plantarflexion/inversion straight leg raise test. An investigation into the effect of cervical flexion and order of component movements on the symptom response. University of South Australia, Adelaide.

Shacklock, M.O., 1995a. Neurodynamics. Physiotherapy 81, 9–16.

Shacklock, M.O., 1995b. Clinical Application of Neurodynamics. In: Shacklock, M.O. (Ed.), Moving in on Pain. Butterworth-Heinemann, Melbourne, pp. 123–131.

Shacklock, M., 2005a. Improving application of neurodynamic (neural tension) testing and treatments: a message to researchers and clinicians. Man. Ther. 10, 175–179.

Shacklock, M.O., 2005b. Clinical Neurodynamics: A new system of musculoskeletal treatment. Elsevier Butterworth-Heinemann. Sydney.

Siddiqui, M., Karadimas, E., Nicol, M., et al., 2006. Influence of X Stop on neural foramina and spinal canal area in spinal stenosis. Spine 31, 2958–2962.

Szabo, R.M., Bay, B.K., Sharkey, N.A., et al., 1994. Median nerve displacement through the carpal canal. J. Hand Surg. 19A, 901–906.

Tal-Akabi, A., Rushton, A., 2000. An investigation to compare the effectiveness of carpal bone mobilisation and neurodynamic mobilisation as methods of treatment for carpal tunnel syndrome. Man. Ther. 5, 214–222.

Tsai, Y.Y., 1995. Tension change in the ulnar nerve by different order of upper limb tension test. Master of Science, Northwestern University, Chicago.

Van der Heide, B., Allison, G.T., Zusman, M., 2001. Pain and muscular responses to a neural tissue provocation test in the upper limb. Man. Ther. 6, 154–162.

Vicenzino, B., Collins, D., Wright, A., 1996. The initial effects of a cervical spine manipulative physiotherapy treatment on the pain and dysfunction of lateral epicondylalgia. Pain 68 (1), 69–74.

Vicenzino, B., Collins, D., Benson, H., et al., 1998. An investigation of the interrelationship between manipulative therapy-induced hypoalgesia and sympathoexcitation. J. Manipulative Physiol. Ther. 21, 448–453.

Vicenzino, B., Cartwright, T., Collins, D., 1999a. An investigation of stress and pain perception during manual therapy in asymptomatic subjects. Eur. J. Pain 3, 13–18.

Vicenzino, B., Neal, R., Collins, D., et al., 1999b. The displacement, velocity and frequency profile of the frontal plane motion produced by the cervical lateral glide treatment technique. Clin. Biomech. 14, 515–521.

Wall, E.J., Massie, J.B., Kwan, M.K., et al., 1992. Experimental stretch neuropathy. J. Bone Joint Surg. 74B, 126–129.

Wilgis, E.F., Murphy, R., 1986. The significance of longitudinal excursion in peripheral nerves. Hand Clin. 2, 761–776.

Woolf, C.J., 2000. Pain. Neurobiol. Dis. 7, 504–510.

Woolf, C.J., 2007. Central sensitization: uncovering the relation between pain and plasticity. Anesthesiology 106, 864–867.

Woolf, C.J., Mannion, R.J., 1999. Neuropathic pain: aetiology, symptoms, mechanisms, and management. Lancet 353, 1959–1964.

Wright, T.W., Glowczewskie Jr., F., Cowin, D., et al., 2001. Ulnar nerve excursion and strain at the elbow and wrist associated with upper extremity motion. J. Hand Surg. [Am.] 26, 655–662.

Yaxley, G., Jull, G., 1991. A modified upper limb tension test: an investigation of responses in normal subjects. Aust. J. Physiother. 37, 143–152.

Young, I.A., Michener, L.A., Cleland, J.A., et al., 2009. Manual therapy, exercise, and traction for patients with cervical radiculopathy: a randomized clinical trial. Phys. Ther. 89, 632–642.

Zochodne, D.W., Ho, L.T., 1991. Stimulation-induced peripheral nerve hyperemia: mediation by fibers innervating vasa nervorum? Brain Res. 546, 113–118.

Zoech, G., Reihsner, R., Beer, R., et al., 1991. Stress and strain in peripheral nerves. Neuro-Orthopedics 10, 73–82.

Zorn, P., Shacklock, M.O., Trott, P., et al., 1995. The effect of sequencing the movements of the upper limb tension test on the area of symptom reproduction. Clinical Solutions. Ninth Biennial Conference of the Manipulative Physiotherapists' Association of Australia, G. Jull. Gold Coast, Queensland, pp. 166–167.

Index

Note: Page numbers followed by *b* indicate boxes, *f* indicate figures and *t* indicate tables.